MOUNTAIN BIKE!
Northern California

MOUNTAIN BIKE!
Northern California

A GUIDE TO THE CLASSIC TRAILS

LINDA GONG AUSTIN

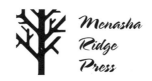

Menasha Ridge Press

© 2000 by Linda Gong Austin
All Rights Reserved
Printed in the United States of America
Published by Menasha Ridge Press
Distributed by the Globe Pequot Press
First edition, second printing, 2001

Library of Congress Cataloging-in-Publication Data:
Austin, Linda Gong.
Mountain bike! Northern California: a guide
to the classic trails / Linda Gong Austin.
p. cm.
Includes index.
ISBN 0-89732-288-6
1. All terrain cycling—California, Northern—Guidebooks.
2. Bicycle trails—California, Northern—Guidebooks.
I. Title
GV1045.5.C22 C2525   2000
917.94—dc21   00-026747
CIP

Photos by the author unless otherwise credited
Maps by Inkspot, a design company™
Cover photo by Dennis Coello
Cover and text design by Suzanne Holt

Menasha Ridge Press
P.O. Box 43673
Birmingham, Alabama 35243
www.menasharidge.com

All trails described in this book are legal for mountain bikes. But rules can change—especially for off-road bicycles, the new kid on the outdoor recreation block. Land-access issues and conflicts between cyclists, hikers, equestrians, and other users can cause the rewriting of recreation regulations on public lands, sometimes resulting in a ban of mountain bike use on specific trails. That's why it's the responsibility of each rider to check and make sure that he or she rides only on trails where mountain biking is permitted.

CAUTION

Outdoor recreational activities are by their very nature potentially hazardous. All participants in such activities must assume the responsibility for their own actions and safety. The information contained in this guidebook cannot replace sound judgment and good decision-making skills, which help reduce risk exposure, nor does the scope of this book allow for disclosure of all the potential hazards and risks involved in such activities.

Learn as much as possible about the outdoor recreational activities in which you participate, prepare for the unexpected, and be cautious. The reward will be a safer and more enjoyable experience.

To my husband Bruce. I love you.

CONTENTS

Map Legend x
Ride Location Map xi
Acknowledgments xii
Foreword xiii
Preface xiv
Ride Recommendations for Special Interests xviii

INTRODUCTION 1
Trail Description Outline 1
Abbreviations 3
Ride Configurations 3
Topographic Maps 4
Trail Etiquette 5
Hitting the Trail 7
Cell Phones 9

THE NORTH COAST 11
1 Grasshopper Peak Loop 12
2 Peavine Road Loop 17
3 Avenue of the Giants Road Ride 20
4 Arcata Community Forest 24
5 Ossagon–Gold Bluff Loop 28
6 Lost Man Creek–Holter Ridge Bike Trail 34
7 Coastal Trail—Last Chance Section 38
8 Howland Hill–Stout Grove 44
9 Gasquet Toll Road 48
Other Area Rides 54
Some Local Bicycle Shops and Organizations 56

SHASTA CASCADE 57
Whiskeytown: Wheeling through History 58
10 Clikapudi Trail 62
11 Waters Gulch Loop 66
12 Boulder Creek Loop 69
13 Mt. Shasta Mine Loop 72
14 The Chimney 76
15 Upper and Lower Ice Box Loop 79

16 Great Water Ditch Trail and El Dorado Mine Loop   83
Other Area Rides   90
Some Local Bicycle Shops   93

THE MENDOCINO COAST   94

17 Manly Gulch Loop   95
18 Caspar Creek–640–630 Loop   99
19 Fern Canyon Trail—Van Damme State Park   102
20 Fern Canyon Trail—Russian Gulch State Park   106
21 MacKerricher Ten Mile Coastal Trail   110
Other Area Rides   114
Some Local Bicycle Shops and Related Businesses   117

THE WINE COUNTRY   118

22 Boggs Mountain Demonstration Forest   119
23 Mt. St. Helena North Peak   124
24 Oat Hill Mine Road   127
25 Annadel State Park Loops   131
Other Area Rides   138
Some Local Bicycle Shops   140

THE GOLD RUSH COUNTRY OF THE WESTERN SIERRAS   141

26 American River Bike Path   142
27 Salmon Falls Out-and-Back   147
28 Olmstead Loop   151
29 Quarry Road Out-and-Back   155
30 Stagecoach–Lake Clementine Loop   159
31 Sly Park–Jenkinson Lake Loop   164
32 Big Boulder Trail Loop   169
33 South Yuba Primitive Camp Loop   173
34 Bullards Bar Loop   177
35 Chimney Rock Trail   180
36 North Yuba River Trail   183
37 Forest City's Pliocene–Sandusky Loop   187
Other Area Rides   194
Some Local Bicycle Shops and Organizations   198

AROUND LAKE TAHOE   199

38 Hole-In-The-Ground Trail   200
39 Sardine Valley Loop   205
40 Backside Loop at Northstar   208
41 TRT–Cinder Cone Loop   212
Ski Resorts Become Mountain Bike Parks in the Summer   217
42 TRT–WST–Paige Meadows Point-to-Point   219

43 Paige Meadows Ride   224
44 Tahoe City Bike Paths   229
45 General Creek Easy Loop   234
46 Fallen Leaf Lake Easy Loop   238
47 Angora Lakes Out-and-Back   241
48 Pope Baldwin Bike Path   245
49 Burnside Lake Out-and-Back   247
50 Genoa Road–TRT Loop   251
51 The Flume–TRT Ride   255
52 TRT: Big Meadows to Kingsbury Grade   261
53 TRT: Big Meadows to Round Lake   269
54 Pine Nut Mountains Loops   273
Other Area Rides   278
Some Local Bicycle Shops and Organizations   280

THE HIGH COUNTRY OF THE EASTERN SIERRAS   281
55 Yosemite National Park Bike Trail   282
56 Black Point at Mono Lake Ride   286
57 South Tufa Out-and-Back   291
58 Hartley Springs Loop   294
59 Inyo Craters Loop   299
60 Easy Shady Rest Ride   304
61 Knolls Loop   307
62 Horseshoe Lake Loop   311
63 Mountain View   315
64 Off The Top—Mammoth Mountain Bike Park   319
65 Paper Route & Big Ring—Mammoth Mountain Bike Park   324
66 Hot Creek Hatchery Road to the Hot Springs   327
Other Area Rides   331
Some Local Bicycle Shops and Related Businesses   333

THE EAST BAY AREA   334
67 Mt. Diablo–Mitchell Canyon Loop   335
68 Shell Ridge–Stage Road Dirt Ride   341
69 Black Diamond Mines Loop   346
70 Briones Crest Loop   351
71 Tilden–Wildcat Canyon Loop   356
72 East–West Ridge Loop   362
73 Lafayette–Moraga Trail   368
Other Area Rides   372
Some Local Bicycle Shops and Organizations   375

THE NORTH BAY AREA—MARIN COUNTY   377
From Repack to the World: Twenty Years   378
74 Angel Island Double Loop   379

75 Tennessee Valley Double Loop 384
76 Mt. Tam Loop via Old Railroad–Eldridge Grades 390
77 Bolinas Ridge Fire Road 396
78 Barnabe Peak Loop and Devil's Gulch 400
79 Pine Mountain–Repack Loop 405
80 China Camp Shoreline—Ridge Loop 411
Other Area Rides 417
Some Local Bicycle Shops and Organizations 418

THE WEST BAY AREA 420

81 Tour of San Francisco and the Golden Gate 421
82 Sawyer Camp Trail 428
83 Purisima Creek Redwoods—Short Loop 430
84 El Corte de Madera Creek Loop 435
Other Area Rides 440
Some Local Bicycle Shops and Organizations 442

THE SOUTH BAY AND SANTA CRUZ COUNTY 443

85 Monte Bello–Stevens Creek Loop 444
86 Henry Coe Middle Ridge Loop 448
87 Pacheco State Park Loop 453
88 Big Basin: Gazos Creek–Chalk Mountain Ride 459
89 Big Basin: Skyline-to-the-Sea Trail (Waddell Creek) 464
90 Henry Cowell State Park Ramble 468
91 Wilder Ranch: Grey Whale Loop 472
92 Wilder Ranch: Old Cove Bluff Trail 477
93 Nisene Marks–Sand Point Ride 480
Other Area Rides 486
Some Local Bicycle Shops and Organizations 489

THE MONTEREY PENINSULA AND BIG SUR 490

94 Toro Park–Ollason Peak Loop 491
95 Fort Ord: Guidotti–Goat Trail Loop 497
96 Fort Ord: Mudhen Lake–Rim Trail Ramble 503
97 Monterey Recreation Trail 508
98 17-Mile Drive to Carmel Road Ride 516
99 Old Coast Road 521
100 Andrew Molera: Creamery-Ridge Ride 525
Other Area Rides 530
Some Local Bicycle Shops 532

Appendix 533
Glossary 535
Index 541
About the Author 556

AMERICA BY MOUNTAIN BIKE! · Map Legend

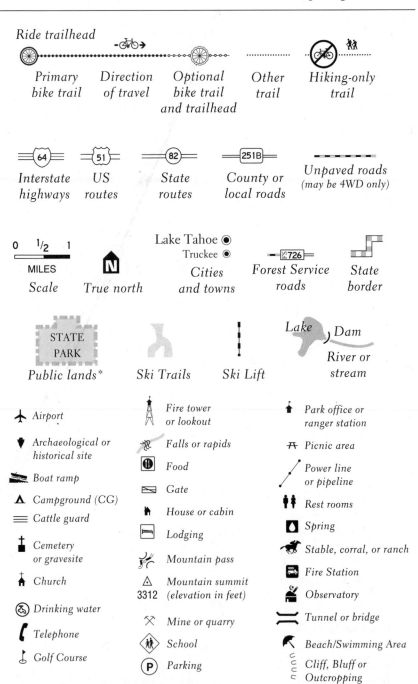

Ride trailhead

Primary bike trail | **Direction of travel** | **Optional bike trail and trailhead** | **Other trail** | **Hiking-only trail**

Interstate highways (64) | **US routes** (51) | **State routes** (82) | **County or local roads** (251B) | **Unpaved roads** (may be 4WD only)

0 1/2 1
MILES
Scale

N
True north

Lake Tahoe ◉
Truckee ◉
Cities and towns

726
Forest Service roads

State border

STATE PARK
Public lands*

Ski Trails

Ski Lift

Lake) Dam
River or stream

Airport

Archaeological or historical site

Boat ramp

Campground (CG)

Cattle guard

Cemetery or gravesite

Church

Drinking water

Telephone

Golf Course

Fire tower or lookout

Falls or rapids

Food

Gate

House or cabin

Lodging

Mountain pass

Mountain summit
3312 (elevation in feet)

Mine or quarry

School

(P) Parking

Park office or ranger station

Picnic area

Power line or pipeline

Rest rooms

Spring

Stable, corral, or ranch

Fire Station

Observatory

Tunnel or bridge

Beach/Swimming Area

Cliff, Bluff or Outcropping

* Remember, private property exists in and around our national forests.

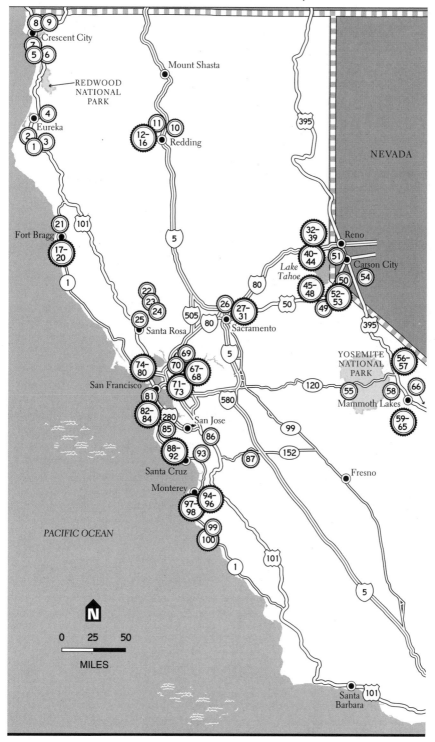

ACKNOWLEDGMENTS

The opportunity to compile a book of this nature is rare. It was a kick to say "I'm going to work" and really mean riding my bike through gorgeous regions of Northern California. Pedaling was the easy part. Sitting in front of a computer, poring over my millions of notes, and writing wasn't nearly as much fun. Truth is, this project was akin to the highest, steepest, longest, and most arduous mountain I've had to pedal up. I was privileged to have the help and support of a number of people, cyclists and noncyclists alike. Some of them generously offered their time and information on rides located in their areas. Others simply offered encouragement, understanding, and patience, especially when I needed it the most. This project was made possible by the following people, and to them I offer sincere thanks:

To all the rangers, land managers, and office personnel at the numerous state parks, national forests, and other recreation areas, many of whom took the time to gather valuable information and offered their personal remarks—your help provided the backbone for this book. To Tom Harrison of Tom Harrison Maps in San Rafael; Dick Powell of the Bicycle Outfitter in Los Altos; Ray Houghton of Mendocino Mountain Bike Tours in Mendocino; Ranger Phil Rovai of Redwood National and State Parks; Don Pass, Director of Recreation at Smith River National Recreation Area; John Stein of Sports Cottage in Redding; John Shuman, author of *Mountain Biking Whiskeytown*; Clinton Kane, park ranger of Whiskeytown-Shasta-Trinity National Recreation Area; Greg Williams of Yuba Expeditions in Nevada City; Lisa Lutz, Ian McDonald, Laura and Zachi Anderson and the Forest City Trail Council in Forest City; Peter Underwood of Olympic Bike Shop in Tahoe City; Greg Forsyth of CyclePaths in Tahoe City; Julie Maurer and David Schotzko of Northstar-at-Tahoe; Keith Hart of Carson Valley Schwinn in Gardnerville, Nevada; David Jones, park aid at Big Basin Redwoods State Park in Boulder Creek; Clark at Pacheco State Park; Jacquie Phelan of WOMBATS; John Foss, the Unicyclone extraordinaire; Greg Garcia; my cousin Bob Gong; Nancy Howden; Andy Steiner; Mary Lou and Keely Scates; Emmanuelle and Dominique Grenier; Terry and Linda Gong; Ron Lautzenheiser, Rod Hiapusio and Paul Malenke (for finding my car keys!); and Jay Seward. A special thank you to Georgena Terry of Terry Precision Cycling in Macedon, New York; Joe Breeze of Joe Breeze Cycles in Marin County; Clay White of Manuscript Ink and his band of hard-working editors; and all the cartographers, layout and production staff at Menasha. Heartfelt gratitude and appreciation goes to Dennis Coello, Molly Merkle, Bob Sehlinger, and Menasha Ridge Press who gave me the opportunity and for having immense patience, faith, and confidence in me—you guys are the best. Finally, I owe an enormous debt of gratitude to Bruce, my husband and primary support system. He lived and breathed this monster project with me throughout the entire process. This achievement is as much his effort as it is mine. I am one lucky girl, thanks to him.

FOREWORD

Welcome to North America by Mountain Bike, a 20-plus-book series designed to provide all-terrain bikers with the information they need to find and ride great trails everywhere. Whether you're new to the sport and don't know where to pedal, or an experienced mountain biker who wants to learn the classic trails in another region, this series is for you. Drop a few bucks for the book, spend an hour with the detailed maps and route descriptions, and you're prepared for the finest in off-road cycling.

My role as editor of this series was simple: First, find a mountain biker who knows the area and loves to ride. Second, ask that person to spend a year researching the most popular and very best rides around. And third, have that rider describe each trail in terms of difficulty, scenery, condition, elevation change, and all other categories of information that are important to trail riders. "Pretend you've just completed a ride and met up with fellow mountain bikers at the trailhead," I told each author. "Imagine their questions, be clear in your answers."

As I said, the editorial process—that of sending out riders and reading the submitted chapters—is a snap. But the work involved in finding, riding, and writing about each trail is enormous. In some instances our authors' tasks are made easier by the information contributed by local bike shops or cycling clubs, or even by the writers of local "where-to" guides. Credit for these contributions is provided, when appropriate, in each chapter, and our sincere thanks goes to all who have helped.

But the overwhelming majority of trails are discovered and pedaled by our authors themselves, then compared with dozens of other routes to determine if they qualify as "classic"—that area's best in scenery and cycling fun. If you've ever had the experience of pioneering a route from outdated topographic maps, or entering a bike shop to request information from local riders who would much prefer to keep their favorite trails secret, or know how it is to double- and triple-check data to be positive your trail info is correct, then you have an idea of how each of our authors has labored to bring about these books. You and I, and all mountain bikers, are the richer for their efforts.

You'll get more out of this book if you take a moment to read the Introduction explaining how to read the trail listings. The "Topographic Maps" section will help you understand how useful topos will be on a ride, and will also tell you where to get them. And though this is a "where-to," not a "how-to" guide, those of you who have not traveled the backcountry might find "Hitting the Trail" of particular value.

In addition to the material above, newcomers to mountain biking might want to spend a minute with the glossary, page 535, so that terms like hardpack, single-track, and water bars won't throw you when you come across them in the text.

All the best.

Dennis Coello
St. Louis

PREFACE

Welcome to Northern California! Whether you're a longtime resident or transplant, you'll find the state's diverse collection of environments impressive. And what better way to see them than by bike? Known for its ancient redwoods, thick and lush forests, high mountain ranges and glacial peaks, powerful canyon-carving rivers, agriculturally rich valleys, and spectacular coastline, there's plenty to discover even if you've lived here all your life. Check it out! The foggy north coast is contrasted by the blazingly hot inland country. Then there's the sprawling metropolis of the Greater Bay Area, saved from itself by forward-thinking regional park districts, which encompasses numerous, year-round accessible trails. How about that emerald gem in the sky, Lake Tahoe, straddling the California-Nevada state line, surrounded by national forests, wildernesses, and snow-capped peaks? Strike it rich along the Gold Rush Country of the western Sierra Nevada range, home to a Mother Lode of mountain bike trails. Yosemite National Park is pure gold, even though bicycling is limited within the park. The desert landscape of Mono Lake offers an intriguing environment, just as earthquake-riddled Mammoth Lakes a few miles south. On the coast, sitting on the north-south boundary is the magnificent Monterey Peninsula and the often-photographed dramatic Big Sur coastline.

Pure and simple, this book is for the person who, first and foremost, appreciates the natural beauty of the great outdoors and, secondly, wishes to enjoy it by mountain bike. Mountain biking can be a leisurely form of exercise, a mode of transportation for sightseeing, an extreme personal challenge, or a combination of all of these, and it can vary from one day to the next. It's whatever you want it to be. Whether you're an uninitiated newcomer who is contemplating taking up the sport, a well-seasoned recreational rider like me, or a hard-core expert-level rider who lives and breathes dirt, I think you'll find lots of useful data on these pages. In the name of enhancing your riding enjoyment, I often present relevant background information on the topics like geology, history, or local politics. In researching and detailing the trail descriptions, my intention is to give you as much information as possible so that you have a good idea of what to expect and to help you avoid getting lost.

Now, if you're an advanced or expert rider, you may think my reporting takes all the fun out of mountain biking because the joy of the sport is exploring and discovering the outdoors on your own. For those of you who prefer that approach, check out the trail suggestions listed at the end of each regional chapter. I did not personally pedal these routes due to lack of time or ability. They were culled from a slew of recommendations from other bikers. Approximate mileages and very brief trail descriptions are offered. So, if you're looking for a demanding experience, arm yourself with the appropriate topo map(s), talk to a ranger, and go explore! I invite you to give me your comments via U.S. mail or email at austinmtnbike@hotmail.com.

Let me debunk a myth right off the bat: Mountain biking is not just for highly skilled, bionic riders. I'm living proof of it. My height is a towering five-foot-nothing (as a friend likes to put it) and I ride a smaller than average bike (specifically designed by Georgena Terry for petite women riders, using 24" wheels). And I'm forty-something. Having ridden hundreds of miles on my Terry bike, I often encounter hikers and other trail users who marvel at my so-called prowess. (I'm saddened by the fact that women are especially impressed. On the other hand, it gives me a chance to tell them that if I can do it, they can, too.) Truth is, I consider myself a mere recreational rider, one who has decent—but not bionic—stamina (I confess: I love spinach but am not particularly fond of Wheaties). I rate my technical bike handling skills as intermediate. That means my skills are slightly above average, which allows me to maneuver around or through reasonable obstacles, like rocks and boulders, dips, tree roots, as well as negotiate narrow trails, drop-offs, a variety of trail conditions, and vehicular traffic. Perhaps one of the best, if not most important tools I have in my repertoire of skills is this: Knowing the limits of my ability. Sometimes that translates into "I have no business trying to ride that trail" after previewing a trail description or having talked with someone who has ridden it. Sometimes it translates into "time to get off and walk, Linda" when I encounter a particularly difficult spot. Bottom line is, having a few key skills will enable you to enjoy many miles of terrific mountain bike trails. Something else to keep in mind when you're being tested on a trail (or in life for that matter): Attitude is everything. How you mentally deal with aerobic and technical challenges directly affects your safety and enjoyment.

LEVELS RATING: A SUBJECTIVE CATEGORIZATION

Of the 100 trail descriptions in this book, I personally rode 84 of them. The rest were generously and enthusiastically contributed by persons whom I regard as the best knowledgeable source in that particular area. The ones I didn't pedal were either due to being under snow, lack of time, or because I felt they were way too difficult for my ability. Nevertheless, all the rides described in this book are rated according to the following scale:

Aerobic Rating

Easy: Minimal exertion required. Generally flat terrain. Tempered by total mileage.
Moderate: Some exertion involved. May involve some gentle hills and perhaps steep but very brief, not overly long stretches of climbing. Influenced by total mileage and difficulty of terrain.
Moderately strenuous: This is often a workout. Definitely includes climbing hills, either steep and brief, sustained, or a series of substantial ups and downs. Influenced by total mileage, altitude, and difficulty of terrain.
Strenuous: Usually heart-pounding, thigh-burning hills, often over very rugged terrain. Influenced by total mileage and altitude.
Very strenuous: Take the "Strenuous" description and intensify it with steeper hills and much more rugged terrain. Often at significantly higher altitude. Synonymous with "epic ride."

Technical Skills Rating

Not technical (nontechnical): Rider is able to control direction of travel, maneuver around occasional obstacles, comfortably share the path with other trail users, and use brakes effectively and properly. Generally means smooth, wide dirt trails or dirt roads, or paved multi-use paths. Cyclists who possess only this skill are considered true beginners (same as novice in my book).

Mildy technical: Same as above except that it generally includes more small obstacles, such as rocks, tree roots, potholes, and irregular trail surface. Generally means wide single-track trails and smooth dirt roads which are usually suitable for two-wheel-drive passenger vehicles. Strong, somewhat experienced beginners can handle these trails comfortably.

Intermediate: Rider is able to maneuver around, through or hop over obstacles of all sizes, including closely placed boulders, loose rock, abrupt and irregular terrain, trees, and exposed roots. Cyclists should also be comfortable pedaling narrow, twisty paths in between trees and boulders, and skirting drop-offs safely. Usually involves doing all this while pedaling up and down moderately steep terrain. Generally means double-tracks and narrow single-tracks as well as rugged dirt roads which are suitable for two-wheel-drive and four-wheel-drive vehicles. Rider should be able to read a topo map, have a good sense of direction, and not freak out from a momentary loss of direction or convoluted trail finding. Strong beginners with the right attitude may enjoy these trails.

Advanced: Rider is able to handle more intensely rugged types of trails with higher concentrations of obstacles of all sizes; possesses quicker bike-handling skills required to "clean" the trail (that is, maneuver around obstacles without much difficulty). Generally involves riding up and down severely irregular and steep terrain and/or dropping down boulders (stair-steps) in the trail. Advanced riders know how to read topo maps and have a good sense of direction. Accepts getting lost and finding a way out as part of the mountain biking experience.

Expert: Take the "Advanced" level and apply the descriptive word "extreme" to every aspect of it. Unafraid to explore new paths encountered on the ride.

HOW DID I CHOOSE THE RIDES FEATURED IN THIS BOOK?

My goal was to include something for everyone, from novices to expertly skilled, from wimps to ironmen and ironwomen. And I wanted to include rides that young families could enjoy, generally free from motor vehicle traffic as much as possible, and as long (or short) as the kiddies' little legs and lungs could handle. To me, a family ride is often suitable for freewheeling youngsters with or without training wheels, parent towing a kid trailer, and alley-cat riders (child seat with working pedals and wheel, attached behind adult rider's seat post). I solicited trail recommendations from bike shops, forest rangers and land managers, and fellow cyclists. I consulted trail guidebooks, maps and searched the Internet. Often times, a state or local park may contain many other bikeable trails than the one or two I have chosen to feature in the book. Once you try those featured rides, I think you'll have a good idea of the lay of the land and you'll soon be exploring other trails within that park on your own. Lastly, a personal requirement was that trailheads for all rides in this book must be accessible by two-wheel-drive passenger vehicle.

The rides featured in this book do not represent the "Best" rides in Northern California. Far be it from me to tell you which rides you will like. The fact is, your ability, fitness level and personal preference has a lot to do with your enjoyment of any ride. Frankly, some of the rides which I think are boring may be perfect for many riders, while those I found to be extremely difficult and not much fun would be awesome to others. So, in choosing a ride, I suggest you read through the descriptions and decide which ones appeal to you. Then, you decide which ones are the best rides in California.

WHAT EXACTLY IS A "TRAIL"?

In my ride descriptions, I often use trail figuratively, not just literally. What that means is I use trail to refer to the bicycle route itself that is being described; that is, the specific line of travel from start to finish. And that route might be composed of a combination of single-tracks, fire roads, double-tracks, etc. Literally speaking though, trail refers to a physically narrow pathway, usually dirt and unpaved, like a single-track. But the fact of the matter is, trail oftentimes refers to a dirt road or a paved narrow path designed specifically for multi-use by bikers, baby-strollers, rollerbladers and the like. While researching printed material and in talking with fellow cyclists and rangers, terms are often loosely and generally applied when describing or identifying routes. Those terms are: road, trail, fire road, dirt road, jeep road, gravel road, service road, single-track, and double-track.

So what's the big deal? Not much really. When you're out there pedaling, you can ride them all (assuming they're legal, of course). Nonetheless, it's a big deal to me because I want to convey descriptions that are accurate. Fire roads, by their nature, are service roads, which in turn are often gravel roads, and nearly all the time dirt roads. A jeep road, as designated on a map, implies four-wheel-drive vehicle with high clearance. In the field, however, sometimes a regular passenger vehicle can handle that jeep road. A stretch of dirt road is sometimes described as a double-track in that the grass growing between the tire tracks make the road seem like a dual single-track. Then there's the dirt road that degenerates into a double-track, then becomes a wide single-track before becoming a dirt road again. Huh? Sound confusing? The fact of the matter is, names are not always consistent with what is in the field or used in casual conversations with one another. Sometimes a reliable map labels a path a trail when in reality it's a wide dirt road. Undoubtedly when a map tells you trail and you find yourself on a dirt road, you're liable to think "Is this the trail or did I miss a turn?"

So, at the risk of over-simplification, here's the nomenclature I use throughout the book: A path that's accessible by a single vehicle of at least normal width, I call a dirt road, which includes fire roads, service roads and some double-tracks. The kicker is sometimes dirt roads become more narrow than one-car width, then widen again. Single-track refers to a narrow path that accommodates single-file riders only. For a path that is consistently slightly less than one-car width (usually due to overgrowth), I generally refer to it as a wide single-track which can tightly accommodate two riders across. On rare occasions, I use the term jeep road to describe a dirt road that truly requires a vehicle with high clearance and is extremely and deeply irregular in surface.

Enough said. Happy trails!

**Wildflower Show
(timing is everything)**
52 TRT: Big Meadows to Kingsbury
      Grade
53 TRT: Big Meadows to Round Lake
69 Black Diamond Mines Loop
87 Pacheco State Park Loop
89 Big Basin: Skyline-to-the-Sea Trail
      (Waddell Creek)
91 Wilder Ranch: Grey Whale Loop

Great Single-track Trails
      Any bike-legal portion of the Tahoe
        Rim Trail (TRT)
10 Clikipudi Trail
16 Great Water Ditch Trail
22 Boggs Mountain Demonstration
      Forest
27 Salmon Falls Out-and-Back
30 Stagecoach–Lake Clementine Loop
31 Sly Park–Jenkinson Lake Loop
32 Big Boulder Trail Loop
33 South Yuba Primitive Camp Loop
34 Bullards Bar Loop
35 Chimney Rock Trail
36 North Yuba River Trail
38 Hole-In-The-Ground Trail
51 The Flume–TRT Ride
62 Horseshoe Lake Loop
64 Off the Top—Mammoth Mountain
      Bike Park
80 China Camp Shoreline—
      Ridge Loop
84 El Corte de Madera Creek Loop
86 Henry Coe Middle Ridge Loop

Wildlife
5   Ossagon–Gold Bluff Loop
81 Tour of San Francisco and the
      Golden Gate (well, not really wild-
      life but you're bound to see some
      interesting species of humans)
92 Wilder Ranch: Old Cove Bluff Trail
      (during whale migration season)
97 Monterey Recreation Trail
98 17-Mile Drive to Carmel Road Ride

Geological Landscape
55 Yosemite National Park Bike Trail

56 Black Point at Mono Lake Ride
57 South Tufa Out-and-Back
59 Inyo Craters Loop
66 Hot Creek Hatchery Road to the
      Hot Springs
85 Monte Bello–Stevens Creek Loop

**Very Easy Rides/
Great Family Outing**
59 Inyo Craters Loop
55 Yosemite National Park Bike Trail
74 Angel Island Double Loop
97 Monterey Recreation Trail
92 Wilder Ranch: Old Cove Bluff Trail
82 Sawyer Camp Trail
57 South Tufa Out-and-Back
73 Lafayette–Moraga Trail
19 Fern Canyon Trail—
      Van Damme State Park
20 Fern Canyon Trail—
      Russian Gulch State Park
21 MacKerricher Ten Mile
      Coastal Trail
5   Ossagon–Gold Bluff Loop (portions)
7   Coastal Trail—Last Chance Section
39 Sardine Valley Loop
25 Annadel State Park Loops (portions)
26 American River Bike Path
44 Tahoe City Bike Paths
45 General Creek Easy Loop
48 Pope Baldwin Bike Path
60 Easy Shady Rest Ride

Incredible View
      Most bike-legal portions of the Tahoe
        Rim Trail (TRT)
30 Stagecoach–Lake Clementine Loop
38 Hole-In-The-Ground Trail
51 The Flume–TRT Ride
52 TRT: Big Meadows to
      Kingsbury Grade
53 TRT: Big Meadows to Round Lake
64 Off the Top—Mammoth Mountain
      Bike Park
67 Mt. Diablo–Mitchell Canyon Loop
74 Angel Island Double Loop
75 Tennessee Valley Double Loop
76 Mt. Tam Loop via Old Railroad–
      Eldridge Grades

81 Tour of San Francisco and the
       Golden Gate
92 Wilder Ranch: Old Cove Bluff Trail
98 17-Mile Drive to Carmel Road Ride

Meeting Other Riders
25 Annadel State Park Loops
30 Stagecoach–Lake Clementine Loop
51 The Flume–TRT Ride
65 Paper Route & Big Ring
64 Off the Top—Mammoth Mountain
       Bike Park
72 East–West Ridge Loop
76 Mt. Tam Loop via Old Railroad–
       Eldridge Grades
80 China Camp Shoreline—
       Ridge Loop
83 Purisima Creek Redwoods—
       Short Loop
84 El Corte de Madera Creek Loop
85 Monte Bello–Stevens Creek Loop
91 Wilder Ranch: Gray Whale Loop
93 Nisene Marks–Sand Point Ride

Tough Climbs
1   Grasshopper Peak Loop
14 The Chimney
17 Manly Gulch Loop
18 Caspar Creek–640–630 Loop
32 Big Boulder Trail Loop
33 South Yuba Primitive Camp Loop
34 Bullards Bar Loop
35 Chimney Rock Trail
36 North Yuba River Trail (Halls
       Ranch–Fiddle Creek option)
52 TRT: Big Meadows to Kingsbury
       Grade
54 Pine Nut Mountains Loops
       (pro/expert loop)
67 Mt. Diablo–Mitchell Canyon Loop
100 Andrew Molera: Creamery-
       Ridge Ride

All-Day Epic Rides
32 Big Boulder Trail Loop
33 South Yuba Primitive Camp Loop
34 Bullards Bar Loop
35 Chimney Rock Trail
42 TRT–WST–Paige Meadows
       Point-to-Point

51 The Flume–TRT Ride
52 TRT: Big Meadows to Kingsbury
       Grade
67 Combine Mt. Diablo–Mitchell
       Canyon Loop
68 Shell Ridge–Stage Road Dirt Ride
69 Black Diamond Mines Loop
75 Combine Tennessee Valley
       Double Loop
76 Mt. Tam Loop via Old Railroad–
       Eldridge Grades
77 Bolinas Ridge Fire Road
78 Barnabe Peak Loop and Devil's
       Gulch
86 Henry Coe Middle Ridge Loop and
       many trails in the state park

Extremely Technical Rides
24 Oat Hill Mine Road
41 TRT–Cinder Cone Loop
67 Mt. Diablo–Mitchell Canyon Loop
       (downhill portion)

**Exceptional Dirt Road/
Fire Road Rides**
1   Grasshopper Peak Loop
8   Howland Hill–Stout Grove
9   Gasquet Toll Road
12 Boulder Creek Loop
56 Black Point at Mono Lake Ride
57 South Tufa Out-and-Back
59 Inyo Craters Loop
61 Knolls Loop
67 Mt. Diablo–Mitchell Canyon Loop
69 Black Diamond Mines Loop
74 Angel Island Double Loop
75 Tennessee Valley Double Loop
76 Mt. Tam Loop via Old Railroad–
       Eldridge Grades
77 Bolinas Ridge Fire Road
88 Big Basin: Gazos Creek–Chalk
       Mountain Ride
91 Wilder Ranch: Grey Whale Loop
95 Ft. Ord: Guidotti–Goat Trail Loop
96 Ft. Ord: Mudhen Lake–Rim
       Trail Ramble
    Tour de Skunk (annual scheduled
       biking event in Jackson State Park
       Demo Forest, Mendocino County)

INTRODUCTION

TRAIL DESCRIPTION OUTLINE

Each trail in this book begins with key information that includes length, configuration, aerobic and technical difficulty, trail conditions, scenery, and special comments. Additional description is contained in 11 individual categories. The following will help you to understand all of the information provided.

Trail name: Trail names are as designated on United States Geological Survey (USGS) or Forest Service or other maps, and/or by local custom.

At a Glance Information

Length/configuration: The overall length of a trail is described in miles, unless stated otherwise. The configuration is a description of the shape of each trail— whether the trail is a loop, out-and-back (that is, along the same route), figure eight, trapezoid, isosceles triangle, decahedron . . . (just kidding), or if it connects with another trail described in the book. See the Glossary for definitions of *point-to-point* and *combination.*

Aerobic difficulty: This provides a description of the degree of physical exertion required to complete the ride.

Technical difficulty: This provides a description of the technical skill required to pedal a ride. Trails are often described here in terms of being paved, unpaved, sandy, hard-packed, washboarded, two- or four-wheel-drive, single-track or double-track. All terms that might be unfamiliar to the first-time mountain biker are defined in the Glossary.

   Note: For both the aerobic and technical difficulty categories, authors were asked to keep in mind the fact that all riders are not equal, and thus to gauge the trail in terms of how the middle-of-the-road rider—someone between the newcomer and Ned Overend—could handle the route. In addition to the ratings described on page xv, comments about the trail's length, condition, and elevation change will also assist you in determining the difficulty of any trail relative to your own abilities.

Scenery: Here you will find a general description of the natural surroundings during the seasons most riders pedal the trail and a suggestion of what is to be found at special times (like great fall foliage or cactus in bloom).

Special comments: Unique elements of the ride are mentioned.

General location: This category describes where the trail is located in reference to a nearby town or other landmark.

Elevation change: Unless stated otherwise, the figure provided is the total change in elevation as measured from high point to low point. Total gain, that is, the cumulative total feet in which the trail ascends, is difficult to measure accurately but suffice it to say that it generally exceeds the simple difference between high and low points. In an effort to give you a sense of how much climbing is involved in a particular ride, brief but general descriptive phrases are used in conjunction with elevation change.

Season: This is the best time of year to pedal the route, taking into account trail conditions (for example, when it will not be muddy), riding comfort (when the weather is too hot, cold, or wet), and local hunting seasons.

Note: Because the opening and closing dates of deer, elk, moose, and antelope seasons often change from year to year, riders should check with the local Fish and Wildlife Department or call a sporting goods store (or any place that sells hunting licenses) in a nearby town before heading out. Wear bright clothes in the fall, and don't wear suede jackets while in the saddle. Hunter's-orange tape on the helmet is also a good idea.

Services: This category is of primary importance in guides for paved-road tourers and is far less crucial to most mountain bike trail descriptions because there are usually no services whatsoever to be found. Authors have noted when water is available on desert or long mountain routes and have listed the availability of food, lodging, campgrounds, and bike shops. If all these services are present, you will find only the words, "All services available in . . ."

Hazards: Special hazards like hunting season, rattlesnakes, mountain lions, bears, ticks, poison oak, earthquake, lightning, other trail users, and vehicular traffic are noted here. Other hazards which are considered a regular part of a ride, such as steep cliffs, boulder stair-steps, or scree on steep downhill sections are discussed in the "Notes on the trail" section.

Rescue index: Determining how far one is from help on a particular trail can be difficult due to the backcountry nature of most mountain bike rides. Authors therefore state the proximity of homes or Forest Service outposts, nearby roads where one might hitch a ride, or the likelihood of other bikers being encountered on the trail. Phone numbers of local sheriff departments or hospitals have not been provided because phones are almost never available. If you are able to reach a phone, the local operator will connect you with emergency services.

Land status: This category provides information regarding whether the trail crosses land operated by the Forest Service, the Bureau of Land Management, or a city, state, or national park; whether it crosses private land whose owner (at the time the author did the research) has allowed mountain bikers right of passage; and so on. A note regarding fees for land usage: There is no standard by which use-fees are charged. Some land agencies charge a fee to park within designated areas, others charge a fee regardless of where you park your car. Some areas are free year-round, others only during the off-season or during the week. Some parks charge a day-use fee, regardless if you park a car or not. Though most national forests do not charge a day-use fee, be prepared to pay something, generally between $2 to $16, depending on your intended usage. Yosemite National Park charges almost $20 per car, even if you're just driving through to get to the Eastern Sierras. State parks almost always charge a day-use fee at the very least.

Note: Authors have been extremely careful to offer only those routes that are open to bikers and are legal to ride. However, because land ownership changes over time, and because the land-use controversy created by mountain bikes still has not completely subsided, it is the duty of each cyclist to look for and heed signs warning against trail use. Don't expect this book to get you off the hook when you're facing some small-town judge for pedaling past a "Biking Prohibited" sign erected the day before you arrived. Look for these signs, read them, and heed the advice. And remember, there's always another trail.

Maps: The maps in this book have been produced with great care and, in conjunction with the trail-following suggestions, will help you stay on course. But as every experienced mountain biker knows, things can get tricky in the backcountry. It is therefore strongly suggested that you avail yourself of the detailed information found in the USGS (United States Geological Survey) 7.5 minute series topographic maps. In some cases, authors have found that specific Forest Service or other maps may be more useful than the USGS quads, and they tell how to obtain them.

Finding the trail: Detailed information on how to reach the trailhead and where to park your car is provided here.

Sources of additional information: Here you will find the address and/or phone number of a bike shop, governmental agency, or other source from which trail information can be obtained.

Notes on the trail: This is where you are guided carefully through any portions of the trail that are particularly difficult to follow. The author also may add information about the route that does not fit easily in the other categories. This category will not be present for those rides where the route is easy to follow.

ABBREVIATIONS

The following road-designation abbreviations are used in the *Mountain Bike!* series:

CR	County Road	I-	Interstate
FR	Farm Route	IR	Indian Route
FS	Forest Service road	US	United States highway

State highways are designated with the appropriate two-letter state abbreviation, followed by the road number. Example: CA 89 = California State Highway 89; NV 28 = Nevada State Highway 28.

RIDE CONFIGURATIONS

Combination: This type of route may combine two or more configurations. For example, a point-to-point route may integrate a scenic loop or an out-and-back spur midway through the ride. Likewise, an out-and-back may have a loop at its farthest point (this configuration looks like a cherry with a stem attached; the stem is the out-and-back, the fruit is the terminus loop). Or a loop route may have multiple out-and-back spurs and/or loops to the side. Mileage for a combination route is for the total distance to complete the ride.

Loop: This route configuration is characterized by riding from the designated trailhead to a distant point, then returning to the trailhead via a different route (or simply continuing on the same in a circle route) without doubling back. You always move forward across new terrain but return to the starting point when finished. Mileage is for the entire loop from the trailhead back to trailhead.

Out-and-back: A ride where you will return on the same trail you pedaled out. While this might sound far more boring than a loop route, many trails look very different when pedaled in the opposite direction.

Point-to-point: A vehicle shuttle (or similar assistance) is required for this type of route, which is ridden from the designated trailhead to a distant location, or endpoint, where the route ends. Total mileage is for the one-way trip from the trailhead to endpoint.

Spur: A road or trail that intersects the main trail you're following.

Ride Configurations contributed by Gregg Bromka

TOPOGRAPHIC MAPS

The maps in this book, when used in conjunction with the route directions present in each chapter, will in most instances be sufficient to get you to the trail and keep you on it. However, you will find superior detail and valuable information in the USGS 7.5 minute series topographic maps. Recognizing how indispensable these are to bikers and hikers alike, many bike shops and sporting goods stores now carry topos of the local area.

If you're brand new to mountain biking you might be wondering, "What's a topographic map?" In short, these differ from standard "flat" maps in that they indicate not only linear distance but elevation as well. One glance at a topo will show you the difference, for contour lines are spread across the map like dozens of intricate spider webs. Each contour line represents a particular elevation, and at the base of each topo a particular contour interval designation is given. Yes, it sounds confusing if you're new to the lingo, but it truly is a simple and wonderfully helpful system. Keep reading.

Let's assume that the 7.5 minute series topo before us says "Contour Interval 40 feet," that the short trail we'll be pedaling is two inches in length on the map, and that it crosses five contour lines from its beginning to end. What do we know? Well, because the linear scale of this series is 2,000 feet to the inch (roughly 2 $\frac{3}{4}$ inches representing 1 mile), we know our trail is approximately $\frac{4}{5}$ of a mile long (2 inches × 2,000 feet). But we also know we'll be climbing or descending 200 vertical feet (5 contour lines × 40 feet each) over that distance. And the elevation designations written on occasional contour lines will tell us if we're heading up or down.

The authors of this series warn their readers of upcoming terrain, but only a detailed topo gives you the information you need to pinpoint your position on a map, steer yourself toward optional trails and roads nearby, and to see at a glance if you'll be pedaling hard to take them. It's a lot of information for a very low cost. In fact, the only drawback with topos is their size—several feet square. I've tried rolling them into tubes, folding them carefully, even cutting them into blocks and photocopying the pieces. Any of these systems is a pain, but no matter how you pack the maps you'll be happy they're along. And you'll be even happier if you pack a compass as well.

In addition to local bike shops and sporting goods stores, you'll find topos at major universities and some public libraries, where you might try photocopying the ones you need to avoid the cost of buying them. But if you want your own and can't find them locally, contact:

USGS Map Sales
Box 25286
Denver, CO 80225
(888) ASK-USGS (275-8747)
http://mapping.usgs.gov/esic/to_order.html/

VISA and MasterCard are accepted. Ask for an index while you're at it, plus a price list and a copy of the booklet *Topographic Maps*. In minutes you'll be reading them like a pro.

A second excellent series of maps available to mountain bikers is that put out by the United States Forest Service. If your trail runs through an area designated as a national forest, look in the phone book (white pages) under the United States Government listings, find the Department of Agriculture heading, and run your finger down that section until you find the Forest Service. Give them a call, and they'll provide the address of the regional Forest Service office, from which you can obtain the appropriate map.

TRAIL ETIQUETTE

Pick up almost any mountain bike magazine these days and you'll find articles and letters to the editor about trail conflict. For example, you'll find hikers' tales of being blindsided by speeding mountain bikers, complaints from mountain bikers about being blamed for trail damage that was really caused by horse or cattle traffic, and cries from bikers about those "kamikaze" riders who through their antics threaten to close even more trails to all of us.

The authors of this series have been very careful to guide you to only those trails that are open to mountain biking (or at least were open at the time of their research), and without exception have warned of the damage done to our sport through injudicious riding. We can all benefit from glancing over the following International Mountain Bicycling Association (IMBA) Rules of the Trail before saddling up.

1. *Ride on open trails only.* Respect trail and road closures (ask if not sure), avoid possible trespass on private land, obtain permits and authorization as may be required. Federal and state wilderness areas are closed to cycling.

2. *Leave no trace.* Be sensitive to the dirt beneath you. Even on open trails, you should not ride under conditions where you will leave evidence of your passing, such as on certain soils shortly after rain. Observe the different types of soils and trail construction; practice low-impact cycling. This also means staying on the trail and not creating any new ones. Be sure to pack out at least as much as you pack in.

3. *Control your bicycle!* Inattention for even a second can cause disaster. Excessive speed can maim and threaten people; there is no excuse for it!

4. *Always yield the trail.* Make known your approach well in advance. A friendly greeting (or a bell) is considerate and works well; startling someone may cause loss of trail access. Show your respect when passing others by slowing to a walk or even stopping. Anticipate that other trail users may be around corners or in blind spots.

5. *Never spook animals.* All animals are startled by an unannounced approach, a sudden movement, or a loud noise. This can be dangerous for you, for others,

and for the animals. Give animals extra room and time to adjust to you. In passing, use special care and follow the directions of horseback riders (ask if uncertain). Running cattle and disturbing wild animals is a serious offense. Leave gates as you found them or as marked.

6. *Plan ahead.* Know your equipment, your ability, and the area in which you are riding—and prepare accordingly. Be self-sufficient at all times. Wear a helmet, keep your machine in good condition, and carry necessary supplies for changes in weather or other conditions. A well-executed trip is a satisfaction to you and not a burden or offense to others.

For more information, contact IMBA, P.O. Box 7578, Boulder, CO 80306, (303) 545-9011.

Additionally, the following Code of Ethics by the National Off-Road Biking Association (NORBA) is worthy of your attention.

1. I will yield the right of way to other non-motorized recreationists. I realize that people judge all cyclists by my actions.

2. I will slow down and use caution when approaching or overtaking another and will make my presence known well in advance.

3. I will maintain control of my speed at all times and will approach turns in anticipation of someone around the bend.

4. I will stay on designated trails to avoid trampling native vegetation and minimize potential erosion to trails by not using muddy trails or shortcutting switchbacks.

5. I will not disturb wildlife or livestock.

6. I will not litter. I will pack out what I pack in, and pack out more than my share if possible.

7. I will respect public and private property, including trail use and no trespassing signs; I will leave gates as I found them.

8. I will always be self-sufficient and my destination and travel speed will be determined by my ability, my equipment, the terrain, and present and potential weather conditions.

9. I will not travel solo when bike-packing in remote areas.

10. I will leave word of my destination and when I plan to return.

11. I will practice minimum impact bicycling by "taking only pictures and memories and leaving only waffle prints."

12. I will always wear a helmet when I ride.

Worthy of mention are the following suggestions based on a list by Utah's Wasatch-Cache National Forest and the *Tread Lightly!* program advocated by the National Forest Service and Bureau of Land Management.

1. *Study a forest map before you ride.* Currently, bicycles are permitted on roads and developed trails which are designated bikes permitted. If your route crosses private land, it is your responsibility to obtain right-of-way permission from the landowner.

2. *Stay out of designated wilderness areas.* By law, all vehicles, including mountain bikes are not allowed.

3. *Stay off of roads and trails "put to bed."* These may be resource roads no longer used for logging or mining, or they may be steep trails being replaced by easier ones. So that the path returns to its natural state, they're usually blocked or signed closed to protect new vegetation.

4. *Keep groups small.* Riding in large groups degrades the outdoor experience for others, can disturb wildlife, and usually leads to greater resource damage.

5. *Avoid riding on wet trails.* Bicycle tires leave ruts in wet trails. These ruts concentrate runoff and accelerate erosion. Postponing a ride when the trails are wet will preserve the trails for future use.

6. *Stay on roads and trails.* Riding cross-country destroys vegetation and damages the soil. Resist the urge to pioneer a new road or trail, or to cut across a switchback. Avoid riding through meadows, steep hillsides or along stream banks and lakeshores because the terrain is easily scarred by churning wheels.

7. *Always yield to others.* Trails are shared by hikers, horses, and bicycles. Move off the trail to allow horses to pass and stop to allow hikers adequate room to share the trail. Simply yelling "Bicycle!" is not acceptable.

8. *Control your speed.* Excessive speed endangers yourself and other forest users.

9. *Avoid wheel lock-up and spin-out.* Steep terrain is especially vulnerable to trail wear. Locking brakes on steep descents or when stopping needlessly damages trails. If a slope is steep enough to require locking wheels and skidding, dismount and walk your bicycle. Likewise, if an ascent is so steep that your rear wheel slips and spins, dismount and walk your bicycle.

10. *Protect waterbars and switchbacks.* Waterbars, the rock and log drains built to direct water off trails, protect trails from erosion. When you encounter a waterbar, ride directly over the top or dismount and walk your bicycle. Riding around the ends of waterbars destroys their effectiveness and speeds erosion. Skidding around switchback corners shortens trail life. Slow down for switchback corners and keep your wheels rolling.

11. *If you abuse it, you lose it.* Mountain bikers are relative newcomers to the forest and must prove themselves responsible trail users. By following the guidelines above, and by participating in trail maintenance service projects, bicyclists can help avoid closures that would prevent them from using trails.

12. *Know your bicycle handling limitations.*

You get the drift. So that everyone can continue riding our bikes through some of our country's most beautiful places, I urge you to follow the codes above and not be the "one bad apple" that spoils it for the rest of us.

HITTING THE TRAIL

Once again, because this is a "where-to," not a "how-to" guide, the following will be brief. If you're a veteran trail rider, these suggestions might serve to remind you of something you've forgotten to pack. If you're a newcomer, they might convince you to think twice before hitting the backcountry unprepared.

Water: I've heard the questions dozens of times. "How much is enough? One bottle? Two? Three?! But think of all that extra weight!" Well, one simple physiological fact should convince you to err on the side of excess when it comes to deciding how much water to pack: A human working hard in 90-degree temperature needs approximately ten quarts of fluids every day. Ten quarts. That's two and a half gallons— 12 large water bottles or 16 small ones. And, with water weighing in at approximately 8 pounds per gallon, a one-day supply comes to a whopping 20 pounds.

In other words, pack along two or three bottles even for short rides. And make sure you can purify the water found along the trail on longer routes. When writing of those routes where this could be of critical importance, each author has provided information on where water can be found near the trail—if it can be found at all. But drink it untreated and you run the risk of disease. (See *giardia* in the Glossary.)

One sure way to kill the protozoans, bacteria, and viruses in water is to boil it. Right. That's just how you want to spend your time on a bike ride. Besides, who wants to carry a stove or denude the countryside stoking bonfires to boil water?

Luckily, there is a better way. Many riders pack along the inexpensive and only slightly distasteful tetraglycine hydroperiodide tablets (sold under the names Potable Aqua, Globaline, and Coughlan's, among others). Some invest in portable, lightweight purifiers that filter out the crud. Unfortunately, both iodine *and* filtering are now required to be absolutely sure you've killed all the nasties you can't see. Tablets or iodine drops by themselves will knock off the well-known *giardia*, once called "beaver fever" for its transmission to the water through the feces of infected beavers. One to four weeks after ingestion, giardia will have you bloated, vomiting, shivering with chills, and living in the bathroom. (Though you won't care while you're suffering, beavers are getting a bum rap, for other animals are carriers also.)

But now there's another parasite we must worry about—*cryptosporidium.* "Crypto" brings on symptoms very similar to *giardia*, but unlike that fellow protozoan it's equipped with a shell sufficiently strong to protect it against the chemical killers that stop giardia cold. This means we're either back to boiling or on to using a water filter to screen out both *giardia* and crypto, plus the iodine to knock off viruses. All of which sounds like a time-consuming pain, but really isn't. Some water filters come equipped with an iodine chamber to guarantee full protection. Or you can simply add a pill or drops to the water you've just filtered (if you aren't allergic to iodine, of course). The pleasures of backcountry biking—and the displeasure of getting sick— make this relatively minor effort worth every one of the few minutes involved.

Tools: Ever since my first cross-country tour in 1965 I've been kidded about the number of tools I pack on the trail. And so I will exit entirely from this discussion by providing a list compiled by two mechanic (and mountain biker) friends of mine. After all, since they make their livings fixing bikes, and get their kicks by riding them, who could be a better source?

These two suggest the following as an absolute minimum:

tire levers	spare tube and patch kit
air pump	Allen wrenches (3, 4, 5, and 6 mm)
spoke wrench	six-inch crescent (adjustable-end) wrench
chain rivet tool	small flat-blade screwdriver

On the trail, their personal tool pouches contain these additional items:

channel locks (small)
air gauge
tire valve cap (the metal kind, with a valve-stem remover)

baling wire (ten or so inches, for temporary repairs)
duct tape (small roll for temporary repairs or tire boot)
boot material (small piece of old tire or a large tube patch)
spare chain link
rear derailleur pulley
spare nuts and bolts
paper towel and tube of waterless hand cleaner

First-Aid kit: My personal kit contains the following, sealed inside double Ziploc bags:

sunscreen
aspirin
butterfly-closure bandages
Band-Aids
snakebite kit
gauze (one roll)
gauze compress pads (a half-dozen 4" × 4")
ace bandages or Spenco joint wraps
Benadryl (an antihistamine, in case of allergic reactions)
water purification tablets/water filter (on long rides)
Moleskin/Spenco "Second Skin"
hydrogen peroxide, iodine, or Mercurochrome (some kind of antiseptic)
matches or pocket cigarette lighter
whistle (more effective in signaling rescuers than your voice)

Final considerations: The authors of this series have done a good job suggesting that specific items be packed for certain trails—rain gear in particular seasons, a hat and gloves for mountain passes, or shades for desert jaunts. Heed their warnings, and think ahead. Good luck.

Dennis Coello

CELL PHONES

Why do we go into the wilderness? Many visitors enjoy wild places, away from civilization. Many backcountry visitors seek the classic wilderness values of risk, solitude, and challenge. Use of cell phones, for anything other than serious emergencies, detracts from the character of wilderness. And keep in mind that it is next to impossible for a dispatcher to give directions to a lost person calling on a cell phone. Route-finding and safety skills are paramount in the wild. Cell phone coverage is very patchy in much of the interior and coastal areas of Northern California. There may be a chance to reach a cell site by climbing to a ridge top but remember, you may be hitting a cell site hundreds of miles from your location. Knowledge of one's location is vital to the success of any rescue. Also, if you're expecting a call back, don't move—sometimes just a foot or two makes a difference in getting a call through to a cell phone in the wilderness. From the backcountry, report only serious emergencies by calling 911. Remember, phone batteries drain, and when your phone is dead, you're on your own again. That said, do not depend on a cell phone to help you in an emergency.

Linda Austin

THE NORTH COAST

The North Coast is a vast territory, extending from the Oregon state line south along the Pacific to Fort Bragg. Veiled in year-round fog, often dampened—even soaked—by rain most of the year, the region is completely dominated by the mountainous Coastal Range. Within this long strip of territory is the remaining belt of giant redwoods that used to blanket the entire California coast, from Santa Cruz to Oregon. When the Gold Rush of the mid-1800s caused population to swell, miners became a ready market for support services and suppliers such as saloons, pack-mule drivers, ocean-bound shippers, sawmills, railways, and the like. After the Rush, many towns including San Francisco continued to flourish. Demand for building materials grew. Logging companies realized "gold in them thar trees" and ruthlessly mined the old-growth forests. Today, after countless political and ecological debates, and court rulings, the whining sound of chainsaws has somewhat diminished and because of that, so too has the area's economy and population. But the trade-off was more than the preservation of "a bunch of old trees." At stake were—and still are—species that depend on the ecology of the forest for survival, such as wild salmon and spotted owls, to say nothing of the flora, erosion, and floods. The battle to save what's left of the redwoods and all its dependents is far from over, and continues on in court and legislative halls.

To understand what the hoopla is all about, you need to meet real, live ancient redwood trees, in their damp environment, enveloped by the ubiquitous mythical fog. And what better way to see it than on a bike, riding underneath the canopies of towering branches, sort of like pedaling through Mother Nature's cathedral. Found in Humboldt, Del Norte, and Siskiyou counties, these rides bring you up close and personal with the world's oldest living life forms. Rides for every ability can be found, from the mountainous redwood forests to the coastal flatlands that were once inhabited by Native American tribes. Not to be missed are the free-roaming Roosevelt elk in Redwoods National and State Park.

RIDE 1 · Grasshopper Peak Loop

AT A GLANCE

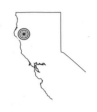

Length/configuration: 17.2-mile loop, counterclockwise; fire roads

Aerobic difficulty: Very strenuous due to elevation gain and killer hill

Technical difficulty: Mildly technical

Scenery: Old-growth coastal redwoods and views of nearby mountain ranges shrouded in fog

Special comments: The first half of this routing replaces the previously popular Bull Creek Road, which was almost completely washed out during the El Niño winter storms in early 1998.

E ver met a living organism that's more than 2,000 years old? What better place to meet these ancient ones than biking through a portion of the 52,000-acre Humboldt Redwoods State Park? Grasshopper Peak Loop, 17.2 miles of mildly technical dirt fire roads, leads you through some of the world's oldest old-growth redwood forests with trees fatter than a Volkswagen Beetle and taller than the Statue of Liberty. But be forewarned: This is a challenging ride. The first 10.2 miles is an unrelenting uphill climb, severely steep in some places. After that, even if you pushed your bike some of the way up Grasshopper Peak, you will have indeed earned your right to enjoy a fast seven-mile descent without cranking the pedal much, if at all.

So what's all the controversy surrounding old coastal redwood trees, the stuff that backyard decks are made of? Why not cut 'em down if they're a replenishable resource? To say that these trees are among the oldest living organisms on earth—some more than 2,000 years old—might give you an idea. To say these are the very same trees that predate Christ might help you put them into perspective. To say that they are some of the world's tallest living structures, growing to more than 360 feet, might help you understand their power of natural survival. To say they play a crucial role in an area's many interrelated ecosystems might give you a sense of their profound influence. To say that we as human beings do not totally understand the complexity of how these trees came to be, yet are willing to destroy these possibly irreplaceable components of the landscape in the name of short-term commercial gain and immediate livelihood might help you to understand the hubbub that has garnered ongoing national attention. But few words can truly describe the majesty of the redwood trees, quietly transforming an otherwise wet, foggy, and dreary northern California coast into a humbling statement of surrealistic, raw beauty that only Mother Earth can speak. You simply have to see the old-growth redwood forest in person in order to appreciate it.

General location: About 30 miles southeast of Eureka.

Elevation change: 2,900 feet; starting elevation and low point about 200 feet; high point 3,100 feet. A huge, brutal hill climb followed by a bulletlike, uninterrupted descent.

RIDE 1 · Grasshopper Peak Loop
RIDE 2 · Peavine Road Loop

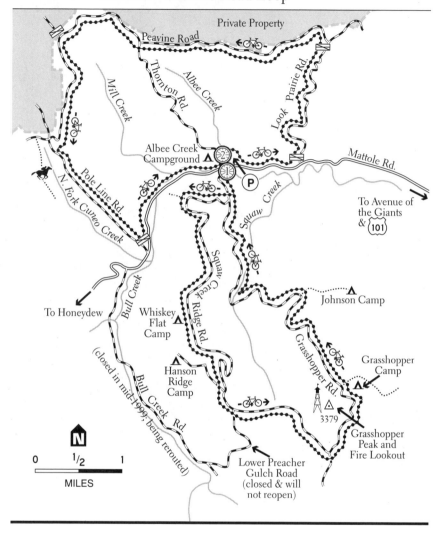

Season: Year-round, though usually sunny in the fall and apt to be foggy and somewhat wet during the rest of the year.

Services: Campsites, water, toilet, solar showers, and pay phone at Albee Creek campground. Trail camps available. Water available at the fire lookout during the summer. Other services in the nearest town of Redcrest or Weott.

Hazards: Occasional poison oak. Some vehicular traffic on Mattole Road.

Rescue index: Grasshopper Road is popular with hikers in the summer, but because of the steepness and the distance, you may not encounter many other trail

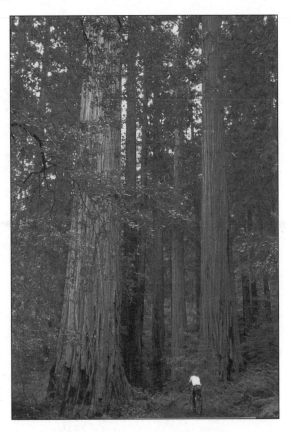

Bruce is dwarfed by stately redwoods while pedaling up Squaw Creek Ridge Road.

users during other times of the year. In the summer, you may find backpackers at any of the primitive campsites who may be of help. Otherwise, you'll have to make your own way back down the trail to Mattole Road and into the Albee Creek campground where you'll find a pay phone and, during the summer, a ranger on duty during the day.

Land status: Humboldt Redwoods State Park.

Maps: *Humboldt Redwoods State Park,* official park map, available at Burlington Visitor Center located on the Avenue of the Giants; USGS Bull Creek and Weott 7.5 minute series.

Finding the trail: From Eureka, travel south on US 101 for about 30 miles to the Mattole Road exit, marked as Rockefeller Forest and Founders Tree (this is also the second exit for the Avenue of the Giants). Take this exit and head south. In about 3.75 miles, go past Founders Grove (site of the impressive Founders Tree) and continue south until you're able to turn right. At this right, go over the Eel River and underneath US 101. You immediately reach a well-signed intersection. Follow the sign to the far left that directs you to Mattole Road and Albee Creek campground. You reach the campground in about 5 miles. Park in either the campground day-use lot or in a dirt pulloff next to the Grasshopper Road trailhead off Mattole, located a few yards beyond the campground entrance.

Sources of additional information:

Humboldt Redwoods State Park
P.O. Box 100
Weott, CA 95571
(707) 946-2409
Tremendous amounts of information,
including maps, available at the state

park's Burlington Visitor Center located on Avenue of the Giants.

North Coast Redwoods District
California State Parks
3431 Fort Ave.
Eureka, CA 95503

Notes on the trail: From the Albee Creek campground, hang a right onto Mattole Road and ride west for about 0.3 mile. Look for the gated fire road on the left, signed "Fire Lookout 7 miles." Though it's not signed as such, this is Grasshopper Road, a one-car width dirt road, and it is the most direct route to Grasshopper Peak and its fire lookout (elevation 3,379 feet). The trailhead here sits at about 200 feet. The bike route described here leads up to Grasshopper Peak in 10.2 miles via Squaw Creek Ridge Road and Upper Preacher Gulch Road. All fire roads throughout the route are basically hard-packed dirt with some loose gravel.

Mileages referenced here are based on starting at the intersection of Mattole Road and Grasshopper Road. Go through the gate and immediately begin a fairly steep climb through the pine and redwood forest. In fact, for the next 10.2 miles, it's a slow uphill grind, varying from 4–9% grade. There are some level sections as well as descents. Problem is, they never seem long enough for your heart to stop pounding so hard. The slow pace, on the other hand, gives you a chance to see and smell the old-growth redwood forest.

At about 0.7 mile and some 600 feet higher, you reach the signed fork of Grasshopper Road and Squaw Creek Ridge Road. Begin the counterclockwise loop by taking the right fork, following Squaw Creek Road as it continues climbing up, though not as steeply as before. (If you want a harder workout, ride the route in the other direction, going up Grasshopper Road first, then ending on Squaw Creek Ridge Road. The climbing is unrelenting!) After 2 miles, you reach a ridge while continuing your uphill grind. Look through the trees, across a ravine, and you might be able to see the lookout at Grasshopper Peak off in the southeast.

Old- and young-growth redwoods are not the only trees living on these slopes. Take a breather when you see trees with chocolate-colored bark peeling like paint. Run your hand over the blond wood which the peeling bark has revealed, and marvel at how incredibly smooth it feels, like a baby's bottom. That's a madrone tree. Take a whiff of pine as your lungs suck in precious air.

At just over 6 miles, after a couple of closely placed, wide switchbacks, you reach an elevation of 2,075 feet, having climbed about 1,875 feet from Mattole Road. You've pedaled into a slightly different ecosystem, as evident by the open forest of mixed conifers and oaks. Hardly any redwoods live in this neighborhood since they prefer elevations below 2,000 feet. Look left, due east, and you're rewarded with an expansive view of the ridge on the other side of the Squaw Creek drainage. You can even see the lookout. At about 6.3 miles, you reach the signed intersection of Hanson Ridge Road leading off on your right. There's a trail camp down Hanson and, for the romantically inclined, it's a great spot to catch a sunset.

For the next 0.3 mile, enjoy a gradual descent as Squaw Creek Ridge Road traverses a slope which drains down on your right (south) into Bull Creek. If you cruise quietly and slowly, you might see deer leisurely grazing in the meadow on the downhill side. At the end of this short descent, you come to a signed intersection with Preacher Gulch Road and Bull Creek Road. Thanks to El Niño's winter wallop, Bull Creek and Lower Preacher Gulch Roads are now closed, the roads almost completely washed out. Mother Nature spoke, and the California Department of Parks listened by undertaking the Watershed Rehabilitation Project. The project's objective is to reduce erosion primarily through the removal of 40-year-old logging roads and creek crossings in hopes that sedimentation will be slowed, thereby encouraging ecosystem recovery on nearby hillsides and areas adjacent to lower Bull Creek.

Here at this intersection with Lower Preacher Gulch Road, the elevation is just over 2,000 feet and you've pedaled about 6.7 miles from Mattole Road. Get ready, because here comes the final 3.5-mile push up to the highest point of the ride. Take a deep breath and turn left onto Preacher Gulch. You will immediately begin climbing a 10% grade hill through the pine and madrone forest. After 0.3 mile of grunting and grinding, you reach the ridge and a merciful, slightly descending stretch. Enjoy it while you can, dropping 334 feet in 0.6 mile to an elevation of 1,876 feet. Next is a roller-coaster section running you past a small stand of redwoods. Some sections are so steep that you might have to dismount and push your tired steed uphill. Tell your riding buddies you're stopping to smell the wild irises and laurel trees alongside the road. And try not to break the serenity of the forest with your heavy breathing.

At 8.7 miles, elevation about 2,500 feet, you reach a signed intersection with Grieg and Bull Creek Roads on the right and Grasshopper Road on your left. From here, you have 1.5 miles to go to reach the high point of the loop, namely, the walking path that leads to the lookout on Grasshopper Peak.

Turn left onto Grasshopper Road and force yourself up the grueling steep climb. After a way too brief gentle descent, climb again, level out, then climb one more time, reaching the intersection with Grasshopper Camp Trail and the lookout walking trail. You made it! At about 10.2 miles, this is the highest point of the ride at elevation 3,100 feet. To reach the lookout located at 3,379 feet, leave your bike and stroll up the walking path directly across the main dirt road from Grasshopper Camp Trail (no bikes allowed). Incidentally, here at this intersection, there is a trail campsite among the tan oak trees and a pit toilet. Walk the short distance up to the lookout and, on clear days, you can see the Kings Range National Conservation Area, the Lost Coast along the Pacific Ocean, glimpses of Eureka to the north, and Fort Bragg to the south. Sunsets can be magnificent here too.

Now comes your well-deserved reward: A fast 7-mile descent, all the way down to Mattole Road via Grasshopper Road. The wide dirt road is generally smooth with some loose rock, gravel, and probably some rain runoff ruts. Steep descents, ranging from 4–9% grades are on tap for this slightly curvy blast downhill. By now, you are undoubtedly aching to let your trusty bike run loose. By all means, let 'er rip, knowing that as you zip pass more redwood groves, you had already paid homage to the older, more impressive groves while grunting up Squaw Creek Ridge Road during your first 6 tortuous miles. Grasshopper is the most popular dirt road in the state park, so stay alert for other trail users on this road, including off-highway vehicles going to and from the lookout. Easy to follow, the road leads you down the hill, pass Johnson Trail (to another trail camp) and over a well-made wooden bridge over Squaw Creek. At about 6.2 miles, you close the loop by passing Squaw Creek Ridge Road on your left. Continue down Grasshopper Road for another mile, go through the gate, and finally reach Mattole Road. Make your way back to your parked car or campsite in Albee Creek campground and begin celebrating your day spent among the "ancient ones."

RIDE 2 · Peavine Road Loop

AT A GLANCE

Length/configuration: 16.6-mile loop, counterclockwise; fire, gravel, and paved roads

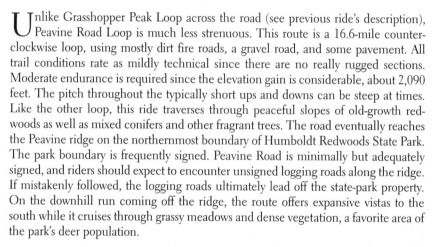

Aerobic difficulty: Moderately strenuous due to climbing

Technical difficulty: Mildly technical

Scenery: Mixed conifer and redwood forest, expansive view looking south toward Grasshopper Peak and its adjacent mountain ranges

Special comments: Loop ride through old-growth redwood forest

Unlike Grasshopper Peak Loop across the road (see previous ride's description), Peavine Road Loop is much less strenuous. This route is a 16.6-mile counterclockwise loop, using mostly dirt fire roads, a gravel road, and some pavement. All trail conditions rate as mildly technical since there are no really rugged sections. Moderate endurance is required since the elevation gain is considerable, about 2,090 feet. The pitch throughout the typically short ups and downs can be steep at times. Like the other loop, this ride traverses through peaceful slopes of old-growth redwoods as well as mixed conifers and other fragrant trees. The road eventually reaches the Peavine ridge on the northernmost boundary of Humboldt Redwoods State Park. The park boundary is frequently signed. Peavine Road is minimally but adequately signed, and riders should expect to encounter unsigned logging roads along the ridge. If mistakenly followed, the logging roads ultimately lead off the state-park property. On the downhill run coming off the ridge, the route offers expansive vistas to the south while it cruises through grassy meadows and dense vegetation, a favorite area of the park's deer population.

General location: About 30 miles southeast of Eureka.

Elevation change: 2,090 feet; starting elevation and low point 405 feet; high point 2,495 feet. A big hill climb; rolling ridge riding; and a long, fast descent.

Season: Year-round, though usually sunny in the fall and apt to be foggy and somewhat wet throughout rest of the year.

Services: Campsites, water, toilet, solar showers, and pay phone at Albee Creek campground, the nearest maintained campground in the park. Trail camps available. Other services in the nearest towns of Redcrest or Weott.

Hazards: Virtually none although a map is highly recommended due to a number of private, unsigned logging roads accessible along Peavine Road. Along the northern boundary, listen up and watch out for occasional logging-truck traffic and falling trees. Occasional poison oak. Some vehicular traffic on Mattole Road.

Rescue index: Because of the steepness and the distance, you're not likely to encounter many other trail users. For emergency help, you'll have to make your way back down the trail to Mattole Road and into the Albee Creek campground where you'll find a pay phone and, during the summer, a ranger on duty during the day. You may find assistance from loggers along the northern boundary of the park.

Land status: Humboldt Redwoods State Park.

Maps: *Humboldt Redwoods State Park*, official park map, available at Burlington Visitor Center located on the Avenue of the Giants; USGS Bull Creek and Weott 7.5 minute series.

Finding the trail: From Eureka, travel south on US 101, for about 30 miles to the Mattole Road exit, marked as Rockefeller Forest and Founders Tree, (this is also the second exit for the Avenue of the Giants). Take this exit and head south. In about 3.75 miles, go past Founders Grove (site of the impressive Founders Tree) and continue south until you're able to turn right. At this right, go over the Eel River and underneath US 101. You immediately reach a well-signed intersection. Follow the sign to the far left directing to Mattole Road and Albee Creek campground. You reach the campground in about 5 miles. Park in the campground day-use lot.

Sources of additional information: See sources of additional information for Ride 1.

Notes on the trail: Starting from Albee Creek campground, go back out to Mattole Road and turn left, pedaling east for about 0.8 mile, toward the Big Tree Area. Look for a brown sign on the left side of the paved road identifying Look Prairie Road, which will have a large gate across it. Turn left, riding around the gate and onto Look Prairie, a one-car-width dirt road that may be a bit overgrown and may look like a double-track. Beginning elevation here at the gate is about 405 feet. For the next 4 miles, the steepness varies between 2–8% grade with some relief in the way of short stretches of level and sometimes descending terrain.

The road begins with an easy climb, leading you in and out of the shade, passing a few surviving old-growth redwoods and mixed conifers, skirting open meadows of grassy, rolling hills. Lush undergrowth combined with California laurel trees here envelop you in a subtly spicy aroma. In late spring and early summer, wild irises and miniature flowering plants that resemble tiny rosebushes dot the trailside. When you take a breather, literally stopping to smell the roses, take a closer look at the color scheme on the irises: a blush of pale pink and purple fading to white and then into yellow throats streaked with brilliant red veins.

Continue the gradual uphill climb. At about 1.6 miles, you ride past a water trough on your right, tucked underneath several trees, overlooking a grassy meadow and the distant mountain range. Soon, you reenter the forest and begin seeing a few redwoods as large in diameter as an old Volkswagen Beetle. At almost 2.5 miles, ride pass a huge fallen spruce tree that's been cleanly sawed through at the base, with "Eel River #1" faintly carved into the cut. Elevation here is about 1,240 feet, a gain of approximately 835 feet since the gate at Look Prairie Road. Push on, continuing the moderate climb up to the ridge, passing more old-growth redwoods as well as oak, mixed conifers, California laurel, and, eventually, madrone trees.

Finally, at about 4.4 miles, you reach an unsigned **T** intersection with another dirt road going both left and right. You've reached the ridge. Though not identified, this is Peavine Road, a narrow fire road ranging from 12 to 20 feet across. There is, however, a single wooden post with equestrian and hiker symbols along with an arrow pointing to the left. Hang a left here, since turning right will take you to the park boundary and into private property. Incidentally, from this point on, you will see more of these single post signs with the symbols accompanied by a directional arrow. (Who knows? Maybe someday little biker symbols will be added.)

Follow Peavine Road due west, grinding up and zipping down short and sometimes steep hills. Keep in mind that Peavine basically skirts the northern boundary

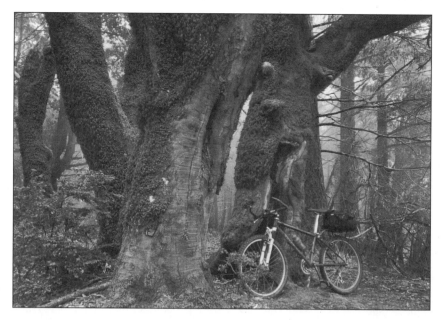

One of many impressively sized old-growth trees alongside Look Prairie Road.

of the state park, now on your right. You will pass other dirt roads connecting to Peavine, mostly coming in from private property on your right (from the north). On the other side of the boundary is privately owned timberland; many of these roads are logging roads. So, when in doubt, stay straight, bearing left (the exception is signed Albee Creek Trail, referred to as Thornton Road on the map and described later). Also, look for a single wooden signpost marked with the familiar equestrian and hiker symbols and the directional arrow.

At almost 5 miles, you reach the highest point of the loop, at an elevation of approximately 2,495 feet. The forest here is of mixed conifers with fewer redwoods, though there are some old-growth trees scattered here and there. From this point, the road continues its familiar roller-coaster ride punctuated by a few steep but short ups and downs, while generally and imperceptibly losing elevation. At about 5.5 miles, the Peavine Road is joined by another dirt road, coming in from behind your right shoulder. This intersection is marked by the familiar single wooden signpost with the hiker and equestrian symbols and directional arrow. Follow the arrow as it points straight ahead. On your right, due north, is a great view across a deep canyon. In less than 200 yards, where the road forks again, take the left fork, bypassing the jeep road on the right.

The next wooden signpost is planted at about 6.3 miles. Follow its arrow as it points up a short but steep hill. Pedal about 1.5 miles farther, and the road traverses the southern slope of the ridge, skirting a steep drop-off along the Albee Creek drainage for a short distance. At about 8 miles, you reach a small clearing and find an intersection with a narrow path leading downhill to the south on your left. A faded, weathered wooden sign here says "Albee Creek" with arrows pointing in both directions. (It doesn't identify this trail as Thornton Road as labeled on the state park map.) In any case, bypass this trail and stay on the main dirt road, still heading west, straight ahead. About 0.7 mile after passing the Albee Creek trail, you come to a T intersection with a well-traveled dirt road. Look for the familiar wooden signpost and follow the arrow to the left, due southwest. (The right turn puts you on a wide logging road which leads out of the state park.) Having made the left turn, you gradually descend the smooth dirt road, about two cars wide. Though the road is not identified, you're still on Peavine Road.

About a mile farther from the left turn, you reach a junction with a smaller dirt road leading off to your left. It's marked with the hiker/equestrian signpost and the trusty directional arrow. By now, you've pedaled approximately 10 miles from the beginning of the ride. Follow the narrow road, passing a cairn on your right, through a stand of large madrone trees, all the while enjoying a sweet and easy downhill cruise.

At almost 12 miles, now at elevation 1,700 feet, you reach a locked metal gate across the road. Go around the gate and continue down the road. In about 100 yards, you reach a T intersection with a gravel road. The wooden signpost directs you to the left. Though there is no sign identifying this road, trust me, it's Pole Line Road. What makes me so sure? The power line overhead, running adjacent to the well-maintained gravel road gives it away. So make a left here onto the wide, hard-packed, gravel road, and in almost 200 yards, pass a sign marked Pole Line Road. From this point, it's practically a straight shot down to Mattole Road with a few blind curves thrown in for fun. The fast downhill leads you over wide, open, grassy meadows and rolling hills, giving you a good view of Grasshopper Peak and its adjacent mountain ranges. Consider this before you blast downhill: Deer love to hang out here. So, if you want to see deer on this stretch, ride slowly so that the noise of the gravel under your tires doesn't scare them off.

After a 2.3-mile, 1,115-foot descent, you reach a locked gate next to paved Mattole Road. Hang a left onto Mattole, shift into higher gear, and cruise the adequate shoulder for just over 2 miles back to your car at Albee Creek campground.

RIDE 3 · Avenue of the Giants Road Ride

AT A GLANCE

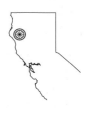

Length/configuration: 18.2-mile out-and-back (9.1 miles each way); paved road

Aerobic difficulty: Easy

Technical difficulty: Not technical, though you should be accustomed to riding a very narrow shoulder on busy vehicle roads

Scenery: Incredibly huge old-growth redwood trees with towering canopies. The ubiquitous misty fog adds to the surreal experience.

Special comments: Not recommended for children because of frequent vehicle traffic

If you've never been in a forest of old-growth redwoods, you're about to be in awe—and humbled—by the sheer size of these remarkable trees. Sure, you could see this stretch of redwoods by car, contorting your torso and neck as you peer up through your windshield. But believe me, the emotional impact is more profound

RIDE 3 · Avenue of the Giants Road Ride

when you're out from the shelter of your car, pedaling your bike. If you want an easy, nontechnical ride while communing with these ancient giants, this ride is for you.

This road ride is an 18.2-mile out-and-back (9.1 miles each way) that shares an easy, fairly flat 4.2-mile stretch of the popular Avenue of the Giants road with motor vehicles. The last outer 4.9 miles travels over paved Mattole Road and leads you to the trailheads of two spectacular and strenuous off-road rides which run through more old-growth forests (Peavine Road Loop and Squaw Creek–Grasshopper Peak Loop). This ride begins at the Burlington Visitor Center and campground in Humboldt Redwoods State Park. You will undoubtedly want to spend some time at the Visitor Center, learn-

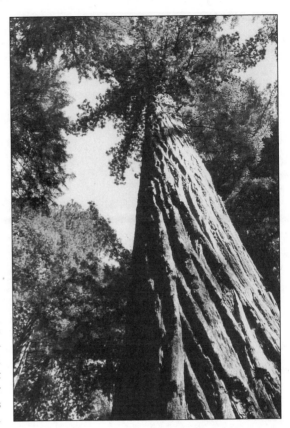

Towering redwoods block most of the sunlight from the ground below. Wearing bright clothing and clear or yellow glasses is recommended.

ing about the redwood ecology from slide shows, displays, books, and mementos. For the ride, consider bringing a picnic to enjoy in the serenity of the forest because the route takes you past Founders and Rockefeller Groves, ending at Big Tree on Mattole Road. Definitely bring along a bike lock as each stop offers walking-only trails—some self-guided, some long, some short—that lead you pass notable ancient trees such as the Dyerville Giant and the Giant Tree. Both trees are referred to as champion coast redwood, as certified by the American Forestry Association based on circumference, height, and size of crown. Not exactly a mountain-biking experience, but then, there's more to life than just shredding and bombing down dirt trails.

General location: About 45 miles southeast of Eureka and 25 miles north of Garberville on US 101.

Elevation change: Negligible. Average elevation is about 200 feet. Softly rolling terrain.

Season: Year-round. Rainfall likely November through April.

Services: Drinking water, toilets, pay phone, and lots of volunteer staff at the Burlington Visitor Center. Several developed campgrounds are available along the Avenue of the Giants as well as on Mattole Road. Burlington campground is open all year.

Hazards: Watch out for motorists who drive 25 to 40 mph while gawking at the redwoods. The shoulder on the road is narrow and nonexistent in some places. Towering redwoods grow close together, resulting in thick canopies that effectively block much of the sunlight from illuminating the road below. Because the roadway is always in the dark, you should wear bright, light-colored clothing in order to be more visible to motorists. If you're in the habit of wearing protective eyewear, consider yellow or clear lenses.

Rescue index: The road is a popular route for tourists, which means you can flag down a passing motorist for help.

Land status: Humboldt Redwoods State Park.

Maps: *Humboldt Redwoods State Park*, official park map, published by the California State Parks, available at the Burlington Visitor Center; *Redwoods Wait for You on the Avenue of the Giants*, a leaflet containing a map, published by Avenue of the Giants Association; USGS Weott and Bull Creek 7.5 minute series.

Finding the trail: From Garberville, travel north on US 101 for about 7 miles toward Phillipsville. Take the Avenue of the Giants exit located here and follow it north through Miranda and Myers Flat. In about 14.5 miles, you reach Burlington Visitor Center on your right. Park and start riding here. From Eureka, travel south on US 101, bypassing the first Avenue of the Giants exit in Pepperwood. In about 30 miles you reach Redcrest and another exit onto Avenue of the Giants. Take this exit and continue south. In about 3.75 miles, you pass Founders Grove. At this point, you can continue south to Burlington Visitor Center, in which case you'd be driving part of the pedaling route. If you'd rather not drive farther, park at Founders and begin riding in any direction on the route. Otherwise, continue heading south on the Avenue for 4.3 miles to the Visitor Center.

Sources of additional information: See sources of additional information for Ride 1.

Notes on the trail: Before hopping on your saddle, consider bringing a bike lock, just in case you want to check out any of the self-guided nature walks. From the Burlington Visitor Center to Founders Grove, Avenue of the Giants is paralleled by the south fork of the Eel River on the west, and by US 101 in the distance on the east. After Founders Grove, Mattole Road leads you past the Rockefeller Forest on the way to the Big Tree Area, home of the Giant Tree and Flat Iron Tree. Watch out for vehicles and stay to the right as much as possible. Keep your caution radar on as there is never a generous shoulder on which to ride. The shoulder is either the width of the painted stripe on the edge of the road or nonexistent. The ascents are generally mild with a couple of slightly more demanding but short hills, no more than 200 yards in length, followed by gentle descents. Elevation of both roads ranges from 150 to 200 feet.

Begin your exploration by pedaling north on Avenue of the Giants. The road from the Burlington Visitor Center to the Founders Grove takes you gradually uphill, through the tiny town of Weott, reached at just under 2 miles. High-water marks of the flood of 1964 can be seen here. The devastating flood has been partly attributed to the fact that much of the Eel River watershed had been logged, leaving much of the earth unanchored. With several days of heavy rainfall, the runoff came rushing down unchecked into the river, carrying with it silt that ultimately filled the once deep channels. Combine that moment with high tide at the mouth of the river some 36 miles north, and the water of the swollen river couldn't dissipate. As a result, the water level rose. Weott, as well as Myers Flat to the south and Pepperwood to the north, were ravaged, and lives were lost. The high-water mark of the flood is at the corner of Avenue of the Giants and Newton Road.

Continue following Avenue of the Giants as it leaves Weott and threads through the redwood forest. About a mile up, check out Dungan Grove. Here, you'll find a curious sight: a redwood with an incredibly huge burl at its base, located on the east side of the road. It's a popular photo op.

Pedal almost 1.5 miles more and you reach Founders Grove, now 4.3 miles from the Visitor Center. There's an easy 20-minute self-guided nature trail here. Worth checking out is the Dyerville Giant, the former reigning champion redwood. This tree is huge, unbelievably huge. Even though it toppled in 1991, it still has a remarkable massiveness about it. When standing, it towered approximately 370 feet. That's taller than giant sequoias, the Statue of Liberty, and the dome of the Capitol in Washington.

OK, enough gawking. Hop back in the saddle and continue north on Avenue of the Giants for almost a half mile, following the road as it leads you onto a bridge over the Eel River and then underneath US 101. Immediately on the other side of the underpass is an intersection. Follow the signs to Albee Creek campground, making a hard left onto Mattole Road, also known as Bull Creek Road. The road travels westward, parallel to Bull Creek on your left. It remains fairly flat, curving and alternating between sunlight and shade. Traffic on Mattole Road, which does not have a shoulder, is much less than Avenue of the Giants. About 1.2 miles after the underpass, Mattole leads you into Rockefeller Forest, one of the largest groves in the state park.

Stay on Mattole for almost 3.3 miles and then turn left into the Big Trees Area, home to the new reigning champion, the Giant Tree. At this point, you've pedaled 9.1 miles from the Visitor Center. There are picnic tables and pit toilets here. If the footbridge is in place, you can walk to the other side of Bull Creek and check out the Flat Iron Tree. (Not all trails here allow bikes; please heed posted signs.) When you've had your fill here, turn around and go back the way you came.

On your way back, if you're interested in another self-guided trail, check out the Rockefeller Loop Trail. It's about 3.3 miles from Big Trees, on the creek side of the road, just before Bull Creek and the Eel River join. Pretty cool way to experience redwoods, don't you think? Motorists don't know what they're missing.

RIDE 4 · Arcata Community Forest

AT A GLANCE

Length/configuration: 4.2-mile loop; clockwise on gravel/dirt roads

Aerobic difficulty: Easy to moderate due to a few steep but very short hills

Technical difficulty: Mild with a few brief stretches of slightly intermediate terrain due to narrowness and water bars

Scenery: Lush, cool natural landscape with a few old-growth redwoods surrounded by young-growth specimens; a gem right in town!

Special comments: The network of trails in the Community Forest offers numerous routing possibilities, some of which can be moderately strenuous. Portions of the trail are suitable for children and kid-trailers.

How many communities do you know that have a real forest right in their own backyards? I don't know about you, but when I was a youngster—reading *Hansel and Gretel, Little Red Riding Hood,* and *Goldilocks and the Three Bears*—this was the kind of forest I envisioned. The Arcata Community Forest is the stuff of childhood fantasies, all contained in a 620-acre dense, lush forest of young- and old-growth redwoods, Douglas fir, and spruce. It's shaded by thick canopies towering overhead and smothered with lots of big, leafy ferns and tall understory. Leave it to progressive Arcata to maintain a forest right in town, open to walkers, equestrians, and bikers.

Even though bikes are allowed on only 7 miles of trail, lots of configurations and many riding directions are possible within this network of gravel/dirt roads with a few stretches of single-tracks thrown in for variety. Though the loop described here is a mere 4.2 miles long, the quality of trail, endurance, and technical skill required is representative of the entire forest trail system. This loop offers plenty of sometimes steep but short ups and downs on generally 8-foot-wide gravel/dirt roads—a great roller-coaster ride for bikers who are at least moderately strong. Technical skill required on this loop range from nontechnical to slightly intermediate. Strong riders can get a real workout grinding up Ridge Road, climbing almost 1,050 feet in nearly two miles from a point offered as an option off the loop. And if you crave more mileage, consider adding other configurations and riding in the opposite direction from which you came.

I highly recommend using the map produced by the City of Arcata, Environmental Services Department, especially if this is your first visit to the forest or if you're not yet well-acquainted with the territory (see "Sources of additional information" below). Even though the Community Forest covers a relatively small area and there are signs at most intersections, it's easy to become disoriented in this network of trails. But not to worry, lots of friendly walkers and bikers enjoy the forest typically in the early evening after work and are happy to offer directions.

General location: In the eastern section of the city of Arcata, about 6 miles north of Eureka.

Elevation change: 235 feet; starting elevation and low point 50 feet; high point 285 feet. Option to add 815 feet for a total elevation change of 1,050 feet. Lots of little hills. Numerous configurations are possible.

Season: Year-round, though the winter is apt to be damp.

Services: All services available in Arcata.

Hazards: Other trail users, including dog walkers. Merciless bloodsucking mosquitoes live here.

Rescue index: The main trails are popular with walkers, joggers, and other bikers. Residences border portions of the Community Forest, so you're sure to find someone who may be of help.

Land status: City of Arcata.

Maps: *Mountain Cycling in the Arcata Community Forest,* published by the city of Arcata.

RIDE 4 · Arcata Community Forest

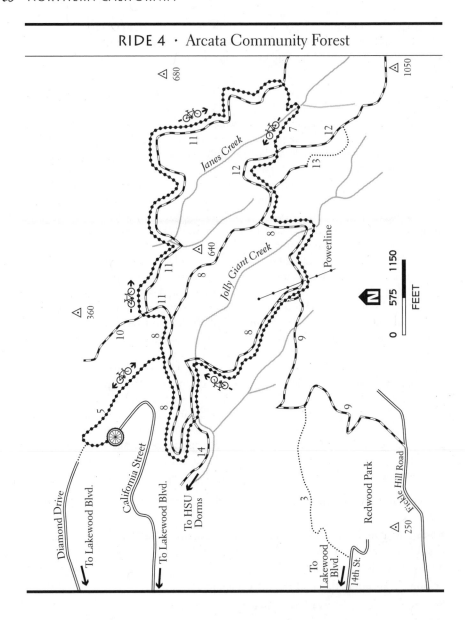

Finding the trail: There are several points from which to access the forest trail system. The ride described here uses the following access point: From within the city of Arcata, take the Sunset Avenue exit off southbound US 101 or the 14th Street exit off of northbound US 101. From either exit, proceed toward Humboldt State University on the east side of US 101. (Both Sunset and 14th run east-west and intersect L. K. Wood Boulevard, a north-south frontage road on the east side of US 101; 14th Street is about 0.5 mile south of Sunset.) From either exit, make your way onto L. K. Wood and turn north onto it. Immediately north of the Sunset and L. K. Wood intersection, turn right onto California Avenue and head east, uphill. Follow California as it climbs

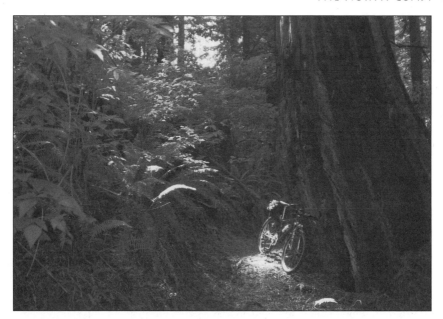

What a great backyard the city of Arcata has.

and winds it way past lovely homes. Check out the huge redwood stumps that have been integrated in the nicely landscaped lawns—evidence that gigantic old-growth coastal redwoods once thrived here. In 1.3 miles, California Avenue ends in a cul-de-sac, running into the trailhead. This trail is made up of wood chips and is actually a narrow public easement that threads between two residences on its way to the Arcata Community Forest. Park on the street and begin your ride here.

Alternate access point: Take the same exit off of US 101 as described previously. This time, follow 14th Street to its end as it as it winds past Humboldt State University, due south and east. Park and begin riding east through Redwood Park on a single-track on your way to the Community Forest.

Sources of additional information:

City of Arcata
Environmental Services Department
736 F St.
Arcata, CA 95521
(707) 822-8184

Notes on the trail: Starting at the end of California Avenue, hop on your bike and crunch your way over the 5-foot-wide wood chip trail, threading between several homes. You may think you're riding through someone's property, but this connector trail is actually a public easement. In a few yards, the trail leads you into the Arcata Community Forest. Go right onto the dirt trail, which initially skirts the backyards of several homes and then begins cruising through the dense, lush, and shady forest.

At 0.5 mile, you arrive at a **T** intersection with a wider, one-car-width gravel and dirt trail. The trail you've been on is signed the California Trail, while the wider trail running left and right is not identified. Make a left here, cruising past a wooden water tank; in a few yards, you reach another signed intersection. This time, it's identified, and the wide trail you're on is signed number "8" and the other number "11," which refers to Community Forest Loop Road and Janes Creek Road respectively, as labeled on the Community Forest map which I recommended you should have. (In the field, trails are signed by number, not the actual name, probably because numbers are easier to post than full names.)

Hang a left onto 11 and begin a roller-coaster adventure for almost 2 miles. Some sections of 11 are somewhat steep at an 8% grade. But never fear. Those climbs are short and there are level stretches. After climbing almost 400 feet, you reach the intersection of trail number 7, Upper Janes Creek Trail, a wide gravel and dirt single-track. Turn right onto 7 and try not to squash those benign little banana slugs while you fly down a moderately steep downhill. Cross a small wooden bridge over Janes Creek and immediately make a hard right, following the trail as it descends over widely spaced water logs. Continue over another creek on a wooden bridge and ride or walk over a series of more water logs. The trail soon climbs gradually out of the ravine. After about 100 yards, the single-track widens to about 5 feet and the steepness softens. In a few more yards, you come to an intersection with gravel/dirt road number 12 (Ridge Road) going both left and right. At this point, you've pedaled 2.5 miles since starting at the California Avenue trailhead. For those of you aching to climb some more, hang a left here and proceed to climb about 700 feet in almost 1.5 miles to reach the high point of the Community Forest.

Otherwise, turn right onto 12 and enjoy a gradual descent. Almost immediately, bypass trail number 13 (Ridge Loop Road) on your left. Continue on 12, and before you know it, you arrive at the intersection with trail number 8 (Community Forest Loop Road) running both left and right. The right turn here shortens this already brief loop by climbing over a moderately steep hill. It returns you to the California Avenue trailhead in less than 2 miles. Instead, turn left and continue the sweet descent and ride past a wooden bench sitting directly underneath power lines. In a few yards later, the road splits. The left split is trail number 9 and leads to the 14th Street access point via Redwood Park. Bypass 9, bear right, and stay on 8. Cruise past trails 16 and 15, both walking-only paths. Go down a bit farther and you reach the intersection with trail number 14 (Jolly Giant Road) which comes in from the Humboldt State University dorms. Stay on 8 as it climbs gradually for a few yards. By now, you skirt the property of several homes and then reach 5, the California Trail, at which point you've just closed the loop. If you've had enough or run out of time, make a left onto the California Trail and retrace the gravel/dirt trail back to your car. Otherwise, ride the circuit again, maybe this time in the opposite direction, or check out some of the other roads you bypassed.

RIDE 5 · Ossagon–Gold Bluff Loop

AT A GLANCE

Length/configuration: 19.4-mile loop; counterclockwise; pavement, single-track and dirt road (reverse direction rideable)

Aerobic difficulty: Easy with a short section of moderate climbing

Technical difficulty: Mildly technical with sections of narrow and slightly rugged single-track

Scenery: Majestic redwoods, verdant forest environment, several hidden waterfalls, sea-level views of the ocean and coastal grassy flatlands replete with herds of Roosevelt elk

Special comments: Portions accessible for young children and kid-trailers—check with a ranger for trail conditions.

No matter what kind of rider you are—beginner or expert, recreational or hard-core, young or old—this 19.4-mile loop in Redwood National Park and State Parks is sure to please. Not a technically challenging ride, the route has you zipping along on smooth pavement, sweet single-tracks and hard-packed, fast dirt roads. The ride is mostly easy, spiced with only a few yards here and there of steep climbing.

Trust me, even if you're an expert rider, you'll like the loop. How can this be? Blame it on the environment: it offers lots to see and experience, like old-growth redwood forests, hidden waterfalls, coastal prairie lands, towering bluffs, and the Pacific Ocean. You can even park your bike and enjoy a picnic at the beach. And there's Roosevelt elk—herds of them, freely roaming the park. You'd have to be asleep to not see any of these guys. Basically aloof, these wild mammals are the largest in the park. Some of them are bigger and weigh more than you, standing about five feet at shoulder height and weighing close to 1,000 pounds or more. (Aloof doesn't mean it's safe to approach them. Leave them be and give them a wide berth.)

The loop can be ridden clockwise or counterclockwise, starting from the Elk Prairie campground in Prairie Creek Redwoods State Park. Since it's so close to several other bike routes, consider using splendid Elk Prairie as a base camp. And get this: unlike other national parks, mountain bikes are allowed off pavement on designated dirt trails!

Say what? "Redwood National and State Parks" sound confusing? Is it a national park or a state park? Yes and no. Is it one park or many? Yes and no. The truth is, in 1968, Redwood National Park was created by the National Park System, a branch of the U.S. Department of the Interior, making it federally protected land. But what makes it unique is that it encompasses three of California's long-established state parks which all predate the National Park designation, having been formed in the 1920s. Those parks are Prairie Creek Redwoods (1923), Del Norte Coast Redwoods (1925), and Jedediah Smith Redwoods (1929). With the awareness generated by the Save-the-Redwoods League (founded in 1918), the state parks were originally created to protect ancient redwoods and the environments they support, including watersheds and the indigenous flora and fauna. In 1980, the entire park was deemed a UNESCO World Heritage Site by the United Nations, which basically recognizes and supports preservation and protection of the park from global development for the benefit of the people of the world. In 1994, the National Park Service and the California Department of Parks and Recreation formally agreed to cooperative management of the parks. Lands adjacent to each state park were subsequently acquired, linking all territories. Today, as a result, Redwood National and State Parks is an oddly shaped narrow strip of land running north and south along the Pacific Ocean, encompassing over 105,500 acres—a happy result of gerrymandering, to say the least. Spend some time here, even if it's for a day. You will begin to understand the importance and beauty of this region.

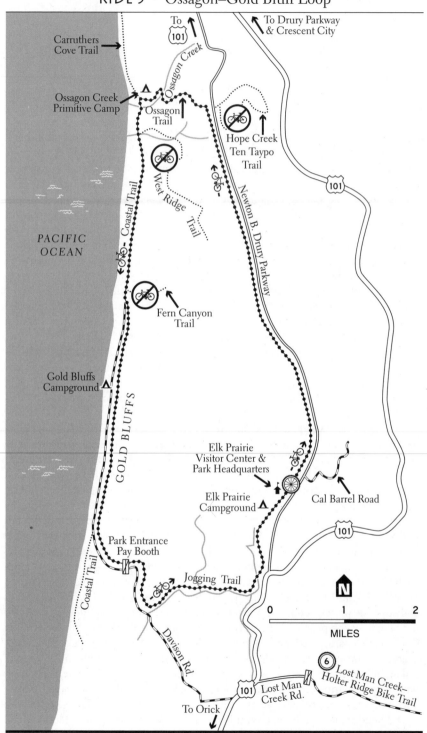

Carruthers
Cove Trail →

To
101

To Drury Parkway
& Crescent City

Ossagon
Creek

Ossagon Creek
Primitive Camp

Ossagon
Trail

101

Hope Creek
Ten Taypo
Trail

West Ridge Trail

Coastal Trail

Newton B. Drury Parkway

PACIFIC
OCEAN

Fern Canyon
Trail

Gold Bluffs
Campground

GOLD BLUFFS

Elk Prairie
Visitor Center &
Park Headquarters

Cal Barrel Road

Elk Prairie
Campground

101

Park Entrance
Pay Booth

Jogging Trail

N

0   1   2

MILES

Coastal Trail

Davison Rd.

6 Lost Man Creek–
Holter Ridge Bike Trail

101   Lost Man
Creek Rd.

To Orick

General location: About 38 miles south of Crescent City and about 45 miles north of Eureka on US 101.

Elevation change: 870 feet; starting elevation 150 feet; high point 870 feet; low point sea level. Easy, soft climb on pavement followed by mostly flat riding.

Season: Trail accessible year-round, though the weather is likely to be wet with fog and rain in the winter and spring. Summer tends to be cool.

Services: Drinking water, rest rooms, and pay phone at the visitor center in Elk Prairie campground. An enjoyable campfire program is presented by the park rangers each evening during the summer. Food, lodging, and gas available among the tiny towns of Orick, Klamath, and Requa, located to the north and south along Drury Parkway. All other services available in Crescent City, about 38 miles north on US 101.

Hazards: Occasional patches of poison oak. Expect to share the paved road with some traffic, including RVs and campers, especially during the summer months. Fortunately, there's a decently wide shoulder, varying from 1 to 3 feet. You may encounter a Roosevelt elk or two on the single-track portion of the Coastal Trail. Though generally aloof, these large herbivores are wild and unpredictable. So, don't approach them; give them a wide berth instead. Avoid prolonged eye-to-eye contact as your stare may provoke a defensive charge.

Rescue index: The entire loop is one of the more popular routes in the park, especially during the summer, so you're likely to find someone who may be of assistance. In the off-season, you might find help in either Gold Bluffs or Elk Prairie campgrounds. You can always flag down a passing motorist on the main road, Drury Parkway.

Land status: Prairie Creek Redwoods State Park, a part of Redwood National and State Parks. The entire park is cooperatively managed by the U.S. Department of the Interior, the National Park Service, and the California Department of Parks and Recreation.

Maps: *Redwood National Park–North Coast State Parks, Smith River NRA,* published by Trails Illustrated™, P.O. Box 4357, Evergreen, CO 80437, www.trailsillustrated.com; *Redwood National Park Trail Guide,* published by Redwood Natural History Association; USGS Orick and Fern Canyon 7.5 minute series.

Finding the trail: This counterclockwise loop begins and ends in the Elk Prairie campground at the Prairie Creek Redwoods State Park Visitor Center. There's a day-use small parking lot nearby (don't park in front of the visitor center). If you want to check out other rides in the vicinity, Elk Prairie makes an ideal base camp. From Orick: On northbound US 101, drive about 4.5 miles to the Newton B. Drury Parkway turnoff. Take the Parkway heading north for about 0.5 mile. Slow your speed and watch out for free-roaming Roosevelt elk on this stretch. Travel past an open, grassy meadow on the west side of the road (your left)—a favorite spot for elk. On the far end of the meadow is the Elk Prairie campground entrance, also on your left. Turn into the campground and park in the designated day-use area near the entry kiosk. From Crescent City: Drive south on US 101 for about 30.5 miles to the Newton B. Drury Parkway turnoff. Continue south on the Parkway for about 7.5 miles to the Elk Prairie campground entrance on your right. Turn into the campground and park in the designated day-use area near the entry kiosk.

Sources of additional information:

Prairie Creek Redwoods State Park
Elk Prairie Campground
  and Visitor Center
On Newton B. Drury Parkway
Orick, CA 95555
(707) 488-2171 or
  (707) 464-6101 ext. 5301
http://cal-parks.ca.gov

North Coast Redwood Interpretive
  Association
Redwood National Park
  Information Center
P.O. Box 234
Orick, CA 95555
(707) 488-2171
One mile south of Orick on US 101

Notes on the trail: This loop is described in a counterclockwise direction, even though the park's interpretive signs describe it clockwise. Though the loop can be ridden in both directions, I prefer the counterclockwise routing because I'd rather climb on pavement and descend on dirt.

If you have young children, I recommend riding in the clockwise direction. It's easily accessible from within Elk Prairie campground and you're immediately on the easiest portion of the loop. Just ride the 4-mile-long, easy trail, (formerly known as the "Jogging Trail"). Go south from the campground, turning around and retracing your path when the kids are good and tired. Kid-trailers may be suitable on this trail, but check with the park service for current conditions. This route keeps you and the kiddies off Drury Parkway, the park's main thoroughfare.

From the visitor center, exit the campground by pedaling east on the main road back out to Drury Parkway. Turn left (north) onto the Parkway, cautiously crossing over two lanes of traffic to the right shoulder. For the next 5.7 miles, relax and enjoy your surroundings as you gently gain about 505 feet before reaching the Ossagon Trail intersection. The ascent is easy, interspersed with short level sections. The shoulder is adequately 1 to 3 feet wide, generally free of ruts and cracks. Black and white metal mile markers dot the roadside. The speed limit on this portion of the Parkway is 45 mph and for the most part, the traffic is bearable, even though there's an occasional speedster, or humongous RV. The towering old-growth redwoods are magnificent, their canopies casting shade onto the forest floor, occasionally fractured by a stream of sunlight. The ground is richly carpeted with ferns, sorrel, and other lush, green underbrush. The hidden birds chirp their songs, and tiny, cheerful roadside waterfalls applaud as you cruise past. If you can bear to stop your momentum, check out the excellent interpretive signs along the way—they offer insight into the area's cultural past along with information about the local flora and fauna. They're placed next to walking-only trails leading off on your left and right.

Keep an eye out for the signed National Council of Garden Club Grove on your right, near mile marker 132.74, about 5.7 miles from your starting point. Also on your right is the trailhead to Hope Creek Ten Taypo Trail, a hiking-only trail. At this point, look left across Drury Parkway, and you see another excellent interpretive sign with Ossagon Trail alongside it. Watch for traffic and cross over to the left (west side) of the parkway. The sign explains the cultural heritage of the Yurok Indians who once inhabited the area.

Say good-bye to the parkway, and begin enjoying Ossagon Trail, a gorgeous single-track trail. Immediately cross a small, wooden bridge. The sign here says Carruthers Cove Trail is reached in 1.6 miles—that's the junction you want. (What it doesn't say is that Carruthers Cove Trail and the Coastal Trail at that point are one and the same—a slight inconsistency, which I explain later.) The hard-packed dirt trail, about 4 feet wide, traverses the northerly slope of a hill covered with old-growth redwood and mixed conifer trees. The hill gently slopes down on your right into a tiny creek. Immediately you begin climbing a steep but short section. The steepness soon mellows though still climbs. About 0.5 mile from the Ossagon Trailhead, you reach the high point of the loop at about 870 feet, gaining 115 feet from the parkway, approximately 6.2 miles from the visitor center.

A lesser hiking trail peels off behind you on the right. Bypass it, staying on the more defined, wider trail, heading west toward the ocean. The trail narrows and the fun downhill begins, descending steeply through tall bush and stands of Alder trees. Trail conditions get a bit technical here with rain-rutted sections, some loose rocks the size of tennis balls, and exposed roots—*use extreme caution.* Beginners should walk this short section. Can you believe that this fabulous trail in a national park is legal? Enjoy it but keep your speed in check: this is an immensely popular trail with hikers. And because there are more hikers than bikers, they have more clout! Irate hikers, having almost been flattened by inconsiderate bikers, have registered complaints with the park service. Let's preserve our rare opportunity to ride this gorgeous area by respecting other trail users.

Continue on the narrow single-track as it descends toward a creek. At 7 miles, cross the creek on a well-made wooden footbridge. Dismount and immediately walk up a set of about 20 steep steps, carrying your bike. Ossagon Trail continues at the top of the stairs, traveling basically flat terrain, still in the tall bushes, past Alder and spruce trees. Eventually, the trail descends again, steeply in some sections with the creek now on your left. At about 7.5 miles, you emerge from the thick of the forest and come into a small clearing of a grassy marsh. The trail is slightly sandy but it's still rideable and it may be somewhat faint here.

Finding your trail may be a bit convoluted here. It's difficult to describe and existing maps only add to the confusion. Why is this? According to park rangers, this is the general area where Butler Creek camp, a primitive walk-in site used to be located. During the past winters, Butler Creek would swell and wash out the camp. Each year, the camp (the obvious indicator being a picnic table) would be relocated in this vicinity. In midsummer 1998, the campsite was re-established at a more stable area closer to Ossagon Creek and the site renamed Ossagon Creek Camp. So, when you reach this area, you may need to do a bit of scouting to find the Coastal Trail leading south. New trail markers have been installed and clearly mark the route. Look for a sign at a kind of T intersection in the slightly sandy and grassy marsh. The Coastal Trail runs both south and north (left and right, respectively). Truth be told, this right-hand Coastal Trail is the same as Carruthers Cove Trail. In any case, you have indeed reached the Coastal Trail in 1.6 miles as promised by the sign back at the Ossagon Trailhead. You're on the right track. Continue on the loop by hanging a left here, heading south.

From this point on, the Coastal Trail parallels the shoreline and ocean on your right. The single-track trail continues to be rideable, eventually leading you back into the forested slope. Just within the forest, the narrow single-track trail becomes a fun roller-coaster ride, remaining basically at sea level. In less than a mile, about 8.2 miles from the visitor center, you reach a set of about 20 steps leading up on your left. At the top of the stairs is a big brown sign indicating Westridge Trail, Friendship Trail, and Zig Zag Trail, all of which are off-limits to bikes. Follow signed Coastal Trail as it continues on the other side of the stairs. Continue the fun roller-coaster single-track through the forest, skirting the edge of the open coastal prairie off on your right.

As you cruise along, the trail is bounded on both sides by thick bushes and trees. Be alert, especially as you round blind curves—you may come face to face with a elk standing in the trail. I did! We were about 30 yards apart when we simultaneously laid eyes on each other. I stood in my tracks for about 10 minutes, unable to go around him. He eventually ambled off the trail, heading back down into the prairie. Continue on and at a little over a mile from the stairs, you pass Gold Dust Falls, tucked inside the forest just a short hike from the Coastal Trail (bikes are not allowed on the short hiking trail). About 300 feet farther, you pass another small waterfall. In almost 1.5 miles farther, (about 10.7 miles from the starting point), the single-track ends in a dirt parking area near the Fern Canyon Trailhead (hiking only). Go past the picnic tables here and continue on the Coastal Trail, now a two-car width, smooth, sometimes dusty dirt road. Though it's not actually signed here, this is Davison Road, heading south and paralleling the shoreline.

For the next 3.4 miles, Davison Road is flat, exposed riding at sea level. The shoreline parallels the road on your right while Gold Bluffs looms overhead on your left. Along the way, bypass Gold Bluffs Beach campground (water and rest rooms here) and, slightly farther, a picnic day-use area.

At about 3.6 miles since the dirt road began, pass a state park entry kiosk and begin curving inland, climbing back into the forest and its welcoming shade. Most of the climbing is moderate, ending with a somewhat steeper 400-yard climb. After that, it's a fast descent, still on hard-packed Davison Road. Stay alert for cars. At just over a mile from the kiosk, keep a sharp eye out for a dirt single-track leading off on the left, at the crest of a fast right-hand curve. Marked simply by a tiny "Trail" sign and biker symbol, it's easy to miss, especially if you're zipping around the curve.

The trail from Davison Road is approximately 4 miles and leads into the campground. (This is the stretch that's suitable for young children and possibly kid-trailers—check with a ranger.) It gently descends over basically nontechnical terrain, though the trail can become muddy and a bit sloppy after a storm. From Davison Road, the trail takes you through a small-scale gorge, bordered by a vertical slope on one side and tall bushes and trees on the other. In about a mile, the terrain opens up and the trail takes you through the tall, cool forest. Go past Elk Prairie Trail and in a few yards, the dirt trail ends, running into the pavement near the Hike-Bike campsites. The paved road is the park's main road and it leads you past the meadow—a favorite grazing area of resident elk—on your way back to your car.

RIDE 6 · Lost Man Creek–Holter Ridge Bike Trail

AT A GLANCE

Length/configuration: 21.5-mile out-and-back (10.75 miles each way); dirt roads with optional 0.3-mile spur on pavement to an overlook. Alternate route: 20-mile loop using paved roads

Aerobic difficulty: Moderately strenuous due to elevation gain

Technical difficulty: Not technical

Scenery: Splendid old-growth redwoods, especially beautiful when the ethereal fog looms overhead.

Special comments: Suitable for young children and kid-trailers when ridden as a much shorter out-and-back. Worth checking out is nearby Lady Bird Johnson Grove off Bald Hills Road.

L ong before the national park system acquired this chunk of land to the north and south of Lost Man Creek, logging companies blazed a road east from Prairie Creek up to Holter Ridge. Today, those dirt logging roads remain as park service roads, closed to unauthorized vehicle use. Unlike other dirt roads in the national park system, Lost Man Creek and Holter Ridge Roads are open to mountain bikers. Though the trails are not glorious, thrilling single-tracks, the serene scenery makes it a worthy outing. You can pedal this route as a 21-mile out-and-back (10.5 miles each way) with an optional 0.3-mile spur to the Prairie Creek Overlook. An alternate return route is a 20-mile loop, which includes a 15%-grade steep descent on the well-traveled, paved Bald Hills Road and a short stretch on US 101. The out-and-back, the loop, and the spur are nontechnical—suitable for beginners with little technical skill, though confidence in riding with fast, roaring traffic is required on the loop. Elevation gain, on the other hand, makes this ride moderately strenuous, steadily climbing 2,150 feet in 10.3 miles, punctuated by sometimes steep roller-coaster terrain through the forested ridge.

Ah, but there's something about being enveloped—indeed, dominated—by towering redwoods shrouded in an omnipresent ethereal fog, set in a spectacularly green, thickly carpeted forest floor. Occasionally, the fog thins for a moment, revealing an unexpected blue sky, and sunlight hits the forest floor. It's a humbling blanket of solitude, calming despite the moderately strenuous journey involved. For those of you who like the kind of ride that chases all thoughts from your mind, leaving you with just the sound of your breathing, this is the place for you. The sound of the dirt and gravel, and occasional fallen tree limbs crunch underneath your tires. The music of gurgling Lost Man Creek faintly diminishes as you climb the ridge, while the sound of your breathing intensifies. But listen closely to the life of the forest. You might hear the high-pitched seagull-like call of a threatened species, the marbled murrelet, a tiny bird believed to be indigenous to the old-growth forest. Enjoy experiencing the ride.

General location: About 38 miles south of Crescent City and about 45 miles north of Eureka on US 101.

Elevation change: 2,140 feet; starting elevation and low point 100 feet; high point 2,240 feet. Gradual climb up to the ridge followed by rolling terrain and gradual, long descent; you do it in reverse for the return.

Season: Trail accessible year-round, though the weather is likely to be wet with fog and rain in the winter and spring, making the trail slightly muddy. Summer tends to be cool.

Services: Picnic tables and pit toilet at the Lost Man Creek Trailhead. Drinking water, rest rooms, and pay phone at the visitor center in beautiful Elk Prairie campground, located on Drury Parkway almost 3 miles from the trailhead. Food, lodging, and gas in the tiny towns of Orick, Klamath, and Requa, located to the north and

RIDE 6 · Lost Man Creek–Holter Ridge Bike Trail

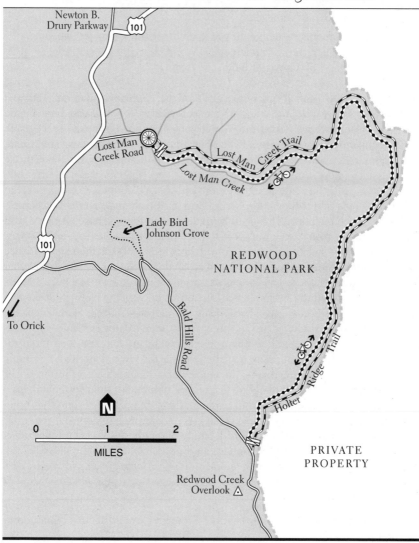

Newton B.
Drury Parkway
101

Lost Man
Creek Road

Lost Man Creek Trail

Lost Man Creek

Lady Bird
Johnson Grove

REDWOOD
NATIONAL PARK

Bald Hills Road

To Orick

Holter Ridge Trail

N

0   1   2

MILES

PRIVATE
PROPERTY

Redwood Creek
Overlook △

south along Drury Parkway. All other services available in Crescent City, about 38 miles north on US 101.

Hazards: Occasional patches of poison oak. Though rarely seen, be alert and prepared for encounters with black bears and mountain lions. If you choose the loop route, expect nonexistent shoulders while you share the narrow, two-lane road with a fair amount of traffic, including massive logging trucks.

Rescue index: Of all the trails in Redwood National and State Parks, this route is the least used, even in the summer. Be self-sufficient. For emergency help, make your own way down to one of several well-traveled paved roads (US 101 or Bald Hills Road) and flag down a motorist.

Land status: Redwood National and State Parks. The entire park is cooperatively managed by the U.S. Department of the Interior, National Park Service, and the California Department of Parks and Recreation.

Maps: *Redwood National Park–North Coast State Parks, Smith River NRA*, published by Trails Illustrated™, P.O. Box 4357, Evergreen, CO 80437, www.trailsillustrated.com; *Redwood National Park Trail Guide*, published by Redwood Natural History Association; USGS Orick and Holter Ridge 7.5 minute series.

Finding the trail: From the Elk Prairie campground in Prairie Creek State Park to Lost Man Creek Road: The trailhead is located approximately 3 miles from the state park entrance and can be reached by bike or car. Leave the campground on the main road and turn right onto southbound Newton B. Drury Parkway. Slow your speed and watch out for free-roaming Roosevelt elk on this stretch. Travel south for almost 0.5 mile, at which point the parkway merges into southbound US 101. Continue south on US 101 for another 1.5 miles to the Lost Man Creek Road turnoff, a signed dirt road on your left (east side). Go 0.9 mile up Lost Man Creek Road to the parking area. The bike route begins at the locked gate spanning the dirt road. From Orick: Drive about 3 miles north on US 101 to Lost Man Creek Road, which leads off on your right. Follow the directions on this dirt road as previously described.

Sources of additional information: See sources of additional information for Ride 5.

Notes on the trail: The only sign you see proclaiming Lost Man Creek Road is where it intersects with US 101. The only sign you see identifying Holter Ridge Road is at the farthest end of the bike trail, at its intersection with Bald Hills Road. Throughout the trail, single wooden mile markers dot the trail in approximately 1-mile increments (when compared to my cyclometer readings, the mile markers sometimes varied from 0.1 to 0.3 mile more). Nevertheless, this route is easy to follow because all other trails that intersect it are lesser paths and are usually signed "Not a Trail." Both Lost Man Creek and Holter Ridge Roads are well-defined roads, generally one-car width, packed gravel and dirt, often with scattered fir needles and leaves. Lucky for us, because when the weather's damp (which is most of the time), the trail remains fairly rideable with no deep, momentum-stopping muddy areas. If you ride early in the year, check with a ranger for trail conditions, especially for trees downed by storms.

Begin by pedaling past the locked gate and the World Heritage sign, heading due east. Starting elevation here is about 100 feet. You're immediately welcomed by majestically towering redwoods, their girth almost the size of old Volkswagen Beetles. In about 0.5 mile, cross a well-made wooden bridge. Pedal a few more yards, cross over another bridge and get ready: the steady climb out of the creek drainage up to Holter Ridge begins. The trail begins a gradual climb with some level spots and less steep sections over mostly nontechnical terrain. If you're lucky, this is where you'd hear—or if you're really lucky, spot—a marbled murrelet, a designated threatened species. Researchers believe that these little stealthy guys like to nest in old-growth forests exclusively. When I rode this stretch of the route, I caught a glimpse of a little black bear in the distance, lumbering off the trail, probably trailing mama bear. (If you're fortunate to spot wildlife, particularly marbled murrelets, black bears, and mountain lions, please report your sighting to the park service by filling out a wildlife sighting card at any of the park's visitor center or entry kiosk.)

At about 3 miles from the trailhead and about 1,100 feet higher, the trail imperceptibly curves to the southeast (your right) and begins skirting the eastern boundary of the National Park. Look left through the thick forest, and you can see a bit of sky; if it's not too foggy, you can see a distant ridge. Continue the moderate climb to the ridge top, often mellowed by level and sometimes descending short stretches. The trail now becomes Holter Ridge Road, though it's not signed as such here. For the next 7.4 miles, the terrain is a roller-coaster ride, with steep but short ascents with a few level, even brief descending stretches. You see fewer old-growth redwoods here but plenty of second-growth as well as other deciduous trees and dense underbrush. Occasionally, you see tiny National Park boundary signs off the trail on your left, on the east side of the dirt road.

As you approach 10 miles, you may hear a truck roaring down Bald Hills Road in the distance. A steep (about 9% grade) hill looms ahead and, after surmounting it at about 10.3 miles, you reach the high point of the ride, having climbed approximately 2,150 feet from the trailhead to 2,250 feet. The next 0.3 mile is a fast and welcome descent to Bald Hills Road.

Upon reaching Bald Hills Road, you have several choices to make. If it's a clear day, go check out the Redwood Creek Overlook because you'll have an expansive 180-degree view of the coastline and the canyon carved by Redwood Creek. To get there, go left onto Bald Hills Road, descending gently for 0.3 mile. There are picnic tables here, making it a fine spot for a breather and snack. After enjoying the view, turn around and retrace your path to the Holter Ridge Road intersection.

The other choice to make here is deciding how to return to the Lost Man Creek Road trailhead. You can go back the way you came or make a loop via Bald Hills Road and US 101. If you opt for the loop, know that there's likely to be a significant amount of traffic on Bald Hills Road, including roaring logging trucks, all the way down to US 101. And while it's virtually all downhill from here, it's extremely steep in some sections, about 15% grade. About 3.5 miles down the road, you reach Lady Bird Johnson Grove, a mystical forest of enormous old-growth redwoods with an excellent 1-mile walking-only interpretive path. (You'll definitely want to lock your bike since they are not allowed on the walking trail.) Back on Bald Hills Road, continue down for 2.7 miles more and then go right onto US 101, using *extreme caution* as the traffic really zooms here and the shoulder is almost nonexistent. Endure this stretch for 2.2 miles to Lost Man Creek Road, turn right, leave the traffic behind, and ride almost a mile back to your car at the trailhead.

Unless you're pressed for time, I personally recommend the out-and-back route, retracing your path on Holter Ridge and Lost Man Creek Roads. The descent is just as fun and no traffic. I would rather face a chance encounter with a bear than a logging truck. Then, once back at your car, visit Lady Bird Johnson Grove by driving 2.7 miles up Bald Hills Road from US 101.

RIDE 7 · Coastal Trail—Last Chance Section

AT A GLANCE

Length/configuration: 13-mile out-and-back (6.5 miles each way); paved, wide dirt single-track. Options: 16.4-mile out-and-back, (8.2 miles each way); paved, wide dirt single-track. Or 17.8-mile loop, same trail conditions with a long stretch on US 101. Or 8.2-mile point-to-point all-dirt ride.

Aerobic difficulty: Easy (the longer out-and-back and point-to-point routes are moderate; loop is strenuous due to elevation gain and traffic)

Technical difficulty: Not technical (the longer out-and-back, point-to-point, and loop all include 1.2 miles of steep, intermediately technical terrain)

Scenery: Incredibly gorgeous redwood forest on a slope facing the Pacific Ocean

Special comments: This trail can be ridden as an out-and-back in two lengths or a point-to-point, depending on the amount of technical terrain and climbing you wish to ride.

Mother Nature humored us by letting us pave paradise. She allowed us to run US 101 through this gorgeous stretch of the California coastline back in the 1930s. Then, in the late 1960s, disliking what we did, she stepped in with a flurry of storms and began reclaiming her land. By 1970, this stretch of US 101 was closed to cars, forcing us parasites to reroute the road to present-day US 101. But, are we lucky or what? She also reintroduced paradise. Today, the old stretch has healed itself, becoming a portion of California's most gorgeous coastline.

Making use of old US 101, this paved path is the Last Chance section of the 20-mile Coastal Trail, and one of two sections that allows bikes. It traverses dense slopes of surreal foggy redwood forests, smothered in lush, cool understory—hard to believe that a busy highway once blazed through here. Though you have several options in which to configure your ride, the route described here is the shorter 13-mile out-and-back (6.5 miles each way), starting at the south trailhead which accesses the easiest portion of the Coastal Trail. It's mostly flat, nontechnical, and generally one-car width across though some sections have become narrow single-track due to tall overgrown bushes. The gentle terrain is suitable for young children—you can turn around when the kiddies have had enough.

Stronger riders looking for more of an aerobic challenge can ride the longer 16.4-mile out-and-back (8.2 miles each way), or the 17.8-mile loop, both of which begin at Enderts Beach Overlook, the north trailhead. The first 1.2 miles of the out-and-back from Enderts is a wide dirt single-track trail, intermediately technical due to a steep 8% grade climb over rocky terrain. The loop can be ridden clockwise or in reverse, and includes 8 miles on present-day US 101 and 1.6 miles on Enderts Beach Road.

General location: The south trailhead is about 14 miles north of the Klamath River on US 101 and approximately 10 miles south of Crescent City. The north trailhead at Enderts Beach Overlook is almost 24 miles north of the Klamath River, approximately 3.6 miles south of Crescent City off US 101.

Elevation change: Short out-and-back: 240 feet change from the south trailhead to the turnaround point at 6.5 miles; involves an almost imperceptible ascent. Long out-and-back, point-to-point, and loop: 960 feet change. The south trailhead starts at about 800 feet and the north elevation at Enderts Beach Overlook starts at about 80 feet. The high point of the entire route is roughly 1,040 feet. Riding south to north, trail ascends softly, then drops steeply to Enderts Beach. North to south involves an initial 1.5-mile steep climb, then tapers off as it approaches south trailhead.

Season: Trail accessible year-round, though the weather is likely to be wet with fog and rain during the winter and spring. Summer tends to be cool.

Services: Basically none, although there is a primitive camp at Nickel Creek near the north trailhead. All services available in Crescent City, about 3.6 miles or 10 miles north on US 101 from the north and south trailheads, respectively. Water available at Mill Creek campground off US 101 between the north and south trailheads.

Hazards: There are 2 small dirt pulloffs at which to park at the south trailhead, either on the east side or west side of US 101. If you park in the east side pulloff, you'll have to run across 2 lanes of US 101 in order to pick up the trail. You'll need to be extremely alert when crossing because traffic can be busy and fast, and curves in the highway limit your visibility. If you have children with you, the west side pulloff is highly recommended. (See "Finding the trail" for more details about these 2 parking areas.) If you park and begin at the north trailhead at Enderts Beach Overlook, do not leave any valuables in your locked car.

Rescue index: The section of the Coastal Trail around the south trailhead (the easy out-and-back) is remote. For that reason, you need to be self-sufficient since you may not see other trail users if you need emergency assistance. The 2 to 3 miles closest to the north trailhead at Enderts Beach Overlook is immensely more popular with other trail users and beachgoers, and thus improves your chances of finding help, especially during the summer.

Land status: Del Norte Coast Redwoods State Park, a part of Redwood National and State Parks. The entire park is cooperatively managed by the U.S. Department of the Interior, the National Park Service, and the California Department of Parks and Recreation.

Maps: *Del Norte Coast Redwoods State Park*, published by North Coast Redwood Interpretive Association; *Redwood National Park–North Coast State Parks, Smith River NRA*, published by National Geographic Maps/Trails Illustrated™; USGS Sister Rocks and Childs Hill 7.5-minute series.

Finding the trail: You have a choice of starting points, depending on how much climbing you're willing to tackle. If you want to ride the easy, nontechnical 13-mile out-and-back (6.5 miles each way), begin at the south trailhead on US 101. If the 8.2-mile point-to-point is your chosen configuration, begin at the south trailhead, leaving the ending shuttle car at the north trailhead at Enderts Beach Overlook. (It's easier and more thrilling to descend the rocky technical section than to ascend it.) If you want to ride the entire trail as a 16.4-mile out-and-back (8.2 miles each way), begin at either the south or the north trailhead at Enderts Beach Overlook. The easiest trail access point is the north end, thanks to a parking lot at the Overlook. Starting there, however, means you'll have to tackle the short but steep and intermediately technical section. Beginners and not-so-strong riders will undoubtedly dismount and push their bike over this 1.2-mile section.

Getting to the south trailhead: Park at 1 of 2 small dirt pulloffs. One is on the west side of US 101 and is recommended if you have children with you. The other is on the east side of US 101 and requires you to run across 2 lanes of frequently fast traffic. (Be extremely alert as the curves in the road limit your visibility.) Both pulloffs are not well marked and are easy to miss when driving, especially when traffic is breathing down your neck. Depending on your driving direction on US 101, park in whichever pulloff is on your right. That way, you avoid stopping traffic and crossing a lane of oncoming traffic. To reach the south trailhead from Crescent City, drive south on US 101 for about 10 miles. Look for milepost marker 15.6 or the more visible white sign saying "Turn off headlights." Immediately after that, go pass the east side dirt pulloff on your left (there may be a small sign marked "C.T." here, short for Coastal Trail). Continue about 300 yards to the west side pulloff—it'll appear just as you drive out from underneath the tree canopy. The west side pulloff is exactly at the south end of the bike route and you'll know it by the gate closing off the trail, about 40 yards set back from the highway. Park here, well off the highway and as close to the edge of the narrow clearing as possible. If you choose to park at the east side pulloff, the narrow, single-track connector trail to old US 101 is barely visible. Fortunately, a small "C.T." sign marks the path. In fact, the east side pulloff is where the Coastal Trail crosses from the east to the west side of US 101. The south trailhead is about 14 miles north of the Klamath River. If you see the sign "Turn on Headlights," you've just passed both pulloffs and the south trailhead.

Getting to the north trailhead: Travel south on US 101 from Crescent City for 1.6 miles; turn right onto Enderts Beach Road. Go about 1.6 miles to the Overlook and parking lot. If you're coming from the Klamath River in the south on northbound US 101, go past the south trailhead at about 14 miles, and continue about 22 miles to Enderts Beach Road. Turn left here and follow Enderts Beach Road 1.6 miles to the Overlook and parking lot.

Sources of additional information:

North Coast Redwood Interpretive Association
Redwood National Park Information Center
P.O. Box 234
Orick, CA 95555
(707) 488-2171
Located one mile south of Orick on US 101

Notes on the trail: No matter which trailhead you choose as your starting point, this route is easy to follow since the direction is basically north-south, following the rugged shoreline, staying about 700 to 900 feet above sea level. The following trail description is based on starting from the east side parking area at the south trailhead.

From the east side pulloff next to the Coastal Trail, cautiously cross US 101 to a very narrow single-track dirt trail that climbs abruptly from the pavement. It may be hard to see at first since it's shady and overgrown with lush bushes here. This tiny stretch is the continuation of the Coastal Trail and is rideable, though the incline and narrowness may cause you to lose momentum, forcing you to dismount and walk. The trail leads south, then makes a sharp right curve toward the north, rounding a berm. You catch a glimpse of the ocean and immediately you're in amazing silence, totally insulated from US 101 and its traffic noise, thanks to the soundproofing effect of the dense forest and abundant vegetation. You can barely hear the crashing waves of the ocean far below. Follow the single-track and it soon dumps you onto a wider dirt trail; go right onto it. You're now on old, dilapidated US 101. (From the west side parking area, there's only one way to go and that's through the gate, heading north.)

It's hard to believe that traffic once roared through here because your surrounding landscape is incredibly dense with vegetation, carpeted with huge ferns, sorrel, salal, moss, and more. The fog permeates the old-growth redwoods, creating a truly ethereal world. You feel miles away from civilization except for the mostly consistent stretches of paved asphalt, still decorated with white highway stripes and old wooden mile marker posts painted black and white. It's amazing how Mother Nature can

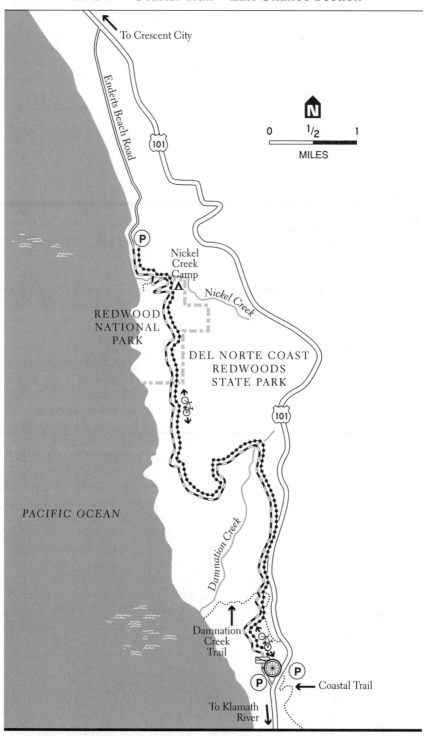

To Crescent City

Enderts Beach Road

101

N

0   1/2   1

MILES

P

Nickel
Creek
Camp

Nickel Creek

REDWOOD
NATIONAL
PARK

DEL NORTE COAST
REDWOODS
STATE PARK

101

PACIFIC OCEAN

Damnation Creek

Damnation
Creek
Trail

P

P

Coastal Trail

To Klamath
River

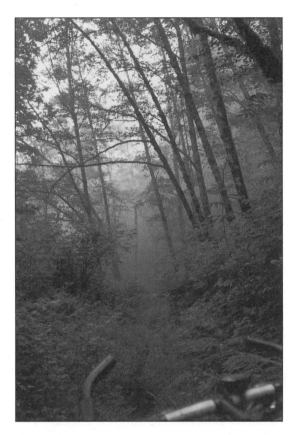

Portions of this route are
likely to be beautifully
overgrown.

sometimes reclaim territory with such intensity and beauty, eradicating the scars we
inflict. Alternating between dirt and asphalt, the trail is mostly covered with fallen
leaves, redwood needles, and debris left from storms. For the most part, you're riding
a dirt, sometimes wide, single-track trail past wet, overgrown ferns and the like.

The trail is basically flat riding, with mild descents and ascents as it traverses a
west-facing slope. At about a mile from the starting point, you past a grove of ancient
redwoods, signed with a plaque honoring Henry Solon Gray, forester, educator, and
administrator. A few yards farther, Damnation Creek Trail, a hiking-only trail, intersects on your right and in 0.1 mile, it peels off on both your left and right (again).
Stay on old US 101.

At just over 3 miles, the road has crumbled down the slope. A single-track dirt trail
continues around this washout, leading you over a creek on a well-made wooden footbridge. Old US 101 resumes on the other side of the bridge. From this point on, the
trail resembles a dirt single-track, but every now and then, you see pavement again.
Where does the pavement end? Hard to say due to the dense vegetation but I think it
ends at around 4.5 miles. At almost 5 miles, the trail narrows significantly due to tall,
overgrown, incredibly thick, and leafy bushes. Persevere and the dirt single-track trail
soon re-establishes itself as it skirts a few yards of bushy drop-off on your left.

At 5.7 miles, you come to a sign indicating that you're about to enter Redwood
National Park, Nickel Creek campground 2 miles, and Enderts Beach parking area

2.5 miles. From the south trailhead, you've been pedaling through Del Norte Coast Redwoods State Park. Enter the national park and continue on the dirt trail. The path widens and your glimpses of the ocean are completely eliminated now due to the tall vegetation and slightly higher slope on your left. The trail begins climbing mildly. At about 6 miles, it levels and then begins to descend gently, this time for a longer duration, almost a half-mile long. For those of you choosing the shorter out-and-back, turn around here and retrace your path back to the south trailhead.

For the longer out-and-back, continue north toward Enderts Beach. Eventually, the trail descends more steeply and the terrain becomes somewhat more technically challenging due to loose rocks and ruts. This challenging section drops roughly 500 feet in less than a mile toward Nickel Creek, leading you through several rocky switchbacks along the way. The path mellows after you cross the creek and past the trail leading to Nickel Creek Primitive Camp. A bit farther, a trail signed Enderts Beach takes off on your left. (It's a great beach with tide pools, worth checking out if you have the time or interest.) For the next 0.5 mile, the trail widens significantly, skirting a completely exposed, sheer drop-off into the ocean, which is about 100 to 150 feet below. Views of the Pacific are thrilling along this stretch. When you reach the Enderts Beach Overlook parking lot at approximately 8.2 miles, you're rewarded with a view of Crescent City, jutting out into the ocean. There's a picnic table here and it's a great spot to relax and have a snack. After that, turn around and retrace your path back to the south trailhead. Take comfort in the fact that the steep section which you just descended and must now surmount is only 1.2 miles long.

For gutsy loop riders, continue down Enderts Beach Road (a narrow paved road) for about 1.6 miles to US 101. Turn right onto US 101 and begin a moderate climb (approximately 8% grade) on the narrow shoulder, reaching the Crescent City Vista Point after about 1.2 miles. Take a breather here and check out the view. Continue on US 101 for another 6.8 miles to the south trailhead and your parked car. And watch out for traffic!

RIDE 8 · Howland Hill–Stout Grove

AT A GLANCE

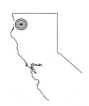

Length/configuration: 10-mile out-and-back (5 miles each way); dirt road. Optional 4.5 miles on Little Bald Hills Road, a dirt road.

Aerobic difficulty: Easy (option is reportedly moderate due to some steep climbs)

Technical difficulty: Not technical (option is reportedly intermediate due to somewhat rocky terrain)

Scenery: Gigantic ancient redwoods along a creek drainage, especially ethereal when the fog permeates the treetops. Stout Grove, at the top of the ride, offers a walking-only path that showcases astonishing stands of old-growth redwoods, including the 345-foot tall Stout Tree.

Special comments: Suitable for strong, young children. Kid-trailers not recommended.

Forming the northern anchor of Redwood National and State Parks, Jedediah Smith Redwoods State Park encompasses more than 9,600 acres, where many of the world's oldest redwood trees are located. They're incredibly huge and you see plenty of them on this easy 10-mile out-and-back (5 miles each way) ride, using a well-traveled narrow, dirt vehicle road, frequented by motor tourists. In the early 1900s, Howland Hills Road was a thoroughfare for logging operations. Before that, it was the stagecoach route to Oregon. Today, the hard-packed, nontechnical, dirt road skirts the Mill Creek drainage, mildly ascending through ethereal stands of old redwoods. It's a timeless wonderland for adults and children, and, indeed, it was the extraterrestrial setting for the Ewoks scene in the third *Star Wars* movie, *Return of the Jedi*.

Long before Jedi Knights, though, there was Jedediah Smith, the legendary mountain man who, as a young pup in the 1820s, explored these northwestern territories on numerous expeditions, paving the way, so to speak, to the settlement of California and Oregon. The young explorer gained a reputation as an extraordinary outdoorsman, having survived a gory grizzly bear attack (not in this area!) that left him mortally wounded. As a businessman, he was a fur trapper and partner in the Rocky Mountain Fur Company, a profession which, arguably, was a major contributing factor in opening up the far western territories at that time. But thousands of years before Smith, the region was revered by American Indians, including the Tolowa tribe who inhabited the areas which now make up most of the state park. They lived off the bounty of the land, rivers, and sea, living in fine split-plank wooden structures along the coast and the rivers. Today, several tribes have outlasted Smith, living in and on nearby reservations, struggling to hold on to their traditions and language.

By the way, at the top of Howland Hill is Stout Grove. It's a must-see, about a 30-minute walk through astonishing stands of old-growth redwoods. In 1929, through the efforts of concerned citizens and the Save-the-Redwoods League, funds were raised to purchase and preserve these ancient trees. Look for the Stout Tree, a redwood measuring 345 feet tall. Right before your eyes, it's a living organism that's taller than the Capitol dome in Washington, D.C., or the Statue of Liberty. Gawking allowed.

General location: On the eastern edge of Crescent City, about 3 miles away.

Elevation change: 420 feet; starting elevation 200 feet; high point 530 feet; low point 110 feet. Soft, gradual climb with plenty of level stretches.

Season: Year-round. Summer ranges from 45 to 85 degrees. Winter and spring are likely to be wet with fog and rain, and the road may be muddy. Call ahead to the park service to check road conditions.

Services: None found on the trail. All services available in Crescent City, about 3 miles away.

Hazards: Expect some vehicular traffic, especially during the summer. Fortunately, most motorists drive slowly since they're admiring the redwood forest. If you visit Stout Grove, bring a lock since bikes are not allowed on the walking path.

Rescue index: This designated auto route which leads to popular Stout Grove is well-traveled in the summer, making your chances of getting help from a passing motorist very good. In the off-season, particularly during the week, make your way back down Howland Hill Road to the residential neighborhood, which you passed on your way to the trailhead.

Land status: Jedediah Smith Redwoods State Park, a part of Redwood National and State Parks. The entire park is cooperatively managed by the U.S. Department of the

RIDE 8 · Howland Hill–Stout Grove

Interior, the National Park Service, and the California Department of Parks and Recreation.

Maps: *Redwood National Park–North Coast State Parks, Smith River NRA*, published by National Geographic Maps/Trails Illustrated™; *Redwood National Park Trail Guide*, published by Redwood Natural History Association; USGS Crescent City and Hiouchi 7.5 minute series.

Finding the trail: From Crescent City, head south on US 101 to the eastern edge of town. At a **T** intersection, look for Elk Valley Road and turn left onto it. About a mile from US 101, you reach the intersection of Howland Hill Road, which leads to Stout Grove. Take this road, turning right, and follow it through a residential neighborhood. Stay on Howland Hill, passing Humboldt Street on the right, and later, Elk Valley Casino on the left. (If you're looking for more miles to pedal, you can park in this vicinity and begin riding.) The road gradually ascends and in just over 2 miles from US 101, you enter Jedediah Smith Redwoods State Park. Stay on the paved road as it narrows and in a short distance, it becomes gravel and dirt. At almost 3 miles from US 101, you reach a large, white metal gate that's likely to be open. On your right is a lesser dirt road with another metal gate, probably locked—don't park here. Instead, park in the small pulloff, on the north side of the main road (your left) and begin your ride here.

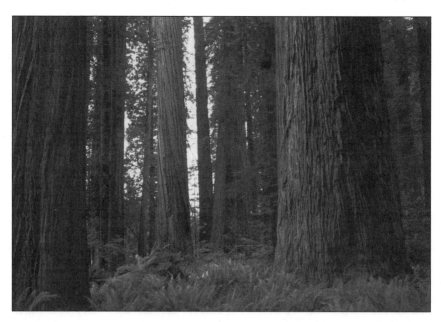

A lush blanket of ferns and stately redwoods create a serene scene easily accessed by most beginners.

Sources of additional information:

North Coast Redwood Interpretive
Association
Redwood National Park Information
Center
P.O. Box 234
Orick, CA 95555
(707) 488-2171
One mile south of Orick on US 101

Jedediah Smith Redwoods State Park
1375 Elk Valley Road at US 199
Crescent City, CA 95531
(707) 464-6101
http://cal-parks.ca.gov

Notes on the trail: Following this route is a no-brainer: you simply stay on Howland Hill Road all the way up to Stout Grove, reaching it in about 5 miles from the white metal gate. The dirt road climbs gently, no more than a 4% grade. The short stretches of flat and subtle descents make for a fun, mild roller-coaster ride. Except for an occasional car, relax and enjoy the ride.

As you begin pedaling, the hill slopes gently down on your right into Mill Creek. You immediately cruise past incredibly tall, old-growth redwoods. The trees are dense here, and the towering canopies of the redwoods filter most of the sunlight. The mostly shaded forest floor is smothered with all kinds of green understory, including ferns, redwood sorrel, and wild rhododendron. Consider yourself lucky if the forest is shrouded in fog during your outing. That's when the forest takes on an ethereal, fantastical quality.

Cruise past the Boy Scout Tree trailhead and shortly thereafter, Mill Creek Trail (both of which are off-limits to bikes). Just before crossing the creek, look for a fallen redwood on the left side of the road. It's been sawed through and the diameter revealed is enormous—about 13 to 15 feet across! Continue on, crossing the creek on a concrete bridge that has seen better days. At just over 4 miles, you come to an intersection with a paved road leading off on your left—it's one of two ways to access Stout Grove. To reach the top of Howland Hill and the other entrance to Stout Grove, bypass the road on your left and continue pedaling up the easy hill for a few more yards, staying on the dirt road. The road levels, and there you find the Stout Grove Trail, a walking-only trail. (Optional side-trip: Across the road from this trail is a another dirt road that climbs sharply. That's Little Bald Hills Road on which bikes are allowed. It reportedly climbs steeply for a short distance, then mellows as it traverses rugged terrain for about 4.5 miles to the park boundary. Check it out if you're up for some exploring.)

A must-do is a stroll through Stout Grove where you find ancient groves of redwoods, including 345-foot tall Stout Tree. Photo opportunities abound. When you feel sufficiently humbled, turn around and return the way you came.

RIDE 9 · Gasquet Toll Road

AT A GLANCE

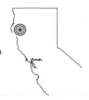

Length/configuration: 18-mile point-to-point; maintained dirt roads and some pavement. Loop option: 25.7-mile loop on dirt and pavement, rideable clockwise or reverse.

Aerobic difficulty: Moderately strenuous due to elevation gain. Elk Camp option reportedly strenuous.

Technical difficulty: Mild to intermediate due to generally somewhat rocky terrain. Elk Camp option reportedly advanced/expert level.

Scenery: Panoramic views of snow-capped Siskiyou mountain range and the canyon carved by the Middle Fork of the Smith River.

Special comments: Strong, adventurous beginners with basic technical skills may enjoy this ride. Brawny riders looking to do some exploring can tackle Elk Camp Ridge Trail, a reportedly more technically challenging trail accessible off Patrick Creek Road.

Though the trail is a maintained, mild to intermediately technical county road, the elevation gain, length, and scenery make Gasquet Toll Road an enjoyable workout. And depending on your biking prowess, this adventure can be custom-tailored to suit your fancy. You can ride it as an 18-mile point-to-point (requiring a shuttle car arrangement). If you're a strong rider who doesn't mind sharing the road with vehicles, consider the 25.7-mile loop, which includes a 7.8-mile stretch on US 199, pedaling clockwise or in reverse direction. For advanced/expert riders, Gasquet Toll Road provides several connecting trails to Elk Camp Ridge Trail, making for an all-dirt configuration worthy of exploration by the adventurous. According to Don Pass, the director of recreation planner (great title, no?) at Smith River NRA headquarters, Elk

RIDE 9 · Gasquet Toll Road

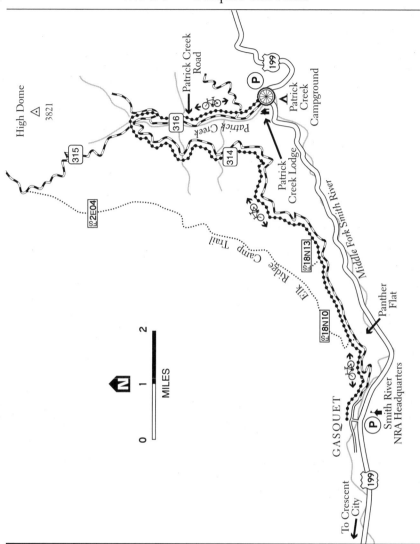

Camp Ridge Trail is a technically challenging single-track with steep, rugged sections (personally, I have not yet pedaled it). Whatever configuration you choose, you will be rewarded with dramatic views of deeply carved Smith River canyon and the surrounding mountain ridges, some of which are likely to be patched with melting snow during early summer.

Smith River is California's one and only truly wild river; it doesn't have any dams. With the establishment of Smith River National Recreation Area which encompasses the North, Middle, and South Forks, Smith River will remain undammed thanks to environmental protections in place that prohibit new mining claims and strictly limit logging activity. Forming the northern end of the long and narrow Six

Rivers National Forest, Smith River NRA is one of four ranger districts operating here. Six major waterways drain or pass through the Forest: Smith, Klamath, Trinity, Mad, Van Duzen, and Eel Rivers, hence its name.

The little town of Gasquet (pronounced *gas-key*) was born in the crazed, fortune-seeking era of the Gold Rush. In 1853, Horace Gasquet, a savvy Frenchman, realized that his gold was not in the mines but in supplying the miners with goods and services. Not only did he find prosperity in the transportation of goods to and from Crescent City, he developed service businesses as well, such as a general store, restaurant, and resort. Enterprising Horace gave birth to the bustling town of Gasquet Flat, now present-day Gasquet. Wanting to expand transportation service into Oregon, Horace, with the help of Chinese immigrants, built the road (which we now ride) from Gasquet Flat, up along the East Fork of Patrick Creek, over the ridge to Shelly Creek, ending in Waldo, Oregon. And, being the enterprising businessman that he was, tolls were charged on anything that moved: persons, wagons, horses, and livestock. Today, the road is maintained by the U.S. Department of Agriculture in its national forest and recreation area program. That means you and I, as taxpayers, fund the maintenance of the former toll road. So, enjoy your ride.

General location: About 19 to 25 miles east of Crescent City on US 199, depending on the starting point you choose.

Elevation change: Point-to-point starting at Patrick Creek at US 199: 1,585 feet gain and 2,050 feet loss. Starting elevation is 865 feet; high point 2,450 feet; low point and ending elevation 400 feet. No abrupt or steep hills, just a long, gradual climb followed by long, easy descent. (Loop: 2,050 feet gain and loss; same starting point as point-to-point.)

Season: May through October, recommend checking with ranger station for snow levels and road condition.

Services: None on the trail. Some services in Gasquet and Hiouchi. All services in Crescent City. Guests staying at Patrick Creek Lodge & Historical Inn (next to trailhead) can get help from the owners in setting up a shuttle car. Several campgrounds nearby: Patrick Creek, Grassy Flat, and Panther Flat, all with water and rest rooms. Patrick Creek campground, built in the 1930s by the Civilian Conservation Corps, is an enduring example of artistically crafted steps, rock walls, rest rooms, and a sunken campfire circle.

Hazards: Watch out for falling rock along portions of the trail. Occasional vehicular traffic while pedaling the dirt road portion. Loop riders: expect a lot of fast traffic on US 199. Area somewhat popular with hunters in the fall. A detailed topo map is a must for explorers of Elk Camp option.

Rescue index: Gasquet Toll Road is designated as a Backroads Discovery auto route and sees light traffic. Elk Camp Ridge Trail is more rugged and with far less trail users. You need to be self-sufficient, no matter which route you choose. For emergency help, make your way back down the trail to US 199 or Gasquet instead of waiting for someone to come along.

Land status: Smith River National Recreation Area, one of four ranger districts in the Six River National Forest.

Maps: *Redwood National Park–North Coast State Parks, Smith River NRA,* published by National Geographic Maps/Trails Illustrated™; USGS Gasquet, Shelly Creek Ridge, High Plateau Mountain 7.5 minute series.

Finding the trail: From Crescent City, travel east on US 199 for almost 19 miles to the small town of Gasquet. Look for the tiny Gasquet Post Office and market on the left at the intersection of Middle Fork Gasquet Road and US 199. If you see the Smith River National Recreation Visitor Center (worth a visit) on your left, you've just missed it. For point-to-point riders, leave your finishing shuttle car either near the post office, or if space is unavailable, park at the Visitor Center. To reach the starting point of the ride for the point-to-point and loop, continue east on US 199 for 7.7 miles to Patrick Creek Lodge & Historical Inn on the left, located alongside Patrick Creek. Across the highway from the Inn is Patrick Creek campground on the south side of US 199. Turn right into the campground and park in the picnic day-use area.

From the California/Oregon state line, travel south on US 199 for about 19 miles to Patrick Creek. Immediately after the creek, turn left into Patrick Creek campground and park in the picnic day-use area. This is the starting place for the point-to-point and loop rides. Point-to-point riders, set up your end shuttle car by continuing southwest on US 199 for about 7.7 miles. On your right is the Smith River National Recreation Visitor Center (worth a visit). You can park here or a short distance farther near the Gasquet post office (preferred, but space is limited), located at the intersection of Middle Fork Gasquet Road and US 199.

Once in Patrick Creek campground, you reach the beginning of the ride by pedaling back out to US 199. Turn right, taking the bridge over the creek, and make an immediate left onto an unsigned dirt road, County Road 316. Be careful as traffic is fast and furious; you might have to dismount and patiently wait for a safe opening in the traffic before crossing both lanes. You're now on Patrick Creek Road. Begin your cycling adventure here.

Sources of additional information:

Patrick Creek Lodge & Historical Inn
13950 Hwy 199
Gasquet, CA 95543
(707) 457-3323
This is located next to Patrick Creek and the trailhead. Originally built in 1926 and renovated in 1988 by Bill and Cindy Grier, the lodge has a cozy restaurant and bar, serving outstanding food, including Sunday brunch. Rustically elegant lodging in a beautiful setting—they even do weddings here! If you're an overnight guest and you want to ride this route as a point-to-point, they can help arrange your end-shuttle car, with some advance notice, of course.

Smith River NRA Headquarters
Six Rivers National Forest
Gasquet Ranger Station
P.O. Box 228
Gasquet, CA 95543
(707) 457-3131

Six Rivers National Forest
1330 Bayshore Way
Eureka, CA 95501
(707) 442-1721
A great source for surrounding national forest maps and some topos.

Notes on the trail: For both the point-to-point and loop, this is an easy route to follow. You basically stay on two well-defined, maintained dirt roads: Patrick Creek Road and Gasquet Toll Road. As part of the NRAs Backroad Discovery Tours, the entire route is suitable for passenger vehicles. An informative leaflet corresponding to interpretive sites along the route is available at the Smith River NRA Headquarters on US 199 in Gasquet. Both dirt roads generally measure one car width across, wider in some places. The terrain is hard-packed dirt with some semi-buried rocks and boulders, occasionally strewn with loose rocks varying in size from golf balls to cantaloupes. Though the

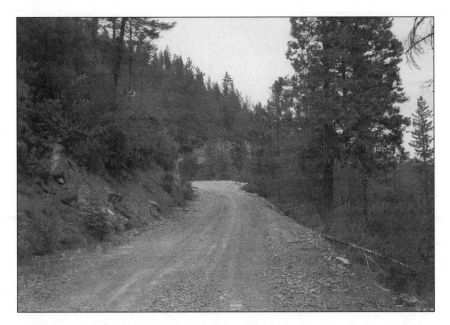

Today, this former historic stagecoach road is toll-free.

roads skirt drop-offs in some stretches (some treacherously deep), the road is comfort-ably wide. Ascents are generally gradual with some level sections.

Start pedaling up Patrick Creek Road, away from US 199. The ride begins with gen-tle climbing, following Patrick Creek upstream, gradually gaining elevation, cruising in and out of the shady forest. Bypass all other trails and smaller roads leading off both sides of your road. Looking left across Patrick Creek, you notice that part of the facing mountain side has slid due to its extreme angle and fractured bedrock, and triggered by rainfall. At about a mile, bypass a semi-paved gravel road leading off on the right.

Continue the gradual climb, still paralleling Patrick Creek, which is flowing about 20 to 50 yards down on your left. At about 2.2 miles, the road crosses a bridge over Eleven Mile Creek and shortly after, the climb steepens a bit. Just beyond 3 miles, you reach a signed intersection: Gasquet Toll Road with Patrick Creek to the left and Shelly Creek to the right. Bear left, following the Toll Road toward the creek which, in a half mile you cross over on an old concrete bridge. You immediately reach another intersection, this time with CR 315 to Elk Camp Ridge Trail.

Brawny riders: Here's a trail worth exploring and it's all on dirt. Though I have not personally ridden it, Don Pass, the director of recreation planner at the NRA head-quarter reports that it is 8.2 miles of technically challenging, somewhat steep ascents and descents on mostly single-track. It eventually rejoins Gasquet Toll Road. To reach the trailhead to Elk Camp Ridge Trail, take CR 315 for almost 3 miles, then go left onto Elk Camp Ridge Trail. Make sure you have a detailed topo map.

For the rest of us mortals, however, continue on Gasquet Toll Road. A short dis-tance beyond the creek is the site of the original Patrick Creek Lodge. In the late 1800s, it served as a stagecoach station for tired drivers, travelers, and horses. After the lodge was moved and rebuilt at its present location on US 199 in 1926, this spot was subsequently mined. What remains are three settling ponds. As you continue to climb out of the ravine, the road becomes slightly steeper than ever before, with, at times, short, level stretches, sometimes descending. The road is rockier and more exposed with fewer shady patches but the views of the Smith River canyon and the mountain ranges in the Siskiyou Wilderness toward the south become more expansive. Pink blossomed wild azalea bushes, scrub bushes, and chocolate-colored madrone and conifer trees decorate the slopes while the road skirts sections of steep drop-offs. Power lines appear overhead intermittently.

At almost 5.5 miles, another trail signed 18N13 runs up the slope on your right. Bypass it, continuing the gradual climb. In about a mile, check out the view of High Dome behind you, toward the north/northeast. It's a rounded mountain topped by a meadow that attracts a variety of wildlife, including deer and bear. The road soon begins a gentle up and down cruise, gaining elevation. At about 9.5 miles, you reach the high point of the Toll Road—a gain of about 1,585 feet from the starting point. Go under power lines again and at about 10 miles, another trail intersects the Toll Road. It's signed to Elk Camp Ridge Trail (2E04) in 2.5 miles. For those of you who accepted the first challenge, this is where you would rejoin Gasquet Toll Road.

Continue on the Toll Road as it skirts a deep drop-off, referred to as Danger Point. Imagine two stagecoaches trying to pass on this stretch of road. It's a long way down Smith River canyon and the name says it all. That said, control your speed because the road begins to descend, slightly steeper in some stretches. At around 13.5 miles, check out the view to the west. The mountain nearest you across the canyon south of Smith River is French Hill, so named for the large number of French workers who mined it in the 1800s. On the other side of the river, farther toward the west is Signal Peak, elevation 2,055 feet, scarred with a distinctive rock slide.

The Toll Road continues to descend through an area that was burned in the Panther Fire of 1996 and scars were still visible two years later. At just over 17 miles, the dirt road becomes pavement as you cruise past the Gasquet Transfer Station. In a short distance, you reach the intersection of Old Gasquet Toll Road and North Fork Road. Go left onto North Fork, passing the Mountain School for children located on your left. Cross Horace Gasquet Bridge and bear left onto Middle Fork Gasquet Road. In a few yards, the road intersects US 199 at the Gasquet post office. Find your end-shuttle car here, or if you parked at the Visitor Center, turn left, paralleling US 199 via side roads and make your way back to your car. If the loop is your plan, then cautiously turn left onto US 199 and ride the shoulder, climbing about 465 feet in 9.7 miles back to the Patrick Creek campground and your car.

OTHER AREA RIDES

BEAR BASIN BUTTE LOOKOUT: How would you like a room with awe-inspiring vistas, sitting atop a butte at 5,303 feet, feeling like the king or queen of three national forests, a wilderness area, and a national recreation area that surround you? Miles of dirt roads and trails beckon you and your bike to come play, leading through conifer forests and bear grass, past rhododendrons and wildflowers set against a blue sky. It can be yours for about $50 a night and advance reservations. I'm talking about "camping out" at the Bear Basin Fire Lookout and Pierson Cabin in the Smith River National Recreation Area within the Six Rivers National Forest, located about 21 miles east of Gasquet. Sitting at 5,303 feet, think of the solitude, the sunrises and sunsets, and the lack of crowds (except for your friends, of course).

In 1935, the Civilian Conservation Corps (CCC)—one of President Roosevelt's plans to spur economic recovery during the Great Depression—built the 30-foot tall Camp Six Lookout on French Hill, a peak south of Gasquet. In 1996, the lookout was dismantled and reconstructed at its present site on Bear Basin Butte, 9 miles to the east of French Hill. Now, rising only 6 feet above its rock base, it is accompanied by Pierson Cabin, a recently built 1930s-style structure modeled after a CCC cabin design. Thanks to the Six Rivers National Forest and generous contribution of labor and materials from Pierson Building Center of Eureka, California, you have a unique opportunity to enjoy the area.

Both the lookout and the cabin are available for rent. Not a shabby place for a base camp—a precursor to a long week of fun and exploration. In the cabin, amenities provided are few but adequate: a wood-burning stove, several double beds, chairs, lots of counter space for your gear, a large window framing the Siskiyou Mountains, and six smaller screened windows. Picnic tables and privy are outside. The lookout, some 250 feet away from the cabin, is sparsely furnished with a single bed, chairs, bookcase, and a firefinder. What it may lack in the comforts of home, it makes up with windows that yield a 360-degree view. After all, this is a fire lookout. In fact, during periods of extreme fire danger, the USFS firefighters may use the lookout and firefinder; they only ask for the occupants' cooperation. Both the privy and cabin are wheelchair accessible. You must bring your own supply of water, cooking equipment, among many other items. Never fear, though, setting up camp has never been so painless. The lookout is easily accessible by passenger vehicles via a mostly chip-sealed and gravel county road, about a 10.5-mile stretch. Sorry, there's no maid service but a broom, carpet sweeper, and other cleaning supplies are furnished.

Interested? The rental season is usually Memorial Weekend to September 30. But don't dally. According to Don Pass, the director of recreation planner at Smith River NRA, reservations for the Lookout and Cabin are booked many months in advance, sometimes solidly booked way in advance of May. Reservations are accepted after January 1 for the current year and not a moment sooner.

For more information, contact:

Smith River National Recreation
   Area
10600 Highway 199
P.O. Box 228
Gasquet, CA 95543
(707) 457-3131

Six Rivers National Forest
1330 Bayshore Way
Eureka, CA 95501
(707) 442-1721

TISH TANG A TANG RIDGE: Intermediate to advanced terrain, 5-plus-mile rides, in Six Rivers National Forest. Site of the annual Tish Tang Tangle, a NORBA-sanctioned race.

Finding the trail: From Eureka, follow US 101 north to Arcata, then go east on CA 299 to Willow Creek. From within Willow Creek, still in CA 299, take Country Club Drive to Patterson Road, then follow signs to Horse Linto Road and ultimately Horse Linto Campground.

Maps: USGS Tish Tang Point and Hoopla 7.5 minute series.

For more information, contact:

Tish Tang Tangle
Mountain Bike Race Series
P.O. Box 1162
Willow Creek, CA 95573

Six Rivers National Forest
1330 Bayshore Way
Eureka, CA 95501
(707) 442-1721

PONY PEAK RIDE: Advanced-level ride on maintained and unmaintained dirt roads; 20- to 33-mile loop or point-to-point; Klamath National Forest.

Finding the trail: From Eureka, follow US 101 north to Arcata, then go east on CA 299 to Willow Creek and CA 96; turn right. Follow CA 96 north roughly 55 to 60 miles toward Pony Peak and Three Creeks. Park your end-shuttle near Pony Peak Road (14N39). To reach the starting point, travel about 10 to 15 miles farther to Bear Peak Road (15N19), about a mile south of the town of Clear Creek. Follow Bear Peak Road west for about 7 miles to where the pavement ends. Begin your ride here. Loop riders: Same starting point but close the loop by pedaling north on Klamath River Highway (CA 96) back toward Bear Peak Road.

Maps: USGS Bear Peak and Dillon Mountain 7.5 minute series.

For more information, contact:

Klamath National Forest
1312 Fairlane Rd.
Yreka, CA 96097
(916) 842-6131

Happy Camp Ranger District in
   Happy Camp
(916) 493-2243

HAPPY CAMP CAMPGROUND RIDES: Moderate to advanced terrain; 7- to 20-mile rides; Six Rivers and Shasta-Trinity National Forests.

Finding the trail: From Eureka, go north on US 101 to Arcata, then go east on CA 299 to Hawkins Bar. From within Hawkins Bar, follow Denney Road to Wallen

Ranch Road, which turns into Forest Service Route 4. Stay on FS 4 for about 8 miles to FS 7N04; go right. Follow FS 7N04 for 2 miles to FS 6N10; go right. Continue for almost 3 miles to FS 6N24; go left and follow it about 0.25 mile to Happy Camp Campground.

Maps: USGS Salyer 7.5 minute series.

For more information, contact:

Six Rivers National Forest
1330 Bayshore Way
Eureka, CA 95501
(707) 442-1721

Shasta-Trinity National Forest
2400 Washington Ave.
Redding, CA 96001
(916) 246-5222

SOME LOCAL BICYCLE SHOPS
& ORGANIZATIONS

Life Cycle
1593 G St.
Arcata, CA 95521
(707) 822-7755

Pro Sport Center
McKinleyville Shopping Center
508 Myrtle Ave.
Eureka, CA 95501
(707) 443-6328

Sport & Cycle
1621 Broadway St.
Eureka, CA 95501
(707) 444-9274

Henderson Center Bicycles
2811 F St.
Eureka, CA 95501
(707) 443-9861

Back Country Bicycles
1329 Northcrest Dr.
Crescent City, CA 95531
(707) 465-3995

Save-the-Redwoods League
114 Sansome St., Room 605
San Francisco, CA 94104

Redwood Natural History
 Association
1111 Second St.
Crescent City, CA 95531
(707) 464-9150

Redwood National and State Parks
 Headquarters
1111 Second St.
Crescent City, CA 95531
(707) 464-6101
http://www.nps.gov/redw/

SHASTA CASCADE

Though there are a gazillion bikeable trails in three national forests between the Oregon boundary to the busy city of Redding, the rides in this chapter are located around Lake Shasta and Whiskeytown, one of the most outstanding mountain biking areas in the state. With fast and easy access via Interstate Five, the Whiskeytown–Lake Shasta region is growing in popularity, thanks to a variety of bike trails. This area offers numerous challenges for the serious mountain biker as well as a few easy and gently moderate routes for the recreational cyclist. Temperatures often soar into the high 90s and low 100s during the summer and the area is typically dry with low humidity. The sweltering heat doesn't deter riders though. It's common practice for locals to stay indoors during the day and ride either early morning or very late afternoon, when the day has cooled. And like the rest of Northern California steeped in Gold Rush lore and historic mining towns, the mountainous Shasta Cascade region is no exception. As a cyclist, another bit of history that you may enjoy reading about centers around the now retired Whiskeytown Downhill Race.

When I began my research of the Whiskeytown and Lake Shasta region, asking many local folks for information and suggestions about mountain biking trails, I was referred to one person frequently. "Oh, the guy you need to talk to is John Stein," they all said. And they spoke of him with either great respect or unshakable awe. "Who is this guy?" I thought to myself. "Some crazy bike fanatic with dreadlocks who pedals everywhere?" I happened to run across a very entertaining and informative article he had written about the area, which appeared in *Northern California Trails*, a semi-monthly publication, and what a mighty fine piece of writing it was. So, I tracked him down. He was neither crazy nor biked everywhere, and he didn't even have a ponytail. John, as it turned out, is a normal guy, with a job as bike shop manager at the Sports Cottage in Redding. Holy 49er! I had hit a modern-day Mother Lode in a region steeped in gold rush history. This guy had an incredible wealth of information, having been around when the mountain biking craze originally hit way back when. And so, it is with great honor and appreciation that John's story is reprinted here with the permission of him and Eric Moore, publisher of *Northern California Trails*. (Eric has replaced NCT with *Trails Online*, the electronic version of the printed piece. Check them out on the Web at www.trailsonline.com.) I think you'll find it a good introduction to the riding this region has to offer. Enjoy. —L.A.

WHISKEYTOWN: WHEELING THROUGH HISTORY
BY JOHN STEIN

The elevation was 4,500 feet and the time was a chilly 7 a.m. I found myself surrounded this fine June morning by 66 cyclists herded behind a chalk line awaiting the start of the first mountain bike race held north of Marin County. The year was 1981. The event was the first annual Whiskeytown Downhill, brainchild of Gary Larson, owner of the Chain Gang Bike Shop in Redding.

Gary saw his first mountain bike at the previous year's trade show and with a premonition, felt this could turn into something big. With a motorcycle racing background, he conceived the notion of a point-to-point race, over all sorts of terrain, with classes, trophies, winners, and a celebratory bash to finish. But what if no one showed up?

They showed. And now, 67 of us slowly thawed out following a 25-mile shuttle ride in trucks, vans, and anything that could hold the unexpected throng. The field was certainly varied. Gary Fisher brought along a Marin contingent, representing the serious omen of talent that was to continue through the present time. Shaved legs! And the few pairs of black shorts on the line. On the start line was a long blond-haired gentleman taking pulls off a bottle of Jack Daniel's. Mingling with us were the BMX riders, complete with leathers and full-face helmets. Jacquie Phelan even had a few women cohorts to race with.

Then, there I was, straddling a borrowed bike. Six-speeds, drum brakes, and a cro-moly frame. What had I gotten my skinny road-racer rear end into?

Off we went. Immediately, the BMX guys got the hole shot, only to bog down and walk seconds later as the road steepened. We maneuvered through the traffic and the talent sorted itself. By the top of the first ascent, we were strung out and gravity took over. Unseen by oxygen-starved bodies were the stunning views of Mt. Shasta and the Sacramento Valley far below.

Brakes working, I white-knuckled my way down into Crystal Creek, passed by riders far more comfortable on decomposed granite than I. This is fun. I needed my own bike.

West Whiskeytown

Today, the western fringe of the Whiskeytown National Recreation Area is a wild, little-used treasure. The high ballies here are a geologic phenomenon of granite bubbles pushed up through the earth's crust, heights reaching altitudes of over 6,200 feet at Shasta Bally. Called batholiths, these mountains resemble many parts of the Sierra.

High enough to capture moisture from the Pacific storm tracks, they are generally snow-covered from December to April. This makes for a prime growing area for towering pines and low manzanita shrubs. Wildlife is truly wild. The bears encountered up here cannot be called campground bears. Their tracks are found everywhere, and a trip to Bully Choop offers very real chances of sightings.

The best views are along the county line between Shasta and Trinity, and use of a regional map will provide a key to the log vistas. The Trinity Alps dominate the western skyline, jagged spires reaching above all else around. The highest points harbor year-round snowfields, and are impressive even from this distance. To the north is majestic Mt. Shasta. Heading from Coggins Park into Crystal Creek, the road tops a small rise, and there it is. I never fail to pause here and admire the view, as it is stunning the first or fiftieth time you see it. Lassen Peak rises above the valley to the east, southernmost sentinel of the Cascade Range. Southward sprawls the Sacramento Valley, and on a clear day, the Sutter Buttes can be seen.

Bicycling these mountains requires a commitment of time and toil. The decomposed granite can be a delight when the soil is moist or a frustrating sand pile in dry times. The key is to lower the air pressure a bit, a light touch on the bars, and relax. When you learn the techniques, you'll seek out all the high roads. Old logging roads interlace the region, and you'll have them all to yourself. This is a high elevation escape from summer's heat, so bring water, as that is lacking from the ridge lines.

The winter rains of 1983 came in with a vengeance. Water-soaked ground which could hold no more came sliding down. Could the race still be held? The park service's maintenance crews had a Herculean task ahead of them, and the prospect of the course being returned to its normal groomed state was bleak. It was time to reconnoiter and assess the damage. Three of us started up the Boulder Creek climb only to encounter a 10-foot deep washout on the access to our favorite trail. So much for getting a crew to checkpoint three this year.

Rob Tatham and I lowered our bikes into the abyss and jumped in. Multiple fallen trees hindered our progress and a bit of scrambling got us into the heart of Boulder Creek. The trail was altered from its previous state but we had a ball exploring the changes. We made it through with a minimum of trauma. It was clear that this year all support in this drainage would have to be done by bike and by foot. A true mountain bike race would follow.

The Whiskeytown event had blossomed into a field of over 250 this year [1983]. Gone were the naive riders on the BMX bikes. By gosh, real bikes were here to stay. I was astride my shiny Stumpjumper with all of 15 speeds, but now, when I was passed, it was by lycra-clad pros.

Finish-line stories were consistent with all sorts of adventures related about the rope safety line above the biggest washout at Mill Creek, a thrilling traverse over a slide that could swallow a mobile home and still have room to spare. Bunny-hopping skills grew in the retelling. We all were winners that year.

The Middle Ground

The region spanning Crystal Creek to Whiskeytown Dam today is the historical heart of the park. Miners from France wandered here as early as 1849, with the discovery of gold along Clear Creek. Others soon followed and mining camps grew along every stream. Legend tells of a keg of whiskey that fell into a creek, certainly a disaster at the time. Whiskey Creek was named and the camp established here was called Whiskeytown.

Mining was everything and a tour of the area is worthwhile. Before the railroad created Redding, Old Shasta was the county seat and commercial hub of the north state. Now, a state park along CA 299, a visit to the museum there gives an appreciation for the hard lives the miners faced.

The Tower House district was an important stopping point for the traveler heading to the mines in Trinity County. Skillfully restored, the visitor is welcome to wander about and return to the sights of the past. A few outbuildings and the nearby El Dorado Mine give a real flavor to this quiet spot.

The town of French Gulch lies three miles north of CA 299 and is a living reminder of a typical mining town, much as Whiskeytown must have been before being inundated by the creation of the lake in 1963. Bicycling in this area is excellent. The Mill Creek road connects Crystal Creek to Boulder Creek and it's aptly named "wall" won't disappoint those looking for a challenge, and perhaps a walk. Look for the Mill Creek trail on your visitor's map for a wilderness quality trip. The deep pine forest here is shady, cool, and a botanist's delight. Mill Creek is crossed at least 14 times and speed demons will not enjoy this technical trail. Good.

Over on Boulder Creek is the faster descent as a very old logging road drops to Whiskeytown Lake. This road long ago degraded into a trail and is some of the finest riding around. An old logging camp is passed quickly, so keep an eye out for it. A sunnier area than others, you'll notice the scragglier grey pine growing among the oaks. A shock fork is a pleasure on the downhill as it was named Boulder Creek for a reason.

Brandy Creek is the front country visitor's favorite spot. A maintained swimming area, snack bars, and RV camping are the focal point here. Most users aren't aware of the shady retreats awaiting upstream. A ride up to the headwaters of the creek can lead to a natural water slide, and a little-used single-track leads back down. Shady and cool, a nice retreat from summer's heat waves.

These areas are all below the normal snow levels and are favorites year-round. Watch out for high water during storms and spring runoff from the higher ground, especially on Boulder Creek. This is prime poison oak land, so beware the pretty little oaks! Bring your own water or be prepared to treat it.

The heat was intense and the 1986 Whiskeytown Downhill was well under way. The late morning temperature was already hovering in the 90s and only a handful of the day's 500 entries had finished. As I made the final granny gear climb above the Mt. Shasta Mine trail, I could hear the music and party starting a short distance away at Horse Camp. I didn't think I could sweat anymore and the cool water at the checkpoints was more than welcome.

As I crested the ridge, I paused, partly to catch my breath and ease the burning in my legs, and partly to reflect on my brief part in Whiskeytown history. Looking around me, I could look down on the Kennedy Memorial at Whiskeytown Dam. When the great man dedicated the facilities, could he have known the pleasures that would follow? Could anyone measure the environmental awareness local children would learn at the nearby school camp? Could anyone get rid of the cramp in my leg? No, so I continued.

A precipitous trail wound down into a narrow canyon, following the remains of an old-time miner's mule path, still using the retaining walls placed there over a hundred years earlier. An overheated racer lay in a shallow creek, no longer concerned with placing but literally surviving. A shared water bottle and we both proceeded.

At last, we crossed beneath the Mountain Goat banner marking the finish and received fluids and good wishes. Some guy named Ned Overend had won an hour earlier, but the biggest applause at the award ceremony was given to the best-dressed winners. With the improbable name of Team Blondini, these four friends rode the entire 38 miles dressed in tights, capes, and balloons floating behind their bikes.

The crowd dispersed, heading home. Some were to race at more events now on the calendar, others to tend to wounds and repairs but all were to have memories of today.

Below the Dam

Ask locals where they ride now and you'll hear of a variety of trails. The common thread is that most of them start in the Clear Creek canyon below the dam. The reasons for this soon become obvious.

This region is easily accessible from Redding, lots of parking and an incredible variety of trails to meet the needs of novice and expert alike. An overview will show a bit of a basin and while certainly not flat, the steepest hills can be avoided if so desired. This is also the busiest locale for other users as well and encounters with equestrians and hikers is most likely here.

This was mining country in the early days. I find wandering the small, unknown trails to be very satisfying, finding the occasional old mining claim with its rock work still intact. Gold-panning is allowed with a permit and, in the spring, is fun while the small seasonal streams still flow. Portions of an old water ditch are now maintained in places as a trail. The Great Water Ditch was a system that conveyed the needed water for mining operations, a serpentine distance of 43 miles from the Tower House area almost to Redding and to Centerville on Placer Road. The work involved is hard to conceive. Imagine yourself digging with hand tools even a small portion of this during your visit.

The Mt. Shasta Mine trail leads to its namesake and is one example of a successful operation open into this century. Watch for many branches leading from this area. Trails are so prolific here that a single map can't begin to show them all. Simply go and explore. Most users park at Peltier Valley parking one mile below the dam on the paved road.

Lodgepole pines seem to grow in profusion down here and, bear in mind, they cast little shade. Summer riding is best done in mornings and evenings. My favorite season is spring. The flowers are in bloom and trail dust is minimal.

This is also a very active mountain lion habitat. Signs are posted at all trailheads and sightings are rare but not unheard of. To date, lions have not been considered a major hazard but keeping an eye open while riding along is advised.

The Peltier Valley area is found east of Clear Creek with the same access point as the Mt. Shasta Mine trail. Only a mile away in distance, this side of the canyon has its own distinctive feel. Steeper initially, one climbs suddenly back up into the pine trees and running water. There are lots of deep shade and ferns and, in the heat of the summer, the secret swimming holes are fine fun.

Trails are numerous and one can create loops to match abilities. Locals have created and maintain many of these systems. Equestrians formed the earliest work forces and now the mountain bikers are returning the favor.

The riding season is year-round in this area with the least amount of use during the winter months. Most of the soils are forgiving of wet weather use and drain well. The park service has been installing aggressive water bars on the steeper terrain.

It has been over 10 years since the Whiskeytown Downhill was last held, a victim of its own success. Five hundred riders proved to be the saturation point of the small finishing area in the woods. Parking and access was limited, raising safety concerns by the park service. Alternative venues weren't attractive to Gary, fearing a loss of the flavor of the race. Racing was now common on nearly every weekend during the season and long courses were not conducive to attracting sponsors. It was time to go out a winner.

I rode out there again last night. I was the old-timer, riding with my sons and friends. A new generation of people using the land, discovering anew treasures more valuable than the gold wrestled from the hard ground. We rode past the Whiskeytown cemetery in the autumn dusk. What stories could these ghosts tell us? Do they sense our passing through? I like to think so. Thanks, guys, for building this ditch. That rock cabin looks good, your apple trees are still there. Sure appreciate that mule trail we just rode down. Now, it's time to go.

—*John Stein*

General Information

Whiskeytown National Recreation Area is located eight miles west of Redding along CA 299. It is administered by the National Park Service which controls the day to day running of the unit. Redding offers all services for travelers. Two fine hospitals are available if you ride faster than your ability. There are few restrictions on bicycle use in the park: Please refrain from riding on the Shasta Divide Trail, Davis Gulch Trail, and the exercise loop at Oak Bottom. Be courteous to other users. Beginning mountain bikers will enjoy the Mt. Shasta Mine area, Oak Bottom, and the Tower House Historic District. Advanced riders must do Boulder Creek, Buckhorn Bally, and Peltier Valley. No one enjoys Shasta Bally. Being the highest point in the park, it's a thigh-burning, lung-searing climb that hurts every inch of the way. The definitive guide to the bicycle trails in the park is *Mountain Biking Whiskeytown* by John Shuman.

RIDE 10 · Clikapudi Trail

AT A GLANCE

Length/configuration: 7.25-mile loop, counterclockwise; single-track and a few yards on pavement

Aerobic difficulty: Moderate to moderately strenuous; varied terrain

Technical difficulty: Intermediate; some switchbacks, rocky ledges, twisty narrow portions

Scenery: Along the shore of Lake Shasta

Special comments: Try to stop once in a while to see your surroundings. Bald eagles nest nearby and make an occasional appearance.

The following trail description was contributed by John Stein, reprinted with his permission. Did you read his historical tale of mountain biking in Whiskeytown presented in the introduction of this chapter? Read it before you ride. And if you happen to visit Sports Cottage, a bike and sporting goods store in Redding, you might see him there. He's the bike shop manager. Tell him how much you enjoyed reading his tale. Thank you, John. —L.A.

Lake Shasta is a magnet for tourism in Northern California and is well-known for its boating and fishing. Considering the 365 miles of shoreline, there are few bikeable trails in the area. The Clikapudi Trail is an exception. This 7.25-mile loop is almost all single-track and a local favorite of mountain bikers, runners, and equestrians. Ridden counterclockwise, it's pleasantly rolling and features two minor climbs of about a quarter mile each, easily scaled with little effort by all but the most novice. The first two miles are very level and will let beginners decide to continue or opt for a pavement return to the car. There are a few technical sections that test even an expert's skills but can be passed safely by a dismount.

The loop will eventually encircle a small mountain, and I find it interesting to watch the vegetation change with increased shade and moisture on the north slope. Springtime flower displays can be awesome, and winter storms have been host to some

RIDE 10 · Clikapudi Trail

classic rides. If you're like most visitors who arrive in summer, be prepared for warm to very hot conditions. We ride in mornings and evenings during the hottest days.

You will pass by ancient Native American village sites, fine swimming holes, beautiful oak knolls, and even be able to find quartz crystals if you look carefully enough. Treat the land gently and enjoy your Lake Shasta adventure.

General location: On the southern shore of Lake Shasta, 15 miles northeast of Redding; 150 miles north of Sacramento on Interstate 5.

Elevation change: 400 feet; starting elevation and low point 1,000 feet; high point 1,400 feet. Varied terrain with lots of short ups and downs.

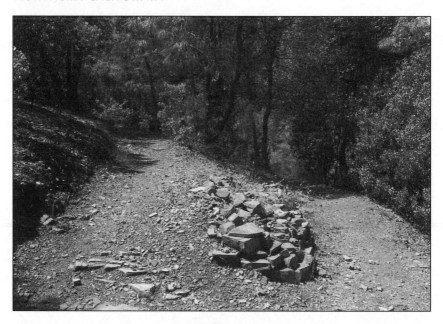

An easy hairpin turn adds variety to the Clikapudi Trail.

Season: Year-round.

Services: Drinking water and rest rooms are located at the Jones Valley boat launch parking lot. A fee is required to park here, but at this time, free parking is allowed along the shoulder of the access road. A fee campground is 1.5 miles to the west and features an alternative trailhead.

Hazards: Poison oak is visible and is a good reason to stay on the trail. Expect other trail users at any time and exercise proper trail etiquette.

Rescue index: The trail sees moderate use in the summer, less in cooler times. The nearest phone is at the market at Jones Valley Market, about 3 miles to the west.

Land status: Shasta-Trinity National Forest.

Maps: Shasta-Trinity National Forest visitors map, also *Trails of Lake Shasta* brochure from the forest service.

Finding the trail: From I-5, 3 miles north of Redding, take Oasis Road east. There will be National Forest information signs at the major intersections beyond this point. Follow the signs to the Jones Valley boat ramp, about 12 miles past I-5. Turn right onto Bear Mountain Road, then left onto Dry Creek Road to the end of the road at the parking lot. There is a well-marked trailhead sign at the southeast corner of the lot, and a less well-marked sign at the southwest corner. The southwest sign is the most common starting point for this loop. Note that there is a fee for parking at the lot but currently no charge to park along the shoulder of the access road.

Sources of additional information:

Shasta-Trinity National Forest
2400 Washington St.
Redding, CA 96001
(530) 246-5222

Sports Cottage
2665 Park Marina Dr.
Redding, CA 96001
(530) 241-3115

Notes on the trail: In the southern corner of the Jones Valley boat ramp parking lot, look for the small trailhead sign. It's located immediately to your far left as you enter the lot. (The more visible trailhead immediately on your right near the lot entrance is where you will finish, in case you're worried about your route-finding skills.) The initial section of single-track starts smooth and fast, staying that way for the first 1.6 miles. With no serious climbs, this is a fine introduction to single-track for first-timers.

Watch for an intersection at 1.6 miles, as you'll want to turn very hard left up the hill. If you don't see this turn, you will reach a campground; if so, turn around and pay the penalty of great single-track until you find the uphill turn.

This hill is short and dumps you onto the paved road on which you've just driven to the trailhead. There are no signs, so turn right on the pavement for maybe 100 yards and watch for the unmarked trail climbing a gully on your left (south). This is the first major climb of the day, and the challenge isn't so much the elevation as it is the ability to ride up the switchbacks without dabbing a foot down. This 0.25 mile passes quickly enough.

Prepare yourself for the nicest part of the loop: a quick switchback lies just down the hill, then follows a long smooth downhill with gentle turns, lots of swooping drops, and a racing sense of speed. Eventually, the trail drops onto a jeep road entering from the south.

At this point, you can decide to continue across on the trail or turn left and follow the jeep road. Both will intertwine a few times and are fun either way. You are now in a good-sized meadow following Clikapudi Creek and if you keep bearing to the left, the single-track will again leave the road on its way downstream to Lake Shasta. Look for a couple of fenced-off areas—these are old village sites from the Wintun culture. What a nice place this must have been to live in.

The single-track is again at lake level and now is in the northern exposure forest with its deeper shade and lush growth. Watch for a couple of tricky sections here. Ride at your own risk over an occasional rocky ledge. While they are rideable, the prudent rider will accept limitations and simply walk over the obstacles. *Voila!* Even novices can thus ride advanced trails.

A picnic table along the way is a nice place to regroup and even take a swim if it's hot. Is it summer? It's hot. Enjoy. The trail will continue along the shore for a bit then enter a cove and start the second climb of the day. If you were to walk along this creek's edge into the shoreline, you might be fortunate and find a few quartz crystals. This can be worth a stop after recent rains, as the amount found can be surprising. Size is small but of nice quality.

This hill is a bit steeper than the first but soon done with. A small shortcut veers steeply to the left at the top of the knoll. This has become the dominant trail but the original continues to the right and is a pleasant route. Either way, you're at the top and it's downhill to the shoreline again. Once at the lake, you might expect to meet fishermen and other day-users, as you are a short distance from the main parking lot. One shift into low gear and you are done. Another awesome day on a bike.

RIDE 11 · Waters Gulch Loop

AT A GLANCE

Length/configuration: 3.75-mile loop, clockwise; single-track and pavement. (Option for strong riders: 7-mile out-and-back on single-track only, 3.5 miles each way)

Aerobic difficulty: Easy to moderate

Technical difficulty: Mildly technical

Scenery: Pine and oak forest along and above Lake Shasta, broad views of surrounding mountains

Special comments: While very smooth, care must be taken above one short section of cliffs. Children should be under close supervision at this point, and be comfortable with single-track technique.

The following description is another fine contribution from John Stein, reprinted with his permission. Sincere thanks, John. —L.A.

This is a short classic that is perfect for travelers needing an excuse to stretch their legs. Located just a mile from I-5, access is easy and fast. Don't let the short distance make you pass this one up, or you'll miss the best trail on Lake Shasta. You can ride this either as a 3.75-mile loop, ridden counterclockwise. If you're looking for more of a workout and an all-dirt ride, pedal the route as an out-and-back, totaling 7 miles round-trip.

I love this trail. It has everything I look for: smooth downhills, steep enough climbs, and scenery that's hard to beat. Wildlife abounds out here, with bear scat replacing the more urban dog-doo of more popular trails. Two of us spent nearly an hour watching a bald eagle circling overhead, just keeping an eye on us. Nearby shore areas are closed seasonally for nesting reasons.

The trail forms three-quarters of a loop, dropping to the shoreline in an exhilarating beginning, climbing above acrophobia-inducing drop-offs, finishing in a gentle drop through a beautiful oak forest to a final stream crossing at the pavement. Largely unused, don't expect company during your stay.

General location: 15 miles north of Redding, 1 mile off I-5. Redding is about 150 miles north of Sacramento.

Elevation change: 200 feet; starting elevation 1,100 feet; high point 1,270 feet; low point 1,070 feet. Short and quick ups and downs.

Season: Year-round.

Services: No services at the trail but rest rooms and water are available at the Packers Bay boat launch just 0.25 mile away. Use of the facilities may not be available in the off-season and parking here requires a small fee. Arrive with full bottles of water to be on the safe side.

Hazards: One drop-off makes me watch my step, otherwise a smooth treadway exists. Walk across the bridges as the spacing of the planks are the perfect size to catch

RIDE 11 · Waters Gulch Loop

a wheel. Poison oak can sometimes encroach upon the trail; take all precautions to avoid it. Bears are common at Lake Shasta with scat encountered along the trail.

Rescue index: Low usage makes help from other users unlikely, although boaters might be hailed from shore. The closest phones are at Bridge Bay Resort, about 3 miles south on I-5.

Land status: Shasta-Trinity National Forest.

Maps: *Trails of Lake Shasta* brochure from the national forest service.

Finding the trail: Southbound travelers should look for the Packers Bay exit, about 10 miles south of the town of Lakehead. From Redding, you must take the Shasta

Caverns exit, 3 miles north of Bridge Bay, then return southbound on I-5 for 1 mile to the Packers Bay exit. Proceed 1 mile down the Packers Bay road and park at the small trailhead lot (space for about 10 cars) on the right. If you miss this lot, you'll arrive at the Packers Bay lot, a fine alternative that allows you to finish on a downhill instead of a climb.

Sources of additional information:

Shasta-Trinity National Forest
2400 Washington St.
Redding, CA 96001
(530) 246-5222

Sports Cottage
2665 Park Marina Dr.
Redding, CA 96001
(530) 241-3115

Notes on the trail: Watch for the obvious trailhead at the west end of the small parking lot. (A second trail shares the spot, climbing steeply up to the left. It soon ends at benches overlooking Lake Shasta, a great spot to watch sunsets and a nice addition to the Waters Gulch Trail.) The trail proceeds down from the lot and is quite smooth and fast. Control your speed around the occasional blind corner and be aware of the drop to Waters Gulch on the right. This first half mile is among the best trails I've ridden and is enjoyed by all. A tree forces a hard left switchback down to the creek, bringing speeds back down to a walking pace. A bench invites contemplation of this beautiful spot, with its towering trees and lush undergrowth. Don't tarry long if the mosquitoes are hungry!

The next few hundred yards are fun. The trail starts a small climb up to a few large blocks of rock and the ensuing dismount is well-timed as the exposure above the creek is increasing dramatically. Finally, you step over the final obstacles and the creek is now a vertical 75 feet below you, complete with a small waterfall. Enjoy it or suffer as you desire.

Soon enough, you'll remount and drop down to Lake Shasta's shoreline. Now, the trail maintains a level profile for about a mile, crossing several small bridges. Their timbers are spaced perfectly to capture your wheels, so walking is wise.

The big climb of a mile follows and you can expect a rise of about 200 feet. The trail is now on a sunnier aspect and small scrub oaks may scratch at your legs. Don't panic, as poison oak is not seen here—yet. Use caution if you're susceptible, though.

At the top is another bench set in an oak forest and while the view of the lake is blocked by trees, the sky is open. Perhaps you too will be visited by the neighborhood bald eagle here. It's quite a sight.

When it's time to proceed, the trail runs smoothly down to the lake, a mile away. The trail here is twistier than the first drop and speeds are slower. Excellent **S**-turns lure you on and all too soon, a creek at the bottom is crossed, albeit without a bridge. Watch for big rocks in the stream bed. It would be a shame to fall with just a hundred yards left to the pavement. After this creek, you climb slightly onto Packers Bay Road, with a huge parking lot to the right. Turn left and climb the paved road the 0.25 mile back up to your starting point. (Strong riders can always turn around and go back the way they came.) It is an easy climb, so spin to keep loose. A second lap is tempting and just as enjoyable as the first.

RIDE 12 · Boulder Creek Loop

AT A GLANCE

Length/configuration: 8.5-mile loop, counterclockwise; single-track and dirt roads

Aerobic difficulty: Moderately strenuous with a mile of very strenuous climbing

Technical difficulty: Intermediate due to somewhat rocky terrain

Scenery: Deep shade along Boulder Creek, views of Whiskeytown Lake and Shasta Bally

Special comments: A steep introductory climb weeds out the casual user. If you persevere, the rewards are worth the effort. Adventurous beginners may enjoy this loop, but pre-teen riders usually don't.

This classic Whiskeytown ride description is another fine contribution by John Stein. Thanks, John, a fun read and great ride.   —L.A.

Whiskeytown is special in the National Park Service, having allowed—and even encouraged—mountain bike use dating from the 1981 running of the now defunct Whiskeytown Downhill race. The few off-limit trails are far outnumbered by miles of legal single-track and backcountry roads.

Beginners enjoy the area below the dam, following old trails from the gold rush days, while more advanced riders challenge themselves in Peltier Valley and the higher roads. Boulder Creek is arguably the classic Whiskeytown trail. The tough climb eliminates the casual rider, but the long, fast downhills more than make up for the sweat.

Isolated from the major population centers, you can expect little or no company while on this trail. Self-reliance is a must, so carry appropriate repair items and a first-aid kit. While spring and autumn are wonderful times to ride the loop, most riders find themselves here in the heat of summer. It's very warm here, so plan on early starts or evening rides and you should do fine. Along the way, you'll enjoy shady tree-covered stream crossings, a fern-graced waterfall, and the best downhills around.

General location: 15 miles west of Redding; about 150 miles north of Sacramento.

Elevation change: 1,100 feet; starting elevation 1,220 feet; high point 2,320 feet. Lots of short hills, some rolling, some abrupt.

Season: Year-round, occasional snowfall doesn't stay.

Services: Drinking water, rest rooms, and picnic facilities at Judge Carr Powerhouse. Camping and pay phones at Oak Bottom, 2 miles to the east on the north shore of Whiskeytown Lake. Day-use fee is currently required, available at various locations including Oak Bottom.

Hazards: Poison oak is prevalent but is avoided by staying on the trail. Spring snowmelt may make the creek crossings unsafe.

RIDE 12 · Boulder Creek Loop

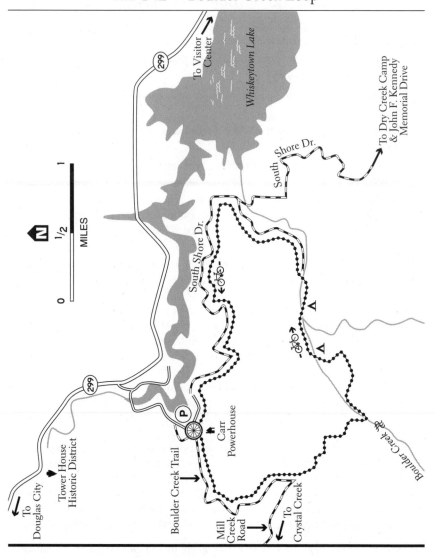

Rescue index: Don't expect passersby on a regular basis. In case of emergency, you should make your way back to the trailhead and then CA 299 where you can flag down a motorist. The nearest phone is at Oak Bottom, where 911 will contact the park rangers.

Land status: Whiskeytown Unit of the Whiskeytown-Shasta-Trinity National Recreation Area.

Maps: Whiskeytown Unit color flier available at Whiskeytown Visitors Center; USGS Whiskeytown 7.5 minute series.

Finding the trail: From Redding, travel west on CA 299 for 15 miles toward the northwest end of Whiskeytown Lake. Turn left at the Judge Carr Powerhouse sign. Follow the paved road to the Powerhouse and its picnic area. Park here. (Incidentally, you'll go past the Whiskeytown Visitor Information Center Overlook located at the intersection of CA 299 and J. F. Kennedy Memorial Drive at 8 miles on your way to the lake's end.)

Sources of additional information:

Whiskeytown Unit
Whiskeytown-Shasta-Trinity National
   Recreation Area
P.O. Box 188
Whiskeytown, CA 96095
(916) 241-6584

Sports Cottage
2665 Park Marina Dr.
Redding, CA 96001
(530) 241-3115

Notes on the trail: Fill your bottles at the picnic area. If it's warm, you'll need plenty, and all water along the trail should be treated before use. Ride the paved road back toward the highway not more than 0.1 mile. Look for a gravel road to your left marked as the road to Crystal Creek and follow that. A wide, well-maintained road easily climbs, leading to a false sense of strength and ability. Pass a water system of tanks and pipes and be prepared for a major turn.

Just beyond the tank is a level wide spot with a vague jeep road leading up past a gate that may be locked. This is your turn, despite the beautiful civilized road that continues up to the left. TURN RIGHT! If you're going to get lost, this is the place.

You should be in low gear at this point if still on route. Perhaps you're walking? Excellent. One foot in front of the other is a common technique for this climb. Repeat as necessary. You will gain about a thousand feet of elevation in the next mile. At just under a mile, you may even want my home address to discuss this climb, but by then there's only one more turn and you're at the top. This summit has seen hundreds of riders and is a fine place to regroup and spin yarns.

FINALLY, a downhill. Hard to believe it's only been about 1.5 miles to this point, but you're about halfway through the time commitment for the loop. Almost too soon the jeep road splits at a Y. Watch for it, as some speedsters will not see the well-marked left turn signed as Boulder Creek. If you cross a bridge at all, you are a really fast rider, and that's a good thing because you have to turn around and climb back up to the Y.

The trail-wise rider that turned left at the Y can now roll with just one low gear surprise that's over just as you decide to commit to a climb. The trail just crossed into a north slope forest and the shadows deepen with the increased tree canopy. This section of trail is closed to motorized use, but at one time was a logging road. Weather and time is softening the road into a true single-track, and you have to look for clues to see this heritage.

A short downhill roller coaster drops into the first crossing of Boulder Creek. Ride it if you must. I walk through it because I know my shoes will get wet eventually. There are deeper crossings ahead. (Stop. There is a hint of a bushwhacked trail upstream that simply must be followed the hundred yards to its end at a stunning waterfall. Ferns, mist, white granite sand, the gentle rush of water, a wading pool at the bottom.) Upon climbing out of the creek's shade, look directly behind you at 6,200-foot Shasta Bally. Often snow-capped into May, this is the source of Boulder Creek. Don't miss it.

E-tickets don't exist at Disneyland anymore, and when they disappeared, this is where they went.[1] The next 2 miles are the reason I mountain bike. Jumps, berms, creek crossings, boulders and boulders, and sweet downhill single-track all blur into an indistinguishable experience that just made the big climb worthwhile. And then it keeps going. How many creek crossings were there? Doesn't matter. Your shoes are already wet.

At about 6 miles, there is a rude reacquaintance with the civilized world in the form of a chain-link gate. Pass this to the side and now you are on South Shore Drive, a two-wheel-drive road that circles the lake. Turn left, but be aware that for the first time today, you'll have to be looking for an occasional car or two.

South Shore Drive is currently a well-graded dirt road. There is a climb that has to be finished under your own power, but it's not too bad as you can look down at Whiskeytown Lake far below, a beautiful blue-green gem of a reservoir. Part of the Central Valley Project, its waters actually are transported via tunnel from the Trinity River many miles away. Because of this, it is almost never drawn down like a typical man-made lake.

The final summit is easily attained and a fast rush down to the lake soon follows. Though this is fast riding with long straights that beg for maximum speeds, an occasional blind corner should be given its due respect for oncoming cars. One last up-slope that barely forces a downshift and you arrive at a section of blacktop that leads down to the picnic area. Though 8.5 miles have elapsed, it feels like 20.

RIDE 13 · Mt. Shasta Mine Loop

AT A GLANCE

Length/configuration: 3.1-mile loop, clockwise; jeep road and single-track

Aerobic difficulty: Easy with a few moderately rugged sections of brief climbing

Technical difficulty: Mildly technical with some intermediate narrow, rutted and rocky sections

Scenery: Oak and mixed conifer forests, small creeks, and peaceful old Whiskeytown cemetery. Glimpses of Whiskeytown Lake and Shasta Bally.

Special comments: Perfect for beginners wanting to develop their technical bike-handling skills. Some spots may require walking.

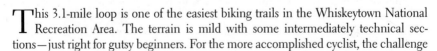

This 3.1-mile loop is one of the easiest biking trails in the Whiskeytown National Recreation Area. The terrain is mild with some intermediately technical sections—just right for gutsy beginners. For the more accomplished cyclist, the challenge

[1]"E-tickets" used to refer to certain amusement park rides at Disneyland in southern California. Rides were rated from A to E, with A rides being the most tame and E rides the most excellent thrill in the park. Paid admission came with a book full of assorted tickets. For thrill-seekers, however, there never seemed to be enough E-tickets in the book. Needless to say, those tickets were highly prized, traded, . . . and scalped. Nowadays, tickets are no longer used, having been replaced by a park policy of unlimited ride opportunities—and long lines.

is to ride the entire short loop without stopping. One of the park's more popular routes for both bikers and hikers, this loop is composed of mostly single-track trails, ranging from one to four feet wide, skirting short stretches along Onofrio Gulch, a few sections of shallow drop-offs and plenty of short ups and downs.

Before, during, or after your ride, you can try your luck at gold-panning along Onofrio Gulch, much like the miners did in the mid-1800s. The first and easiest method favored by the prospectors was placer mining, the skimming of gold from streams and creeks, requiring only a suitable pan, the proper wrist action, maybe a pack mule, and lots of patience. When the rewards from placer mining dwindled, other methods took hold, including hard-rock mining which involved carving deep shafts into the hillsides. Hydraulic mining, based on highly pressurized water, lead to the building of miles of flumes, which allowed miners to work year-round through the dry season. Shasta Mine was one of several mines in the area that produced significant amounts of gold. By the turn of the century, the gold played out and the local population dwindled. In 1945, as part of the Central Valley Project, Shasta Dam was completed, creating Whiskeytown Lake. Before water filled the canyon, the Whiskeytown Cemetery was relocated to its present-day location just below the dam. The bike trail runs alongside it. (The dam was dedicated in 1963 by John F. Kennedy. There's a monument at the dedication site, including a tape recording of his speech—you passed this site on your way to the trailhead.) Today, the "gold" mined from these hills is the water regulated by Shasta Dam, which supplies continuous agricultural water to the Central Valley and arid southern California. Still, gold-panning is allowed for fun, requiring only a permit from the Whiskeytown NRA. So, grab a pan and saddle up your trusty two-wheeled steed. Who knows, you might find gold in "them-thar hills!"

General location: Almost 11 miles northwest of Redding; about 163 miles north of Sacramento on I-5.

Elevation change: 450 feet; starting elevation and low point 1,150 feet; high point 1,600 feet.

Season: Year-round, though winter-swollen Onofrio Gulch may infringe on a small stretch of the route

Services: Water, phone, and rest rooms at the Whiskeytown Visitor Information Center Overlook at the intersection of CA 299 and J. F. Kennedy Memorial Drive, about 2.2 miles from the trailhead. Day-use fee required for parking at the trailhead. Self-serve machines at the Visitor Information Center and at various major-use sites collect fees and dispense receipts. Receipts must be displayed on your car window. All other services in Redding, about 11 miles away. Developed campgrounds at numerous locations within the vicinity.

Hazards: Hikers and equestrians frequent this trail. Occasional poison oak. Stay alert for ticks, rattlesnakes, and rarely seen mountain lions and bears. Hunting is allowed in the fall. High fire danger between May and November.

Rescue index: This is a short loop and its easy access attracts a moderate number of trail users during weekends in the summer. Be prepared, and in case of emergency, plan to make you own way back to the trailhead, adjacent to paved Paige Bar Road.

Land status: Whiskeytown Unit of the Whiskeytown-Shasta-Trinity National Recreation Area.

Maps: Whiskeytown Unit color flier available at Whiskeytown Visitors Center; USGS Igo 7.5 minute series.

RIDE 13 · Mt. Shasta Mine Loop

Finding the trail: From Redding, travel northwest on CA 299 for 8 miles to the Whiskeytown Visitor Information Center Overlook located at the intersection with J. F. Kennedy Memorial Drive. Go left onto J. F. K. Memorial Drive, following the lake edge due southwest for about 1.6 miles to the intersection with Paige Bar Road and the Kennedy Memorial. Don't go over the dam; instead, bear left, heading south on Paige Bar. Continue for about 1.2 miles, at which point you reach a wide, open dirt parking area located on the left side of the road (east), across from Peltier Valley Road, a jeep road. Park here.

Sources of additional information: See sources of additional information for Ride 12.

Notes on the trail: From the parking area off Paige Bar Road, begin riding toward the rest rooms located on the southeastern end of the parking area. There's a sign here, identifying the Mt. Shasta Mine Loop Trail as well as Mt. Shasta Mine 1.2 miles; Onofrio Gulch 1.5 miles; Loop Distance 3.1 miles. (Since we're biking the loop in a clockwise loop, the mine is reached in 2 miles.) Just behind the rest room, pick up the dirt single-track trail, following it down and up over a berm to a dirt jeep road. Hang a left onto the dirt road, ignoring the single-track which continues straight across the dirt road (you'll be returning on that trail). After the initial left, this clockwise routing basically follows trails which peel off to the right. (Of course, if you're up for exploring, do check out the other intersecting trails.)

The dirt road is a semi-packed dirt and gravel path, about 1-car width across. It's mildly technical with just enough loose rock ranging from golf ball to cantaloupe sizes to keep you alert. Within the first 0.5 mile, the road climbs moderately, varying from level to 7% grade, with short stretches of level terrain in a sparse forest of pine and manzanita. At 0.4 mile, having climbed 280 feet from the trailhead, you catch a view of Whiskeytown Lake on your left (north). The road becomes more rugged with larger, loose rocks and some shallow patches of sand. After a markedly steeper but brief climb, check out Shasta Bally sitting at 6,209 feet directly behind you in the west—it's the highest point in the Whiskeytown National Recreation Area. Such geological protuberances are a result of bubbles pushing through the earth's crust eons ago.

At almost a mile, having climbed approximately 490 feet from the trailhead to about 1,550 feet, you reach the high point of this short loop. Here, the jeep road forks with a wide single-track trail descending on the right. Follow the right trail which is signed with hiker and equestrian symbols and an arrow pointing to it (bikes allowed). This downhill stretch is steep, about a 7 to 9% grade, spiced by intermediately technical terrain, thanks to rain ruts, exposed tree roots, land loose rocks. Following the trail becomes a bit difficult here with stretches of wide run-off resembling the trail. In several places, the trail splits only to rejoin in a few yards. Choose whichever split you like as one may be more technically challenging than the other.

At about 1.2 miles from the trailhead, having dropped about 95 feet in 0.2 mile, the single-track levels, becoming less technical as it approaches tiny Onofrio Gulch on your left. (For the next half mile or so, your number of wet crossings will depend on recent storms which may or may not have produced minor branches of the creek, intertwining with the trail.) Continue paralleling the creek and the trail soon begins to gradually rise and fall, skirting shallow drop-offs in a few spots. Go through the creek at about 1.6 miles and in a few yards, you reach a T intersection marked with a brown carsonite sign stating "Trail" with arrows in both directions. Go right, crossing a branch of the creek. (The left trail crosses the creek as well and leads to Mule Train Road.) The single-track widens, climbing moderately and becoming a bit rocky again, eventually leading you away from the creek.

At 2 miles from the parking lot, about 50 yards from the trail, you catch a glimpse of the cyclone fence closing off Mt. Shasta Mine. There's not much to see of the mine—it's basically a 465-foot-deep hole in the ground. During it's hey-day of gold mining between 1897 and 1905, at least 90 men labored here in the summer heat. By 1926, the gold played out and the mine was abandoned. (The abandoned mine shaft is fenced in due to dangerous conditions—please stay out.)

Follow the single-track as it continues to climb moderately. Trail conditions have mellowed considerably, leading you through a forest of lodgepole pine. The trail soon descends and at 2.6 miles, you reach a fork with another wide single-track. The left fork is simply signed "Trail," indicated by an arrow. (Following that left fork will lead you to paved Paige Bar Road in a short distance.) Take the right fork, a wide single-track, following it as it ascends and descends. In a few yards, you reach another signed fork. Look straight ahead through the trees, toward the left, and you see Paige Bar Road. Hang a right here, following the dirt trail. Bypass any lesser trails leading off your more well-defined wide single-track trail, still paralleling Paige Bar off in the distance on your left.

At almost 3 miles, you pass what appear to be two, small semi-buried, old concrete pillars which probably served as a foundation for a sign or gate at one time. Just a few yards beyond the pillars and up a rise, is the relocated Whiskeytown Cemetery. A stroll through the grounds reveals a few old gravesites, marked with tombstones dating back to 1860. The single-track trail continues behind the cemetery toward your right, winding through the sparse forest. Cross a loose, black gravel trail and continue climbing on the dirt single-track through the woods. After a few yards of steep climbing, the trail gradually descends and before you know it, you close the loop by intersecting the same jeep road on which you started, next to the parking area. Total miles on this short but pleasant loop is 3.1 miles.

RIDE 14 · The Chimney

AT A GLANCE

Length/configuration: 8.3-mile out-and-back with a loop (about 2.4 miles each way with a 3.5-mile counter-clockwise loop); dirt road and single-track

Aerobic difficulty: Moderately strenuous with a very strenuous short section at the Chimney

Technical difficulty: Intermediate due to rocky conditions; some tough sections may have to be walked

Scenery: Lush, green creekside environment including waterfalls

Special comments: This ride gets its name from a deep trough cut into a steep embankment caused by a washout draining into Brandy Creek. Not recommended for timid beginners. A short side trip leads to waterfalls and great swimming holes.

Thanks to John Shuman for contributing the following ride description. He's the author of the definitive booklet on trails in the region, *Mountain Biking Whiskeytown*. Unfortunately, finding a copy of it in bookstores and bike shops in Redding is as rare as finding gold nuggets in a stream; it is out-of-print. Keep your fingers crossed, though, John is planning to update and reprint it.   —L.A.

The Chimney is one of my favorite Whiskeytown rides. It is challenging but still manageable enough where I would drag one of my more adventuresome beginning rider friends along. The upper Brandy Creek area has some of the nicest scenery around. The valley that houses it is always lush and green, a perfect retreat during the hot summer months. Other than being an action-packed bike ride, there is a great system of waterfalls to visit. The long stretch of cascading falls with pools and natural water slides makes a great weekend destination to get away from it all.

General location: About 13 miles northwest of Redding; about 165 miles north of Sacramento just west of I-5.

Elevation change: 1,220 feet; starting elevation and low point about 1,280 feet; high point about 2,500 feet. Begins as moderate climb, becoming tougher and steeper to the Chimney, then mostly downhill thereafter.

Season: Year-round, although winter storms may make some creek crossings impassable.

Services: Water, phone, and rest rooms at Brandy Creek marina and campground as well at the Whiskeytown Visitor Information Center Overlook at the intersection of CA 299 and J. F. Kennedy Memorial Drive, about 4 miles from the trailhead. All other services in Redding, about 13 miles away.

Hazards: Watch out for poison oak.

Rescue index: The single-track portions, which are the more technical sections, attract fewer trail users. For that reason, you need to be self-reliant during emergency situations and make your way back to Shasta Bally Road, the main dirt road, where you might be able to flag down a passing motorist. You'll find a phone and, most likely, other people who may be of help at the Brandy Creek marina.

Land status: Whiskeytown Unit of the Whiskeytown-Shasta-Trinity National Recreation Area.

Maps: A good map of this route does not exist. The best map available is found in *Mountain Biking Whiskeytown*, by John Shuman, the definitive booklet on trails in the region. If you find a copy of this rare booklet in any local bike shop, consider yourself lucky as it is temporarily out of print. USGS Igo 7.5 minute series (trails not completely shown, but then it's better than no map).

Finding the trail: From Redding, travel northwest on CA 299 for 8 miles to the Whiskeytown Visitor Information Center Overlook located at the intersection with J. F. Kennedy Memorial Drive. Go left onto J. F. K. Memorial Drive, following the lake edge due southwest, going past its intersection with Paige Bar Road and the Kennedy Memorial. Stay straight on J. F. K. Memorial Drive and continue another 2.6 miles to Brandy Creek marina and campground. After you pass the beach access, you come to the bridge crossing the creek itself. Just before the bridge is a dirt parking lot on the left side where Shasta Bally Road joins the main road. This is the parking spot of choice. If this is full, just park at the Brandy Creek Beach parking. Begin your ride from here.

Sources of additional information:

Whiskeytown Unit, Whiskeytown-Shasta-Trinity National Recreation Area
P.O. Box 188
Whiskeytown, CA 96095
(916) 241-6584
Visitor Information Center located at J.F.K. Mem. Drive and CA 299

Notes on the trail: Begin by riding up Shasta Bally Road, a well-maintained dirt road. At just over a mile, go past the left turn toward Peltier Valley, staying straight. After another mile of mellow climbing on Shasta Bally, go straight slightly bearing

RIDE 14 · The Chimney

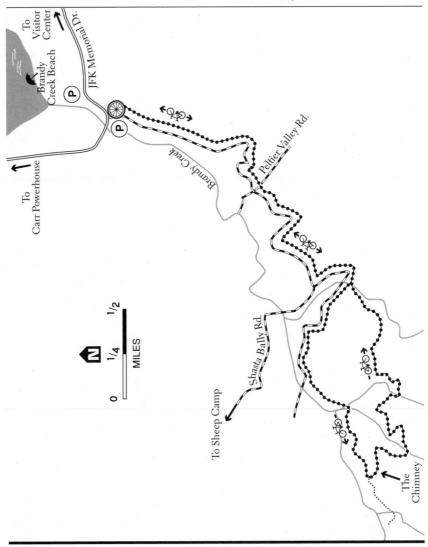

left at the Sheep Camp intersection toward the Chimney. (Staying right on the main dirt road takes you to Sheep Camp and eventually Shasta Bally. Incidentally, for those of you aching for major climbing, consider riding up to Shasta Bally. From this point, it's 5.6 miles up Shasta Bally Road which becomes more of a rugged four-wheel-drive road before reaching the summit at 6,209 feet.)

Continue climbing the road for another mile. Ride until the road opens up and then climbs a much steeper section. Just at the top of the hill before the road drops back down and crosses Brandy Creek, there will be a small trail on the left. It cuts up the bank and you may have to carry your bike up. Here is where the single-track starts.

After 0.3 mile on the single-track, the trail crosses a huge washed-out section along the stream and continues on the right. When you reach the top of a small hill, the trail seems to disappear. Follow it left and it will soon reappear. At almost a mile from the beginning of the single-track, you reach the Chimney. On the left-hand side of the trail, keep on the lookout for a washed-out trough cut deeply into a steep embankment. This is really tricky to find the first time through. To give you a clue, it will be just after completing a steeper section where the trail flattens out and turns right following the contour. On the right side will be a drop-off where a small stream has cut a ravine. (Good luck!) Look for an orange arrow spray-painted on a rock here and follow its direction. When you find it, carry your bike up. It's steep and loose, so be careful. If you want to check out the waterfalls and do some exploring, don't climb up yet. Instead, continue along the original trail.

The waterfall side trip: Staying on the original trail, continue past the Chimney turnoff for about a half mile. At this point, the trail will drop all the way to the creek and become unrideable. Throw your bike into the bushes and walk from here. There is interesting stuff both upstream and downstream. Upstream, in a flat spot of the creek, there is an island of sorts. Farther on up are some good swimming pools and sunbathing rocks. Have fun and don't leave any trash behind.

After braving the Chimney, the trail remains steep for a short while but soon becomes rideable. This is where the downhill begins. A bit farther, the trail crosses seasonal streams in several spots. These streams usually create ravines that must be walked over. Many spots look unrideable but experienced riders can find challenge in discovering a way to do the impossible. It's definitely rideable—you just need the right skills and mental focus.

At about 5 miles from the start, the trail merges with an old four-wheel-drive road. Hang a left onto this road, which is old and overgrown and may not even seem like a road. Soon after this turn, there is a stream crossing and it's rideable. After the crossing, the trail really starts to get fast and fun. Watch the ruts and use them to your advantage in banking the turns. In a short while, the trail forks. Both ways end up in the same place. Try both of them. In a short while, the trail becomes particularly rutted. One outstanding feature is the Mound of Mutilation. During a straightaway, there is a great bump in the trail. If you dare, get some speed and go for some air! It's better to favor the right side. There are more ruts but you avoid a stump behind the jump on the left side which would be painful to crash into.

At approximately 6 miles, you connect back into a familiar dirt road. Go right, retracing the way you came up. Don't forget to try the Ice Box on the way down (see the following trail description).

RIDE 15 · Upper and Lower Ice Box Loop

AT A GLANCE

Length/configuration: 5-mile loop, clockwise; dirt road and single-track

Aerobic difficulty: Easy to moderate due to little climbing and some rough sections

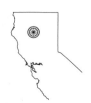

Technical difficulty: Intermediate due to tight turns and some sections of very rocky terrain

Scenery: Lush, green creekside environment

Special comments: Combine this ride with the previous one, the Chimney. Many dirt roads which intersect points of the loop offer a bail-out option if the terrain proves too technical for your liking.

This is another great ride contributed by John Shuman. His definitive booklet on trails in the region, *Mountain Biking Whiskeytown* describes many more trails but, unfortunately, it's temporarily out-of-print. Many thanks, John, for this submission. —L.A

This is a fantastic short loop that offers some great technical fun and only a modest amount of climbing effort. It's an excellent way to spice up the other rides in the area if used as an add-on. The single-track portion can be ridden both up and down. Many ride up it on the way to the Chimney and take the road down on the way back.

General location: About 13 miles northwest of Redding; about 165 miles north of Sacramento just west of I-5.

Elevation change: 700 feet; starting elevation and low point about 1,280 feet; high point about 1,980 feet. Steady, moderate climb, then a descent varied with dips and flat sections.

Season: Year-round, although winter storms may make some creek crossings impassable.

Services: Water, phone, and rest rooms at Brandy Creek marina and campground as well at the Whiskeytown Visitor Information Center Overlook at the intersection of CA 299 and J. F. Kennedy Memorial Drive, about 4 miles from the trailhead. All other services in Redding, about 13 miles away.

Hazards: Watch out for poison oak. Dead Man's Elbow is a tight turn on a steep downhill section of Lower Ice Box, and lots of speedsters have crashed and burned trying to negotiate it.

Rescue index: The single-track portion, which features the more technical sections, attracts some trail users, especially during the summer months. Still, you should be self-reliant during emergency situations and make your way back to the main dirt road, Shasta Bally Road, where you might be able to flag down a passing motorist. You'll find a phone and, most likely, other people who may be of help at the Brandy Creek beach and marina.

Land status: Whiskeytown Unit of the Whiskeytown-Shasta-Trinity National Recreation Area.

Maps: A good map of this route does not exist. The best map available is found in *Mountain Biking Whiskeytown*, by John Shuman, the definitive booklet on trails in the region. If you find a copy of this rare booklet in any local bike shop, consider yourself lucky as it is out-of-print. USGS Igo 7.5 minute series. (It's better than no map.)

Finding the trail: From Redding, travel northwest on CA 299 for 8 miles to the Whiskeytown Visitor Information Center Overlook located at the intersection with J. F. Kennedy Memorial Drive. Go left onto J. F. K. Memorial Drive, following the lake edge due southwest, going past its intersection with Paige Bar Road and the

RIDE 15 · Upper and Lower Ice Box Loop

Kennedy Memorial. Stay straight on J. F. K. Memorial Drive and continue another 2.6 miles to Brandy Creek marina and campground. After you pass the beach access, you come to the bridge crossing the creek itself. Just before the bridge is a dirt parking lot on the left side where Shasta Bally Road joins the main road. This is the parking spot of choice. If this is full, park at the nearby Brandy Creek Beach parking. Begin your ride from here.

Sources of additional information: See sources of additional information for Ride 14.

Notes on the trail: From either the dirt pulloff next to the bridge or the Brandy Creek beach parking lot, start by riding up Shasta Bally Road. It's a nice, gentle climb and in about a half mile, you bypass a set of turnoffs. About 0.25 mile after the Peltier Valley

Road junction, continue past a signed single-track trail on your right (you'll come back to this point later). Keep going straight. In another 0.25 mile, about 2 miles from where you started, keep an eye out for a small trail leading off on the right—it's just before you come to a fork in the main dirt road. That's the beginning of Lower Ice Box and may be hard to see the first time, even though there's a trail marker there. Not to worry. You'll return to this spot later, after your run on Upper Icebox. Bypass the Lower Ice Box trailhead, staying on the main dirt road for about 50 yards to the fork where there's a sign for Sheep Camp to the right. Stay straight, bearing left on the dirt road for about another half mile. (Incidentally, this road leads to the single-track trailhead of the Chimney; see the previous trail description.) Watch for a trail marker on the right of the road, planted next to a single-track leading down a drainage. This is the beginning of Upper Ice Box, also known as the Freezer.

Go right onto Upper Ice Box and enjoy a fun half-mile stretch before it dumps you onto Shasta Bally Road. Turn right here and in a few yards, you're back at the fork near Sheep Camp turnoff and the Lower Ice Box trailhead. Keep an eye out for the trail marker on the left side of Shasta Bally Road. When you find it, jump onto the single-track which is Lower Ice Box, also known as the Fridge.

The top part of Lower Ice Box is a technical section. It's fairly narrow with lots of little obstacles. The pinnacle of this technical workout is Dead Man's Elbow (or just the Elbow). This is a steep downhill section with a sharp right-hand turn at the bottom. If you look, you will see a dead-end trail which is developing due to all the people who go crashing through the forest after not being able to make the turn. The rider who can make this corner is well on the way to becoming a master over his or her steed. Just before you come back out onto Shasta Bally Road, you have some challenging roots and ledges to get up and over.

Having survived that, go left and down the hill about 0.1 mile. Lower Ice Box continues off on the left. There is a raised turn-out of sorts with a parking area on the top. The trail can be found behind it. It starts with some fun switchbacks and quickly turns into a series of challenging drops. Make sure your seat is low and be ready to eject off the bike if you get into trouble. About 0.2 mile from leaving the parking area, the trail flattens out. Stay left if there is any question as to which way to go. You should come around the left side of a pond. Follow the trail right and over the dam of the pond. Then, go left onto the road which appears on the other side. In a few yards, you reach a 4-way intersection. Take the smallest option which is straight ahead. This is my favorite section of Lower Ice Box. It consists of some interesting turns which are really fun to hit at speed.

In less than a half mile from the 4-way intersection, the trail meets another intersection after descending a trench with a technical drop-off at the end. Go right. [If you are coming up from the other direction, you will be going left up a washed-out section which is hard to identify as a trail. Keep a sharp eye out or you will miss it. It is just after the road narrows into a trail; 0.8 mile from the bottom if you have a computer.] Coming down the hill, the trail will widen into a road which has some good rocks to jump. These are nice round rocks sunk into the dirt which make great mini-ramps.

About 0.25 mile farther, the trail crosses the stream twice. Sometimes they're dry in the summer. Then, the trail drops into a clearing of sorts. It looks like there is a road to the left but it disappears. Go right and immediately cross another small, sometimes dry stream. A short way after this, there is a fork. The main road goes right and the single-track trail drops to the left along the creek. Follow the trail and it eventually leads you to a washed-out section. The trail disappears, but if you keep your eyes open, you will see it on the left as it enters the forest. Follow the trail and it brings you out onto a road. Go left, into the clearing, and in a few yards, hidden behind a dirt pile on the right, the trail continues. Go down the trail into the Boulderland Playground section of Lower Ice Box. There are many turnoffs and variations here. Don't worry about getting lost though, all roads lead home from here. The parking lot will appear shortly.

RIDE 16 · Great Water Ditch Trail and El Dorado Mine Loop

AT A GLANCE

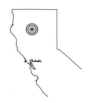

Length/configuration: Part 1: 5-mile out-and-back (2.5 miles each way). Part 2: 4.8 mile loop (with some out-and-backs); mostly single-track, some dirt and paved road

Aerobic difficulty: Easy to moderate due to brief climbs

Technical difficulty: Mildly technical with intermediate section in the middle

Scenery: Shady riding along the lake's edge. Wooded hillsides and drainages, including the haunted Deer Forest. Tower House Historic District includes the El Dorado Mine and other gold rush–era buildings.

Special comments: Part 1 suited for beginners. Part 2 suited for advanced beginners and intermediates.

Part One consists of the Great Ditch Trail and is a five-mile out-and-back (2.5 miles each way). This is a great trail for beginners to hone their single-track riding skills. It's mildly technical, basically flat and smooth, following the edge of Whiskeytown Lake. Except for a short stretch that parallels busy and loud CA 299, the route is generally a sweet cruise weaving through the shady forest and tall vegetation.

Part Two is the El Dorado Mine Loop, a sort of a double loop with some out-and-back stretches. I'm not going to try and explain the route's configuration—better for you to look at the map. Suffice it to say that the complete mileage on this routing is 4.8 miles and combines the Clear Creek Vista Trail through Haunted Deer Forest and several Ditch Trails. Short? Perhaps, but the splendid, well-groomed single-tracks that lead up and down creek drainages and hug steep forested slopes are not to be missed. There are no major climbs, making these trails perfect for cruising. Riders ranging from adventurous beginners or better will have fun here. Less-experienced riders can skip a steep downhill section to change the difficulty of the ride from intermediate to advanced beginner.

Not only are these great riding trails but there's the added bonus of some interesting historical sites worth exploring. The ride takes you to the Tower House Historical District, which is a good place to learn about the gold rush days. As for the unattractive name "Ditch Trail," we have Levi Tower, Charles Camden, and the Clear Creek Ditch Company to thank. The two were enterprising business associates (and best buds) back in the mid-1800s. Like thousands of other folks, they were lured by the prospect of gold in the creeks and, later, in the hillsides. When the effectiveness of

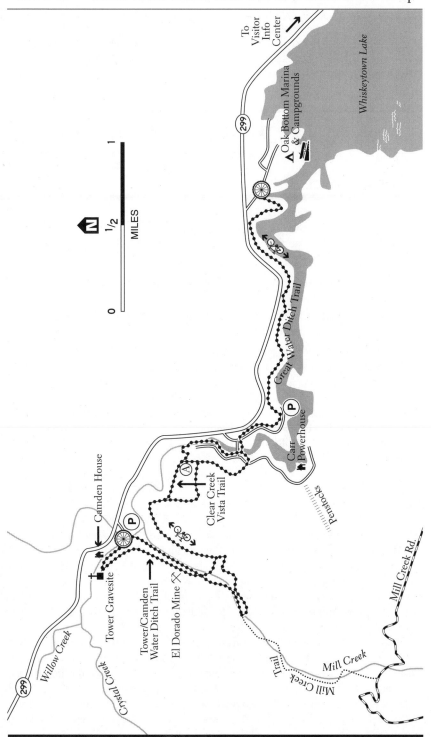

To Visitor Info Center

Whiskeytown Lake

299

Oak Bottom Marina & Campgrounds

Great Water Ditch Trail

N

MILES

0   ½   1

Carr Powerhouse

P

Penstocks

Camden House

Clear Creek Vista Trail

A

P

Tower Gravesite

Tower/Camden Water Ditch Trail

El Dorado Mine

299

Willow Creek

Crystal Creek

Mill Creek Trail

Mill Creek

Mill Creek Rd.

placer mining declined (removing gold from creeks and streams), other methods of extracting gold out of the hills were employed. Hard-rock mining answered the yearning by boring deep shafts into the hillsides. To move tons of dirt and gravel, high-pressure water was used via aqueducts, flumes, and ditches. Tower and Camden, along with the Clear Creek Ditch Company, constructed a staggering 41-mile ditch system to provide a continuous flow of water to the mining operations year-round. They eventually switched to "mining" the local population. Tower built a 21-room hotel (the Tower House), several bridges, and ditches to carry water to the various mining operations—all for a fee, of course. Tower raised orchards of fruit trees, thriving on water irrigated from the nearby creeks. In a few short years, Tower House grew in popularity and became widely known as one of California's most splendid hotels, serving guests from afar and local miners alike. In 1919, the house burned clear down to its foundation and was never rebuilt. This bike route follows this historic path and takes you past the El Dorado Mine and Stamp Mill, Tower's gravesite and ends near Camden's "cottage in the garden." When you see Camden's white picket–fenced house, look a few yards northwest of it, to where the Tower House once stood and try to imagine a 3-story hotel bustling with folks and commerce.

Thanks goes to John Shuman for contributing to this ride description. Considered by locals to be one of the most knowledgeable sources of bike trail information, John is the author of *Mountain Biking Whiskeytown*, an out-of-print booklet of the region. He has tentative plans to reprint it, so stay tuned.   —L.A.

General location: About 13 miles northwest of Redding.

Elevation change: 520 feet; starting elevation 1,280 feet; high point 1,800 feet; low point 1,040 feet. Lots of ups and downs with stretches of easy cruising.

Season: Year-round, although winter storms may swell Mill Creek, and crossing it means water up to your knees or thighs. Fortunately, it's not too wide, about 10 to 15 feet across.

Services: Water, phone, rest rooms, and privately operated concession stands at Oak Bottom marina and campground. Water and rest rooms also located in the Tower House District parking lot (the farthest point on the ride).Water, rest rooms, and phone also at the Whiskeytown Visitor Information Center Overlook at the intersection of CA 299 and J. F. K. Memorial Drive, about 2.2 miles from the trailhead. Picnic tables at Judge Francis Carr Powerhouse (albeit under power lines) at the outer end of the out-and-back. All other services in Redding, about 11 miles away. Developed campgrounds at numerous locations within the vicinity.

Hazards: Frequent hikers and equestrians, as this is a popular trail. Scattered poison oak. Crossing winter-swollen Mill Creek can be treacherous. Be cautious in deciding whether to cross. Be alert for an occasional motorist on the paved stretch near the end of the ride. Be alert for ticks, rattlesnakes, and rarely seen mountain lions and bears.

Rescue index: This is a popular route with other trail users, especially in the summer. There are two access points along this out-and-back, which means you're never too far from finding other trail users and motorists who may be of assistance. The historic Tower House District attracts many visitors, especially during the summer months. Though you should always be prepared and self-reliant, you're likely to find other trail users who may be of assistance. During the off-season, don't expect anyone to come along anytime soon; you should make your way back to CA 299 and flag down a passing motorist, or head to Oak Bottom where there is a public phone.

Land status: Whiskeytown Unit of the Whiskeytown-Shasta-Trinity National Recreation Area.

Maps: Whiskeytown Unit (the standard information brochure published by the National Park Service. It's a barely adequate map, but it's better than nothing). USGS Whiskeytown and French Gulch 7.5 minute series.

Finding the trail: From Redding, travel northwest on CA 299 for 8 miles to the Whiskeytown Visitor Information Center Overlook located at the intersection with J. F. Kennedy Memorial Drive. (Incidentally, the Center is worth visiting to find out more about the area.) Continue past the Center on CA 299 for almost 5.5 miles. Turn left, following the sign to the Oak Bottom campgrounds and marina. About 0.2 mile, look for a small paved pulloff on the right side of the road and a small brown sign, "Ditch Trail Access." Park here.

Sources of additional information: See sources of additional information for Ride 14.

Notes on the trail: The Part One out-and-back is fairly easy to follow. From the parking area, start pedaling on the trail signed "Ditch Trail Access." The first 2.3 miles of the out-and-back route is the Great Water Ditch Trail, a wide single-track dirt path. It begins with a slight downhill, and within a few yards, it leads you to a kind of T intersection with a signed hiking trail. Since bikes aren't allowed on the left trail, go right and cross a creek draining into the lake. You're now virtually at water level with the narrow western end of Whiskeytown Lake. It's shady here and the trail is generally hard-packed and mildly technical, if at all. There may be some standing pools of water and muddy patches in the trail if it has been rainy recently.

Within the next 0.4 mile, as the Ditch Trail narrows, you emerge from the shade and begin skirting—literally hugging—the edge of the lake on your left and CA 299 within ten yards off on your right. The trail is quite removed from the highway, and the view of the lake at water level makes it easy to endure the zooming cars and trucks. At 0.7 mile, say "good riddance" to the highway, following the trail as it curves away from the road, still hugging the shoreline. The single-track trail remains well-defined, varying in width about 3 to 6 feet across as it gradually rises above the lake. Bypass any lesser trails leading from your path.

At about 1.5 miles, the Ditch Trail begins paralleling a creek on your left, then crosses it on a well-made footbridge. The trail eventually curves back around and parallels the creek again on your left. In a few yards, pass a small building and tank, then climb up nine wooden steps. A few yards more and you reach a locked gate. Go around the gate, continuing on the wide and fairly smooth single-track trail. Almost immediately, a rutted jeep road crosses your trail. Look left down the road and you'll see a brown carsonite sign pointing to the right toward the continuation of the single-track trail; follow it as it rises and falls. In less than 0.2 mile, cross another jeep road, and once again follow a brown sign directing you straight across the dirt road. The lake is still visible through the trees on your left though about 20 to 30 feet in the distance. At 2.3 miles from the beginning, Great Water Ditch Trail ends at a paved road.

Go right onto the paved road and cruise down and back up an easy hill. Bypass all dirt roads leading down toward the lake on your left. About 0.5 mile since beginning the paved road, you reach the intersection with another wide, paved road. Go left here and follow the road as it crosses over Clear Creek. On the other side of the bridge is a dirt pulloff. This is the beginning of Part Two. Timid beginners should continue following the main paved road for about a half mile all the way to Judge Francis Carr Powerhouse. There are picnic tables at the Powerhouse, albeit in the shadow of gigantic electric towers and power lines. Fishing is reportedly fairly decent here. When you've had enough of the man-made surroundings, turn around and head back the way you came.

For Part Two, from the dirt pulloff alongside the bridge, bear right down a paved road which quickly becomes dirt. In less than a half mile, you come to a clearing. Here are the ruins of several old mining cabins from the gold rush days. Continue straight and the dirt road will turn into a single-track trail. Keep to the left to avoid the sandy riverbed. Eventually, the trail will turn left up the hill and start a series of switchbacks.

You finish most of the climbing at about 0.8 mile from the dirt pulloff and the switchbacks end. Make sure you follow the trail to the right at the top where your trail intersects Clear Creek Vista Trail. At a mile from the starting point, now on Clear Creek Vista, you come to an intersection of several trails. (Call this intersection "A" because on your return, you will come back to this point and take the trail that is now on your left.) Take the one that goes straight, not the first trail that runs uphill on your left nor the other trail that looks like a road that drops downhill steeply to the right. The next 0.3 mile is a great stretch of trail that you can really get moving on. There are plenty of chances to get some air off the speed bump–type formations in the trail. At one point, you cross a set of old mining car rail tracks, a sign that you have almost reached the next turnoff. Just before reaching the base of a power line tower, there will be a steep trail dropping off to the right. Plunge down this to the creek and follow it to the right.

Following a short parallel of Mill Creek, a set of old rock stairs drop to the left into the creek. This is where you cross. There is almost no way to stay dry on this one, so be careful. Turn right on the dirt road (looks like a wide single-track) after the creek crossing.

You're now entering the Tower House Historic District and the wide single-track you're on is the Tower Irrigation Ditch Trail. Pedal a few yards and you reach the site of El Dorado Mine and its Stamp Mill. This was one of the big profitable mines of the Whiskeytown area during the gold rush. The old buildings and equipment are relics from the hard-rock gold mining boom, which began in the late 1880s. After checking out the site, continue on the trail, bearing left. A few yards past the Stamp Mill, the single-track continues up a set of wooden steps on your left while a wider dirt road continues on the right, leading past the Camden Sawmill, Tenant Farm House, and Barn. (The Farm House is still in use as living quarters for a ranger with the National Park Service.) Carry your bike up the steps and continue on the mildly technical single-track. In a few more yards, you reach another set of wooden steps, this time leading down.

Back in the saddle, follow the trail, and in about 0.5 mile, you reach the Tower gravesite. Follow the trail through a tight right curve, now heading back in the opposite direction, only this time paralleling Willow Creek. Get ready, you are about to encounter a few tiny sand traps. In about 0.2 mile, you reach a well-made pedestrian footbridge on your left. It leads across Willow Creek toward the main parking lot. Take a side trip by going over the bridge, and then hang a left to see the remains of the once-magnificent Camden House and outbuildings. Check out the back of the main house. It has one of Shasta County's first indoor rest room, protruding from an upper floor. Plumbing was gravity and a drain pipe, running directly into Willow Creek! (If you go a few yards farther and cross another bridge, and you reach the Tower House Historical District parking lot. Here you'll find picnic tables and rest room facilities—with proper plumbing!)

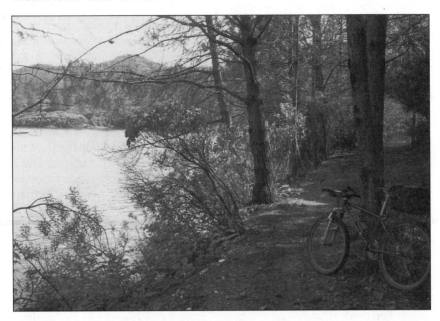

This easy single-track skirts the Whiskeytown Lake shoreline along a few stretches.

When you're finished exploring, retrace your path back over both bridges and intersect with the sand-trap trail again. This time, bear left and follow the dirt road leading back toward El Dorado Mine, as it weaves past the Camden Sawmill, Tenant Farm House, and Barn. Continue past the mine and the first trail that you used to cross the creek. Continue on and look for a small dirt road that crosses the stream again on your left. Cross the stream and follow the road uphill. You know you have gone too far if you find yourself on a single-track before crossing the stream. (If you continue on the single-track, it begins to ascend, becoming Mill Creek Trail. It's favored by strong, intermediately skilled riders and it climbs up to Mill Creek Road and other bike routes.)

After the creek crossing, keep your eyes open for two trails branching off on the left. There will be a lower one that heads down and an upper one that follows the contour. Take the upper one. In a short while, you begin retracing your path on Clear Creek Vista Trail. Remember intersection "A" that you encountered about a mile after the starting point? Keep an eye out for it. This time, turn right and travel uphill. At this point, you're leaving Clear Creek Vista Trail. (Beginning riders may want to skip this section and go straight instead, retracing the path all the way down the switchbacks and back to the starting point.)

In less than a half mile from the intersection, near the top, the trail thins out and turns left. Then, it disappears into an open forest with no underbrush, just a blanket of leaves. You have found the Haunted Deer Forest. (According to John, "Every time I go through here, I either see them off in the distance through the trees or hear them suspiciously rustling somewhere out of sight.") There will be no trail at first, but head straight down the hill through the trees (in the leaf-covered area) and you should come across a trail/rock slide. It is probably a good idea to lower your seat before you start the descent. This is one heck of a ride down. Even the hot shots can end up going over the bars on this one.

   The trail eventually spits you out onto a more reasonable path where you will make a right turn back onto Clear Creek Vista Trail. About 0.3 mile more, just when the trail starts to get steep, there is a trail joining from the right. This means you are almost to the bottom and if you're racing your friends, this is your last chance to make a break for it. The right-hand trail looks like it used to lead somewhere, but it ends after a short while. Bypass the right trail by bearing left. After the descent, there is another mysterious dead-end trail that comes in on the right. Stay left. Just after this, there is another small trail to the right that goes into a clearing. Follow it and, according to John, "In the right-hand side of the clearing is a weird stone creation. What it is I don't know, but it's interesting to look at." After contemplating this for a bit, go back to the main trail and continue following it down to the paved road at the bottom. Take a left on the road and return to the dirt pulloff by the bridge. Retrace your Part One path back to your car at Oak Bottom.

OTHER AREA RIDES

THE RAMS RIDE (RIDE AROUND MT. SHASTA): A moderately technical yet strenuous ride; 65-mile loop on dirt roads and pavement; Shasta-Trinity National Forest and railroad access lands. Super-strong bikers can ride it in a day with an early-morning start. Otherwise, plan a two-day adventure with an overnight campout.

Finding the trail: Loop starts in the town of Mount Shasta on I-5, about 50 miles south of the Oregon state line.

Maps: USGS Mount Shasta, The Whale Back, Juniper flat Hotlum, City of Mount Shasta, McCloud, Elk Springs, Ash Creek Butte 7.5 minute series.

For more information, contact:

Mount Shasta Ranger District
Shasta-Trinity National Forest
204 West Alma
Mount Shasta, CA 96067
(916) 926-4511

Mud Creek Cyclery
316 Chestnut St.
Mount Shasta, CA 96067
(530) 926-1303

CANYON CREEK–BUKER RIDGE LOOP: Moderate ride on maintained dirt road and pavement; 18 miles; Klamath National Forest.

Finding the trail: From Yreka on I-5, follow CA 3 south to Fort Jones. Take Scott River Road about 12 miles to Indian Scotty Campground. Ride begins from the campground.

Maps: USGS Marble Mountain, Grider Valley, and Scott Bar 7.5 minute series.

For more information, contact:

Klamath National Forest
1312 Fairlane Road
Yreka, CA 96097
(916) 842-6131

GUNSIGHT PEAK–HUMBUG CREEK LOOP: A somewhat moderate to strenuous ride requiring intermediate technical skills; dirt roads and double-track; Klamath National Forest.

Finding the trail: From Yreka, following Miner or North Streets, make your way up to Humbug Road. Go right on Humbug and follow it to the Four Corners intersection. Park and begin riding from here.

Maps: USGS Badger Mountain, Indian Creek Baldy, Yreka, and McKinley Mountain 7.5 minute series.

For more information, contact:

Klamath National Forest
1312 Fairlane Road
Yreka, CA 96097
(916) 842-6131

BIZZ JOHNSON TRAIL: This trail is suitable for everyone, from beginners to expert riders, youngsters to adults. You can make it a workout by tackling it as a one-day outing. You can even camp overnight or spend the night in a quaint inn. To some cyclists, this trail is one of the loveliest, traveling through the beautiful Susan River gorge, a conifer forest, a desertlike landscape, and two tunnels. To others, it's boring, being mostly straight and flat, completely devoid of any technical challenge. Your enjoyment depends on your purpose and fitness level. One of the gems of the nationwide Rails-To-Trails Conservancy, this point-to-point route measures 25.4 miles one way, 50.8 miles round-trip, and is chock-full of rail history. Following an old Southern Pacific railroad line, the grade is mellow (elevation gain is about 1,300 feet over the course of 25 miles), and the route is mostly hard-packed, smooth dirt trails along with some pavement. The Lassen Rural Bus runs between the two endpoints of the trail, and they will carry bikes. [For more information, call (916) 257-5697.] From summer to early fall, many events, including mountain-bike rides, are held around this historic trail. The 6 miles immediately outside Susanville is reportedly the prettiest.

Finding the trails: The Bizz Johnson Trail is anchored on the west end by the Mason Station Trailhead just north of Westwood. The east end is anchored by Susanville. Other access points are available off CA 44 and CA 36. To reach Mason Station, from Red Bluff on I-5, follow CA 36 east out of town past Lassen Volcanic National Park. Continue through Chester to Westwood and County Road A-21. Head north (left) on A-21 for about 3 miles to CR 101. Follow CR 101 for about a half mile to the Mason Station Trailhead. Park and begin riding from here. The trail is marked by an informational kiosk and signs. To reach the Susanville Trailhead, continue east through Westwood on CA 36 about 23 miles farther. Once in Susanville, follow Main Street through the historic part of town to Weatherlow Street (at the first stoplight). Go right onto Weatherlow and head south (the road soon becomes Richmond Road). In about a half mile, you reach the Susanville Railroad Depot and Visitor Center. The trail begins at the Depot. Parking is permitted here. For more information, including lodging, camping, and overnight parking information, contact any of the following agencies.

Maps: Trail map, interpretive guide, and free brochure from the Bureau of Land Management office as listed below.

For more information, contact:

Lassen Land and Trails Trust
(916) 257-0456
(Info for special events)

Lassen National Forest
Eagle Lake Ranger District
55 South Sacramento St.
Susanville, CA 96100
(530) 257-2151

Bureau of Land Management
Eagle Lake Field Office
2950 Riverside Dr.
Susanville, CA 96130
(916) 257-0456

SOUTH WARNER WILDERNESS LOOP: Encircling the wilderness area in Modoc National Forest, mostly above 7,000 feet, this 70-mile loop combines mostly dirt and gravel roads, including a long stretch on paved Surprise Valley Road.

Finding the trail: Starting in Eagletown in the valley, the route heads south and then west up into the Warner Mountains via gravel roads 40 and 42 to South Warner Road. The route then heads north via Blue Lake and West Warner Roads. At the northern end of the loop, Parker Creek and Old Granger Creek Roads leads east to paved Surprise Valley Road. Once on the paved road, the route runs south for about 16 miles. High point of this clockwise loop is roughly 2,919 feet on South Warner Road reached within the first one-quarter of the entire ride. After that, there are plenty of steep ups and downs, in addition to the total mileage, that will challenge you. The rewards along the way are views of the wilderness area and the desert valley floor of Surprise Valley, where dry Middle Alkali Lake lies. This is an epic ride, though it's not necessarily technically difficult. You need to start at daybreak if you plan to ride the entire route in one day. Depending on where you begin, you can tackle the ride as a two-day affair (there are campgrounds on the west side of the loop) or enjoy lodging in Eagleville. Assuming you want to begin in the town of Cedarville or Eagleville (basically the low points on the loop), follow CA 299 east from Alturas for about 22 miles to Cedarville. You can park in Cedarville and begin pedaling south on Surprise Valley Road toward Eagleville. Or turn right and head south on Surprise Valley Road for 17 miles to Eagleville. Park and begin riding from there. Best time to ride is late May through June. Thanks goes to Chuck Elliot, owner of Bodfish Bicycles in Chester for suggesting this route.

Maps: USGS Eagleville, Snake Lake, Emerson Peak, Jess Valley, Soup Creek, Shields Creek, Warren Peak, and Eagle Peak 7.5 minute series.

For more information, contact:

Bodfish Bicycles
152 Main St.
P.O. Box 1969
Chester, CA 96020
For more big rides in very remote places, visit Chuck Elliot, the shop owner who has ridden and written about this region of California.

Modoc National Forest
800 W. 12th St.
Alturas, CA 96101
(916) 233-5811

Warner Mountain Ranger District
P.O. Box 220
Cedarville, CA 96014
(916) 279-6116

LITTLE MT. HOFFMAN LOOKOUT: Medicine Lake Highlands is the largest volcano in northern California, measuring roughly 15 miles east to west and 25 miles north to south. Sitting at 7,309 feet with a 360-degree view, Little Mt. Hoffman Lookout is an historic fire lookout built in the 1920s and is available for overnight recreational use. The lookout is located at the northern edge of the Medicine Lake Highlands Volcanic Area in Shasta National Forest. As a cinder cone sitting on the rim of a caldera, Little Mt. Hoffman and the lookout itself offer panoramic views of one of the state's diverse volcanic landscape. If you like checking out cinder cones, craters, and ancient lava flows, consider booking the lookout as a base camp from which to explore nearby sites on your mountain bike. Miles of dirt forest roads offer hours of exploration. There are several self-guided roadside geology tours of the volcanic area measuring roughly 22 miles and 28 miles. Hearty cyclists who don't mind sharing the road with motorists may enjoy it (when ridden as an out-and-back, the round-trip clocks in at 44 miles and 56 miles, respectively). Though this is an under-appreciated area of the state, these roads often experience heavy traffic during the height of the travel season. A little over 20 miles north of the lookout is Lava Beds National Monument, and even though bikes are only allowed on paved vehicle roads, it's a worthy visit.

Finding the area: From Mt. Shasta on I-5, pick up CA 89 a few miles south of town and head east toward McCloud, about 12 miles. Be sure to stop at the McCloud Ranger Station and inquire about the entry status of the Highlands area. From McCloud, continue on CA 89 about 27 miles to CR 15 (Harris Spring Road). Go left (north) onto CR 15 and follow it for a little over 28 miles to the Glass Mountain turnoff (Forest Service Road 43N48). This portion of CR 15, incidentally, is the popular Modoc Volcanic National Scenic Byway, which is the 28-mile self-guided geology tour mentioned above. Turn right (east) on the dirt road toward Glass Mountain and Medicine Lake, following the signs to the lookout, or continue on FS 43N48 to Medicine Lake Headquarters and campgrounds.

For more information, contact:

Shasta-Trinity National Forests
McCloud Ranger District
P.O. Box 1620
McCloud, CA 96057
(916) 964-2184

Modoc National Forest
Doublehead Ranger District
P.O. Box 369
Tulelake, CA 96134
(916) 667-2246

SOME LOCAL BICYCLE SHOPS

Sports Cottage
2665 Park Marina Dr.
Redding, CA 96001
(530) 241-3115

The Fifth Season
426 N. Mount Shasta Blvd.
Mount Shasta, CA 96067
(530) 926-3606

Mud Creek Cyclery
316 Chestnut St.
Mount Shasta, CA 96067
(530) 926-1303

Bodfish Bicycles
152 Main St.
P.O. Box 1969
Chester, CA 96020

THE MENDOCINO COAST

Sitting about 170 miles north of San Francisco along Highway 1, the towns of Mendocino and Fort Bragg are both perched on windy but spectacular headlands overlooking the Pacific. Like the "Odd Couple," these two towns couldn't be more different. Quaint and charming are the words most often used to describe Mendocino, overrun with artists' shops, quaint bed-and-breakfast inns, and tourists. Fort Bragg, on the other hand, is best described as a stepsister, a former logging town that has seen better, more robust economic times. Ironically, Mendocino artisans who are responsible for creating the town's charm have been forced out by high rents, many of whom now live in more mainstream Fort Bragg. Despite the fact that the roads to and from the area either snake up and over the southern end of the Coastal Range or follow curvy but magnificent Highway 1, the tourists keep coming. Don't let the twisty road or tourists stop you. Most of the visitors are sedentary and never leave the pavement, which means you won't be sharing the trail with too many of them. Admittedly, the Mendocino Coast is not a popular mountain biking destination, at least not yet.

Bike trails abound and most of them can be found inside a 20 by 12-mile area between Mendocino and Fort Bragg. Though a small area, it's packed with rich resources, including thick redwood forests, wild coho salmon, and unusual pygmy forests. Drained by numerous rivers and creeks, Mendocino County is mountainous and blessed with verdant vegetation year-round. Within this area is Jackson State Demonstration Forest, the premier playground for serious mountain bikers seeking dirt, short or long mileages, lots of climbing and a fair amount of technical terrain. Located between the two towns, the Demo Forest extends east from Highway 1 through the tiny town of Dunlap. On the mellow side, neophytes and leisurely bikers, perhaps with youngsters in tow, will find that Russian Gulch, Van Damme, and MacKerricher State Parks offer easy riding through lush redwood forests and on an old, shoreline logging road. The five rides in this chapter are all within this small region and it gives you a good taste of what many other trails in Mendocino County and nearby Lake County have to offer.

RIDE 17 · Manly Gulch Loop

AT A GLANCE

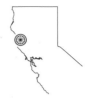

Length/configuration: 6.7-mile loop, counterclockwise; single- and double-track dirt road

Aerobic difficulty: Strenuous due to steep climbing sections

Technical difficulty: Expert due to a narrow trail cut into a steep hillside and several treacherous sections

Scenery: Mixed second- and third-growth redwood forest

Special comments: This is a trail for people with confidence in their technical skills. You will enjoy several tight switchbacks, narrow bridges, tricky technical sections, and even a water crossing or two in the winter.

Unlike most of the other state forests in California, Jackson State Forest is a demonstration forest, managed primarily for its forest products and ongoing study of sound growing practices. Though allowed, recreational use of the forest is not its top priority. In fact, managers at the Jackson Demonstration State Forest headquarters in Fort Bragg advise trail users should call ahead to learn which areas are currently closed to public use. Because logging operations often close access roads and regions and significantly alter the landscape, permanent trails for mountain biking—or hiking—can't really be established with any dependability. Don't expect to see signed trailheads here. While the numerous dirt logging roads that crisscross the forest are generally identified by numbers instead of descriptive or creative names, there are many more spurs that are not identified, even on the official state forest map. Needless to say, biking in Jackson Demonstration State Forest is not recommended for anyone who "freaks out" when lost. On the other hand, if you have a hankering for adventure and have intermediate technical skills and endurance, you will have a good time here.

Enter Ray Houghton. Having pedaled this area, particularly Jackson Demonstration State Forest for over 10 years, what better guide is there than Ray? He knows the region like the back of his hand. Arguably, he's also the best person to talk to about where the great trails are. In 1996, based on a tip from a friend employed at a local bike shop, Ray launched Mendocino Mountain Bike Tours. It seems that the beautiful Mendocino coast attracts lots of folks who want to include biking in their visit. Many seek trail recommendations and some even want to hire a local guide. Today, Mendocino Mountain Bike Tours offers inexpensive personal guide and shuttle services to many of the area's favorite bike trails. Many thanks to Ray for enthusiastically contributing the following trail notes on Manly Gulch Loop.   —L.A.

This is one of those trails that reminds a person why they love mountain biking, from the first sweeping turns down the single-track, over narrow log bridges, through tight switchbacks and technical obstacles, to the last log bridge. All this, set in the beautiful setting of lush, green, redwood forest uniquely indigenous to the California northwest. Manly Gulch Loop is a favorite of mine and many of the local mountain bikers. Although the loop is a short one—6.7 miles—most local riders add miles and

RIDE 17 · Manly Gulch Loop
RIDE 18 · Casper Creek–640–630 Loop

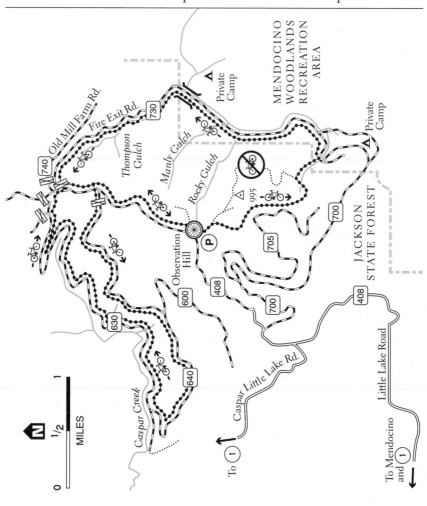

elevation by parking where the pavement ends on Little Lake Road, then pedal up the first dirt road to the single-track trailhead. This not only adds a few more miles and several hundred feet of elevation to the ride, it also leaves you feeling warmed up and ready for the thrilling descent of Manly Gulch. At the trailhead, the single-track runs just over two miles down to the bottom of Manly Gulch. There, the trail winds through a small portion of the historic and beautiful Mendocino Woodlands Recreation Area. After that, the route makes a two-mile, nearly 1,000-foot climb back to Road 408 (also known as Little Lake Road) and eventually back to the trailhead. If you find yourself wanting more mileage when you get back up to 408, look into adding the Caspar Creek–640–630 Loop (Ride 18) to your ride. Incidentally, Manly is also spelled "Manley" on several pieces of literature published by Jackson Demonstration State Forest.

General location: About 7 miles east of the village of Mendocino, about a 3.5-hour drive north of San Francisco.

Elevation change: 960 feet; starting elevation 880 feet; high point 960 feet; low point is sea level. Series of descents into the gulch, followed by a steep climb back out.

Season: Year-round, though sections likely to be muddy from rain and lingering moisture. Logging operations, which generally occur in the summer, may close portions of the forest to public access. Call the Jackson Demonstration State Forest office for current conditions.

Services: No services on this trail. Limited food, gas, lodging, and other services in Mendocino. All other services in Fort Bragg.

Hazards: Jackson Demonstration State Forest allows deer hunting from mid-August through September. Wearing brightly colored clothing during hunting season is strongly advised. Watch out for poison oak, which can be found growing along the trails and roads. Deer ticks in the area are reported to have a 1% infection rate for Lyme disease.

Rescue index: Road 408 at the trailhead is lightly traveled. Still, in an emergency, make your way back up to Road 408 and you might get lucky with a passing motorist. The Forest History Trail (the starting point of this loop) attracts a fair amount of visitors, especially in the summer. In the summer, help may also be found in the Mendocino Woodlands Camp, a popular private campground. During the winter, when the camp is deserted, you might find a caretaker who may be of assistance. (Since this is a private campground, please do not disturb the campers unless it's a true emergency).

Land status: Jackson Demonstration State Forest, managed by the California Department of Forestry and Fire Protection. A portion of the loop lies in the Mendocino Woodlands Recreation Area.

Maps: *Jackson Demonstration State Forest*, published by the California Department of Forestry and Fire Protection.

Finding the trail: From Highway 1 (CA 1), go east on Little Lake Road, which eventually becomes Road 408. Stay on 408 for approximately 5.7 miles, at which point the road splits and the pavement ends. Stay to the left and follow the dirt road up a few short, steep climbs for about 1.3 miles to where the road levels out. Drive another several hundred yards to the Forest History Trail trailhead at mile marker 6.85. Don't expect to find a parking lot here. Instead, look for where the road widens, offering just enough space for several cars to park along the shoulder.

Sources of additional information:

Jackson Demonstration State Forest
California Department of Forestry
  and Fire Protection
802 No. Main St. (Highway 1)
Fort Bragg, CA 95437
(707) 964-5674

Mendocino Mountain Bike Tours
10450 Nichols Lane
Mendocino, CA 95460
(707) 937-3069

Notes on the trail: The start of the loop bike route is marked by a redwood post sign that says "Forest History Trail," which is planted on the other side of the road opposite the trailhead. The trail is easy to see and drops off the right (south side) of the road just beyond the parking area. At the trailhead, you may be lucky to find a box stocked with trail guides. The booklet contains a rough map of the area, describes the trees and plants of this part of the forest, and provides information about the logging and history of the forest.

As you start down the trail, you descend a winding, narrow single-track, making tight turns, weaving past tan oak, madrone, Douglas fir, and, of course, redwood trees. You pass many large redwood stumps, remnants of logging from the turn of the century as well as quite a few trees brought down in the El Niño storms of 1998. At first, the trail winds along down a gradual slope, eventually threading through a group of moss-covered logs to the main trail intersection. Wonderful handcarved signs once marked the trails here. Now, all that remains are naked four- by four-foot posts. If you continue to follow the trail you've been riding, it would take you to the Observation Point, Cook House Gulch, and what is often known as the back side of the Forest History Trail. These trails, however, are designated for foot traffic only. The best route to take at this intersection is the trail that leads off to the left and down to Manly Gulch.

The trail starts off on a gentle slope, levels out and then takes you back up hill for a short while. Not far into it, you encounter your first obstacle, a short bridge made of logs sawn in half and laid lengthwise across a small ravine. Each plank is about eight inches wide. The space between each plank is just wide enough to swallow a bike tire. I always pick the second plank from the left but it's a matter of personal preference. You might want to walk this section—I have taken a nosedive down this ravine myself several times. Just beyond this plank-crossing, around the next bend, the trail seems to vanish through a narrow passage between two trees, a result of a quick turn to the left. It's a steep out-of-the-saddle climb and over a short rise. Just beyond this, around an old-growth redwood stump with a sharp drop-off to the outside and over a short narrow bridge, you reach the final rise. Now starts your descent.

The trail winds down the hillside, around a few large craters left by uprooted trees. Stay alert for you'll need to duck under several fallen trees lying over the trail. Ride past an old watering trough and a bit farther, you encounter your first tight rocky switchback. Soon after the switchback, the trail forks and there is a sign marked "Camp" with arrows pointing down both trails. The best trail for biking is straight ahead. (Taking the left fork will lead you down the other side of the gulch, over some older and questionable bridges and several long portage sections.) Stay on the main trail, and just ahead is a sharp gully which forces you to make a quick hard left before continuing the descent. Be prepared for the first portage section a short way beyond this point. The trail ends abruptly and drops down into a deep gulch without warning.

To the right, walk a crude log bridge over a trail rut and continue descending. One more switchback and a creek crossing later, and you're at the bottom of the gulch. Here you'll begin to ride a level or softly descending section. You reach a point where there may be a small tree lying across the trail—just wheelie over it. However, I advise walking over the bridge that follows. Just beyond the bridge is a short, steep rise with a sharp drop-off. If you are unsure of your skills, walk this section—many people do. What you can't see here is that just over the rise, a good half of the trail washed away in the 1998 storms. After that, you quickly traverse through a log garden. Keep a fair momentum, lift your front wheel at the right time and let it roll over the logs. You'll be through this fun obstacle course and across the creek in no time. Pedal through a few quick ups and downs and cross a well-constructed final log bridge. Soon, you enter the Mendocino Woodlands Recreation Area on a double-track trail that heads toward Road 700.

Stay on the double-track until you come to a **T** intersection with Road 700. It's signed here in the opposite direction, "Trail to Observation Point." Turn left here. Behave yourself now and ride quietly, staying on the dirt road. *This is a privately run camp; please respect the privacy of the people camping in this area.* Follow the road until you cross a bridge. There is a white sign with red letters that says "Fire Exit." Turn left onto this road, which is Road 730, and follow it back up to Road 408.

The climb back up to Road 408 is a steep, 2-mile climb with an elevation gain of about 1,000 feet. It's a long, steady climb that actually does get steeper as you approach the top—you're not just imagining it. The road never really levels out anywhere and proves to be a great workout.

Once at the top, go left onto Road 408 and follow it back to the trailhead, closing the loop after 6.7 miles. Road 408 is open to vehicular traffic, so keep your eyes out for occasional cars, trucks, and motorcycles.

If you're aching for more mileage and riding time, you might want to consider the Casper Creek–640–630 (Ride 18) Loop as you will be passing Road 630 on your way back to the trailhead and your car. Whatever you do, have fun.

RIDE 18 · Caspar Creek–640–630 Loop

AT A GLANCE

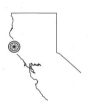

Length/configuration: 11.6-mile loop, clockwise; double-track and dirt logging roads

Aerobic difficulty: Moderate due to climbing

Technical difficulty: Easy to intermediate

Scenery: Mixed second- and third-growth redwood forest with blue ocean views on clear days

Special comments: Suitable for beginners with a moderate level of endurance. Also a good add-on ride to the Manly Gulch Loop.

Caspar Creek–640–630 Loop, an 11.6-mile loop, is in the Jackson Demonstration State Forest. Using mostly logging roads that appear to be double-track trails at times, this clockwise loop is great for beginners with decent endurance and with little technical skills. The following trail description is another fine contribution from Ray Houghton of Mendocino Mountain Bike Tours (read about him in the Manly Gulch Loop description). Thanks again, Ray. —L.A.

This loop takes you down into the watershed that feeds Caspar Creek and can be ridden in either direction. I usually ride down Road 640 and up Road 630 to avoid climbing a steep section on 640, near the bottom toward the creek, where it links to 630. This ride is all on logging roads, but the last time I was enjoying this loop, a good part of 630 had become overgrown to the point of almost being a trail.

However, being an actively logged forest, things like this often change over the course of a year. This is a great loop to add on to the adjacent Manly Gulch Loop.

General location: About 7 miles east of the village of Mendocino, about a 3.5-hour drive north of San Francisco on Highway 1 (CA 1).

Elevation change: 1,040 feet; starting elevation 880 feet; high point 1,200 feet; low point 160 feet. Mix of gentle and abrupt descents into the watershed, followed by climbs back out on a series of gradual hills.

Season: Year-round, though sections likely to be muddy from rain and lingering moisture. Logging operations, which generally occur in the summer, may close portions of the forest to public access. Call the Jackson Demonstration State Forest office for current conditions.

Services: No services on this trail. Limited food, gas, lodging, and other services in Mendocino. All other services in Fort Bragg.

Hazards: Jackson Demonstration State Forest allows deer hunting from mid-August through September. Wearing brightly colored clothing during hunting season is strongly advised. Watch out for poison oak, which can be found growing along the trails and roads. Deer ticks in the area are reported to have a 1% infection rate for Lyme disease. Avoid pinch flats by pumping up those tires.

Rescue index: Road 408 is lightly traveled by motorists. That means you should be self-reliant. In case of an emergency, your best chance for help is to make your way back to Road 408 and the starting point of this loop at near the Forest History Trail. During the summer, the History Trail is somewhat popular with visitors.

Land status: Jackson Demonstration State Forest, managed by the California Department of Forestry and Fire Protection.

Maps: *Jackson Demonstration State Forest*, published by the California Department of Forestry and Fire Protection.

Finding the trail: This ride uses the same starting point as the previous ride, Manly Gulch Loop. From Highway 1 (CA 1), go east on Little Lake Road, which eventually becomes Road 408. Stay on 408 for approximately 5.7 miles, at which point the road splits and the pavement ends. Stay to the left and follow the dirt road up a few short, steep climbs for about 1.3 miles to where the road levels out. Drive another several hundred yards to the Forest History Trail trailhead at mile marker 6.85. Don't expect to find a parking lot here. Instead, look for where the road widens, offering just enough space for several cars to park along the shoulder.

Sources of additional information: See sources of additional information for Ride 17.

Notes on the trail: Leaving from the parking area where the Forest History Trail is located, pedal north on Road 408 for 1.2 miles. For those of you that don't use a cyclometer, it takes between 5 to 10 minutes to get there. Once at Road 640, you see on the left a yellow metal gate with the number 640 painted in black on it. Just ride around the gate to the left and head down the road. The trail follows a series of gentle climbs and gradual descents. Stay alert for water bars in the road during the descents. These water bars are grooves cut into the road in order to divert water off the road and reduce erosion. They are almost always shallower on the uphill side of the road and deeper on the downhill side. They tend to show up when you least expect them.

As you ride along, you see several connecting roads and faint trails mostly leading off to your left. I've explored most of these and found them to be spur roads. These are roads that branch off main logging roads and allow trucks to reach specific areas of the forest. Most of them go on for a mile or two, only to end in a clearing, which trucks use to turn around. So, unless you have the time to get lost for a while and don't mind back-tracking, I'd avoid following any of these side roads. The one exception is Road 600, which leads to some nice trails. Road 600 was decommissioned in 1998 and the CDF (California Department of Forestry) has led me to believe that they plan to clear it and make it into a trail. The last time I looked, it was still impassable, but, like many things in the Jackson Demonstration State Forest, that could change in a season.

You know you're approaching the final downhill because it becomes steeper and longer than the previous ones. The road surface is loose and rocky. If you have the skill, this is a great place to let go and have some high-speed fun. Keep an eye open for water bars. At about 4.7 miles, you come to a junction in the road where the main road makes a tight left turn. Follow the road through the curve. If you miss the turn and go straight instead, the road quickly becomes less traveled. Not to worry. Both roads link up with Road 630 in roughly 100 yards. Turn right when you get to 630, though there will be no number here telling you are on Road 630. In roughly another 100 yards, go through another yellow gate. This one is usually open and will have no other markings. Here is where you begin climbing up and out of the Caspar watershed.

The climb starts with a gentle slope, almost level, rolling up and down for a few miles. The trail is lined with blackberry, thimbleberry, and huckleberry bushes. Who can resist all these enticing berries that line the trail? In late summer, I always like to stop and enjoy a quick snack of sweet, juicy berries.

Through much of the climb, the road looks very lightly used. The way back up is a gradual one. The road rolls up, leveling off and even cruising back down before heading up again. From the beginning of the climb, the road surface is mostly dirt, somewhat overgrown—sometimes to the point of being a single-track trail. The climb out along Road 630 is something that won't overstress a rider of moderate physical fitness.

As you near the top of the climb, the road surface becomes more strewn with gravel and starts to look a bit more traveled. Go past a road that intersects from behind your left shoulder, sort of like a Y junction. Just a bit farther, the road climbs a bit steeper, then levels off slightly, and there's a short, easy downhill on which to quickly catch your breath. Peer through the trees and on a clear day, you can see the Pacific Ocean in the distance. On other days, fog fills the watershed depending on the time of year and even the time of day. Continue on the road as you make your way up to Road 408. You pass another Y junction with a trail coming in from behind your left shoulder. When you pass this intersection, you know that the top of the climb is near. Not far from the Y, go around a bend and meet up with another big yellow gate. Painted on the outside of that gate in black numbers is 630. Here is where you close the loop by linking up with Road 408 again. Turn right onto 408 and retrace your path back to the parking area. On your way back, you go past the road to Old Mill Farm (Road 740) and Road 730 (the fire exit road for the Mendocino Woodlands), both on your left. End your ride at the parking area near the Forest History Trail.

RIDE 19 · Fern Canyon Trail— Van Damme State Park

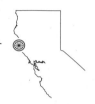

AT A GLANCE

Length/configuration: 4.6-mile out-and-back (2.3 miles each way); paved bike path; optional 15-mile loop, counterclockwise combines the bike path with 12.7 miles of paved vehicle road

Aerobic difficulty: Easy out-and-back. Optional loop is moderate.

Technical difficulty: Both out-and-back and optional loop are not technical

Scenery: Follows Little River through a deep canyon smothered by luxuriant forest of impressively large second-growth redwoods. Worth a look is the Pygmy Forest, site of decades-old but very short cypress and pine trees.

Special comments: The bike path is completely free of vehicles, making the out-and-back a great family ride. Interpretive signs throughout the trail give insight into the life cycle of the indigenous Coho salmon.

Welcome to the Fern Canyon Trail in Van Damme State Park. Like its identically named neighbor just up the road—Fern Canyon Trail in Russian Gulch State Park—both trails hold many similarities. Still, Van Damme's Fern Canyon Trail is deserving of its own stage. For such a short route, it offers much to discover.

Located on the east side of Highway 1 (CA 1), this Fern Canyon Trail is a 4.6-mile out-and-back (2.3 miles each way) paved bike path. Totally devoid of motor vehicles, it's a great outing for families and anyone seeking a serene and leisurely riding experience. The trail offers a journey through a deep, forested canyon, thick with shady second-growth redwoods and conifers. Every now and then your nose catches a delightful whiff that reminds you of Christmas trees. The understory is rich with huge ferns, nettles, and rhododendrons. Running due east, the Fern Canyon path weaves back and forth over Little River, crossing it nine times via footbridges. And thanks to the typical moist weather and the surrounding dense forest, the paved trail often resembles a dirt path, having been blanketed by fallen pine needles and other debris. (If you ride in any season other than summer, call the state park office listed below to check on the status of the trail since stormy weather may have brought down tree limbs. Ask about creek crossings, because footbridges are usually in place only during the summer.)

But hey, there's more than just riding through a lush canyon on this route. Not to be missed are the beautifully illustrated signs and interpretative stops that discuss the life cycle and habitat of the indigenous and rare Coho salmon. Posted throughout the trail are rustic metal cutouts in the shape of salmon and numbered to correspond to an informative color leaflet (available at the trailhead). Though the route was originally used as an old skid road for hauling logs, give thanks the Civilian Conservation Corp (CCC) for laying the groundwork on the trail which we enjoy today. The CCC was a government work program designed to employ thousands of men during the Depression in the late 1930s and early 1940s. Crews worked in this

RIDE 19 · Fern Canyon Trail—Van Damme State Park

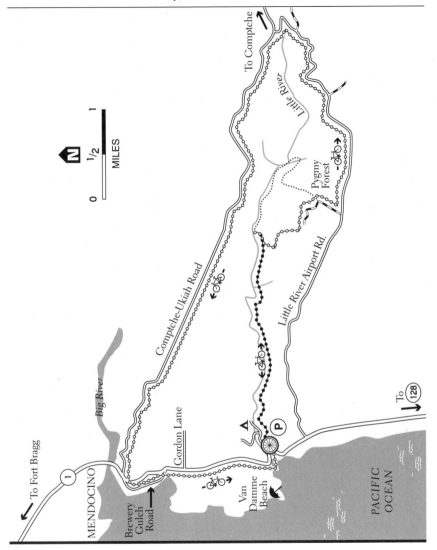

canyon, building campgrounds and trails, including this one. Maintaining a natural landscape was a priority, especially when building numerous rock river crossings. Driven by enthusiasm and the need for work, the crews were unaware of their impact on the migratory habits of wild salmon. The painstakingly laid crossings acted as a dam across the river. Today, state and local parks staff have worked to remove most of these obstacles in an effort to restore salmon habitat. Some of the artistic masonry still exists.

And here's one for *Ripley's Believe It or Not!*: Located just beyond the eastern terminus of the Fern Canyon Trail is the fascinating Pygmy Forest, the result of an amazing interaction of soil, geology, and climate. Here, adjacent to the fertile rain

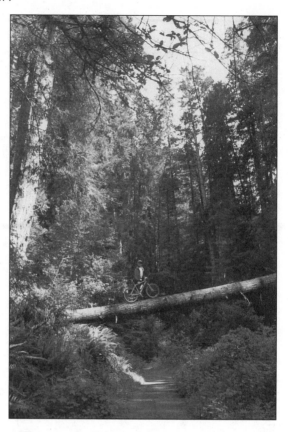

Bruce finds a different
view of the bike path and
Creek Canyon.

forest–like canyon, is a curious display of decades-old but very short cypress and pine trees, stunted by the acidic soil, some measuring less than an inch in diameter. Beginners and leisurely riders will want to turn around here and return to their car via Fern Canyon Trail.

Aching for more of an aerobic workout? At the eastern end of the trail, moderately strong riders wanting to pedal more miles have the opportunity to connect with a paved vehicle road, making the outing a 15-mile counterclockwise loop. From the Pygmy Forest, the trail becomes dirt and climbs steeply out of the canyon for a short distance before hitting a paved road. Once on the road, the route climbs gradually for several miles past sleepy homes tucked in between the redwoods. When you reach the ridge, you're rewarded with views of the Big River watershed and the coastline before descending five miles and nearly 500 feet to Highway 1 and eventually back to your car.

General location: 3 miles south of Mendocino on Highway 1 (CA 1).

Elevation change: 220 feet; starting elevation and low point 20 feet; high point 240 feet. Basically flat. Optional loop: 780-foot change; starting elevation and low point 20 feet; high point 800 feet. Add-on portion climbs moderately up pavement, then descends gradually.

Season: Year-round, though the weather is likely to be wet with fog and rain in the winter and spring months. Small wooden bridges are in place during the summer. At other times of the year, expect to deal with wet creek crossings.

Services: Pay phone, drinking water, picnic tables, and rest rooms available near the trailhead. Campground with showers open year-round (reservations are recommended between May 1 and September 30). All other services in Mendocino and Fort Bragg.

Hazards: Scattered poison oak and stinging nettle along the bike path. Trail crosses Little River about nine times. During the summer months, footbridges are usually in place, giving you a dry creek crossing. In the off-season, the bridges are moved off to one side of the river to protect them from winter runoff damage. Though the trail is accessible year-round, expect wet crossings in the off-season. Use the first crossing as your gauge to determine difficulty, since all subsequent crossings will not be easier. Cyclists who opt for the loop need to be cautious of vehicles, especially on Highway 1 where the shoulder is either narrow or nonexistent, and traffic can be frequent during the summer months.

Rescue index: The route is popular with other trail users during the summer, and you can usually find someone who can offer assistance. In the off-season, weekday users are fewer and the visitor center is likely to be closed. So, in case of emergency, make your way back to Highway 1 or the paved vehicle road at the far end of the paved trail, and flag down a passing motorist. There is a pay phone at the park entrance.

Land status: Van Damme State Park.

Maps: A map can be found in the *Northwind Mendocino Coast Parks Guide*, a free tabloid published annually by the Mendocino Area Parks Association and the California Department of Parks and Recreation. The publication is available at many visitor centers and chambers of commerce throughout coastal Mendocino County. For more information, see the MAPA address listed below in "Sources of additional information."

Finding the trail: Fern Canyon Trail is located on the east side of Highway 1 (CA 1). From Mendocino, drive south on Highway 1, following the rugged coastline as it weaves and descends. At about 3 miles, the road descends steeply to sea level. Here, on the east side of Highway 1, across from Van Damme Beach is the entrance to the State Park. You have a choice of several parking places. Parking is available in the beach parking lot, on the west side of Highway 1. If you have young children, you can avoid crossing Highway 1 by parking inside the state park. Expect to pay a parking fee during the summer.

Sources of additional information:

Mendocino Area Parks Association
P.O. Box 1387
Mendocino, CA 95460
(707) 937-5397

Van Damme State Park
Mendocino District Headquarters
P.O. Box 440
Mendocino, CA 95460
(707) 937-5804

Notes on the trail: This is a fairly easy route to follow. Start pedaling from inside the state park, just past the entry kiosk and continue on the main state park road as it leads due east past the visitor center and camping areas. Cross over a bridge and look for a brown sign indicating Fern Canyon and the beginning of the paved bike path. If you're interested in learning about the Coho salmon in this habitat, pick up a color leaflet at the trailhead. It corresponds to sites along the route.

The trail hugs Little River every inch of the way toward the Pygmy Forest, weaving back and forth across the river. (If you ride in the off-season, don't expect the small footbridges to be in place. Usually, you can easily cross the creek without getting too wet. Keep in mind, though, that if your first wet crossing is difficult, the subsequent other eight crossings will be no easier, if not more challenging.) The winter storms of early 1998 caused significant trail erosion in some places, so expect to encounter some rugged and rutted sections in the otherwise smooth bike path.

No other trails intersect Fern Canyon Trail, until almost 2 miles from the beginning of the paved bike path, at which point, the trail splits. The right path gently descends toward Little River, while the left climbs gradually a for a few yards. The trails rejoin in about 0.1 mile. Follow whichever route you wish. A few yards farther and you reach the end of paved Fern Canyon Trail. Two dirt trails continue beyond. The signed left trail is a hiking-only path and leads to the Pygmy Forest in 2.3 miles. The right trail is unsigned and bikes are allowed. If you have time, leave your bike here and walk the 2.3 miles to the Pygmy Forest. It's worth a look. Then, hop back on your bike and return the way you came.

Optional loop: At the end of the paved trail, take the right unsigned dirt trail (really a narrow jeep road) and follow it as it descends, crossing over Little River and threading past a few pygmy trees. Climb steeply out of the ravine for about 1.7 miles until you reach Little River–Airport Road, a paved, narrow two-lane vehicle road. Watch out for vehicles. There's not much of a shoulder but fortunately, the road is not heavily traveled. Hang a left onto this road and continue a gradual climb. Follow Little River–Airport Road, eventually curving left and right past quiet homes tucked in the shade of the redwood forest. After about 3.3 miles on this road, you reach Comptche-Ukiah Road, another paved, two-lane vehicle road. Turn left onto it, stay alert for traffic, and begin a fun gradual descent, heading northwest toward the ocean. After about 5 miles from this intersection, you reach Highway 1. Directly across the road is Brewery Gulch Road (another paved road that was unsigned the last time I was here). Cautiously go across busy Highway 1 and continue due west on Brewery Gulch Road. The road curves south and steepens significantly, though briefly, as it climbs the bluff, bordered on the west by modest oceanfront homes. What terrific views these homes must have! In less than a mile, Brewery Gulch intersects Highway 1. Go right onto Highway 1, cautiously riding the narrow shoulder. Here comes a fast and fun curvy descent to sea level and Van Damme Beach. Close the loop by making your way back to your car, which you have either parked at the beach parking lot or inside the state park. Traffic can be heavy at times, so be cautious, especially if you need to cross over to the east side of Highway 1.

RIDE 20 · Fern Canyon Trail—
Russian Gulch State Park

AT A GLANCE

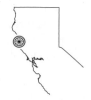

Length/configuration: 3.2-mile out-and-back (1.6 miles each way); roughly paved bike path

Aerobic difficulty: Easy

Technical difficulty: Not technical

Scenery: A lovely deep canyon carved by Russian Gulch, cloaked by dense riparian growth in the shade of second-growth redwoods. The 36-foot-tall Russian Gulch Falls can be accessed via a 0.7 mile hiking-only trail.

Special comments: A short and easy route, perfect for families. Great picnic spot at the end of the paved trail.

Similar to Van Damme State Park's Fern Canyon just a few miles south of here, Russian Gulch State Park's Fern Canyon Trail is paved, flat, easy, and incredibly gorgeous. And because it's free of motor vehicles, it makes a perfect outing for families and anyone wanting a leisurely ride. As a 3.2-mile out-and-back (1.6 miles each way), this trail has virtually no elevation change, and because you stay on the paved trail, you'd really have to work hard to get lost.

Yes, it's a short route, but oh, what a scenic and serene journey it is. The trail hugs Russian Gulch, a small but lively creek flowing through a deep and fragrant riparian canyon. Here you'll find the thick understory is composed of huge leather ferns, large patches of moss, and rhododendron tucked within a dense forest of second-growth redwoods, bay laurel, tan oak, Douglas fir, and big-leaf maple trees, to name a few species. Located at the end of the paved trail, under the canopy of tall redwoods, are several picnic tables and a bike rack. Here, you'll find a hiking-only trail leading to Russian Gulch Falls in less than a mile. The waterfall is a lovely 36-foot spout that plunges into a rocky basin crowded by ferns and moss, particularly impressive in late winter.

General location: 2 miles north of Mendocino and 8 miles south of Fort Bragg on Highway 1 (CA 1).

Elevation change: Negligible change, mostly at sea level.

Season: Year-round, though the weather is likely to be wet with fog and rain in the winter and spring months.

Services: Pay phone, drinking water, picnic tables, and rest rooms inside the park near the main entrance. Campground with hot showers generally open mid-March to mid-October. All other services in Mendocino and Fort Bragg.

Hazards: Occasional poison oak.

Rescue index: Because the route is popular with other trail users, especially in the summer, you're bound to find someone who might be able to offer assistance. There are less users on weekdays, particularly in the off-season, and for that reason, you should make your way back to the trailhead in an emergency situation.

Land status: Russian Gulch State Park.

Maps: A map can be found in the *Northwind Mendocino Coast Parks Guide,* a free tabloid published annually by the Mendocino Area Parks Association and the California Department of Parks and Recreation. The publication is available at many visitor centers and chambers of commerce throughout coastal Mendocino County. For more information, see the MAPA address listed below in "Sources of additional information."

Finding the trail: From Mendocino, drive north on Highway 1 (CA 1) for almost 2 miles to the Russian Gulch State Park entrance, located on the west side (ocean side) of Highway 1. After turning off of Highway 1, make an immediate left into the

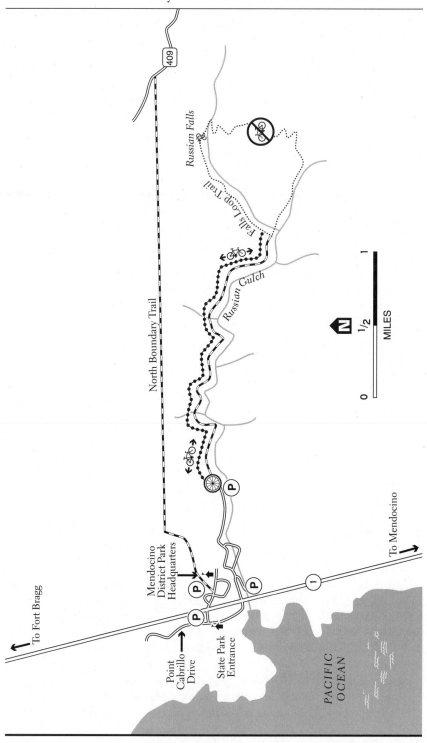

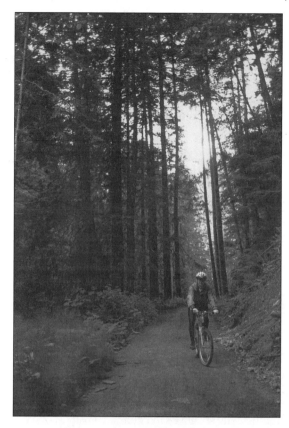

This easy path skirts a rich riparian environment and ends at a hiking trail leading up to Russian Gulch Falls.

state park. Go past the fee kiosk and follow the paved road as it leads under Highway 1, heading east. The road takes you through the campground area and you can park here in the day-use area, or continue east to the end of the road, past Camp 30 and the South Trail wooden bridge, to where the Fern Canyon Trailhead is located. Alternate parking: on the shoulder of the road outside the park kiosk (not on Highway 1). This option adds about a mile of pavement riding to the start of the out-and-back section.

Sources of additional information:

Mendocino Area Parks Association
P.O. Box 1387
Mendocino, CA 95460
(707) 937-5397

Russian Gulch State Park
Mendocino District Headquarters
P.O. Box 440
Mendocino, CA 95460
(707) 937-5804

Notes on the trail: Before setting out, pack a bike lock, just in case you want to visit the waterfall located beyond the far end of the trail and accessed by a short walking-only trail. Being an easy trail to follow, you really don't need a map since the route stays on the paved path. It's only 1.6 miles one way and basically heads due east, always on the north side of Russian Gulch, with no real significant turns or trail junctions. The North Trail, a dirt hiking path, intersects paved Fern Canyon Trail on both ends of the route and is off-limits to bikes. Other than a few minor storm-damaged spots, it's an easy, flat 10- to 15-foot-wide paved trail, free of any water crossings.

When you reach the end of the paved trail at 1.6 miles, you can leave your bike on the bike rack provided and follow the hiking-only trail to the lively 36-foot Russian Gulch Falls. The waterfall is a 0.7 mile hike one way, so you could walk a loop back to your bike for a total distance of 2.3 miles. After enjoying the serene forest, hop back on your bike and return the way you came.

RIDE 21 · MacKerricher Ten Mile Coastal Trail

AT A GLANCE

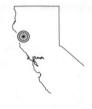

Length/configuration: 7-mile out-and-back (3.5 miles each way); paved trail; optional 14-mile out-and-back (7 miles each way)

Aerobic difficulty: Easy; on paved path; longer option leads to the northern end of the trail, where there's a 1-mile stretch of arduous walking over beach sand to bypass a washout

Technical difficulty: Not technical

Scenery: Picturesque old railroad trestle over Pudding Creek. Bluff riding with great views of the ocean, terrific for whale and harbor seal watching and exploring tide pools, especially at Laguna Point. Terrain includes stretches of environmentally sensitive sand dunes, a small lagoon and popular Lake Cleone.

Special comments: Great outing for families and cyclists wanting a leisurely ride. Lots to hold the interest of youngsters, including a nature walk around the lake and campfire programs in the summer.

The Ten Mile Coastal Trail, also referred to as the Old Haul Road, hugs the shoreline bluffs and dunes from Fort Bragg north to Ten Mile River. The river gets its creative name for the fact that it's 10 miles north of the Noyo River. The Ten Mile Coastal Trail is really a seven-mile out-and-back stretch (3.5 miles each way) of mostly paved trail. Unfortunately, winter storms over the years have washed away an approximate one-mile stretch in the midsection of this route, thus foiling an otherwise pleasant seven-mile northerly trek to Ten Mile River. If you're a hearty rider, you have the option of traversing the washout by foot in order to rejoin the paved trail and continue on to the northern terminus. Otherwise, you can use the washout, reached at about 3.5 miles from the southern starting point, as your turnaround.

The asphalt trail travels north and south, offering panoramic vistas of the ocean and dunes. The southern terminus is the picturesque Pudding Creek railroad trestle, situated on the northern edge of Fort Bragg. Near the midsection of the route is Laguna Point, the site of a Pomo Indian encampment. Loading chutes for logging schooners later took over the site. Today, the Point is a popular place to view the horde of resident harbor seals and the seasonal parade of migrating whales, generally December though April. The dirt trail on the bluff and the boardwalks at Laguna

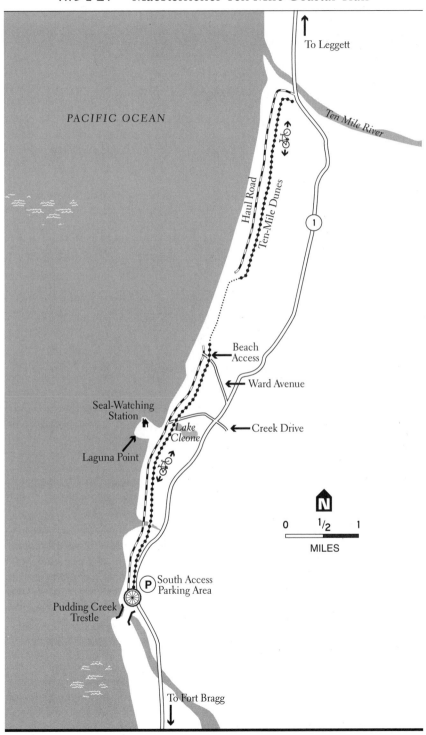

PACIFIC OCEAN

To Leggett

Ten Mile River

Haul Road

Ten-Mile Dunes

1

Beach
Access

Ward Avenue

Seal-Watching
Station

Creek Drive

Lake
Cleone

Laguna Point

N

0   1/2   1
MILES

South Access
Parking Area

P

Pudding Creek
Trestle

To Fort Bragg

Point, however, are off-limits to bikes. Still, it's worth a stroll to explore tide pools and view the rugged, exposed bedrock. Close to the Point is Lake Cleone, a small lake that's popular for fishing and bird-watching. Campgrounds and the park's visitor center are located alongside the lake.

The trail was originally used by American Indians over 140 years ago. As with much of this area, logging operations flourished and dominated land use. The trail became a haul road connecting the loading docks at Laguna Point. In 1915, a railroad was built alongside the trail to transport logs to the mills in Fort Bragg. Thirty-four years later, the rail tracks were removed and the trail paved over to accommodate roaring logging trucks. But, whatever Mother Nature wants, she gets, one way or another. Erosion was (and still is) an ongoing occurrence and in 1983, after a major storm, significant portions of the haul road were washed away by the pounding surf, effectively halting logging transportation. The Georgia Pacific Company, who owned the road at the time, decided not repair the road. The California Department of Parks and Recreations acquired the road between 1992 and 1995, including small portions of the surrounding land and Lake Cleone. The acquisition eventually opened for recreational use as MacKerricher State Park.

Today, the trail remains interrupted by the washed-out section. Restoration of the trail is still under consideration since the area affected involves environmentally sensitive sand dunes that support threatened and endangered species of flora and fauna. Several beautifully illustrated and informative interpretative signs are posted along the trail. No doubt, the fate of an Indian archeological site next to the trail will be impacted. What all this means is that the original project to restore the trail is on hold, pending results of an environmental impact review. Once revisions to the project are accepted, restoration will commence and take from three to five years to complete, using federal, state, and public grant funds.

General location: 3 miles north of Fort Bragg on the west side of Highway 1 (CA 1).

Elevation change: Negligible change, mostly at sea level.

Season: Trail accessible year-round, though the weather is likely to be wet with fog and rain in the winter and spring months.

Services: Drinking water, rest rooms, and beautiful campsites. Small grocery store and gas approximately 0.25 mile north of the park. All other services available in Fort Bragg.

Hazards: None along the designated bike path. Bringing a bike lock is recommended for the times you wish to check out walking-only paths. If you explore the tide pools at Laguna Point, be aware that rocks can be slippery. If you venture out to the beach, watch out for the occasional huge waves capable of sweeping you into the surf—children must be supervised at all times. Windy, blustery days create stinging sand storms, making the ride a bit uncomfortable.

Rescue index: This is a popular route, especially with local folks. Nearby residential neighborhoods line the eastern edge of this narrow strip of coastal park.

Land status: MacKerricher State Park.

Maps: A map can be found in the *Northwind Mendocino Coast Parks Guide*, a free annual tabloid published by the Mendocino Area Parks Association and the California Department of Parks and Recreation. The publication is available at many visitor centers and chambers of commerce throughout coastal Mendocino County. For more information, see the MAPA address listed below.

Finding the trail: You can access the trail at several places: near the southern end of the trail or at the main park entrance at Mill Creek Road and Lake Cleone. To get to the southern access point from Fort Bragg, drive north on Highway 1 (CA 1) to the northern edge of town. Stay on Highway 1, go over Pudding Creek and continue for about a mile. Keep an eye out for a small, unsigned dirt parking lot on the west side of the road, adjacent to a strip of buildings. Look closely and you can see the bike path from Highway 1. If you go past Airport Road, you've gone too far. From Fort Bragg, to reach the park's main entrance, continue as above, going past Airport Road. In a little over 3 miles from Pudding Creek, you reach the main entry to MacKerricher State Park. Turn left into the park, toward the ocean, and park near Lake Cleone or closer to the beach near Laguna Point. Access the trail by heading toward the ocean.

Sources of additional information:

Mendocino Area Parks Association
P.O. Box 1387
Mendocino, CA 95460
(707) 937-5397

California Department of Parks and
    Recreation
Mendocino District Headquarters
P.O. Box 440
Mendocino, CA 95460
(707) 937-5804

Ten Mile Coastal Trail Foundation
P.O. Box 1534
Fort Bragg, CA 95437-1534
(707) 964-9340
www.mcn.org/1/10milecoastaltrail

Notes on the trail: Whichever starting point you choose, you can't get lost since the trail hugs the shoreline and it's a paved path that's about 15 feet wide. Keep in mind that bikes are allowed only on the paved trail (except for the beach at the washed-out section). If you want to explore any of the dirt trails, plan to lock your bike or portage it. Both access points place you on the southern continuous 3-mile stretch of the paved trail, between the Pudding Creek trestle and the washed-out section, with Laguna Point and Lake Cleone in between. You can use the washout and the trestle as your turnaround points.

Optional miles: If you're looking for more miles, drop down to the beach (please stay off the sensitive sand dunes on the inland side of the trail) and trudge past the washed-out section, portaging or cajoling your bike before reconnecting with the paved trail. Once back on the asphalt, continue north and in about 2 miles, go past Ten Mile Beach and Dunes, a state park–designated preserve. At least 12 threatened or endangered species are protected here, including the Howell's spineflower, menzies wallflower, and the western snowy plover and for that reason, you're asked to stay on the trail. (Occasionally, ranger-led groups are allowed onto the dunes.) Keep a sharp eye out for decaying piles of seashells, evidence that coastal Indian tribes once camped here and lived off the bounty of the sea. If you're blessed with a clear day, look northward and you can see the rugged coastline of the Sinkyone Wilderness and the Lost Coast in the distance. At just over 4 miles from the washout, the trail curves inland, paralleling Ten Mile River. By now, the tall grass on the dunes on your left obscures your view of the ocean. In a short distance, the paved trail ends at Highway 1. Turn around and head back on the trail.

OTHER AREA RIDES

TOUR DE SKUNK: This is an annual organized mountain-biking event that benefits the Mendocino Coast Recreation and Park District Community Center. The day's adventure begins in Fort Bragg with a 22-mile train ride on the historic Skunk Train, a steam locomotive. From deep within Jackson Demonstration State Forest, amidst thick redwood forests, bikers disembark and pedal 26 miles back into town, following logging roads and old migratory Native American trails. With enthusiastic cooperation from the state agency, typically restricted areas of the Demonstration Forest are opened for the event. Held in either late September or early October, this fun event is suitable for children and is limited to the first 250 riders that sign up. Cost is about $55 per person (less for children under 18 years) and includes train fare, a continental breakfast, catered lunch, and manned rest stops.

For more information, contact:
Mendocino Coast Recreation and Park District
P.O. Box 907
213 E. Laurel St.
Fort Bragg, CA 95437
(800) 726-2780
www.mcn.org/l/mcrpd/mcrskpgl.htm

NAVARRO RIDGE ROAD: Like most ridges, you can expect ups and downs on Navarro Ridge Road. Originally a stagecoach route, this county road is a combination of little-used narrow pavement, gravel roads, and dirt double-tracks. Not always maintained after a winter storm, don't be surprised to find downed trees in the outer, lesser-used stretches. Expansive views of mountain ranges and deep canyons are rewards on this route. Riding Navarro Ridge is essentially an out-and-back affair, which means you can turn around when you're good and tired. Technically, the road is mild. Aerobically, it can be easy to strenuous, depending on how far you ride. You can also make this a 27-mile loop via CA 128, a well-traveled vehicle road with traffic that runs through "a tunnel of redwoods" in the Navarro River Redwoods State Park. The first 6 miles (almost 12 miles round-trip) is relatively easy on mostly paved, quiet roads, and the climbing is moderate. As you continue farther on Navarro Ridge Road, the brief climbs are more frequent and arduous.

Finding the trail: From Fort Bragg, head south on Highway 1 (CA 1) and go through the towns of Mendocino, Little River, and Albion. Just before CA 128, watch out for Navarro Ridge Road leading east from Highway 1. Park in a nearby wide dirt pulloff on the west side of Highway 1 and begin pedaling from here.

Maps: USGS Elk and Navarro 7.5 minute series.

For more information, contact:

Mendocino County
Department of Transportation
340 Lake Mendocino Dr.
Ukiah, CA 95482
(707) 463-4363

COW MOUNTAIN RECREATION AREA: This 50,000-acre playground is located between Clear Lake and the town of Ukiah, in the Mayacmas Mountains. Lying mostly in eastern Mendocino County, spilling into neighboring Lake County, Cow Mountain is managed by the BLM. Many of the bikeable routes are dirt roads, accessible to motorized vehicles. The area is divided into north and south sections. The southern portion, where the majority of the land is found, caters to OHV recreation, which means if you ride there, you'll have to share the roads with noisy dirt bikes, all-terrain vehicles, and jeeps. Fortunately, the northern section (27,000 acres) is closed to off-highway vehicles and provides over 30 miles of dirt roads, ranging from smooth, mildly technical fire roads to rugged four-wheel-drive jeep trails. Aerobically, the terrain varies from moderate to strenuous.

Finding the trail: To reach the main entrance of the north section, travel north on US 101 toward Ukiah. As you enter Ukiah city limits, take Talmadge Road (CA 222) east to East Side Road, and then turn left onto Mill Creek Road. Follow Mill Creek as it heads east, then southeast for about 4 miles. Look for a trailhead on the left side of the road. Park in any of the pulloffs and begin pedaling on the trail, which is Valley View Trail. You've just driven past the Valley View trailhead if you reach Mendo Rock Road (a dirt fire road). No matter. You can ride up Mendo Rock to Willow Creek Recreation Site where you can pick up Valley View Trail or just continue on the fire road.

For a topo map and more information, contact:

Cow Mountain Recreation Area
Bureau of Land Management
Clear Lake Resource Area
2550 North State St.
Ukiah, CA 95482-3023

Vichy Springs Resort
2605 Vichy Springs Road (same as
   Perkins Street in Ukiah)
Ukiah, CA 95482-3507
(707) 462-9515
This is a 700-acre property located on the western edge of the north section. This historic bed-and-breakfast inn offers lovely rooms and quaint cottages, naturally bubbly mineral baths, and soothing massages. The resort's biking and hiking trails lead directly into Cow Mountain. Mountain bikers are enthusiastically welcomed.

LETTS LAKE RECREATION AREA: The area was settled by the Lett brothers in 1855, both of whom were murdered in 1877 by a squatter who was constructing a cabin on their property. Today, Letts Valley is designated a California Historical Landmark and is listed in the National Register of Historic Places. Located in the southern portion of Mendocino National Forest, just below Snow Mountain Wilderness, this area offers many miles of bikeable dirt roads, usually offering impressive views of the Wilderness Area. Consider setting up a base camp at Letts Lake so that you can ride the following three routes. One of the loveliest yet little-known camping spots in the state, several seasonally maintained campgrounds are available with piped water, vault toilets, and picnic tables. Fishing enthusiasts will be glad to know that the lake is stocked with brook trout. Letts Lake Loop is 7.5 miles on unimproved road and is suitable for beginners with decent endurance. Reportedly well-signed and easy to follow, this route has a few moderate climbs and leads through a conifer forest. A clockwise direction is recommended. Miner Ridge Loop is also 7.5 miles but uses low-maintenance roads, including OHV trails, with a short stretch on paved county road. Steep grades in some spots combined with rocky terrain and ruts demand strong endurance and advanced skills. South End Loop is a longer ride, clocking in at 24 miles on unimproved dirt road. You need strong endurance to do this entire ride in one day. Camping along the way is an option and several sites are available on the route.

Finding the trails: On I-5 next to the town of Maxwell, head west on Maxwell Sites Road, following it through the tiny towns of Sites, Lodoga (on Sites Lodoga Road), and then Stonyford (on Lodoga Stonyford Road). [Incidentally, be sure to stop by the Stonyford Ranger District Office at 5080 Lodoga Stonyford Road and pick up a map and more info on the area's bikeable trails.] In Stonyford, go right (west) to Fouts Springs, following Fouts Springs Road. Pick up Letts Valley Road and continue west and then southwest. Go past Lily Lake and proceed about a mile farther to Upper Letts Lake and its campground. Park in this vicinity. Letts Lake Loop is located immediately south of the lake, and the bike route basically follows Forest Service Road 17N14. Contrary to what the name implies, this ride is not a loop around the lake. Miner Ridge Loop is just east of the Letts Lake and follows designated OHV trails. South End Loop makes a huge circle to the east of Letts Lake. It follows a portion of Letts Lake Loop and encircles Miner Ridge Loop via FS 18N07 (Trough Spring Ridge) to Fouts Springs, County Road M10, and FS 17N02, and closely skirts Lily Lake.

Maps: USGS Fouts Springs 7.5 minute series.

For more information, contact or visit:
Mendocino National Forest
Stonyford Ranger District
5080 Lodoga Stonyford Rd.
Stonyford, CA 95979
(916) 963-3128

SOME LOCAL BICYCLE SHOPS & RELATED BUSINESSES

Mendocino Mountain Bike Tours
10450 Nichols Ln.
Mendocino, CA 95460
(707) 937-3069

Fort Bragg Cyclery
579 South Franklin St.
Fort Bragg, CA 95437
(707) 964-3509

Catch A Canoe & Bicycles, Too!
Coast Highway One at Comptche-
  Ukiah Road, next to The Stanford
  Inn By The Sea
P.O. Box 487
Mendocino, CA 95460
(707) 937-0273
Probably one of the most unique and
fairly well-stocked bike stores you'll
ever see. It sits on a dock floating on
Big River.

THE WINE COUNTRY

When the Franciscan fathers planted the first grapevines in Sonoma Valley, little did they know they were launching the multi-billion dollar industry we know today. Yet, like a cruel stepsister, it is neighboring Napa Valley that enjoys the international reputation, with its numerous award-winning small wineries and fine restaurants. Unlike Napa, Sonoma Valley has far fewer wineries but more fruit and nut orchards, livestock farms, and is much less pretentious. Both snug valleys lie within the Coastal Range and parallel one another, running north to south, separated by a low mountain range. Napa Valley is a narrow valley that stretches 35 miles, anchored in the south by the bustling city of Napa and in the north by the funky but fun, mud-obsessed town of Calistoga (that's mud as in beautifying, rejuvenating mud-baths). Sonoma Valley is also a narrow valley, but covers much less territory, only about 17 miles long. It's anchored by the peaceful towns of Sonoma and Kenwood, south and north ends respectively.

Let's face it. The Wine Country is a mecca for wine lovers, not mountain bikers. Still, you don't have to be a wine lover to enjoy this part of the state. Like its fine wines, bike trails in this region are somewhere between "robust, bold, complex, and full-bodied with a hint of bell pepper" and "light, crisp, and fruity with essence of freshly mowed lawn." Take Oat Hill Mine Road for example. Its gnarly, intensely rocky character is definitely full-bodied and complex—best left to riders with highly developed bike handling skills who have acquired an unshakeable taste for the tough stuff. Mt. St. Helena, on the other hand, offers smooth terrain that doesn't require much more than basic skills and a fair amount of endurance. Generally speaking, a respectable amount of great trails can be found along and in the mountainsides that shape both valleys. Go further west toward coastal Sonoma County along the Russian River and northwest into Lake County near Clear Lake and you open yourself up to more riding adventures. One word of advice: If you want to partake of wine tastings by biking from one winery to the next, I don't recommend doing it during the height of the tourist season, that is, summer and early fall. Traffic on the paved two-lane roads is a nightmare of touring motorists, especially on the weekends.

RIDE 22 · Boggs Mountain Demonstration Forest

AT A GLANCE

Length/configuration: 12.9-mile loop; single-track and fire road

Aerobic difficulty: Moderate; some steep sections

Technical difficulty: Mildly technical; some intermediate sections of narrow single-track

Scenery: Nothing but trees, trees, and more trees. Primarily pine and fir forest. If you're lucky, you might see a black bear.

Special comments: Lots of different routing configurations possible on a number of single-track and fire roads. Well-placed fire roads offer bail-out options for beginners who quickly get their fill of single-tracks. A frequent site for NORBA races.

The primary purpose of Boggs Mountain Demonstration Forest is not recreation but forestry for commercial purposes. But the folks who manage the place enthusiastically welcome outdoor activities so much that you'd think recreation was Boggs' main objective. Among bikers, Boggs is known for its endless miles of pure, sweet, completely rideable single-track trails. Though not a huge chunk of land—it's only 3,493 acres surrounded by private property—the network of single-tracks along with a few fire roads offer many ride configurations. Beginners as well as advanced riders will find lots of agreeable trails here. Collectively, the trails are, for the most part, mildly technical since conditions are semi- and hard-packed dirt with some exposed tree roots and loose bits of rock thrown in for good fun, of course. Aerobically, moderate endurance is required since there are a few strenuously steep but short sections. The 12.9-mile loop described here is a mixture of short ups and downs, giving you a generous taste of the kinds of single-tracks and fire roads in the forest. By all means, make up your own configurations. Most, but not all, trails and fire roads are signed.

So what exactly is a demonstration forest? Sometimes called an experimental forest, these areas are actively managed by the California Department of Forestry. Its objective is to demonstrate and experiment with techniques involving continuous growing and harvesting practices in order to foster wise economic and ecological use of the forest's resources. That includes managing wildlife habitat, watersheds, and, for some areas, allowing public recreation. Sad but true, not all demonstration forests welcome, encourage, or allow recreational use. Boggs, however, is a rarity. It's rumored that a bunch of the forest personnel here like to mountain bike and the trails give them an opportunity to stay in shape while working in the field. Great job, no?

General location: 23 miles north of Calistoga, just beyond the northern edge of the Napa Valley.

Elevation change: 980 feet; starting elevation 2,850 feet; high point 3,700 feet; low point 2,720 feet. Lots of ups and downs interspersed with flat, cruising stretches.

Season: Year-round.

Services: Camping is free. Fifteen campsites at Calso Camp and some group sites at Ridge Camp, all of which include tables and fire rings. Pit toilets at the campgrounds.

RIDE 22 · Boggs Mountain Demonstration Forest

Hazards: Hunting for deer, mountain quail, and tree squirrels permitted in the fall. Few black bears and mountain lions have been sighted.

Rescue index: You need to be self-reliant because the remote location of the forest is only moderately popular with other bikers, even on summer weekends. Weekday users are fewer, particularly in the off-season. During emergencies, you may get lucky and find a forest crew working along the trail. The forest office, located near the heliport as you enter the forest from US 175, is generally staffed during normal working hours. There are private residences outside the northwestern boundary of the forest.

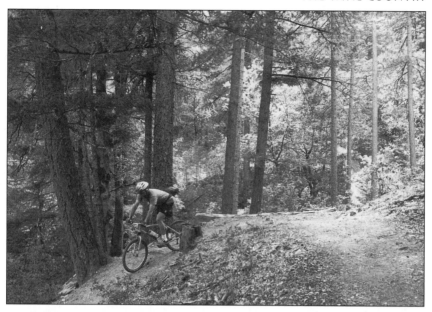

Bruce eases through a moderately tight, descending turn on Jethro's Trail.

Land status: Boggs Mountain Demonstration State Forest.

Maps: *Boggs Mountain Demonstration State Forest* brochure produced by the Department of Forestry, available as you enter the State Forest in a bulletin board box in front of the heliport. If the box is empty, check at Calso Camp down the road or the forest office near the heliport.

Finding the trail: From Calistoga, travel north on US 29 for 16 miles past Robert Louis Stevenson State Park to Middletown. Turn left, due west, onto US 175 for about 7 miles to the town of Cobb (your last chance for food or gas). Continue through Cobb for 0.8 mile and keep an eye peeled for the unsigned paved road to Boggs. Since there is no sign indicating Boggs Mountain State Forest, follow signs to the fire station instead. Look for a blue and white fire station sign posted very close to this entrance road. Turn right onto the paved road, heading southeast. In about 200 yards, you see a brown sign announcing you're entering the state forest. Continue on the road for less than a mile, toward the heliport on your right and the office on your left. Park in the dirt lot here.

Sources of additional information:

Boggs Mountain Demonstration State Forest
P.O. Box 839
Cobb, CA 95426
(707) 928-4378

Notes on the trail: If this is your first time here, you definitely need a map. (See "Maps" above.) You'll find that not all the trails and fire roads in the forest are signed. Generally speaking, nearly all trail junctions shown on the map are actually signed in the forest. So, if you feel a bit lost, never fear, you will stumble upon a signed clue usually in less than a mile.

This loop is described in a clockwise direction and is just one of many biking configurations possible. From the dirt lot, across from the field office, begin pedaling back down the forest entrance road for a few yards. The trail you want is Mac's Trail; look for it on your right. Mac's is a single-track trail that immediately climbs somewhat steeply up the side of the hill, weaving through the trees. The trail is a bit technical here as you ascend through semi-packed dirt mixed with some loose rock of varying sizes along with pine needles and a few exposed tree roots. Then, gradually descend to a junction of three wide single-track trails radiating away from the trail you're on. The trail immediately to your right is the one and only signed trail here (the sign is possibly hidden by bushes) identifying Hobergs Loop Trail, a single-track.

Turn right onto Hobergs and follow it as it ascends a moderate but short hill. Stay on the well-defined single-track and bypass an unsigned fire road within a small clearing. Enjoy a gentle descent for about a half mile (1.5 miles from trailhead), where you reach a major signed intersection with another single-track. Hang a right hairpin turn here, following Boggs Ridge Trail to Vista Point. (Don't expect some sort of viewing platform. Vista Point is just a tiny section of the trail that offers a view of a distant mountain range in the southwest, and unless you're looking for it, you'll blow right past the views.) A couple of hundred yards farther and you reach the junction of fire road 210. Your single-track trail, now called Karen's Trail, continues across 210. Stay with Karen's as it runs up and down the slope of a tiny saddle before intersecting with fire road 210 again. Now, go right on 210, following the wider trail and after a short descent, at 2.6 miles, it becomes a single-track again. There's a sign here marking the re-appearing single-track as Jethro's Trail. Weave and dodge your way around the trees, cruising on the easy trail.

At 3 miles, you reach a major intersection with fire roads 200 and 210 (at this point, 210 is the same as Jethro's trail which you've been riding). Continue straight through on Jethro's to Barry's Trail. It's a bit confusing here, but fortunately there are signs. After a few yards, the trail forks. The right fork is Barry's while the left is Jethro's. Follow Jethro's as it continues to weave through the forest on a slightly descending, mildly technical path. Still on Jethro's, bypass unsigned lesser trails, cross over trickling Mill Creek, and pass a water tank. You reach fire road 300 at almost 4 miles. Go right onto 300 for a short distance and you see Grizzley Trail shooting off on your right. If you want single-track that's more challenging, then jump onto Grizzley for a 0.3-mile exhilarating, sometimes steep, downhill run. Otherwise, stay on 300, which is still a fun, easy, and enjoyable road. Road 300 gently ascends then descends for the next 2.3 miles, bypassing another Grizzley intersection, fire road 400, and John's Trail. Eventually, 300 curves to the right and hooks up with fire road 600. At this point, you've pedaled about 6.3 wonderfully forested miles from the trailhead where your car is parked.

Follow the signs to fire road 600. Just when you might be getting bored with riding an easy fire road, 600 grabs your attention by challenging you with a steep, 9% grade uphill. Lucky you, it's short, about 200 yards, and mildly technical. At the top of the climb, you find Big Springs Trail, another single-track disappearing into the forest on your left. Big Springs requires intermediate technical skill in that it climbs sharply up and down, skirts steep drop-offs in a few places, weaves in and out of trees and around semi-buried rocks in the trail, all while traversing a steep slope. It's guaranteed to keep you from boredom. Not to fret, though, it's short, just under a mile.

Option: Running out of time or just not up for the challenge of Big Springs? Then stay on fire road 600 to reach Bear Bones Trail in almost a mile or fire road 500 in a little over a mile, both as measured from the base of Big Springs. Bear Bones is an easy, mellow, level single-track to which 600 later connects. The main road is 500 and leads out of the Boggs Demonstration Forest—it's the same road on which your car is parked.

From the intersection of fire road 600 and Big Springs Trail, hang a left onto Big Springs and tackle the challenge. After almost a mile of the technical portion, Big Springs dumps you onto a fire road. Turn right onto the fire road. Immediately ahead is Big Springs itself, gurgling out of a tiny pipe that's protruding from the hillside. (Sorry, this is non-potable water.) Here at the springs is the bottom of Charlie's Trail, and from this point, it's an extremely steep uphill. Yup, pedal—or walk—up this section. The loose rock-strewn condition combined with its steepness (11% grade) makes it an extremely technical trail—the stuff that strong, advanced riders love to tackle. Try not to disturb the lovely singing birds or fracture the peace and calm of the forest with your huffing and puffing. Luckily, it's about 200 yards of insane steepness, followed by a gentler grade.

When you reach the top, Charlie's Trail intersects with an unsigned fire road. By now, you have pedaled about 8.2 miles from your car. Hang a right onto the smooth, level fire road and follow it for almost a half mile to another intersection, this time with fire road 541. Take 541 as it leads off to the left, due north. Pedal a short distance and you come to a small, man-made clearing in the forest, which the published map calls "well-pad." The fire road splits here. Follow the dirt road to the left as it skirts a rusty, dilapidated makeshift cable fence for a few yards. The fire road splits again; follow the left fork (the right fork is a lesser-traveled road). The rock-strewn fire road climbs a bit, then levels out and leads right smack into High Point Trail, a very wide, signed single-track. Continue on the easy High Point Trail as it gently climbs to a little more than 3,600 feet at about 9.6 miles. This is the highest point of the loop and in the forest.

Descend High Point Trail for about 0.2 mile, bypassing all lesser trails, until you arrive at a mess of unsigned trails. Stay right—twice—on the fire road and you reach the signed intersection of fire roads 610 and 600. Make your way to 600 by going right onto 610, then stay right as the road becomes 600 heading north. Follow 600 for not quite a half mile and watch for Bear Bones Trail, a single-track trail, leading off on your left, at about 10.2 miles. Hop onto Bear Bones and enjoy a sweet, easy, level ride weaving and dodging through the forest. The trail gradually descends a short distance and intersects with an unsigned fire road and Ball Cap Trail, a signed single-track. Go left on the fire road and in a fairly short distance, come to another signed intersection. The road you're on is fire road 400 and you've just intersected fire road 500, a well-traveled gravel road (the same road on which you drove when entering the state forest). Follow 500 to the right for about 300 yards to the campgrounds.

At the campground, a single-track signed Creek Trail (labeled "Houghton Creek" according to the published map) shoots off downhill on your left. Drop down onto Creek (Houghton) Trail and follow it as it rolls through a more densely forested and bushy area. The trail parallels the intermittently gurgling creek on your right. Basketball-sized boulders in the trail and hanging tree branches require a bit more technical finesse than the previous single-track. Ride or walk over log water bars in the trail and very soon reach a fork in the trail. Watch out for poison oak. Take the right fork as it crosses over the creek, then the hard right following the trail as it climbs steeply out of the creek bed. After climbing through a couple of switchbacks, the single-track intersects with another single-track running left and right of your trail, unsigned. Follow the right trail, the more well-defined single-track. In a few yards, at about 12.5 miles, your trail forks at a huge, seemingly out-of-place round boulder. It's almost the size of a Volkswagen Beetle. Take the left fork toward the boulder and continue on the single-track as it leads you through the dense bushes and trees. In about 200 yards, Creek Trail intersects with fire road 500 again, the wide gravel/dirt road. Go left onto 500 and within a half mile, at 12.9 miles, you close the loop by reaching your parked car.

RIDE 23 · Mt. St. Helena North Peak

AT A GLANCE

Length/configuration: 11.2-mile out-and-back (5.6 miles each way); wide fire road

Aerobic difficulty: Moderately strenuous due to nearly unrelenting gradual climbing all the way to the top

Technical difficulty: Not technical

Scenery: On clear days, incredible panoramic views in all directions, including Mt. Shasta to the north and the snow-capped Sierra Nevadas to the east.

Special comments: If you really want a workout, tow a child in a kid-trailer and impress everyone on the trail.

This 11.2-mile out-and-back (5.6 miles each way) is so easy to follow that you really don't need a map. Just stay on the easy, wide, well-traveled, nontechnical, smooth fire road, and keep grinding up, bypassing the few foot trails (off-limits to bikes) leading away from the road. Signposts along the way measure your progress, or at least remind you of the push you must sustain. Fortunately, the pain is eased by about six switchbacks and the emerging views of the Napa Valley. A high peak of volcanic origin, this nearly mile-high mountain boasts an incredible panoramic view in all directions. On a clear day, you can see San Francisco, the ocean, the snow-capped Sierra Nevadas, Mt. Diablo, and even Mt. Shasta to the north. You're certainly never too far from civilization as you gaze down into the wine country with its sprawling vineyard estates. The only abundant shade on this route is during the first mile. After that, only small spots of shade offer some respite on warm, sunny days.

Mt. St. Helena is the crown jewel of the 4,161-acre Robert Louis Stevenson State Park, named for the author of *Treasure Island* and *Kidnapped*. Stevevson was so inspired by the region that he penned *The Silverado Squatters*, a story about his 1880 stay in Calistoga. He spent his honeymoon in a cabin at the base of Mt. St. Helena, and there is a hiking-only path to what little remains of it. Prior to Stevenson, the Russians came to this region in the early 1800s in search of resources that would help support their settlements in the Alaskan territory. During their brief stay, they unknowingly (albeit arguably) gave birth to a billion dollar industry—they cultivated grapes for winemaking. The Russian's last claim to fame before leaving in the late 1800s is scaling the mountain peak here and naming it Mt. St. Helena, in honor of the empress of Imperial Russia.

General location: 8 miles north of Calistoga, just beyond the northern end of Napa Valley.

RIDE 23 · Mt. St. Helena North Peak

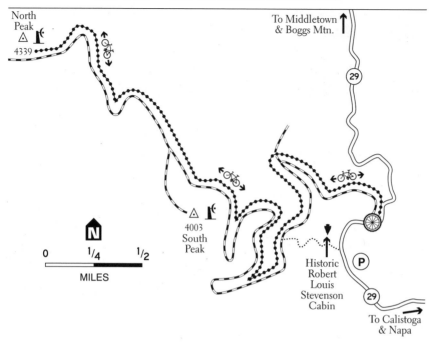

Elevation change: 2,093 feet; starting elevation and low point 2,250 feet; high point 4,343 feet. Basically, one big hill climb with a short level stretch near the top; return is an uninterrupted descent.

Season: Year-round. Winter days are more apt to be free of atmospheric haze, which increases your chances for spectacularly clear views. If you ride in the winter, be prepared—snowflakes at the peak are not unusual.

Services: None on the trail or at the parking areas (but then, there's no fee either). Many services can be found in Calistoga.

Hazards: Watch out for other trail users. After climbing to the North Peak, you'll undoubtedly want to fly all the way back down. Loose gravel on the road makes it hard to stop on a dime and you wouldn't want to run into a hiker or another biker, especially around a curve. If the day is not particularly warm, bring a lightweight jacket to keep you comfortable on your downhill flight.

Rescue index: The route is somewhat popular with other trail users on the weekends, especially in the summer. Weekday users are fewer, particularly in the off-season. Otherwise, for emergency help, you'll have to make your own way back down the trail to CA 29 where you can flag down a passing motorist.

Land status: Robert Louis Stevenson State Park.

Maps: USGS Detert Reservoir and Mount St. Helena 7.5 minute series.

Finding the trail: CA 29 runs through the State Park. From the intersection of CA 29 and the Silverado Trail on the northeast edge of the town of Calistoga, drive north

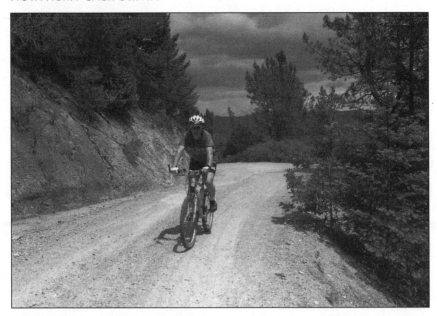

Thoughts of flying downhill is enough to sustain Bruce on this gradual, mostly unrelenting climb on a wide, smooth dirt road to the top.

on CA 29 for 7 winding miles. Park in the small dirt lot on the right (east) side of CA 29. From the dirt lot, pedal up (north) on CA 29. There's not much of a shoulder along this stretch but fortunately, the trailhead is about 400 yards ahead. Along the way, you immediately go past a metal gate closing off a slightly obscure dirt road located on the other side of CA 29. Continue on the shoulder for the final 300 yards, at which point there is another metal gate closing off an obvious fire road, also on the left side of the paved road. The fire road is signed "Authorized vehicles only," and this is the trailhead you want.

Sources of additional information:

Robert Louis Stevenson State Park
3801 N. St. Helena Hwy.
Calistoga, CA 94515
(707) 942-4575

Notes on the trail: The following mileages use the intersection of CA 29 and the fire road as the starting point. Begin by pedaling the fire road as it traverses a shady canyon of fir and deciduous trees. Emerge from the shade as the trail navigates up the south-facing slope of the canyon. Look behind you to the right, and you may catch a glimpse of the South Peak radio towers off in the distance. At about 2 miles, at the crest of a switchback, you reach a rock outcropping overlooking the Napa Valley. It's a popular rock-climbing practice site and you may see some folks honing their skills here. Your ascent remains moderate, about 7% grade, with a few welcoming but far too short flat spots. Slowly, the trail weaves around to the northern slope, due west.

At about 4 miles, another fire road leads off on your left toward the South Peak, marked by several radio towers. (Feeling pretty good? Do a side trip to the South Peak summit, elevation 4,003 feet. It's a short but somewhat steep fire road.)

Continuing on, the main fire road begins a welcomed, gently rolling stretch for almost a half mile. As the road gradually curves to the south at about 4.5 miles, get ready because here comes the last big climb to the North Peak. It's steep—about an 8 to 9% grade. Fortunately, it's a short climb. At 5.6 miles, you've just climbed about 2,150 feet. You're at the top! Elevation here at the North Peak is 4,339 feet. With good timing and a little bit of luck, you're rewarded with a crystal-clear day yielding a spectacular view in all directions. Nevertheless, you've earned the right to scream your head off all the way back down to the trailhead. You'll rarely have to crank the pedal. The descent is so fast, you'll probably make it down in half the time it took to reach the north peak—or less. Enjoy and stay alert for other trail users and loose gravel, especially in the turns.

RIDE 24 · Oat Hill Mine Road

AT A GLANCE

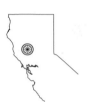

Length/configuration: 8.6-mile out-and-back (4.3 miles each way); wide single-track

Aerobic difficulty: Somewhat strenuous due to extremely rocky terrain

Technical difficulty: Expert due to loose, rough rocks. Expect drops created by boulders planted in the trail.

Scenery: Great, expansive views of the Napa Valley and rock outcroppings overlooking Calistoga

Special comments: Seeing old wagon-wheel ruts carved into a few boulders on the trail is humbling, especially when you feel like the trail is beating the heck out of you.

Few places in the heart of northern California's wine country are open to public use. Nearly every inch of land in this valley of liquid gold is privately owned. This trail, fortunately, is one of those few public places. Locally referred to as a "road," Oat Hill Mine Road is more like a foot trail that varies from four to 15 feet wide. The route was originally created as a wagon road so that miners who worked in the hills could haul supplies to and from the town and valley lying below. Indeed, there are wagon-wheel ruts carved into boulders in the trail. Today, the only traffic the "road" sees are hikers and mountain bikers. Many parts of the once wide road are overgrown with shrubs and tall grass, making the trail look more like a wide single-track trail than a wagon road.

The ride described here is an 8.6-mile out-and-back (4.3 miles each way). The turnaround point is the "campground ruins" (locals call it that because it's a favorite camping spot). In the days before the Napa Valley vineyards became a gold mine, this site was a "halfway house" (that is, the halfway stopping point in land travel). The only evidence of this halfway station are stone foundations. How far into the mountains the miners lived and worked is anybody's guess. The "road" does continue beyond the ruins. What is amazing—and humbling—is the ruggedness of the trail. If you like intensely technical trails, try this one. Virtually every inch of the trail is rock-strewn and full of large, semi-buried boulders, ruts, and roots. Though not in-

RIDE 24 · Oat Hill Mine Road

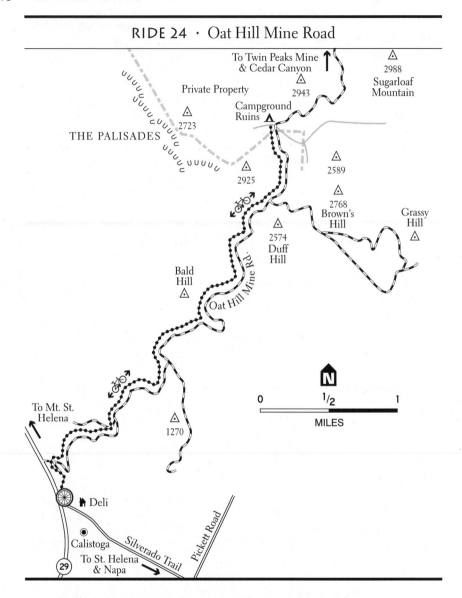

tensely steep, the ride up and down is extremely satisfying for those who like conquering challenging technical routes.

The route travels through some shady stretches of forest but is mostly exposed, particularly as it traverses alongside grassy clearings. You can expect to see a show of wildflowers in the late spring and early summer. Expansive views of the Napa Valley are superb the higher you go. Throughout the ride, keep an eye out for poison oak hidden in the abundant vegetation that smothers both sides of the trail. Not as ubiquitous as the green plant but definitely worthy of your attention are mountain lions. Though sightings, much less attacks, are rare, stay alert anyway.

General location: On the northeastern edge of the small town of Calistoga, located on the northern end of the Napa Valley; 75 miles north of San Francisco.

Elevation change: 1,730 feet; starting elevation and low point 400 feet; high point 2,130 feet. Gradual, rocky climb with a few level stretches.

Season: Year-round.

Services: No services on the trail. Even though this is a short ride, your level of technical skill dictates how long you'll be out there, so bring enough water especially if it's a hot day. Located at the trailhead is a great little deli and juice bar aptly named Trailhead. Housed in an old converted gas station shack, the deli serves breakfast and lunch, as well as to-go sandwiches. If you decide to ride without a map, at least go and check out the USGS topo map posted on their wall. While you're at it, consider filling up your water bottle with some of their fine lemonade, particularly quenching on a hot summer day. All other conveniences can be found in Calistoga, less than a mile away. Take note, though, Trailhead closes in the mid-afternoon. Also across the street from the deli is a pub that serves up ice-cold beer.

Hazards: Poison oak is just about everywhere, especially hazardous as you maneuver around obstacles in the sometimes narrow trail. Mountain lions occasionally spotted in the vicinity.

Rescue index: Since this is a somewhat popular hiking route on the weekends, especially during the summer, other trail users might offer assistance. Otherwise, for emergency help, make your way back down the trail to the main road. A phone is available at the deli and the pub across the street.

Land status: County road through private property. Public access permitted so long as you stay on the road.

Maps: USGS Calistoga and Aetna Springs 7.5 minute series.

Finding the trail: The town of Calistoga is located at the northern end of Napa Valley (the town of Napa anchors the southern end of the valley). On the northeastern edge of Calistoga, the trailhead is located at the intersection of CA 29 and the northern end of the Silverado Trail (the well-known north-south wine road in Napa Valley). It's about a 1.5-mile bike ride from the center of town. If you drive, park in the dirt lot kitty-cornered across CA 29 from Trailhead deli.

Sources of additional information:

Trailhead (a tiny deli/café)
2082 Lake County Highway
(CA 29 at Silverado Trail)
Calistoga, CA 94515
(707) 942-9068

Notes on the trail: The route generally heads east, gradually curving north and then east again. There are no directional signs throughout the route. Basically, stay on the main road, bypassing other lesser-traveled, tiny trails that connect to it. In fact, the area that the trail traverses is private property—another reason to stay on the main road. Though the trail continues beyond the "campground ruins," I advise turning back at this point as the undefined property beyond is private.

Start by finding the trailhead, located just to the left of the Trailhead deli, over a dirt berm. A few yards up the trail is a sign-in ledge awaiting your autograph.

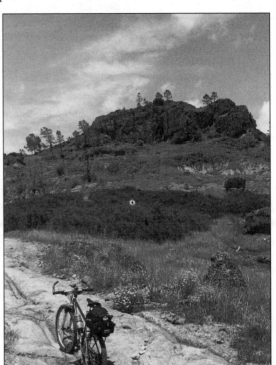

The wagon wheel ruts carved deeply into boulders here convey a sense of the hard labor endured by miners long ago.

Immediately, the trail begins a steep climb over easy ground, although depending on how wet the winter has been, the trail here might be deeply rutted by rain runoff. In a few yards, as you grind up a moderate hill, cautiously follow the narrow single-track as it closely and treacherously parallels a barbed-wire fence for a few yards. On the other side of the fence is a steep drop-off into a tiny vineyard. As the trail continues its moderate climb up the southern slope of the hill, the condition becomes more technical with loose rocks, rain ruts, semi-buried boulders, and exposed tree roots. Expansive views of the Napa Valley to the south begin to emerge.

At about 1.5 miles from the trailhead, you've climbed about 690 feet. The rock-strewn trail becomes more technically difficult, leading you over and around massive semi-buried boulders and ruts. You'll be tempted to skirt this mess by riding the shoulder of the trail but watch out for the pervasive poison oak. After 2.5 miles, a wide, 180-degree view of the Napa Valley appears off on your right, due south.

As the trail begins curving north, keep an eye out for a huge semi-buried, flat boulder in the trail. Hey, this isn't just any boulder. There are wagon wheel ruts carved into it. You've now climbed about 1,000 feet and as you huff and puff along, think how arduous the miners toiled, hauling supplies up and down the trail. Their supplies weighed more than you and your bike combined. Continue on, still climbing and picking your way up the technically rugged but aerobically moderate trail. Soon, you begin to see the Palisades towering in the distance on your left, looking northeast. The Palisades is a tall, broad, brownish-black cliff face, looking westward, majestically over Calistoga.

Take a breather at 3 miles and enjoy the views from a small, flat clearing situated at the base of a rocky outcropping. Here you get a full view of the Palisades. In about a half mile from this landing and about 200 feet higher, you begin approaching the base of more rock outcroppings. At this exposed section of the mountainside, unless you're delirious from the technical challenge, you notice wagon-wheel ruts that are much more obvious than before. Incidentally, the day I was here at this spot, checking out the ruts and munching on a PowerBar, I began hearing what I thought was a huge gust of wind. Then, all of a sudden, whoosh! A glider soared—and roared—so close overhead that I thought I could reach up and touch it. Almost choked on my PowerBar.

The trail now begins heading north, skirting the base of more rock outcroppings looming overhead on your right. A great view of the Napa Valley is below on your left, westward. Continue on the trail, which has now leveled somewhat, and you have a closer look at the Palisades. The trail remains seriously technical, with lots of loose rocks ranging from golf ball to beach ball size. Follow the trail as it leads pass the right side of the Palisades. At about 4.3 miles, you reach the "campground ruins," tucked within a small, shady clearing of trees on your left. You've just climbed 1,730 very technical feet. Elevation here is approximately 2,130 feet.

The ruins is a pleasant, shady area with makeshift benches—a great rest stop. Look closely and you see evidence of what used to be the foundation of a small building. Watch out for poison oak if you go exploring for more ruins here. The trail continues due east into private property so turn around here and retrace your path back to the trailhead. Upon your return, reward yourself for all the pain you endured by indulging in local refreshment at either the Trailhead or the pub across the street from it. Maybe even treat yourself to a soothing massage or a relaxing mud bath in one of Calistoga's many spas.

RIDE 25 · Annadel State Park Loops

AT A GLANCE

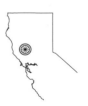

Length/configuration: 16.6 miles, two loops combined; narrow dirt roads with a short stretch on single-track

Aerobic difficulty: Moderately strenuous; includes a few stretches of climbing over bumpy terrain

Technical difficulty: Mostly intermediate though the bigger loop is mostly mild

Scenery: A mixture of oak, Douglas fir, and occasional young redwood trees amid rolling hillsides, interspersed with open meadows and marshland.

Special comments: Though the first 2 miles from the main parking area is suitable for kid-trailers, it would be a workout due to the gradual uphill terrain.

In the 1800s, growing cities like San Francisco quarried tons of cobblestones from this region in order to quench their thirst for building materials. Fast-forward to present times. That same rocky substance became the stuff of mountain bikers' dreams, attracting skilled riders who thrived on intensely difficult trails. In the early to mid-1990s, 5,000-plus-acre Annadel State Park had plenty of technical terrain that consistently challenged the skills of intermediate and advanced level riders. But, not all of the trails were legal. The park was literally becoming a mess of bike paths crisscrossing oak and fragile habitat, intruding on cultural and historic sites and promoting serious erosion problems. In the mid '90s, a campaign was launched by all groups of local trail users—hikers, equestrians, and bikers—along with rangers and the park service, in a concerted effort to save their backyard paradise. Several new multi-use trails were constructed in 1997 to reroute existing trails that cut through meadows and suffered from poor construction and lack of maintenance. Illegal single-tracks were shut down while stretches of hiking-only trails became multi-use. Some trails were preserved for hiking-only. The good news is that more legal bike trails have been opened up. The bad news, according to some hard-core riders, is the taming of once awesomely technical, challenging terrain in order to become more accessible to all users.

Today, maintaining the park is an ongoing process. Though the trails in general survived El Niño storms in early 1998, subsequent storms have forced the closure of some trails in order to halt further damage by trail users and to allow for repair. Keep in mind that if you hope to ride Annadel early in the year, particularly after a wet winter, expect many trails to be closed until spring.

Annadel is still popular with mountain bikers of all abilities and there are sections and trails that are fairly advanced. Legal trails and fire roads are well signed and any that are not should be considered off-limits. The route described below is a 16.6-mile, figure-eight loop that uses mostly narrow fire roads and a stretch of single-track, all of which are generally open year-round. The climbing is moderate, and you gain about 1,190 feet over ascending and descending terrain. The first loop, which widely encircles secluded Lake Ilsanjo, is mostly mildly technical with some spots of intermediate terrain; adventurous beginners are bound to enjoy it. (Several options and configurations are available for an easy return.) Advanced riders will want to tackle the outermost loop, which goes around Ledson Marsh. That loop includes short but intense stretches of technical terrain characterized by semi-buried chunks of rough rock. That kind of terrain, combined with a moderate climb to the marsh, followed by gradual ups and downs, will make you either appreciate the shocks on your bike or wish you had them.

General location: Immediately east of Santa Rosa, about 75 miles north of San Francisco.

Elevation change: 1,020 feet; starting elevation 400 feet; high point 1,420 feet; low point 380 feet. Gradual climb with a few mellow sections in between.

Season: Year-round, though some trails are closed in winter and may not open until spring.

Services: Drinking water at the main parking lot. Pit toilets at a few locations throughout the park. All services in Santa Rosa, about 15 minutes away by car.

Hazards: Scattered poison oak along the trail. The park is popular with equestrians and other bikers. Watch out for other trail users, especially when you're flying down descents on the major multi-use trails.

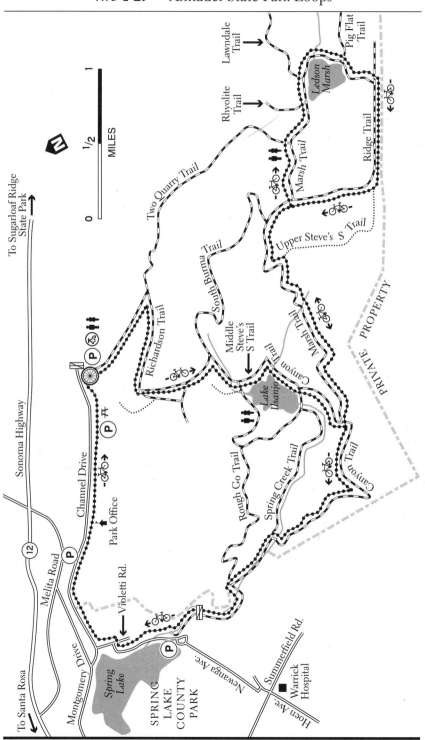

Rescue index: Because the park is adjacent to the well-populated town of Santa Rosa (and immediately next to residential neighborhoods), it sees lots of runners and bikers in the late afternoon. During the weekend, you'll see plenty of trail users, including many equestrians. And so, in case of emergency, you're likely to meet other trail users who may be of help. Rangers and volunteers occasionally patrol the trails during popular hours and days. The southern edge of the park borders residential homes. Spring Lake is a popular park and there is a pay phone near its rest rooms. Otherwise, to get help, you should make your way back down to the ranger station on Channel Drive.

Land status: Annadel State Park.

Maps: *Annadel State Park*, official park map. Though it may be older than 1999 and not reflect current trail status, it's still useful. These maps are generally available at a self-paying wooden dispenser located next to an information kiosk at the ranger station as you enter the park on Channel Drive. Cost is 75¢, but like all other publicly funded park facilities, expect the price to be slightly higher. Maps are also posted on kiosks located along the popular trails throughout the park.

Finding the trail: From the intersection of US 101 and CA 12 (Sonoma Highway) in the city of Santa Rosa, travel east on CA 12. Go past the Sonoma County Fairgrounds. At almost 1.5 miles at a signal light intersection, CA 12 goes a left and becomes Farmers Lane, a busy street that runs through town and past residential neighborhoods. There are plenty of services here, including grocery stores to pick up a snack or water for your ride. Watch for signs to stay on CA 12, now called Farmers Lane. At about 3.5 miles, (just as you pass Santa Rosa Cyclery on your right), turn right onto Montgomery Drive. This 2-way street leads you through a residential area and at almost 5 miles, go right onto Channel Drive. Continue past Violetti Drive, staying straight toward Annadel State Park. You can park in the dirt lot on the left, just before entering the state park, and then pedal about a mile to the trailhead. Otherwise, continue into the park and don't forget to pay the park fee when you register yourself at the ranger station on your right. Continue straight on Channel Drive for not quite a mile to where the pavement ends, next to the main parking lot. You'll find a couple of picnic tables, drinking water, and a pit toilet here as well as the Warren P. Richardson Trailhead.

Sources of additional information:

Annadel State Park
California Department of Parks and
  Recreation
6201 Channel Dr.
Santa Rosa, CA 95409
(707) 539-3911

Notes on the trail: Fire roads at Annadel State Park are referred to as trails. All legal trails throughout the park are well signed, and kiosks posted at a few major intersections may offer more current trail information. Generally speaking, if a trail is unsigned (typically enticing single-tracks), you should consider it off-limits to bikes. Please obey posted signs.

Begin pedaling on the Warren P. Richardson Trail, the trailhead located near the entrance of the parking lot. The first 2 miles toward Lake Ilsanjo is a moderate and steady climb, about a 3% grade. The trail leads you through gnarly oak woodlands, a forest of Douglas firs along with occasional redwood trees, and past open meadows. Richardson is best described as mild because it's basically a smooth, hard-packed dirt and gravel, wide fire road. Along the way, several single-track trails peel off of the main road. Ignore those and stay on the main road. Just over 0.5 mile after the beginning, surrounded by lightly forested rolling hills, Richardson Trail becomes a narrow fire road and takes you past a small marsh. Continue the gradual climb and in almost a mile, Two Quarry Road intersects Richardson on your left. Bypass Two Quarry and follow Richardson as it makes a sharp, steeply ascending right turn around a picnic table and kiosk. Not to worry, the steepness quickly mellows as you continue riding through the shady forest. (Incidentally, adventurous, technically advanced riders equipped with great suspension may enjoy Two Quarry. It's so rocky and bumpy, it's guaranteed to rattle your eyeballs in their sockets. Recommended for advanced riders only.) After a brief downhill stretch, Richardson is intersected by Lower Steve's S Trail, next to a picnic table. Stay left, continuing on Richardson, and in a few yards, bypass Louis Trail.

At two miles from the beginning, you essentially reach the top of Richardson. Here, on your left, is a picnic bench and North Burma Trail taking off on your right. Bear left, staying on Richardson. On your right, on the other side of an open rolling meadow, is Lake Ilsanjo—your destination. Enjoy a sweet descent, losing 155 feet in less than a half mile by the time you reach the lake.

You reach lake level at 2.6 miles at the intersection with Middle Steve's S Trail. The posted sign here tells you that Lake Ilsanjo covers 26 acres and the elevation is 750 feet. (Though Lake Ilsanjo is a secluded lake, it's somewhat popular with anglers hoping to hook large-mouth bass and blue gill.) Immediately on your right is the huge, wide-open meadow that you previously viewed from above. Lower Steve's S Trail peels off into the meadow. Richardson Trail, still a wide, smooth and flat fire road, curves to the right and in the distance, through the clearing, you can see it leading past several outhouses.

Hang a left onto Middle Steve's S Trail and begin a fairly level ride along the eastern side of the lake, heading south. Stay left at unsigned intersections (the right-hand trails lead down to the lake). Middle Steve's is technically mild with a few intermediate spots due to semi-buried chunks of rocks in the trail. At 2.9 miles, you have a wider view of the lake. Here, in this vicinity, Middle Steve's S Trail becomes Canyon Trail. (A couple of years ago, the trail made a split here with Middle Steve's, peeling off to the left and Canyon to the right. The park service has since closed that portion of Middle Steve's, so you most likely will blow right past the trail without noticing it. Until the park service reprints updated versions, the map you're likely to see still shows this split.) At just over 3 miles from the beginning, you reach the junction of Canyon and Rough Go Trail leading off on your right. (If you're a beginner, you should go right onto Rough Go and ride around the western edge of the lake to Richardson Trail. Hang another right onto Richardson. Then, in about a half mile, Richardson returns to the intersection with Middle Steve's S Trail. Then, go left, staying on Richardson, and retrace your path back to the main parking lot. If you're an adventurous beginner out to develop your bike-handling skills, then continue on for another 0.6 mile.) From the Canyon and Rough Go intersection, the rest of the route is mostly mildly technical with some intermediate and advanced stretches of extremely rocky and bumpy terrain. Those conditions, combined with a final climb to the ridge, will challenge your skills.

Continue on Canyon Trail, passing Hunter Spring, (a water trough for horses, non-potable for humans). You reach a signed major intersection with Marsh Trail and Canyon Trail at 3.6 miles. Here begins the route for the optional loop, which consists of some advanced rocky stretches and more moderate climbing. At this intersection, bearing right onto Canyon will give you a fast, mostly easy, almost nontechnical descent all the way back down to Channel Drive and ultimately back to your car. Beginners who are unsure of themselves on the previous, short stretch of bumpy and rocky terrain should choose this route. Intermediate and advanced riders can venture onto the more technical, optional loop by making a hard left onto Marsh Trail.

Marsh Trail begins a moderate climb over somewhat bumpy terrain, thanks to semi-buried chunks of rocks. As you ascend, look left and you have a wide-open view of the small valley in which you rode near Lake Ilsanjo. Eventually, you begin to see a few scattered young redwood trees alongside the Douglas firs, oak, and madrone trees. The climbing levels out when you reach Buick Meadow, a signed wide-open clearing. Bypass South Burma Trail that takes off on your left and stay right on Marsh. The bumpy, intermediate trail soon brings you to the intersection with Ridge Trail, reached at almost 6 miles. This is the beginning of the optional loop around Ledson Marsh, and you have a choice of direction. If flying over bumpy trails that demand bike-handling nimbleness is what you like, then hang a left, staying on Marsh and ride the loop clockwise. If you like moderate, 6% grade climbing over advanced-rated rocky terrain, then stay straight onto Ridge Trail, and ride the loop counterclockwise. Whichever direction you choose, you'll be closing the loop when you arrive at this intersection again after 3.2 miles.

For this trail description, I took the left turn, riding clockwise. Continue on Marsh Trail and begin a gradual uphill climb over somewhat rocky terrain. At 6.3 miles, Two Quarry Road intersects at a right bend in Marsh. There's a pit toilet here. (Advanced and expert riders take note: As its name implies, Two Quarry is extremely rocky and biking it requires solid technical skills. It connects to Richardson Trail about a mile from the main parking lot where you're parked. Remember passing it earlier in the ride?) Bypass Two Quarry, staying right on Marsh. After a few yards of climbing over rocky terrain, the trail descends toward Ledson Marsh, cruising past Rhyolite Trail along the way. Continue around the east side of the Marsh, still on Marsh Trail. The bumpy, wide path gives way to smooth, easy terrain as you past Lawndale Trail and Pig Flat Trail. Stay right past these two trails. When you reach the ridge top, the terrain opens up and you begin to have a view of the rolling hills all around you. To your left is an old stone wall, marking the southern edge of the park boundary. You can make out a few rooftops just beyond this stone fence. Though it's not signed here, you've just begun pedaling Ridge Trail, a narrow fire road. Get ready, the next half mile is guaranteed to rattle your eyeballs. You'll either be thankful for the shocks on your bike or you'll be wishing you had them. In any case, this stretch along the southern park boundary climbs up and down over seriously bumpy terrain before mellowing out a bit at 8.4 miles.

When you reach the junction with Upper Steve's S Trail coming in on the left, stay right on Ridge Trail, following it northward. Still a narrow fire road, the trail continues its gradual and brief up and down attitude. A few spots of rocky terrain keep you alert and, in general, Ridge is mostly descending. At 9.1 miles, you close the loop by reaching the junction of Ridge and Marsh Trails. Get ready. The next 2.3 miles is an exhilarating downhill blast as you retrace your path back to the intersection of Marsh and Canyon Trails, reached at mile 11.4.

Once at Marsh and Canyon, you can return to your car by retracing your entire route down Richardson Trail. Or, if you're like me, choose a different return route by hanging a left onto Canyon Trail. The trail begins by running through oak and fir forest, then opens up, giving you a glimpse of Santa Rosa in the western distance as you cruise down the rolling hillsides. In years past, this stretch of Canyon was rocky, bumpy, downright technical, and not suited to all bikers. After grading, the trail has become a mostly smooth, wide fire road with some rocky and somewhat intermediate sections. While the grade is gentle, you can really pick up speed on this stretch. At almost 13 miles, go over a well-made wooden bridge spanning Spring Creek (which looks more like a man-made flood channel than a creek). The trail you're following now becomes Spring Creek Trail. Turn left onto Spring Creek and continue heading due north. The trail is still a hard-packed, smooth fire road and now parallels the creek on your left. Zip past a spillway on your distant left, and soon thereafter, Rough Go Trail on your right. Ride over another well-made wooden bridge at 13.4 miles. In a few yards, Spring Creek Trail ends as you ride past a metal gate that prevents unauthorized vehicles from accessing the dirt road you've just enjoyed flying down.

Now, in the Spring Lake county park, follow the dirt road that's signed by a "Do Not Enter—Authorized Vehicles Only" sign. Stay on it for a few yards, passing a parking lot, rest room, pay phone, and picnic tables. In a few yards, you reach a paved narrow path. Hang a right and go over a culvert through which Spring Creek runs. Follow the trail as it curves left, paralleling the creek. In a few yards, the paved path becomes a narrow, hard-packed dirt and gravel trail. The trail is unnamed but it's signed "No Equestrians." Go past a set of about 8 wooden steps on your right. Spring Lake is off in the distance on your left. The dirt trail climbs a bit, then descends past a tiny brick building before ending at a paved vehicle road. Turn right onto the road and ride the decently wide shoulder up a steep but short climb. At 14.7 miles, you exit the county park as evidenced by riding past the park entrance pay booth. Immediately hang a left onto Violetti Road. Descend several hundred yards through a residential neighborhood and then turn right onto Channel Drive. Follow Channel Drive back into Annadel State Park. Look right, and upon passing the park office area and self-pay kiosk, keep an eye out for an informational signboard alongside a single-track trailhead. You've just found one of the few legal single-tracks in the park. It parallels Channel Drive all the way to the main dirt parking lot where your car is located. Though this single-track is short—about a mile long—it's somewhat technical. The narrow trail weaves and twists past trees and is spiced with a few abrupt dips. Beginners looking to improve their single-track skills may enjoy this trail. If the single-track is not to your liking, just take any of several bail-out trails onto Channel Drive. Whichever route you take, you finish the ride at the main parking lot at 16.6 miles.

OTHER AREA RIDES

SKYLINE WILDERNESS PARK: Dynamite comes in small packages. Though Skyline Wilderness Park (also simply referred to as Skyline Park) is just an 850-acre park with over 20 miles of bikeable trails, don't expect to find easy trails here; you need skills in the intermediate to advanced level. As the site of World Cup mountain-bike race in the late 1990s, it's home to some of the most technically challenging single-tracks in the Wine Country. As a city-maintained park, a small parking fee is charged, and RV and tent camping is available in the spring and summer. The park is subject to closure relating to fire hazards, heavy storms, as well as at Thanksgiving and Christmas.

Finding the trail: From San Francisco, drive north on CA 29 toward the town of Napa. When CA 29 begins to jog west, bear right onto CA 221/121 (Soscol Avenue). Proceed north and then turn right onto Imola Avenue (Napa State Hospital on the corner). Follow Imola to its end at Skyline Park.

Maps: Generally available at the park kiosk.

For more information, contact:
Skyline Wilderness Park
2201 E. Imola Ave.
Napa, CA 94559-0793
(707) 252-0481

BALD MOUNTAIN LOOP AT SUGARLOAF RIDGE STATE PARK: This strenuous ride on designated fire roads is suited for riders with intermediate to advanced technical skills. The approximately 7-mile, clockwise loop uses these trails in the following order: Stern, Bald Mountain, and Gray Pine. Other bikeable trails in the park are out-and-back roads.

Finding the trail: From San Francisco, drive north on US 101 toward Santa Rosa. Take the CA 12 exit and follow it through Santa Rosa, past Annadel State Park and toward Sonoma. After about 12 miles from Santa Rosa, turn left onto Adobe Canyon Road and follow it to the end into Sugarloaf Ridge State Park. Park in the Visitor Center parking lot and don't forget to pay the parking fee, about $5.

Maps: Sugarloaf Ridge State Park map, available at the visitor center or kiosk for about $1.

For more information, contact:
Sugarloaf Ridge State Park
2605 Adobe Canyon Rd.
Kenwood, CA 95452-9004
(707) 833-5712

WILLOW CREEK ROAD: Willow Creek Road is a 12-mile stretch of mostly un-paved narrow road which connects the tiny towns of Occidental and Bridgehaven at the mouth of the Russian River and Highway 1 (CA 1). You can ride this stretch as an out-and-back, making it 24 miles round-trip. For a 32-mile ride, add on the lightly traveled, scenic paved roads of CA 116 along the Russian River and the Bohemian Highway along Dutch Bill Creek. Riders who don't mind sharing the road with mo-torists can also make a loop via Highway 1 and Coleman Valley Road. Whichever route you choose, expect some steep but short climbs on mildly technical terrain (paved and unpaved). Pedaling from the tiny town of Occidental, head out on Willow Creek Road, a public access road bordered by private property. Follow it to its termination in Sonoma Coast State Beach land. Please respect private property by staying on the road. Pomo Canyon campground is located on Willow Creek Road. Other campgrounds can be found in nearby Sonoma Coast State Beach.

Finding the trail: Located just north of Bodega Bay and slightly inland are four par-alleling roads that run essentially north-south: Highway 1, Bohemian Highway, CA 116, and US 101. The suggested starting point for this ride from Occidental is lo-cated due west of Santa Rosa on Bohemian Highway. From Occidental, drive or pedal west on Coleman Valley Road for about a mile to the Willow Creek Road junction. Begin your cycling adventure by going right (north) onto Willow Creek.

Maps: USGS Duncan Mills and Camp Meeker 7.5 minute series.

For more information, contact:

> Sonoma Coast State Beach
> 3095 Highway One
> Bodega Bay, CA 94923
> (707) 875-3483

ROCKVILLE HILLS PARK: This ride is located just east of the city of Napa and west of Fairfield and Rockville in Solano County. A city park managed by the Solano County Farmlands & Open Space Foundation, this park encompasses more than 600 acres of valleys and steep slopes. Oak hillsides and beautiful rock outcroppings decorate most of the terrain, hence its name. That said, expect a fair amount of rocky and technically challenging single-track trails within its web of bikeable routes. Hours of fun can be had here.

Finding the trail: From the intersection of I-80 and I-680 in the northeast edge of San Francisco Bay, travel north on I-80 and immediately take the Suisun Valley Road exit. Make your way to the north side of I-80 and head toward Rockville. Turn left onto Rockville Road and proceed west about a mile to the park entrance located on your left.

Maps: Check kiosks at major trailheads. In 1999, a local cycling enthusiast posted a map on the Web at http://vader.castles.com/huston/rides.html.

For more information, contact:

> Solano County Farmlands & Open Space Foundation
> P.O. Box 115
> 744 Empire St., Suite 112
> Fairfield, CA 94533
> (707) 421-1351; or (707) 428-7580

SOME LOCAL BICYCLE SHOPS

St. Helena Cyclery
1156 Main St.
Saint Helena, CA 94574
(707) 963-7736

Palisades Mountain Sports
1330-B Gerrard St.
Calistoga, CA 94515
(707) 942-9687

Bicycle Trax
796 Soscol Ave.
Napa, CA 94559
(707) 258-8729

Rincon Cyclery
4927 Sonoma Highway
Santa Rosa, CA 95409-4289
(707) 538-0868

Gianni Cyclery
3798 Bohemian Highway
Occidental, CA 95465
(707) 874-2833

THE GOLD RUSH COUNTRY OF
THE WESTERN SIERRAS

Welcome to the territory that started the Americanization of the West. Gold flecks discovered by John Marshall in January 24, 1848, at his sawmill near Colma in El Dorado County single-handedly ignited the largest human migration in the nation's history. The Gold Rush was born. Native Americans were shamefully mowed down. Respect for rich forest environments and water resources were blindly disregarded. The heady prospect of unlimited wealth attracted·a colorful crowd of dreamers from the eastern states and world-wide, eager to strike it rich, unrestrained by the old social norms they had left behind. Eccentric characters, from audacious "gentleman bandit" Black Bart to provocative "spider dancer" Lola Montez to master "yarn-spinner" Mark Twain, gave birth to a new cultural identity that characterizes the attitude of Californians to this day. Even though the mythical Mother Lode vein of gold was never found, the state's population kept growing, fed by boundless opportunities offered by other natural resources. The West was the place to be.

The Gold Rush Country along the western slope of the Sierra Nevada mountain range stretches from Oroville and Chico down to Bear Valley and Yosemite, and west to Sacramento and the Central Valley. Six major rivers and their subsidiaries drain this region and include the Feather, American, Cosumnes, Mokelumne, Tuolumne, and Merced Rivers. Ranging in elevation from 400 to 8,000 feet, carved by the rivers and eons of erosion, the landscape is mostly granite, mixed with volcanically transformed metamorphic rock. The climate is typically hot and dry during the summer, often reaching the 100s in the lower elevations. Rain usually waters the area from late fall through spring though summer thundershowers are not uncommon. Snow level can drop to 2,500 feet and is not unusual. During the fall, winter, and early spring, mornings often see fog snaking through narrow valleys and river canyons. Four adjoining national forests—Plumas, Tahoe, Eldorado, and Stanislaus—create a solid belt of protected land in which a gazillion mountain biking trails for all abilities abound. We have pack-mule drivers to thank for they laid the groundwork to many of today's single-track trails, some of which are considered world-class. But you needn't possess expert technical skills or amazing stamina to enjoy the Gold Country. Beginner and intermediate riders with decent endurance are sure to strike it rich with lots of suitable routes.

RIDE 26 · American River Bike Path

AT A GLANCE

Length/configuration: 64-mile out-and-back (32 miles each way); paved bike path with a short stretch on paved vehicle road and dirt. With its numerous access points, the trail can be easily shortened.

Aerobic difficulty: Easy; moderately strenuous if riding the entire distance

Technical difficulty: Not technical

Scenery: A thriving riparian environment along the American River, running through suburban communities east of Sacramento. The more scenic eastern end consists of rolling oak woodlands as it gently climbs to Lake Natoma, Nimbus Dam, Folsom Lake, and Folsom Dam.

Special comments: A great family outing, suitable for kid-trailers.

Arguably one of the most successful and beautifully paved bike paths in northern California, this 32-mile gem of a trail stretches from downtown Sacramento eastward to Folsom Dam (64 miles round-trip). Also known as the Jedediah Smith National Recreation Trail, the American River Bike Path is nearly 100% separate from vehicle roads (a mile or two shares the road). The route hugs the American River as it ever so gently gains roughly 450 feet elevation as you ride from west to east. The trail is well maintained and mile markers are posted, starting at zero on the western end. You can start from a dozen access points and ride for as long or short as you like. In between the two trailheads, the path leads through a rich riparian environment, graced by an abundance of birds. You're never far from civilization since the bike path leads past many residential and commercial neighborhoods and city parks (some of which have historical significance).

If you're short on time and low on endurance, pedal the most scenic part by starting from Beal Point in the Folsom State Recreation Area at the eastern end of the route. Ride as far as you want, but know that your return will be a gradual uphill push. If you start at the western end from Discovery Park, the path is generally flat for the first 20 miles or so. Thereafter, the path gains elevation, 7% grade in some stretches, as it cruises past the Nimbus Fish Hatchery, Nimbus Dam, and on up to Beals Point at Folsom Lake. Regardless of where you start on the path, you can really pick up speed, but beware. Park rangers patrol the bikeway, giving warnings or citations for speeding as well as riding on illegal dirt single-tracks.

Near the eastern end, the little town of Folsom (yes, that Folsom in which the state slammer immortalized by country crooner Johnny Cash in "Folsom Prison Blues" is located), is a worthy detour if you're looking for distractions. There, you'll find lots of points of interest, such as the Folsom History Museum, the Folsom Prison Museum, the Gekkeikan Sake brewery with its 60-minute guided tour, the City Zoo, and the Railroad Turntable and Depot. Of course, many eateries abound, including microbreweries, hip coffee shops, and restaurants. At the western end of the path, you can take a one-mile, one-way excursion into Old Town Sacramento, a state historic park and national landmark. There, you'll find several excellent historic museums (the

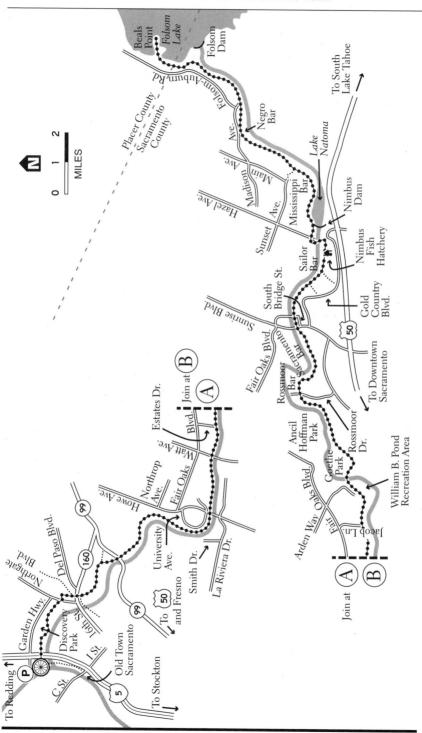

California State Railroad Museum and the Sacramento History Museum) as well as the five-story Delta King, one of California's last original steam paddlewheel ships still sitting in the Sacramento River. Though it's now a luxury, floating hotel, it was quite a decadent palace during the 1920s Prohibition, moving passengers between San Francisco and Sacramento. In the 1940s, it was called into military duty, transporting Navy troops.

General location: Stretches 31 miles east from the heart of Sacramento.

Elevation change: 435 feet; starting elevation and low point 25 feet; high point 460 feet. West to east direction is very mellow climbing becoming slightly steeper at eastern end.

Season: Year-round.

Services: Many rest rooms, drinking fountains, picnic tables, public phones, and emergency call boxes located throughout the bikeway. During the summer months, a well-stocked snack bar is open at Beals Point. All other services located in the suburban neighborhoods adjacent to the path.

Hazards: Sadly, Discovery Park, at the western trailhead, is considered somewhat unsafe for solo women, even in the daylight hours. Riding with a friend is a wise idea. Watch out for vehicular traffic as the bikeway crosses a handful of streets. Especially unnerving is a short 0.25-mile section alongside Hazel Avenue where the fast traffic seems to be hurling directly toward you. If you have youngsters in tow, you may want to walk this stretch—or avoid it entirely. You're likely to encounter "rush hour" traffic of cyclists and joggers during weekdays, generally after 4 p.m.

Rescue index: Emergency call boxes and public pay phones are located throughout the bikeway. Except for the first 6 miles, the route is within 0 to 0.5 mile of residential and commercial neighborhoods. You're likely to meet other trail users who may be of assistance, especially in the late afternoon.

Land status: Folsom Lake State Recreation Area, Sacramento County of Parks and Recreation.

Maps: *Sacramento Bikeway Maps,* published by the Sacramento Metropolitan Air Quality Management District, Mobile Source Division.

Finding the trail: The bikeway can be accessed at numerous locations within commercial or residential neighborhoods. Following is a list of locations with convenient parking:

1. Discovery Park in the city of Sacramento. Located at the western end of the route, at the confluence of the American and Sacramento Rivers, the path's mile marker system starts in this park as mile 0. To get there, traveling northbound or southbound on Interstate 5, take the Richards Boulevard exit located on the south side of the American River. Follow the signs to Discovery Park. Make your way to the west side of I-5 and turn right (north) on Jibboom Street and enter the park at the toll gate (a small day-use fee is charged). Proceed over the American River and park in any of the lots provided. Begin pedaling by picking up the paved bikeway directly underneath I-5.

2. At the end of Kingsford Drive, off Arden Way and Fair Oaks Boulevard, near mile marker 13, north bank; in Sacramento.

3. Arden Way at William B. Pond Recreation Area, near mile marker 13, north bank; in Sacramento.

4. At the end of Rod Beaudry Drive, off Folsom Boulevard, near mile marker 14, south bank; in Sacramento/Rancho Cordova.

5. Rossmoor Drive, off Coloma Road at Folsom Boulevard, near mile marker 17, south bank; in Rancho Cordova.

6. El Mano Drive, off Coloma Road at Folsom Boulevard, near mile marker 18, south bank; in Rancho Cordova.

7. South Bridge Street, off Sunrise Boulevard near Folsom Boulevard, near mile marker 20, south bank; in Rancho Cordova.

8. Nimbus Fish Hatchery on Gold Country Boulevard off Folsom Boulevard, near mile marker 23, south bank; in Folsom.

9. Near the end of Hazel Avenue at mile marker 23, north bank; in Fair Oaks.

10. Intersection of Sunset and Main Avenues near Hazel Avenue, near mile marker 25, north bank; in Folsom.

11. At Negro Bar, off Greenback Lane, near mile marker 28, on the north bank; in Folsom.

12. Folsom Dam Road, at its intersection with Folsom-Auburn Road, near mile marker 30, north bank; in Folsom.

13. Beals Point overlooking Folsom Lake in Folsom. This is the eastern terminus of the paved bikeway in Folsom Lake State Recreation Area. To get there, go east on I-80 toward Auburn. In the suburb of Roseville, take the Douglas Boulevard exit and follow it due east for about 5.3 miles. Turn right onto Auburn-Folsom Road and drive almost 1.7 miles where you make a left turn to Beals Point. Follow the signs to the parking area.

Sources of additional information:

Sacramento Metropolitan Air
  Quality Management District
Mobile Source Division
8411 Jackson Rd.
Sacramento, CA 95826
Fax: (916) 386-2279
Contact this agency for excellent
maps.

Sacramento Area Bicycle Advocates
  (SABA)
909 12th St., Suite 100
Sacramento, CA 95814
www.smart-traveler.com

Notes on the trail: You can begin pedaling at any point on the bikeway. There are several spots worthy of mention and for the sake of this description, the following observations are based on riding west to east, from Sacramento to Folsom Lake.

The bikeway stays on the north bank of the American River for the first 13.5 miles. Near mile 2.8, just before the elevated train tracks, a paved path intersects, running left and right. Stay straight, going underneath the tracks. You may have to pedal a few yards to find the right path since the bushes and trees here are thick and tall, effectively obscuring your view. If you cross over the river, you're off the main route and are now heading into downtown Sacramento.

At almost 8 miles, still on the north bank, another paved path leads south across the river and into California State University–Sacramento. Stay left, keeping the river on your right.

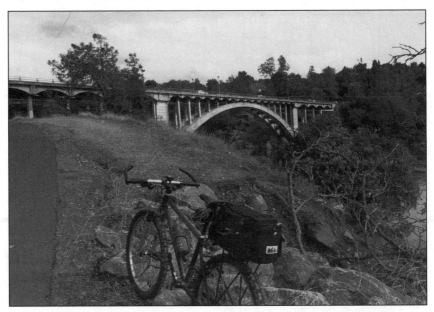

Like a narrow strip of wilderness slicing through urban Sacramento, the American
River is hugged by this paved 32-mile bike path.

The bikeway crosses the river at almost 14 miles. From 14 to almost 23 miles, the
route hugs the river on the south bank, all the way to the Nimbus Fish Hatchery. At
23 miles, the paved path ends at Hazel Avenue. Go left onto Hazel Avenue, a fright-
eningly fast four-lane highway, and proceed to cross over to the north bank. Do not
cross Hazel Avenue. Instead, stay on the west side of Hazel Avenue—yes, you will be
riding against traffic. There's a wide, paved shoulder, about four feet across, and the
distance on this treacherous stretch is less than 0.25 mile. If the traffic barreling and
curving downhill toward you is terrifying (as it was to me), move yourself farther from
the line of traffic by making use of the small dirt shoulder. Dismount and walk if you
need to. Proceed through a fenced, somewhat separated pathway on the bridge over
the river, still on the shoulder of the highway. Once back on ground, follow the dirt
trail as it hairpin turns to the left and descends steeply back under Hazel Avenue. You
might want to dismount and walk this section if you're unaccustomed to such steep
terrain. Now on the north bank, the trail continues to follow the river eastward, toward the Nimbus Dam and Lake Natoma. The dirt trail eventually becomes a paved
bike path again. Along this stretch, at the base of Nimbus Dam, you're likely to see
lots of anglers in tall waders, standing in the water, fishing. This is a popular fishing
spot, and trout, perch, bass, and catfish are the rewards.

Continuing on, go underneath Jedediah Smith Bridge at about mile 28. Cruise
pass condos and apartments as you approach the Folsom-Auburn Road junction.
The path now begins a gentle climb toward the top of Folsom Dam, now coming
into view on your right. Soon after the dam, the paved path ends, dumping you out
onto a vehicle road. Follow the road for a few yards to the entrance of Beals Point, a
large, maintained park. Enjoy a break here. There are drinking water and rest rooms
here. The snack bar is generally open during the summer months. Afterward, return
the same way you came.

RIDE 27 · Salmon Falls Out-and-Back

AT A GLANCE

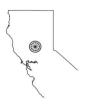

Length/configuration: 19-mile out-and-back (9.5 miles each way); mostly single-track and some dirt roads

Aerobic difficulty: Moderately strenuous; steep but brief ups and downs

Technical difficulty: Intermediate; twisty, sometimes rocky, narrow single-track

Scenery: Trail hugs the shoreline of Folsom Lake and travels through stands of oak and manzanita trees. One of the sweetest, legal single-tracks in the Sacramento area.

Special comments: Strong and adventurous beginners with some experience riding single-tracks might enjoy this challenge. This trail also referred to as Darrington Trail. A nearby single-track called the Sweetwater Trail is worth checking out and is easily accessed from the starting point described at the end of this profile.

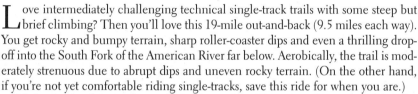

Love intermediately challenging technical single-track trails with some steep but brief climbing? Then you'll love this 19-mile out-and-back (9.5 miles each way). You get rocky and bumpy terrain, sharp roller-coaster dips and even a thrilling drop-off into the South Fork of the American River far below. Aerobically, the trail is moderately strenuous due to abrupt dips and uneven rocky terrain. (On the other hand, if you're not yet comfortable riding single-tracks, save this ride for when you are.)

It's hard to get lost on this trail. On the outbound portion, the trail parallels the South Fork canyon. The canyon widens into Folsom Lake with the water always on your left except for a short stretch which veers inland for a moment. Add a handful of well-placed bike markers at key intersections and the result is a route that's a piece of cake to follow. In the spring and early summer, the rolling hills are gorgeously green and, if you're timing is right, you may see a splattering of spectacular wildflowers. This insanely popular single-track cruises through small meadows, alternating between sun and shade as it leads through groves of manzanita and oak and past thick chaparral. Leisurely and quiet riding may yield a glimpse of jackrabbits, opossum, coyote, gray foxes, and bobcats, to name a few of the resident mammals.

So where is Salmon Falls? Named for a small pair of falls, it is located about a mile west of the Salmon Falls Bridge, about a half mile downstream from Sweetwater Creek. As its name implies, the region was once rich in wild salmon, which provided plenty of food for the Nisenan Indians who lived here. In the late nineteenth century, logging companies began using the South Fork to transport lumber to mills in Folsom and Sacramento. Gigantic logjams formed at the falls. No problem. The American River Land and Lumber Company blasted the falls, effectively clearing the waterway. But in so doing, the natural passageway of salmon to their spawning grounds was nearly destroyed. In the 1920s, the State Fish and Game Department obliterated the remaining passageway, causing the salmon to disappear forever. Today, Folsom Lake and the South Fork yield trout, bass, catfish, and kokanee.

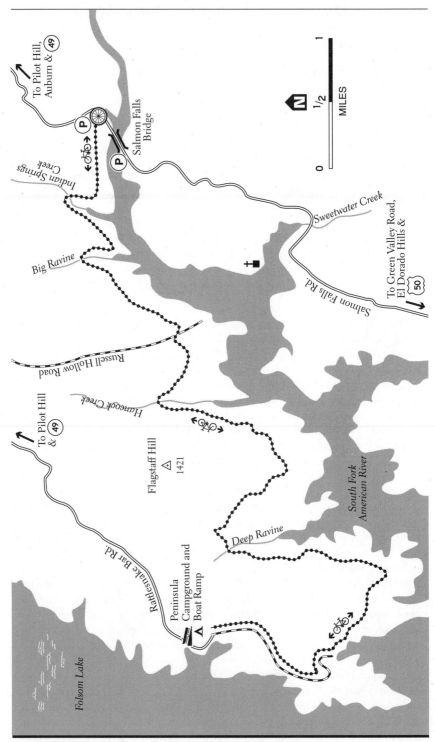

To Pilot Hill, Auburn & (49)

Salmon Falls Bridge

P

P

Indian Springs Creek

Big Ravine

Sweetwater Creek

To Green Valley Road, El Dorado Hills & (50)

Salmon Falls Rd.

Russell Hollow Road

Hancock Creek

Flagstaff Hill △ 1421

To Pilot Hill & (49)

Deep Ravine

South Fork American River

Rattlesnake Bar Rd.

Peninsula Campground and Boat Ramp

Folsom Lake

N

MILES

0   ½   1

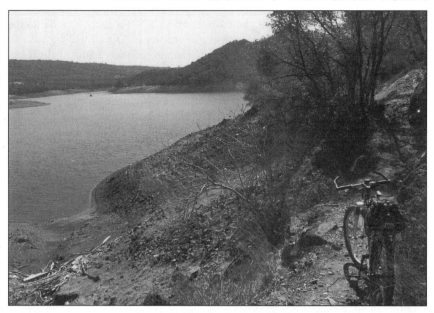

Clinging to a slope along Folsom Lake, this rocky single-track near the trailhead twists and dips as it skirts sections of rugged drop-offs.

General location: About 45 miles east of Sacramento, on the eastern edge of Folsom Lake.

Elevation change: 500 feet; starting elevation and low point 320 feet; high point 820. Lots of roller-coaster terrain with stretches of nearly flat riding.

Season: Year-round, though summers can be extremely hot.

Services: None on the trail. Drinking water and rest rooms at Peninsula Campground located at the far end of the ride. Rest rooms seasonally available at a boat landing across the road from the trailhead (starting point). Most services are in El Dorado Hills, and all services are available in Sacramento.

Hazards: This insanely popular mountain bike route is fairly crowded on the weekends. Watch out for oncoming trail users. Some stretches of the single-track are only wide enough for one cyclist, let alone two in passing mode. Extra caution is required on the portions of the first mile where the trail traverses a steep, exposed wall, twisting and running up and down over somewhat rocky terrain. The fire hazard easily reaches into the extreme range in summer to fall. Stay alert for poison oak and, though rarely seen, rattlesnakes and mountain lions.

Rescue index: During the weekend and possibly late in the afternoon on a sunny day, you're likely to encounter other bikers who may be of help in an emergency. During the summer, you may find help at the Peninsula Campground, located at the outer end of the trail. Salmon Falls Road at the trailhead is frequently traveled, and you may have good luck flagging down a passing motorist.

Land status: Folsom Lake State Recreation Area.

Maps: USGS Pilot Hill and Clarksville 7.5 minute series.

Finding the trail: From Sacramento, travel east on US 50 for about 38 miles to the El Dorado Hills exit. Take the exit and head north on El Dorado Hills Road. Go through Green Valley Road at which point El Dorado becomes Salmon Falls Road. Continue on Salmon Falls Road and in about 6 miles from Green Valley, cross the South Fork of the American River. Immediately after the bridge, look for a small parking lot on your left and park there. Remember to pay the small parking fee here by using the self-pay dispenser. The trailhead is located behind the pay container on the west end of the lot. (For those of you who don't want to cough up a few bucks, you can park in a pulloff area just before crossing the bridge. Then, bike to the trailhead.)

From Auburn (located about 30 miles east of Sacramento on I-80), drive south on CA 49, going through the town of Cool at about 6 miles. Continue on CA 49 and reach the intersection of Rattlesnake Bar Road at 10 miles. Go right onto Rattlesnake and then take an immediate left onto Salmon Falls Road. Follow Salmon Falls for almost 6 miles more to the trailhead, located at a small parking lot on the right side of the road, just before the Salmon Falls Bridge.

Incidentally, you can do this ride starting from the trailhead described below or in reverse from Peninsula Campground, which is accessed by taking Rattlesnake Bar Road due southwest to its end near the lake's edge, about 9 miles from CA 49.

Sources of additional information:

Folsom Lake State Recreation Area
7806 Folsom-Auburn Rd.
Folsom, CA 95630
(916) 988-0205

FATRAC (Folsom-Auburn Trail
Riders Action Coalition)
P.O. Box 6356
Auburn, CA 95604

Notes on the trail: Begin pedaling by hopping onto the single-track trail that leads from the west end of the small Salmon Falls Road parking lot. The trail is mildly technical and hard packed, with some large chunks of rocks accenting your path. Right off the bat, you encounter a series of quick ups and downs that are steep but brief. You might even catch some air through a few dips. Watch out for boulders big enough to catch your pedal as you zip by. In about a mile, the trail widens and broken pavement emerges. Follow a trail marker and go left. Hug a hairpin turn to the left, cross a dry creek, and continue with the compact roller-coaster ride through the sparse forest.

The trail begins to narrow to about 3 feet, bordered on both sides by tall bushes. The trail is not as rocky here and is easy to ride. Cross another tiny dry creek, almost a mile from the last one, about 2.7 miles from the trailhead. Begin turning inland, following the trail as it leads away from the water. A barbed-wire fence starts to parallel your path as you cruise the easy single-track through groves of oak and some pine trees. Few obstacles of semi-buried rocks and trees in the trail keep you on your toes. Other lesser single-tracks lead away from the main trail, heading toward the water. Stay on the main trail pedaling though a meadow. At 3.4 miles, pass a bike marker which indicates to stay on the single-track (which may look like a double-track for at least a few yards). By now, you know that the trail conditions vary between mildly smooth and intermediately rocky terrain.

At 4.4 miles, about a mile from the last bike marker, cross the third dry creek and follow a set of closely spaced bike markers. Cruise pass pine and manzanita trees as you weave toward the lake edge. For almost a half mile, the increasingly rocky trail skirts a slope that drops off directly into the lake. Zip pass a small wooden bench overlooking the lake at 6 miles and about 1.2 miles farther, cross a tiny creek. Follow the single-track as it runs up and down again to another creek crossing at mile 7.5.

You reach the end of the single-track at a fire road, signed (in the other direction) as the Darrington Trail. Take the fire road, going straight through an intersection. Stay on the main fire road and at about 9.7 miles, you reach Peninsula Campground. There are picnic tables here and you might even find a vacant one on which to lean your bike and rest your body. Refill your water bottles before turning around and retracing your fun 9.5 mile roller-coaster path back to your car. Round-trip mileage back to the Salmon Falls Bridge trailhead is 19 miles.

Sweetwater Trail option: For those of you looking for more single-track riding, check out Sweetwater Trail, an 8-mile out-and-back (4 miles each way). It's reportedly much like the Salmon Falls/Darrington Trail, only not as technical. To get there, leave your car at the parking lot and pedal over the Salmon Falls Bridge, heading due southwest (the lake is on your right). Immediately on the other end of the bridge, on the water side of the road is a small parking area. The trailhead is located at this parking area and stays on the water side of the road.

RIDE 28 · Olmstead Loop

AT A GLANCE

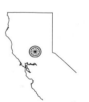

Length/configuration: 9-mile loop, clockwise (or reverse) direction; fire roads, single- and double-tracks

Aerobic difficulty: Moderate; some strenuous stretches due to steep but brief climbing

Technical difficulty: Intermediate; some challenging rugged spots

Scenery: Rolling grassy hills with a pleasant blend of shady oak forests and open meadows

Special comments: This is a great ride for strong beginners. Strong bikers looking for more saddle time often ride this loop twice, going in the opposite direction on the second time.

Olmstead Loop is a technically intermediate, aerobically moderate 9-mile loop that's guaranteed to please all levels of riders, from expert to beginner. It's also one heck of a fun ride up and down rolling grassy hills covered with oaks. Located in the Auburn State Recreation Area, the route is a combination of fire roads, wide single- and double-tracks that run like a roller coaster through short and sometimes steep hills. Not overly taxing, the rises are about 6 to 8% grades—just enough to get you breathing hard. It's the kind of variety that puts the fun in mountain biking. And for those strong riders really aching for a challenge, consider riding from Auburn across the North Fork American River via the Auburn-to-Cool Trail (briefly described at the end of this description).

This gem of a trail is a testament that harmony between equestrians, mountain bikers, and hikers can exist. Dan Olmstead, for whom the loop is named, devoted

RIDE 28 · Olmstead Loop

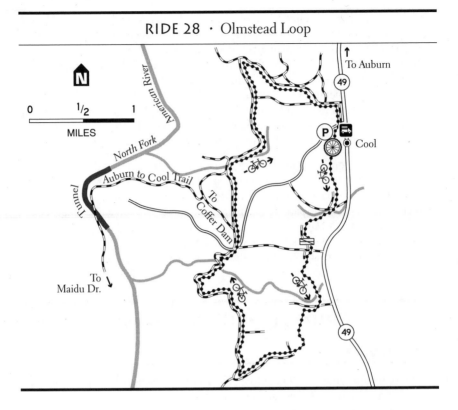

the last years of his short life to establishing that harmony. An avid lover of nature and being outdoors, he bought Auburn Bike & Hike, a retail store in 1979, and soon developed a deep love for mountain biking. As with other regions in the state, the early days of the sport saw numerous conflicts between the different trail users, particularly equestrians and bikers. All trail users were determined to protect and preserve what they enjoyed the most: their valuable outdoor surroundings. Wanting to understand why equestrians were so passionate about their activity, Olmstead participated in a week-long horseback trip. He gained insight and appreciation for horses and their owners. With that understanding, he worked to bring together bikers, equestrians, and hikers so that everyone could enjoy their chosen activity. He was involved in mobilizing people into work parties to maintain and repair trails. And from his tireless effort, Olmstead succeeded in opening this popular horse trail to mountain biking. On February 13, 1993, he succumbed to cancer, the day before this loop held a mountain bike race that he was instrumental in organizing. Today, the race is held each year around February 13 in his memory and has become synonymous with mud, slop, and great fun.

General location: About 39 miles east of Sacramento and south of Auburn.

Elevation change: 280 feet; starting elevation 1,500 feet; high point 1,620 feet; low point 1,220 feet. Mostly rolling hills with some steep climbing stretches.

Season: Early spring to late fall.

Services: Picnic table at the trailhead. No services on the route. A couple of eateries and a convenient store in the town of Cool, about a half mile from the trailhead. All other services in Auburn, about 6 miles north.

Hazards: Watch out for rattlesnakes, especially during the spring and summer. This area of the Auburn State Recreation Area is extremely popular with equestrians, so exercising trail etiquette is vitally important to keeping trails open to bikers. Bring plenty of water, especially during the scorching summer months. Water taken from creeks must be treated. Stay alert for rarely seen mountain lions.

Rescue index: During the weekend, you're bound to see other trail users who may be of assistance. The best and closest place for emergency help is at the trailhead, which is located immediately behind the Cool fire station. On weekdays, don't expect someone to come along on the trail; make your way back to the trailhead for help.

Land status: Auburn State Recreation Area.

Maps: *Olmstead Loop*, published by Sowarwe-Werher, P.O. Box 17, Weimar, CA 95736; USGS Auburn and Pilot Hill 7.5 minute series.

Finding the trail: From Sacramento, drive east on I-80 to Auburn, a little over 30 miles. Take the CA 49 exit and follow it as it twists and turns through Auburn. Staying on CA 49 is a bit of a challenge, so pay attention to signs. As you quickly cruise through town, the road begins winding down into the canyon created by the confluence of the North and Middle Forks of the American River. Go right at a **T** intersection and immediately cross over the North Fork. About 4.5 miles from the bridge, just as you approach the tiny town of Cool, turn right onto a paved road immediately before the fire station. Behind the station is a big dirt parking area. Park and begin your ride from here.

Sources of additional information:

Auburn State Recreation Area
P.O. Box 3266
Auburn, CA 95604
(916) 885-4527; (916) 988-0205

FATRAC (Folsom-Auburn Trail
Riders Action Coalition)
P.O. Box 6356
Auburn, CA 95604
www.jps.net/fatrac/news.html

Notes on the trail: Though you can ride this loop in either direction, the route described here is clockwise. Scattered throughout Olmstead Loop are brown trail markers decorated with mileages and bike symbols. Most of those markers are well placed, although a couple seemed to be slightly off. Nevertheless, this loop is fairly easy to follow.

Begin your fun by picking up the trailhead (look for marker) at the southern end of the parking area. The trail for the next 3 miles alternates between narrow and wide single-track and dirt road. Starting off, the trail leads you through a wide-open, gentle roller-coaster meadow. Cross a stream via a wooden bridge and begin a brief climb. At 1.3 miles, go through a gate, bearing left following a trail marker. (Remember to leave the gate as you found it—open or closed.) A couple of deep ruts punctuate an otherwise hard-packed trail. Go through another gate at 1.5 miles, followed by another creek crossing on a wooden bridge. The trail curves right after the creek, leading you through oak groves interspersed with open, rolling meadows. Check out those bushes by the creek, and you may find juicy wild blackberries.

Look for a trail marker at about 2 miles. Bear left here onto a single-track, leaving the wider single-track that you had been riding. The trail sporadically widens and narrows as you climb a gentle hill. When you reach 2.5 miles (and another marker), look straight ahead and notice four radio towers in the distance. Enjoy a bit of a downhill curvy run amid a wide-open meadow. At about 3.1 miles, the towers are behind your left shoulder. Pass another marker and go through a gate (there's a break in the fence next to the gate and it's obvious that many trail users take advantage of it). At this point, several other lesser single-tracks intersect your trail. Stay straight as you go through the gate and look for another marker a few yards ahead, planted at a split in the trail. By now, the radio towers have completely disappeared from view. Follow the trail, now a wide single-track as it makes a hard hairpin right turn, running up and down an open meadow scattered with oak and conifer trees.

As you enjoy your sweet roller-coaster ride, cruising in and out of the shade, keep a sharp eye out and you might see flocks of wild turkeys scampering through the sparse forest. Go through another sturdy gate at about 4.6 miles and gear down for a brief and steep climb, about 0.2 mile. The trail quickly mellows and resumes its fun up and down attitude. Rain ruts and semi-buried rocks make this stretch technically more interesting. As you approach 5 miles, gear down and let 'er run as you enjoy a fast but short descent. Keep pedaling through a wet creek crossing and immediately climb up a very steep and loose, semi-packed dirt road. If you lose your momentum and/or traction, don't fret—the steepness is less than 0.2 mile. The uphill mellows out a bit and at about 5.4 miles, you've reached the top of the ridge. Here, your trail intersects a paved road, seemingly devoid of auto traffic. If you were to follow the road left, you'll find that after about a mile, the terrain drops steeply, the pavement ends, and an unmaintained dirt road begins, leading down to the south dam abutment. On the other hand, if you go right on this road, it would lead you quickly down to the fire station, reached in about 1.5 miles, (a great shortcut to keep in mind if you get caught in foul weather).

Continue on the Olmstead Loop by crossing the paved road and picking up the dirt trail alongside a marker. At 5.5 miles, you reach a junction with several trails, one of which is signed "Cofferdam trail to Auburn," leading left toward the proposed Auburn Dam (construction halted in 1976). This is also known as the "Auburn to Cool Trail" (ACT). (Those of you aching for some rugged climbing, this reportedly rocky trail descends steeply toward the dam site, at which point you'll have several trail options, all of which lead into the town of Auburn. You can also ride a short distance then turn around and hop back on the Olmstead Loop. Adventurous, strong riders can even access the Olmstead Loop by pedaling from Auburn via the ACT. For the starting point of this arduous routing, see the option at the end of this description.) Bypass the Cofferdam trail, staying straight on the Olmstead Loop and continue the roller-coaster ride on a wide single-track trail. The trail is accented with technical, rocky, and rutted spots, just enough to keep you alert. You reach another marker at about 6 miles and a few feet beyond that, a trail leading off on your left, also toward the proposed dam. (This is another portion of the ACT trail and reconnects with the previous ACT trail bypassed earlier.) Begin a downhill run by bearing right at this intersection and at the following one. Keep that momentum because here comes a somewhat steep stretch that's strewn with some big chunks of rocks and boulders. The wide single-track is still mostly hard-packed. Scattered trees offer some shade.

Reach a level stretch, then descend a short way to a junction with another trail. There's a marker here directing you to bear left. Continue the moderately steep climb to a **T** intersection. Follow the marker indicating the right trail. At almost 8 miles, you reach a flat clearing of gently rolling hills. Look to your right, due southeast, and you can see the trails that make up the first part of the loop—probably with bikers chugging up the slope. Ride a bit farther and bypass a narrow single-track signed "RB," which indicates the Wendell T. Roby Trail, a horse-only path. Follow the usual brown bike markers found in this vicinity and at about 8.4 miles, you reach another **T** intersection. It's likely the trails here are unsigned. Take the left trail (though when in doubt, stay on the wide, multi-use trail, not the enticing single-track) and follow a barbed-wire fence on your right. Gear down. The trail leads through scattered oak trees, and when you reach the top of this short climb, you can see the fire station and your parked car off in the distance. Pick your way through a short and steep loose rock section as you head downhill toward CA 49. At the highway, hang a right and parallel CA 49 for a short distance to the fire station and your car. You close the loop at a little over 9 miles. For more time in the saddle, lots of riders do this loop a second time, going in the opposite direction.

Optional route: From Auburn to the Olmstead Trail via the ACT. In Auburn, pick up the beginning of the ACT at Maidu Drive, across from the former dam construction offices, located along the south edge of town, near the fairgrounds, just before the canyon. Though faded signs declaring "No Public Access" and "Construction Vehicles Only" may still be in place, you are allowed to use these roads and trails. The portion of the trail that drops down into the riverbed and up the south side of the canyon uses paved and gravel roads originally built for trucks working on the dam. (The history of the Auburn Dam project is long and checkered. Though construction was halted in 1976, multimillion dollar concrete abutments still scar the canyon, and erosion and landslides have contributed to the deterioration of roads and trails. Hence, there are numerous trails here and not all of them are marked.) Generally speaking, head down into the riverbed. Go around a gate via a throughway near Shirland Canal. Eventually, pedal to the south side of the North Fork American River by crossing over a half-mile-long tunnel that channels the river through the former Auburn Dam site. Once on the south edge of the canyon, climb up the steep trail on the Auburn-to-Cool Trail. After almost 1.5 miles, the ACT intersects the Olmstead Loop.

RIDE 29 • Quarry Road Out-and-Back

AT A GLANCE

Length/configuration: 10.4-mile out-and-back (5.2 miles each way); dirt road and single-track

Aerobic difficulty: Easy to moderate; mostly flat terrain punctuated by brief, steep inclines

Technical difficulty: Mildly technical with some intermediate spots of rocky terrain and ruts

Scenery: The shady trail hugs a canyon carved by Middle Fork American River. Several spots on the trail drop down to the riverbed, especially welcomed when the weather is close to 100 degrees or more.

Special comments: The first 1.4 miles is suitable for young children. Thereafter, portions of the dirt road may have washed away, falling down into the river. Those sections may require dismounting and walking around the eroded sites.

Following a trail doesn't get any easier than this. Quarry Road closely parallels the Middle Fork of the American River, sometimes at water level, other times about 80 feet up on the canyon walls. Offering dramatic views of the deep river canyon and spots of whitewater flowing through it, the road receives plenty of shade from the oak and pine forest, especially after the first several miles from the trailhead at CA 49. Elevation gain is negligible, even though there's a fair amount of short ups and downs, some of which can be steep for beginners and youngsters. Except for a few moments of moderately rocky or eroded terrain, Quarry Road is basically considered mildly technical. You can make this a leisurely half-day ride or a fast and furious workout by powering through the many brief rises. During the summer when the temperature is hot, the first mile or so from the trailhead is likely to be populated with folks enjoying an afternoon in the river's many accessible swimming holes. Nevertheless, if you want to get away from the crowds, just continue farther on Quarry Road and you'll see fewer people. The turnaround point is at Main Bar, about 5.4 miles out (10.8 miles round-trip). Beyond that, please obey posted "No Bike" signs. A stretch of this route also makes up a portion of the Western States Trail, a much longer equestrian trail. So expect to yield to equestrians, stopping to let them pass or asking for permission before passing them.

Young families often pedal the first several miles of the road, turning around when the kiddies are good and tired. Bear in mind that if you have freewheeling kids with you, close supervision is suggested, because the road may skirt deep drop-offs where winter storms have washed away part of the trail into the river below. Even though the road is about ten feet wide on average, eroded sections will undoubtedly force you to portage your bike over more stable ground before resuming the trail. That said, children need to be confident with their bike-handling abilities.

General location: About 35 miles east of Sacramento, southeast of Auburn, on the south side of the confluence of the North and Middle Forks of the American River.

Elevation change: 280 feet; starting elevation 600 feet; high point 840 feet; low point 560 feet. Outbound direction rolls along with some stretches of moderate climbing.

Season: Year-round.

Services: No water is available on the trail. Pit toilets located about 6 miles from the trailhead.

Hazards: Portions of the trail may have washed away or slid down into the river, forcing you to dismount and walk around them. The outer portion of Quarry Road, roughly after mile 2, is part of the Western States Trail and is frequently used by equestrians. Rain runoffs may produce deep ruts, requiring you to dismount before crossing.

Rescue index: This is a fairly popular route, especially on the weekends. Hot summer temperatures and easy accessibility to the river attract lots of water enthusiasts, and for that reason you're likely to meet other trail users who may be able to offer assistance. Otherwise, no matter where you are on the trail, turn around and head back to the trailhead and CA 49 where you can flag down a passing motorist.

RIDE 29 · Quarry Road Out-and-Back

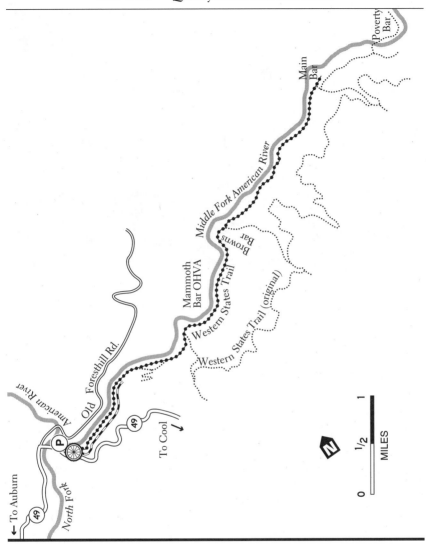

Land status: Auburn State Recreation Area.

Maps: *Auburn State Recreation Area*, published by Sowarwe-Werher, P.O. Box 17, Weimar, CA 95736; USGS Auburn 7.5 minute series.

Finding the trail: From Sacramento, drive east on I-80 to Auburn, about 30 miles. Take the CA 49 exit and follow it as it twists and turns through Auburn. Staying on CA 49 is a bit of a challenge, so pay attention to signs. As quickly as you cruise through town, the road begins winding down into the canyon created by the confluence of the North and Middle Forks of the American River. Go right at a **T** intersection, cross the bridge over the North Fork, and immediately look for a side road

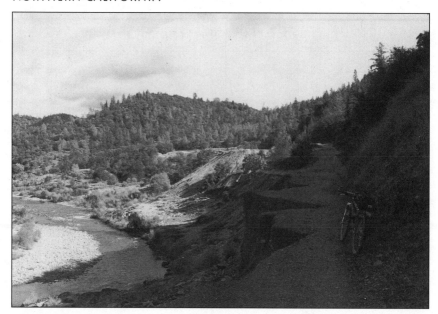

Portions of this road have washed into the river and subsequent storms may force you to portage your bike onto safer ground.

on your left. Turn onto this road, which quickly descends into a dirt parking area. Begin your ride here.

Sources of additional information:

Auburn State Recreation Area
P.O. Box 3266
Auburn, CA 95604
(916) 885-4527; (916) 988-0205

Notes on the trail: The outbound, eastward direction of Quarry Road runs upstream, so closely paralleling the Middle Fork that you think you might fall into the river in some places. Generally speaking, the trail itself is mostly a combination of wide and narrow single-track, composed of stretches of old, broken asphalt, gravel, and hard-packed dirt. While the route is mostly smooth, some sections are somewhat rocky and loose, adding some noise to an otherwise quiet trail. Though elevation gain is negligible, expect the trail to be a roller-coaster ride with some short but steep ups and downs. A brief stretch drops down to the sandy riverbed, leading over and around boulders, their sizes ranging from basketball to almost a Volkswagen Beetle. (If the day is especially hot, you'll be tempted to cool off in the river. You're bound to see some people doing just that.) But even if it's a sunny, sweltering day, you'll be glad to know that Quarry Road is mostly shaded by a thick, cool forest and undergrowth as well as a steep north-facing slope. About five other narrow trails interspersed throughout the route extend uphill (due south) from the main road, few of which are signed.

When you begin the ride, a sign at the trailhead tells you that Poverty Bar is 7.1 miles away. Your turnaround point, however is at Main Bar (not indicated on the sign), at about 5.4 miles, roughly 1.7 miles shy of Poverty Bar. Portions of the trail may have suffered storm damage, washing away into the river. You may want to dismount and walk around these sections, carrying your bike. In any case, stay away from ledges that show signs of recent erosion.

Go through a green metal gate at about 1.8 miles, and if you're lucky, there won't be any dirt motorbikes screaming and piercing the peacefulness across the river at Mammoth Bar, an off-highway vehicle area. You begin to see occasional trail markers identifying Quarry Road as WS Trail, which stands for Western States Trail, a popular, nationally known equestrian route. (Remember to stop and let equestrians and hikers pass, since they have the right of way.) Incidentally, the original WS Trail is higher up and some maps do not label Quarry Road as the alternate WS Trail.

At almost 3 miles, the trail drops down into the riverbed, leading you over a short stretch of large boulders and sandy terrain before climbing out. At about 3.5 miles, cross a tiny creek, and bear left as you bypass Browns Bar Trail. Drop down to the riverbed one more time and then climb a steep 8% incline. You reach Main Bar at just over 5 miles, your turnaround point. There you'll find a couple of pit toilets and a picnic table as well as a trail leading uphill on your right with a sign prohibiting bikes. After enjoying your break, turn around and retrace your path back to the trailhead.

RIDE 30 · Stagecoach–Lake Clementine Loop

AT A GLANCE

Length/configuration: 11.5 miles total; out-and-back with a clockwise loop; single-track, fire roads, and some pavement

Aerobic difficulty: Moderate; some brief, steep climbing

Technical difficulty: Intermediate with a short, treacherous drop-off section

Scenery: Breathtaking views of the deep canyons carved by the North and the Middle Forks of the American River. Rolling, grassy hills sparsely covered with black oak trees.

Special comments: Not recommended for riders prone to vertigo or beginners unaccustomed to single-track riding. Alternate starting point eliminates a 1.8-mile climb at the end of the route described below. An optional, short, technically advanced trail can be added near the Stagecoach trailhead.

This is one of my favorite rides because, in my humble opinion, it offers a bit of what makes mountain biking fun: spectacular scenery, moderate climbing, and fast downhills on intermediately technical single-track. The route leads you down a ridge, then through the canyon carved by the lively North Fork of the American River. Climb another ridge and go bombing down the other side into the canyon of the Middle Fork. It's a gorgeous chunk of territory to enjoy huffing and puffing on your two-wheeled steed, especially on an early fall mornings when the bright sun chases away the fingers of thick fog slowly rising from within the canyons. Plenty of bikers of all abilities come from near and far—confident beginners to hard-core experts. And if you're hoping to make new biking friends, this is a great place.

But don't be fooled by the mention of experts: this route is suitable for intermediate riders. The ride, as described here, is an out-and-back with a big loop attached, totaling 11.5 miles round-trip. Starting with Stagecoach Trail, you follow a screaming fast descent over mildly rocky terrain for 1.8 miles. Though it's a rock-strewn fire road, the high volume of bikers have blazed a relatively smooth single-track trail through it, running over and around rugged sections on the way down toward the confluence of the North and Middle Forks of the American River. When you reach the bottom of Stagecoach, you hop onto the 7.9-mile Lake Clementine Loop trail, pedaling clockwise, climbing a bit on single-track as you skirt the river lying below. After a stretch of paved road, you earn your reward: let 'er rip with a screaming fast downhill over twisty and bumpy technical single-track terrain amid gently rolling hills. If that doesn't get your adrenaline going, maybe this will: Before closing the loop, a short but very narrow portion of the single-track hugs a steep slope with a big, thrilling drop-off right down into the swift Middle Fork of the American River.

Strong beginners and riders who have a fear of heights can avoid the big drop-off section by riding parts of this route as an out-and-back. Advanced and expert riders may want to challenge themselves either on the way down or up Stagecoach by taking the adjacent Manzanita Trail. Reportedly, it's rockier, steeper, and more technically challenging that Stagecoach. Catch it about a mile from the trailhead.

General location: About 30 miles east of Sacramento, on the southeast edge of Auburn, between I-80 and the confluence of the North and Middle Forks of the American River.

Elevation change: 1,400 feet; starting elevation 920 feet; high point 1,640 feet; low point 240 feet. Plenty of big descents and ascents; some flat and mellow stretches in between.

Season: Early spring through late fall.

Services: No water is available on the trail. Pit toilets located about 2.3 miles from the trailhead, at the junction of Old Foresthill Road and Old Lake Clementine Road. All services located in Auburn, about a mile away from the trailhead.

Hazards: Though the Stagecoach Road out-and-back portion is a wide dirt road, a well-used single-track trail has been blazed due to frequent use. So, watch out for the oncoming traffic of bikers bombing down this section as you grind back up it near the end of your ride. There is about a mile of extremely narrow, technical single-track that treacherously hugs a steep slope that drops about 50 yards into the Middle Fork of the American River. Depending on the condition of the trail after winter storms, take extra caution here—dismount and walk where prudent. Keep your eyes out for occasional rattlesnakes and rarely seen mountain lions.

Rescue index: This being a highly popular route, you're likely to meet other trail users, especially other bikers who may offer help. There are several places where the trail crosses vehicle roads and you might be able to flag passing motorists for help. The trailhead is located in a residential neighborhood, and the commercial area of Auburn is about a mile away where you'll find plenty of public phones.

Land status: Auburn State Recreation Area.

Maps: *Stagecoach–Clementine Loop* and *American River Canyon*, both published by Sowarwe-Werher, P.O. Box 17, Weimar, CA 95736; USGS Auburn 7.5 minute series.

Finding the trail: Auburn is located on I-80, a little over 30 miles east of Sacramento. From the Russell Road/Lincoln Way exit off I-80, make your way to the intersection of

RIDE 30 · Stagecoach–Lake Clementine Loop

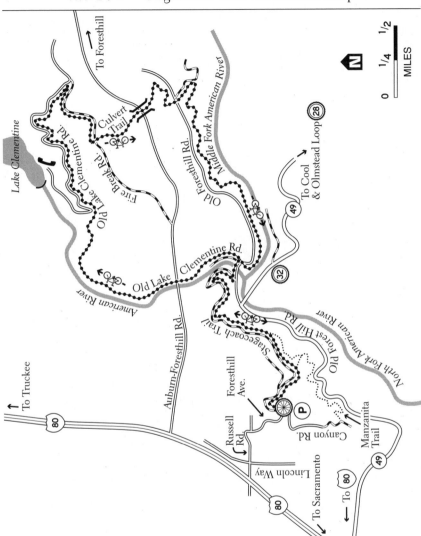

Russell and Lincoln Way on the south side of I-80. Follow Russell due east for almost 0.5 mile, winding through a quiet neighborhood to a sharp right bend in the road, at which point Russell becomes Foresthill Avenue. Exactly at this bend, look for a dirt parking area on the left. This is where you'll find the Stagecoach trailhead. Park here.

Sources of additional information:

Auburn State Recreation Area
P.O. Box 3266
Auburn, CA 95604
(916) 885-4527; (916) 988-0205

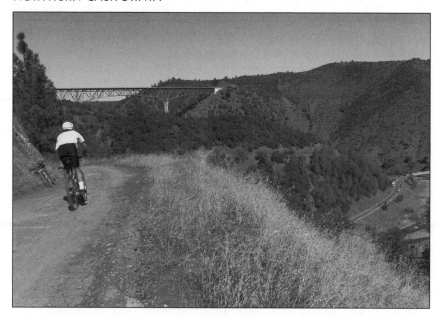

Stagecoach Trail leads down and around to Old Foresthill Bridge at the confluence of the North and Middle Forks of the American River, as seen in the lower right corner.

Notes on the trail: From the parking area off Russell Road, start your ride by accessing Stagecoach Trail on the south edge of the dirt lot. Your warm-up is a hot descent on a wide, rocky fire road. Watch out for oncoming cyclists and trail users grunting their way up Stagecoach, but don't snicker—you'll be climbing this stretch on your return. A narrow and mildly technical trail has been blazed through the rocky road and offers a less jarring, torturous route, unless, of course, you like rattling your eyes in their sockets. (In about a half mile, there's a lesser trail peeling off on your right. It's a short connector to Manzanita Trail, a much more technical alternative to Stagecoach.) At about 1.8 miles, near the bottom of this descent, as you see the modern Foresthill Bridge looming overhead in the near distance, a lesser trail continues straight ahead, and the trail you want makes a right hairpin turn. A few yards after easing your way through the hairpin, you reach Old Foresthill Road, a paved road. You're at the confluence of the North and Middle Forks of the American River. (There's a small dirt parking area here and it's a popular alternate parking place for riders who prefer riding Lake Clementine Loop only and skipping Stagecoach completely.)

Be aware of vehicular traffic as you hang a left onto the paved road. Cross the North Fork on the Old Foresthill Bridge and immediately turn left onto Clementine Road, a dirt road. Begin paralleling the southern edge of the North Fork. The trail quickly becomes a wide single-track as it leads you under the modern Foresthill Bridge looming high overhead. At 2.3 miles, stay left at a junction, and continue to parallel the edge of the river. The trail is mildly technical, punctuated by several spots of slightly challenging terrain. Keep your cool—or enjoy the thrill—as the trail skirts breathtaking drop-offs along some spots. For the most part, the trail is fairly level as it traverses the slope.

At 4 miles, go through a gate, and before you know it, you've reached paved road. Bear right onto the paved road and begin an unrelenting 1.3 miles steep climb (about 8% grade). The road is lightly traveled but still, be alert for cars.

At about 5.4 miles, you reach the top of the paved climb. Look for a couple of huge boulders and a gate on the right side of the road. Say good-bye to the pavement and go through the gate, at which point you see at least three trails leading off in all directions. Take the immediate right trail, a narrow fire road now, and begin a steep climb. The trail soon narrows into a wide single-track. You're now among black oak trees, and their shade is particularly welcome if the day is a scorcher (and believe me, it can get oppressively hot here.) The climbing is short and at 5.6 miles, the single-track levels before forcing you to climb one last brief stretch through a small meadow to the high point of the loop.

Now, at 5.9 miles, you've earned your dessert: get ready for a fun, twisty ride down the north side of the Middle Fork canyon. The single-track is basically mildly technical, and you'll be tempted to bomb down the hill. Let your trusty steed run, but in 0.2 mile keep an eye out for a hard 90-degree turn to the left at about 6.1 miles. This is an easy turn to miss. (If you blow straight pass it, you'll continue a gradual descent on a wide single-track. Eventually, you reach the Auburn-Foresthill Road. You could continue onto the pavement but that's not nearly as fun as single-track. So, grunt back uphill to that missed turn.) Take the hard left and the fun begins. You're now on the Culvert Trail. This single-track twists and turns and, at times, you feel like you're riding a bucking bronco. Whoop and holler your head off, especially as you cruise through a culvert which leads under the Auburn-Foresthill Road. Mind your speed, though. The culvert is 30 to 40 yards, and it's dark!

Once out of the culvert, now on the south side of the busy highway, the next 0.6 mile continues its fun character as before. It's still a hard-packed, single-track, twisty trail with dips and some technical sections. Pure downhill fun. At 7.1 miles, Old Foresthill Road briefly interrupts your fun. (Riders wanting to avoid the drop-off stretch along the Middle Fork can do so by going right on Old Foresthill Road. Ride the shoulder back to the base of Stagecoach Trail.) Cross the road and continue on the wide gravel road where you see a sign indicating that the direction in which you are heading leads to the Mammoth Bar OHV Recreation Area. Stay on the gravel road; in a few yards, at 7.4 miles, turn right onto a gated and signed bike trail (really a wide fire road). Go through the gate and begin descending ever so slightly.

Get ready: here comes the thrilling part of the entire ride. The road is a bit rocky and mildly technical in sections, and you cruise over broken pavement occasionally. Before you know it, you're pedaling a single-track with just enough room for one cyclist. Technically, the trail becomes slightly more challenging with some semi-buried sharp rocks and boulders. Now, these obstacles in the path are generally a piece of cake and fun to maneuver around. But combine that with occasional stretches of severe drop-offs that plunge about 50 yards down into the roaring Middle Fork, and all of a sudden, it's not such a cakewalk anymore. Use extreme caution, especially through sections that show evidence of erosion—you may want to walk through or go around them. But, alas, the thrill is brief and at 9.1 miles, the trail turns away from the drop-off and intersects with Old Foresthill Road, a paved road. You've just closed this loop route and the dirt road directly across the road is where you began the Lake Clementine Loop.

Unless you want to repeat the loop, go left onto the road, crossing the bridge and then hang an immediate right through the gate onto Stagecoach Trail. Here's where you pay for your fun. Remember that fun downhill screamer you took as a warm-up at the beginning of the ride? It's payback time. Shift into low gear and grind all the way back up to your car. Not to worry, though. It's a short two-mile climb with at least one level resting spot. Your finishing mileage is about 11.5 miles.

RIDE 31 · Sly Park–Jenkinson Lake Loop

AT A GLANCE

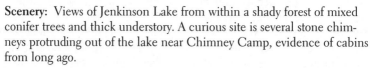

Length/configuration: 9-mile loop, counterclockwise; single- and double-track and pavement

Aerobic difficulty: Moderate; occasional short but steep dips

Technical difficulty: Intermediate; narrow, twisty single-track with some exposed tree roots and spots of drop-offs

Scenery: Views of Jenkinson Lake from within a shady forest of mixed conifer trees and thick understory. A curious site is several stone chimneys protruding out of the lake near Chimney Camp, evidence of cabins from long ago.

Special comments: The first half of this loop is completely uninterrupted sweet, twisty single-track while the second half is a combination of single- and double-tracks and pavement, leading through numerous campgrounds.

This nine-mile counterclockwise loop is known by two names: Sly Park and Jenkinson Lake Loop, the former being the area which contains the loop and the latter being the more descriptive name since the route basically encircles the lake. No matter which name you prefer, general consensus is that it's a really cool trail. Composed mostly of narrow single-track, the trail twists and turns through a dense pine forest and pops up and down short and sometimes steep dips. Throw in a few obstacles like exposed tree roots, spots of rocky terrain, and short stretches of somewhat deep drop-offs, and you have a ride that requires intermediate technical skills. That's not to say beginners with the right attitude and strong endurance won't enjoy the route. Beginners who are out to hone their precision, single-track riding skills may want to dismount and take a couple of steps over extremely technical spots.

On the south side of the lake, the first 3.7 miles is the most fun and challenging. It's gorgeous single-track all the way to Hazel Creek, uninterrupted except for encounters with other trail users. After that, the last 5.3 miles on the north side is mildly technical in that the route is a combination of easy, smooth single- and double-tracks and paved road, interrupted by numerous maintained campgrounds and day-use picnic areas. Other than a couple of brief sections of drop-offs and dips, the real challenge is finding your way through the campgrounds in order to stay on the dirt trail. But not to worry. Throughout the loop, the lake is always in close proximity on your left, and depending on the water level, the trail skirts the lake within several hundred yards.

Like other places along the Sierra Nevada mountain range, Sly Park has its share of history. In 1848, the Mormon Wagon Road was discovered by James Calvin Sly. The road starting from Pleasant Valley through Sly Park meadow near the Hazel Creek area became known as the best route through the Sierra Nevadas for Mormons who were leaving California and heading east to Salt Lake City. Today, the route has been renamed the Mormon Emigrant Trail, part of which is the paved highway that goes over the two dams near this ride's starting point. Of course, prior to Sly, like other parts of California, American Indians from Pleasant Valley—the

RIDE 31 · Sly Park–Jenkinson Lake Loop

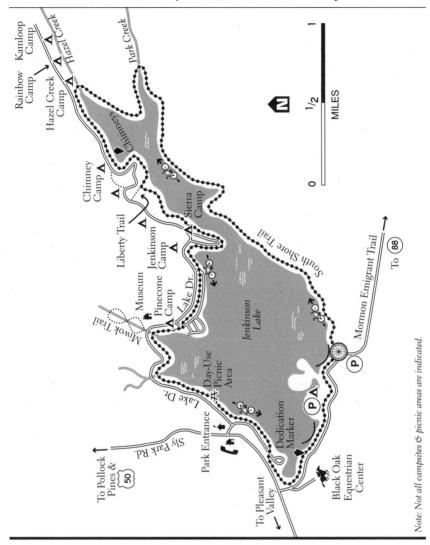

Maidu and Miwok Indians—frequently visited the Hazel Creek area, even after a frontier community was established by the white men. In the early days, there was a hotel, small general store, and a dairy. It was a favorite region in which to drive through thousands of heads of cattle and sheep on their way to summer feeding grounds in the higher elevations. In 1925, the El Dorado Irrigation District was formed, covering approximately 125,000 acres of land and water in this area. Supplying water for irrigation as well as domestic, industrial, and municipal needs was the district's primary goal. In 1955, the two dams on the southwest end of the lake were constructed by the Bureau of Reclamation as part of the Central Valley Project. The lake is named in honor of Walter Jenkinson, the Secretary-Manager of the El Dorado Irrigation District, who died in 1955. Today, Sly Park, in which Jenkinson Lake lies, is an immensely popular, easily accessible summertime destination, offering recreational enjoyment such as boating, fishing, camping, hiking, horseback riding—and mountain biking.

General location: About 42 miles east of Sacramento and 45 miles west of Lake Tahoe off of US 50 near Pollack Pines.

Elevation change: 160 feet; starting elevation 3,400 feet; high and low point negligible. Mostly flat with lots of dips during the first half of loop.

Season: Year-round with occasional fast-melting snow in the winter.

Services: Drinking water, picnic tables, rest rooms, and campsites can be found along the last 5.3 miles of the loop on the north side of the lake. Paddle boat, kayaks, and canoe rentals available near the campgrounds too. There is a public pay phone, grocery store, gas station, and snack bar located on Sly Park Road (also known as Alternate US 50), across from the main Sly Park entrance, near the intersection with the Mormon Emigrant Trail road. From May through September, the James Calvin Sly Museum is open from mid-morning to mid-afternoon, showcasing the history, flora, and fauna of the region. It's located near the Miwok Trail (a hiking-only trail) not far from the main park entrance. All other services available along US 50 in Placerville and outlying eastern suburbs of Sacramento.

Hazards: Be alert for oncoming hikers, equestrians, and bikers, especially on the south side of the lake where the single-track is extremely narrow and twisty. Heed trail designations that separate bikers, hikers, and equestrians. Paved roads that connect the campgrounds are generally less traveled during the week and in the winter, but they see significant traffic during the summer weekends. The last half mile of the loop is on Mormon Emigrant Trail, a well-traveled, two-lane road without a shoulder that has fast cars and logging trucks.

Rescue index: During the summer, you're likely to encounter many other trail users who may be of help, particularly on the north side of the lake near the campgrounds. At other times of the year, you should make your way to the trailhead on the heavily traveled Mormon Emigrant Trail and flag down a passing motorist. The nearest pay phone is across from the main Sly Park entrance on Sly Park Road (also known as Alternate US 50).

Land status: Sly Park Recreation Area, El Dorado Irrigation District.

Maps: *Jenkinson's Lake, Guide #2*, Sierra Foothills Series, published by the Boomerang Design Group, (916) 541-3682; USGS Sly Park 7.5 minute series.

Finding the trail: From Placerville, head east on US 50 toward Pollack Pines and South Lake Tahoe for about 25 miles. Exit at Sly Park Road, also known as Alternate US 50. Go south for 4.7 miles to the Mormon Emigrant Trail, a paved highway on your left. Continue past the main entrance to Sly Park Recreation Area along the way. Turn left onto Mormon Emigrant and proceed over the first dam. You can park in one of two places. The first opportunity is the large parking area on the left side of the road in between the two dam faces. From the dam face parking area, pedal across Alternate US 50 to the right side of the road and continue east on the road. The shoulder is almost nonexistent, and the cars and trucks really zoom here, so be careful. Pedal less than a half mile to the end of the dam face and look for the signed trailhead "Southshore Hiking Trail" on the left side of the road. The other parking location is directly across from this trailhead on the right side of the road. To reach it, drive past the second dam face and immediately turn into a tiny dirt pulloff on the right of the road, next to a green highway sign that lists mileages for Alternate US 50. Though the trailhead sign says "Southshore Hiking Trail," it is the beginning of the loop. Never mind the word "Hiking"—bikes are indeed allowed.

Sources of additional information:

Sly Park Recreation Area—Trail Systems
P.O. Box 577
Pollack Pines, CA 95726
(916) 644-2545

Notes on the trail: Begin pedaling northeast on the Southshore Hiking Trail along the south side of the lake. (Bikes are allowed.) Following the trail on this side of the lake is a piece of cake. Though the narrow single-track is quite curvy, there are no real significant trails intersecting it. Forks are generally signed and direct specific trail users to them, such as equestrians onto one trail and bikers and hikers onto another. The trail weaves through the forest, popping up and down short, sometimes steep dips, and skirts brief sections of drop-offs. At about 3 miles, after you cross Park Creek Bridge, there is a single-track leading off on the right. Bypass it (it ends at a tunnel just up the hill). Continue on and you'll see signs tacked up on trees suggesting that you walk your bike. I'm not sure why this suggestion is warranted, since the trail is not treacherous. I concluded that there are many blind curves in which you can crash head-on with other trail users, so stay alert and keep your speed under control. The narrow single-tracks widens and then narrows again. When you see a signed trail leading to Rainbow and Kamloop Camps, bear left and immediately go over Hazel Creek. After the creek crossing, the single-track dumps you out onto a paved road. Here, you find picnic tables, barbeque pits, drinking water, rest rooms, and campsites 144 and 145. This is Hazel Creek Campground on the north end of the lake. (From this point, the rest of the loop is not as sweet and uninterrupted as the 3.6 miles you just rode. You can turn around here and head back the way you came if you want. Just watch out for oncoming trail users.)

From Hazel Creek Camp, continue on the loop by going left onto the paved road and pedal past the rest rooms. Turn left again onto another paved road. Watch out for speed bumps on this stretch. Following the loop route gets a bit convoluted here. You may find yourself wondering if you're on the right trail or not. Use the lake as your guide—it should always be on your left within several hundred yards from the water line. Of course, this distance will vary depending on how much water is in the lake. Cruise past a signed day-use picnic area and over another speed bump. Look for campsite 133 on your left. A few yards beyond this camp you see the back side of a brown sign, planted on your left. It's directly across the road from camp 132 on your right. The front of this sign says "Chimney" and the single-track leading off behind the sign on the left is the trail you want. Follow this single-track as it cruises gently up and down. It's an easy trail and skirts the lake. Soon, begin a gentle climb up from the water line.

At about 4.7 miles from the start at the dam face parking area, a trail leading to Hilltop Campground peels off on your right. Bypass it as well as the Liberty Nature Trail a few yards farther. Stay on the main single-track. Go across a wooden bridge. The trail soon climbs a few yards up toward a boat ramp. Look for rest rooms and cement steps on the ramp and head for it. There, at the foot of the steps, the single-track resumes. In a few yards, the single-track dumps you out onto the paved boat

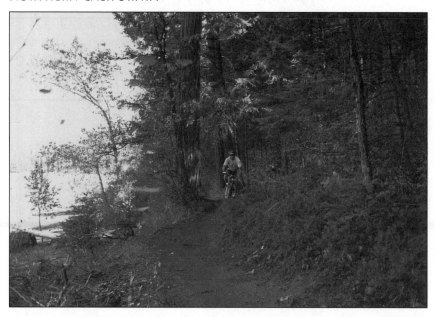

Heads up for oncoming bikers, hikers, and equestrians on this narrow and twisty single-track.

ramp. Go across the boat ramp and find the single-track again. You're now back in the serenity of the forest.

At 5.4 miles, after passing more picnic tables and campsites, the dirt trail hits pavement again and you see the back of a sign. The front of the sign reads "Chimney Sierra Trail," which is the trail you've just been riding. Pedal the pavement toward campgrounds 57 to 66. Make your way to campsite 62. A few yards beyond the 62 signpost, look for the continuation of the single-track on the left. Follow the trail as it dips up and down. Bear left, and eventually you see a tiny wooden bridge, across from the signpost for campsite 63. Cross over the tiny wooden bridge, stay left, and begin a gentle uphill climb. The single-track intersects pavement again at about 5.8 miles.

Follow the road left toward Pinecone campground. Enjoy a fast ride as you zip through the campground — just stay alert for dips in the road. When you reach campsite 1, head toward the rest rooms. Look for the signed Miwok Nature Trail on the right, a single-track. Follow this Nature Trail through the day-use picnic area. The trail here actually is wide and splits, becoming three paralleling trails. Take the trail above the picnic tables, with the tables and the lake on your left. The terrain is smooth and nontechnical. Cross a wooden bridge alongside trees decorated with ugly graffiti. After the bridge, you come to a T intersection; signed to the right is Miwok Nature Trail. Go left, away from the Nature Trail and toward the picnic area. A short distance farther, after a couple of brief, rocky sections, you reach another bridge at about 6.8 miles. Proceed over the bridge, which is named the Craig Taylor bridge, built by the Boy Scouts. A few yards farther, go over another bridge, and immediately go left. If you miss the left, you end up on pavement. Follow the left trail through more picnic areas. The dirt trail is fairly wide and smooth and it cruises past two sets of horseshoe pits. (Incidentally, this is a nice place to let very young children ride as it is well separated from the paved roads that run through the park.) By now, the loop trail is running somewhat close to Sly Park Road now on your right through the trees. You can't really see it, but you can hear car and truck traffic on it.

At 7.7 miles, the wide trail intersects a paved road. Go across the pavement and resume riding the single-track. Down below on your left is a day-use parking lot. A few yards farther, at about 8 miles, the single-track runs downhill then intersects a double-track trail, formerly a paved road as evident by scattered bits of broken asphalt. Go right onto the double-track, heading toward Sly Park Road. Deep within the shade of the forest, keep your eyes peeled for a single-track that drops steeply downhill on the left, between two huge pine trees. Hop on the single-track and enjoy a fun ride of steep but short ups and downs. Exposed tree roots keep you alert.

The single-track ends at a parking lot next to the Mormon Emigrant Trail. (This is the parking area between the two dam faces at which you may or may not have chosen to park.) If you parked at the trailhead on the south side of the road about 0.3 mile down, your challenge is to safely return to your car. The shoulder on the right side of the road is practically nonexistent, and that, in my opinion, makes this the most challenging part of the loop since cars and trucks travel treacherously fast on this road. I suggest riding through the parking lot as far as you can, then cautiously crossing over to the right side of the road. Finish the last few yards to your car by riding the narrow strip of dirt off the edge of the pavement. Back at your car, you complete the loop in 9 miles.

RIDE 32 · Big Boulder Trail Loop

AT A GLANCE

Length/configuration: 33- to 35-mile loop, counterclockwise; single- and double-tracks, dirt roads and pavement (18.5 miles if ridden as a point-to-point)

Aerobic difficulty: Very strenuous due to terrain and distance

Technical difficulty: Advanced due to mostly rocky terrain

Scenery: Gorgeous views of deep, forested canyons carved by Pauley and Butcher Creeks.

Special comments: If you are looking for a ride with some good climbing, outstanding views, fresh single-track, and a bit of adventure, this is the ONE! (Not recommended for beginners.) Big Boulder is a primitive ridgeline trail, which the Forest Service has recently reopened using motorcycle "Green Sticker" funds.

Ask hard-core, expert riders to name their favorite died-and-gone-to-heaven biking regions, and they're likely to name the Downieville area in Sierra County. Downieville is a tiny gold-rush town sitting at the confluence of the Yuba and Downie Rivers. A land of deep canyons carved by the Yuba River (North, Middle, and South Forks) and its many tributaries, this region attracted a colorful cast of characters, from gold miners, saloon hall girls, shopkeepers, to Chinese immigrants—just about anyone looking to make a fortune off the gold fever in the mid-1800s. With the abundance of creeks, placer mining yielded tremendous amounts of gold nuggets, sometimes found just sitting in the streambed, waiting for a lucky soul to come along. Such is how William Downie, the town's namesake, made his fortunes. With miners fueled with a rabid, unfettered drive to strike it rich, one can only imagine the bawdy, bustling town that flourished here. History tells a story about a saloon girl who, in self-defense, mortally stabbed a miner. The trial was swift, and she was hastily found guilty. Justice was equally swift as she was immediately lynched off a bridge over the Yuba River near Downieville.

Today, the Downieville region attracts bikers passionate about the sport, seeking a gold mine of outstanding trails. Nobody knows this region and its dirt trails like Greg Williams. An eighth generation resident of nearby Nevada City, Greg's great, great, great uncles were pack-mule drivers who supplied miners with provisions in the far-reaches of the Sierras. Who would've known that today, a descendent would still find gold, this time in "them thar trails." After five years as the founder and active partner of the now-defunct Coyote Adventures, this twenty-something lad helped launch Yuba Expeditions in 1999. Much like Coyote, Yuba offers a tremendously valuable service to mountain bikers. Yuba's basic van shuttle service (drop-off and pick-up, from $15 to $30 per person), maximizes your riding time, gives you access to many of the region's prime trails, and—the best part of all—makes your day's outing a mostly screaming downhill adventure over inspiring terrain. After you've spent most of the day negotiating with them gnarly trails, it's a small price to pay to avoid miles of arduous climbing back to your car. In fact, what attracts gonzo riders to this area are the incredible vertical descents found on these trails, many of which require a shuttle arrangement. (One such trail is the wildly popular Downieville Downhill, a 15-mile-plus point-to-point, dropping over 4,000 feet before the finish. Unfortunately, this trail, like many others in the area, has suffered significant damage from overuse, and the forest service is hoping to rescue it by diverting bikers to other trails. For that reason, the Downieville Downhill is not included in this book, but if you must ride it, get the lowdown from Greg at Yuba Expeditions.) In addition to the shuttle service, Yuba Expeditions offers guided tours from one day to five days as well as fully arranged tours that include deluxe lodging and camping, all meals, and trail guides. You can even book a vacation package that includes rafting and fly-fishing! Greg's wealth of regional knowledge has made customized tours a hit with groups of all abilities, from both the personal and corporate world. (To contact Yuba Expeditions, see "Sources of additional information" below.)

And so, it is with great honor that four trail descriptions, submitted by Greg Williams are reprinted here with his permission. According to the him, these rides give you a good taste of the region and its numerous trails.

General location: Downieville is about 75 miles north of Auburn; about 60 miles northwest of north shore Lake Tahoe.

Elevation change: About 5,000 feet; starting elevation and low point 2,900 feet; high point 7,900 feet. Lots of long, rugged ascents and descents.

Season: Spring through fall, depending on rate of snow melt.

Services: None on the trail. Most services in Downieville. Water available at Union Flat Campground, at the intersection of CA 49 and Gold Valley Road. All water taken from streams should be treated before drinking. More services available in Nevada City and Auburn.

RIDE 32 · Big Boulder Trail Loop

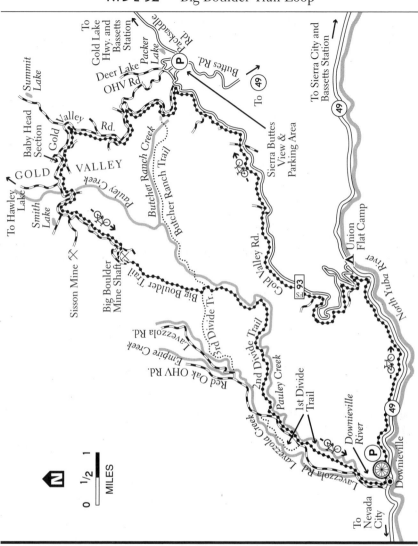

Hazards: Stay alert for rattlesnakes, which reside below 4,000 feet, especially on the first and second Divide Trails. This loop is an epic, highly technical ride, and beginners are not likely to enjoy it. Watch out for occasional vehicular traffic, including OHVs (off-highway vehicles), along the dirt roads. And for your own safety, do not enter any mine shafts or tunnels.

Rescue index: Though sections of this route are accessible by four-wheel-drive vehicles, most portions are fairly remote. Don't expect to meet others on the trail who may be of help during an emergency; you may be waiting a long time. You need to be self-reliant. Cell phones only work from mountaintops. Be sure you ride with a buddy and not alone. There is a medical clinic in Downieville, including other emergency services.

Land status: Tahoe National Forest. Please respect private property.

Maps: USGS Mt. Fillmore, Downieville, Sierra City and Gold Lake 7.5 minute series.

Finding the trail: You can do this ride either as a loop, beginning and ending in Downieville, or as a point-to-point, in which case you need to set up a shuttle or hire the shuttle service of Yuba Expeditions. To do this ride as a point-to-point, you'll need to arrange your shuttle cars. Leave your end car in Downieville. To reach the starting point, load up your bikes and buddy in the other car and leave Downieville by following CA 49 north for a little over 17 miles to Bassetts Station. Make a left onto Gold Lake Highway and drive for about a mile to the first paved road on the left. Turn left and cross Salmon Creek. A few hundred yards beyond this intersection is Packer Lake Road. Take a right on this road and follow it as it meanders through the Lakes Basin. Stay left at the Packer Lake intersection and head up Packsaddle Road. This road becomes steep and narrow as it climbs the ridge. At about 11 miles, keep to the left on the pavement and climb to the Sierra Buttes view/parking area on the left which you immediately reach before the pavement ends. Forest Service Road 93-3 heading west is directly across from this parking area. Park here.

Sources of additional information:

Tahoe National Forest
Downieville Ranger District and
   North Yuba Ranger Station
15624 Highway 49
Camptonville, CA 95922-9797
(916) 288-3231

Yuba Expeditions
P.O. Box 750
Nevada City, CA 95959
(530) 265-8779

Notes on the trail: To do this ride as a counterclockwise loop: Leave Downieville by pedaling north on CA 49 toward Sierra City. At around six miles is Union Flat Campground on the right. Directly across on the left side is Gold Valley Road. Follow it for 12 miles to the paved intersection, reaching it at about 16.5 miles. Turn left at the Y onto FS 93-3 and head toward Butcher Ranch Trail and Gold Valley. The road turns to dirt after a few hundred yards. (Point-to-point riders: This is where you park your car and begin pedaling.) About a mile farther, bypass Butcher Ranch Trail on the left. Stay on FS 93-3, a frequently traveled dirt road, so be aware of cars! After passing two left turns and crossing over a drainage, Gold Valley Road turns to the left, about 20.5 miles since you left Downieville. (A right turn will take you up a steep and rocky climb to Summit Lake.) Stay left on Gold Valley Road. There is a trailhead sign tacked up in one of the trees to the left that says "Pauley Creek 2 miles."

Gold Valley Road descends into Gold Valley heading west. Keep to the right at the first intersection. The road becomes very fast and rocky as it descends into the valley. After a mile or so it becomes much rougher. This section is called Baby Head because of the size of the rocks. This section is fairly short and switches back four times. As soon as the road flattens out, a double-track intersects to the left. (There are several large log rounds at this intersection, at almost 22 miles. If you pass it, you will see an aspen grove on the right.) Turn left onto this double-track heading west toward Pauley Creek.

After crossing the sometimes deep Pauley Creek, there is a short, steep climb, always a challenge with wet tires. After this short climb, a dirt road will intersect on the right. Gear down and prepare to climb a rough and rocky dirt road. Turn right and follow this mile-long climb toward Smith Lake. Stay left at the first intersection and continue climbing for another half mile or so. (Bearing right will drop you down to Smith Lake.) Stay left at the next intersection and continue to climb (a right drops to Sisson Mine). As you are climbing, go around a fallen tree to the right and continue on the double-track as it descends through the saddle. After rolling along for a mile, you'll reach another intersection at a little over 24 miles. (To the left, you can access an incredible view of Pauley and Butcher Creeks.) Stay to the right for Big Boulder Trail. From the ridge top, you can take in outstanding views of the Lavezzola and Empire watersheds. Drop down the rough double-track for approximately 0.5 mile. Continue past the Big Boulder mine shaft on your left. Please be considerate of this historic site.

Welcome to the Big Boulder Trail. The single-track starts soon after the mine shaft, so gear down and prepare for a steep climb. Once atop the climb, you'll begin to descend this 130-year-old trail. Twisting and turning its way through the trees, this trail redefines the word "single-track" as it drops to the famed 3rd Divide Trail, which you reach after 26 miles. From here, you can stay right and descend this roller coaster of a trail to its end at Lavezzola Road. Those of you wanting even more tasty single-tracks, turn left for the short climb to the top of 3rd Divide and descend a short distance to 2nd Divide Trail. Turn right and follow this rugged trail as it climbs and descends to Lavezzola Road. Steep cliff edges and technically rocky sections definitely make this an advanced route. With either option, turn left at Lavezzola Road and continue down toward Downieville. Before reaching town, you will want to take a left onto 1st Divide Trail, which pops you out like toast onto Main Street in town. The speed limit in town is 15 mph. Please stop at all stop signs.

RIDE 33 · South Yuba Primitive Camp Loop

AT A GLANCE

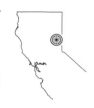

Length/configuration: 19-mile-plus loop, clockwise; dirt road and single-tracks

Aerobic difficulty: Strenuous due to often rugged terrain

Technical difficulty: Intermediate through advanced; dirt roads are rough in some stretches; steep single-track descents are lined with poison oak in some places

Scenery: Gorgeous river canyon of pine forests and a ride around Malakoff Diggins State Historic Park, site of hydraulic mining during the gold-rush era.

Special comments: Bring your snorkel and flippers for this one. Endless swimming holes are the highlights for this ride. Pack a lunch and a water filter on hot days.

If anyone knows where the great swimming holes and single-tracks are, it's Greg Williams of Yuba Expeditions. South Yuba Primitive Camp Loop is a great route that takes you back into the gold-rush era before dumping you down screaming single-track descents. This clockwise loop rides a variety of terrain, from rugged dirt roads to extreme rocky single-track descents to tight switchbacks. A great summertime ride, the stretch along the South Yuba River entices you with swimming holes. Depending on how much you explore side trails, this clockwise loop is at least 19 miles in length. The route starts off by climbing up to Malakoff Diggins State Historic Park, site of horrific hydraulic mining practices that transformed the landscape into a barren moonscape, all in the quest for gold. This now-historic site is a strangely interesting monument that shows what greed can do to a tremendously pristine environment. Such is the result of gold frenzy in the mid-1800s. If you're into gold-rush history, check out the town of North Bloomfield, which is located on this loop. Much of the town has been restored to resemble its mid-1800s character.

The South Yuba Trail is becoming a gold mine in and of itself. What was formerly known as the South Yuba River Project, this treasure trove of white water, history, and scenic vistas became the South Yuba River State Park in November 1998. Co-managed by the Bureau of Land Management, South Yuba River State Park, and Tahoe National Park, the park encloses the 20-plus miles of South Yuba Trail, stretching east from Englebright Reservoir into the Tahoe National Forest. Plans are in store to extend the trail farther east of the town of Washington and into the single-track mecca of Grouse Ridge. That will add 10 more miles to the already 20-plus miles of single-track that make up South Yuba Trail. The loop described here exposes you to over seven miles of this tasty trail. (Incidentally, hearty riders looking for an all-day affair with the South Yuba Trail can partake of an awesome point-to-point ride from Grouse Ridge descending all the way down to Purdon Crossing on the South Yuba River. You'll need to arrange a shuttle. Better yet, to maximize riding time, book the shuttle services of Yuba Expeditions.)

Thanks, Greg, for submitting this trail description. Yuba Expeditions, the local source for trail information, offers guided mountain bike tours, shuttle, and drop-off services at trailheads, and week-long vacation adventures. For more information, see "Sources of additional information" below.

General location: Nevada City is about 28 miles north of Auburn; about 60 miles northwest of north shore Lake Tahoe.

Elevation change: About 2,000 feet; starting elevation 2,600 feet; high point 4,550 feet; low point 2,550 feet. Long, gradual climb; fast, steep descent with a few flat stretches; roller coaster before climbing back up trailhead.

Season: Year-round, though snow may linger during the winter months.

Services: South Yuba Camp at the trailhead (not the Primitive Camp) has piped water, pit toilets, picnic tables, and fire grills. All other services available in Nevada City and Grass Valley.

Hazards: Poison oak, especially along Missouri Bar and South Yuba Trails. North Bloomfield Road sees some traffic as it leads to popular Malakoff Diggins State Historic Park and the town of North Bloomfield.

Rescue index: During the summer months, you're likely to see hikers and other mountain bikers on the single-track trails who may be of assistance. All other times of the year, you should make your way back North Bloomfield Road where you might be able to flag down a passing motorist. If not, you may be able to find help in the town of North Bloomfield as well as at Malakoff Diggins State Historic Park. Regardless of the time of year, you should be self-reliant and not expect other trail users to come along.

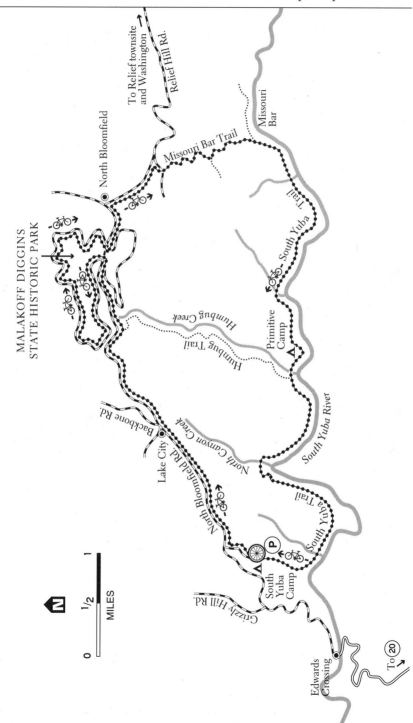

MALAKOFF DIGGINS
STATE HISTORIC PARK

To Relief townsite
and Washington

Relief Hill Rd.

North Bloomfield

Missouri Bar Trail

Missouri
Bar

South Yuba
Trail

Humbug Creek

Humbug Trail

Primitive
Camp

South Yuba River

Backbone Rd.

Lake City

North Canyon Creek

North Bloomfield Rd.

South Yuba Trail

P

South
Yuba
Camp

Grizzly Hill Rd.

Edwards
Crossing

To 20

N

MILES
0   1/2   1

Land status: Bureau of Land Management.

Maps: USGS Nevada City, North Bloomfield, and Washington 7.5 minute series.

Finding the trail: From the intersection of CA 49 and CA 20 in Nevada City, head west toward Downieville on CA 49 for about 0.3 mile. Go right onto North Bloomfield Road and follow it up to the top of the hill where the road splits. Keep to the right and follow North Bloomfield for more than 8 miles to Edward's Crossing. Continue across the bridge and the road turns to dirt. Follow it for another 2 miles to the top where the road splits again. Keep to the right, and the road descends for a short distance. As North Bloomfield Road starts to climb, the signed turn-off for South Yuba Primitive Camp is on the right. Pull into the camping area, bear left and park.

Sources of additional information:

Bureau of Land Management
Folsom Field Office
North Bloomfield Rd.
South Yuba, CA 95991
(916) 985-4474

Tahoe National Forest
Downieville Ranger District and
    North Yuba Ranger Station
15624 Highway 49
Camptonville, CA 95922-9797
(916) 288-3231

South Yuba River State Park
17660 Pleasant Valley Rd.
Penn Valley, CA 95946
(530) 432-2546

Yuba Expeditions
P.O. Box 750
Nevada City, CA 95959
(530) 265-8779

Malakoff Diggins State Historic Park
23579 North Bloomfield Rd.
Nevada City, CA 95959
(530) 265-2740

Grass Valley/Nevada County
Chamber of Commerce
248 Mill St.
Grass Valley, CA 95945
(530) 273-4667
Call or write for information and
maps on mountain biking trails in
the region.

Notes on the trail: From the primitive camp, pedal back out to North Bloomfield Road and go right, heading east. Continue to climb for roughly two miles to Lake City. Once you reach the site of Lake City, the road splits. Stay right and head toward Malakoff Diggings State Historic Park and the town of North Bloomfield. As you descend, keep an eye out for the Rim Trail on your left at about 4 miles. Rim Trail leads you out and around the historic hydraulic diggings site, through pine and cedar forests.

At just over 8 miles, after your historic tour of the mining site, hop back onto North Bloomfield Road and continue heading east. In less than a mile, you reach the town of North Bloomfield. Take a right (sort of due south) toward the town of Washington; this road is signed. Follow this dirt road over a wooden bridge, climbing for about a mile. (If you're up to it, there is a cool trail to check out a few feet beyond the wooden bridge. It's signed and will take you to an old ranch site before connecting back with the main road.)

As you climb the road, at about 10 miles, you see a sign indicating the direction to Missouri Bar Trail. Take a right turn onto this road and in a short distance, catch

Missouri Bar Trail on the left. Hang on! Missouri Bar descends more than 1,200 feet in a mile and a half! A brake check is a must at the top. And try not to take a nose-dive into the poison oak.

When you reach the river, turn right onto South Yuba Trail and follow it, heading downstream. There are a few trails that will take you down to the river, providing access to nice swimming holes. You reach Primitive Camp in about 3 miles from Missouri Bar Trail. Though the route tends to get a little confusing near the camp with all of the side trails, just keep heading downstream. The trail is also washed out in a couple of spots, so expect to portage your bike for a short distance.

Once you cross over Humbug Creek, less than a half mile from Primitive Camp, there is a nice picnic area to catch some sunshine. The trail splits here. For this ride, continue downstream. Do not take Humbug Trail as it is extremely steep and technical. The South Yuba Trail becomes amazingly fun along this section as it serpentines through the rugged canyon. Cross North Canyon Creek at roughly 16 miles. After a few miles, the trail will pop you out onto a dirt road. Head up the road for a half mile, and a single-track takes off on the left. It is signed for nonmotorized use. Take this trail, and it will take you back to your car. Ending mileage is approximately 19 miles. Enjoy!

RIDE 34 · Bullards Bar Loop

AT A GLANCE

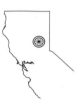

Length/configuration: 28.5-mile loop within a loop, counterclockwise; pavement, single-track and dirt roads

Aerobic difficulty: Strenuous due to steepness

Technical difficulty: Intermediate to advanced due to rugged, steep terrain

Scenery: Endless rolling single-track with inspiring lake views, old-growth forests and great swimming possibilities.

Special comments: For first-time single-track riders, the section of Bullards Bar Trail between the Sunset Vista Point and Dark Day is great for building confidence and improving your skills.

This is another great ride submitted by Greg Williams of Yuba Expeditions. (See previous ride, Big Boulder Loop, for more info about Greg and his bike touring company). Sandwiched between the south shore of Bullards Bar Reservoir and Marysville Road, many configurations of varying distances can be ridden—you can make this an all-day or half-day affair. Thanks Greg!

General location: The reservoir is about 73 miles north of Auburn; about 66 miles northwest of north shore Lake Tahoe, on the southern shore of Bullards Bar Reservoir.

Elevation change: 2,000 feet gain and loss. Lots of ups and downs with stretches of mellow riding.

Season: Year-round.

Services: Campsites, water, flush and pit toilets, picnic tables, and fire pits at Dark Day Camp and Schoolhouse Camp, walk-in and drive-in camps, respectively. Grocery store, gas, eatery, and phone at nearby Emerald Cove Marina and near the intersection of Old Camptonville Road and Marysville Road. Many more services in Nevada City and Grass Valley. A good selection of maps and information about the area at the Downieville Ranger Station located at the corner of CA 49 and Marysville Road (you pass it on the way to the beginning trailhead).

Hazards: Stay alert for rattlesnakes and poison oak. Expect to share the trail with hikers and other bikers. Marysville Road is heavily traveled, so exercise caution when pedaling it.

Rescue index: During the summer months, you're likely to meet other trail users near the campgrounds who may be of help. Marysville Road is well traveled, and you might be able to flag down a passing motorist for assistance. A U.S. Forest ranger station is located near the intersection of CA 49 and Marysville Road.

Land status: Tahoe National Forest.

Maps: USGS Camptonville and Challenge 7.5 minute series.

Finding the trail: From I-80 and CA 49 in Auburn, take CA 49 north and continue through Grass Valley and Nevada City. At about 50 miles from I-80, following signs for New Bullards Bar Reservoir, look for Marysville Road on your left. (The U.S. Forest Service–Downieville Ranger District station is at this intersection, and it's worth stopping to find out more biking information and to purchase maps.) Turn left onto Marysville Road and follow it for 5 miles to the Sunset Vista Point. Park here.

Sources of additional information:

Yuba Expeditions
P.O. Box 750
Nevada City, CA 95959
(530) 265-8779

Tahoe National Forest
Downieville Ranger District and
North Yuba Ranger Station
15624 Highway 49
Camptonville, CA 95922-9797
(916) 288-3231

Notes on the trail: Pedaling from Sunset Vista Point, take a left onto Marysville Road heading back toward CA 49. After a short pavement spin of about a mile, turn left into Schoolhouse Campground. Immediately on your right is the trailhead for 8-Ball Trail, and it's signed Dark Day (road and campground). Take this trail as it contours Marysville Road heading northeast. The trail crosses over the paved road (which leads into Dark Day campground) and eventually dumps you out at the Old Scaling Station, about 2.7 miles from the vista point. Take a left onto the pavement and in a few yards, bypass 7-Ball Trailhead on your left, and turn left onto Marysville Road.

Spin up the road for almost a mile, and on your left is Rebel Ridge Trail, signed to Bullards Bar Trail. Take this left, following it as it starts out on a dirt road and soon turns off onto single-track. Rebel Ridge switches back taking you down to the Bullards Bar Trail. Once you reach the lake edge and intersect Bullards Bar Trail at about 4.5 miles, turn left and contour the lake for a few miles to 7-Ball Trail. Take a left onto 7-Ball and head back out of the lake basin to the ridge. At the top you will be at the Old Scaling Station again.

Go left onto Marysville Road and continue past Rebel Ridge to Jaynes Lane. A little over 8 miles, take a left on Jaynes and go by the burnt remains of Doc Willy's.

RIDE 34 · Bullards Bar Loop

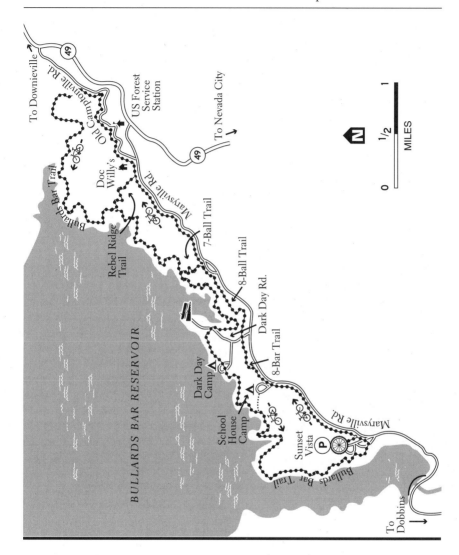

Turn left onto Old Camptonville Road and start climbing through the trailer park community. Be prepared to get barked at—fortunately, these trailer folks have fences. Climb Old Camptonville Road for just under 2 miles to the Bullards Bar Trailhead, which will be on your left. You reach this trailhead roughly 10 miles since the beginning at the vista point. The descent to the lake starts here. This is a screamer 2-mile downhill plunge with large jumps at the top followed by numerous high-speed sweeping turns. Oh yeah!

Near the bottom, the trail narrows down a bit and starts to weave its way along the lakeside for more than 11 miles. After passing by Rebel Ridge and 7-Ball, you will reach the Dark Day boat ramp, roughly 16.5 miles. Cross directly over the pavement and take the short section of trail to the camping area. Turn right on the paved road. At the parking lot, stay left and the Bullards Bar Trail picks up again. This lower section of trail is a bit wider and faster than the previous. Follow the trail for another 5 miles and it will eventually drop you onto an old paved road. Turn left and start climbing for less than a mile back to your car at the Vista Point. Total distance is about 28.5 miles.

RIDE 35 · Chimney Rock Trail

AT A GLANCE

Length/configuration: 28- to 29-mile loop, clockwise; dirt roads and single-tracks. (Option: 20-mile point-to-point with a shuttle arrangement.)

Aerobic difficulty: Strenuous, due to climbing at elevation

Technical difficulty: Advanced

Scenery: Forested canyon country created by creeks and populated by old-growth trees. Magnificent volcanic rock formations and 360-degree panoramic views.

Special comments: A lot of climbing at a high elevation (the high point sits at almost 7,000 feet). At the Saddleback Lookout intersection, there is a spring from which to fill your water bottles. This is a must on a hot day. To shorten this ride to about 20 miles, call Yuba Expeditions for shuttle service or set it up yourself.

Like many of the other outstanding trails in the Downieville region, Chimney Rock Trail is not for wimps. You need both advanced bike-handling skills and good stamina, no matter if you tackle this ride as a 28-mile clockwise loop or a 16- to 20-mile point-to-point (in which case you'll need to arrange a shuttle car or use the drop-off service of Yuba Expeditions). Ridden clockwise, the route climbs from the town of Downieville, sitting at 2,900 feet, to about 7,000 feet. It's a lot of hard work, but fortunately the route rewards with long and sweet descents. There are also tremendous panoramic vistas and dramatic volcanic rock formations, as well as magnificent old-growth timber and lush environments indigenous to creek canyons and drainages. Splendid lunch sites abound. Be sure to bring plenty of food and water with you. While you grind up the trail, just think how good that brewski will taste when you get done with this epic ride—and Downieville has plenty of watering holes and eateries.

Sincere thanks to Greg Williams of Yuba Expeditions for submitting this ride description. Not only is Yuba Expeditions the local source for trail information, it offers guided mountain bike tours, shuttle, and drop-off services at trailheads, and week-long vacation adventures.

General location: Downieville is about 75 miles north of Auburn; about 60 miles northwest of north shore Lake Tahoe.

Elevation change: 5,000 feet; starting elevation and low point 2,200 feet; high point 7,200 feet. A monster ride with lots of climbing and downhills.

Season: Spring through fall. During the summer, it's best to begin early in the morning to avoid the afternoon heat.

Services: Water from a spring can be found at Saddleback Lookout (a fire lookout station), about 8 to 9 miles into the loop ride. Other than this spring, there are no services on the route. Water taken from streams found throughout the ride should be treated before drinking. Most services in Downieville.

Hazards: Watch out for rattlesnakes, poison oak, and bees. Expect to share the trail with hikers and other bikers. Dirt roads see occasional vehicular traffic.

Rescue index: Occasionally, you may meet other trail users on this route. Still, you need to be self-reliant. Don't ride alone; ride with a buddy. There is a medical clinic and other emergency services in Downieville. Portions of the loop are accessible by four-wheel-drive vehicles.

Land status: Tahoe National Forest.

Maps: USGS Downieville and Mt. Fillmore 7.5 minute series.

Finding the trail: To do this ride as a point-to-point: Leave your end car in Downieville and load up your bikes and buddies in the starting car and head west on CA 49 toward Nevada City for about 2 miles to Saddleback Road, a dirt road. If you have a four-wheel-drive with good clearance, you can turn right onto Saddleback Road and head up as far as you would like. For those with two-wheel-drive cars, continue out on CA 49 for about 10 miles more to Cal-Ida Road, a paved road also referred to as County Road 490, located on the right immediately after Fiddle Creek Campground. Follow Cal-Ida Road for about 20 miles to Saddleback Road, (pavement ends and dirt road begins about 17 miles into Cal-Ida). The road intersects Saddleback Road just south of the Saddleback fire lookout. Park and start pedaling here. For loop riders: begin and end your ride in Downieville.

Sources of additional information:

Yuba Expeditions
P.O. Box 750
Nevada City, CA 95959
(530) 265-8779

Tahoe National Forest
Downieville Ranger District and
North Yuba Ranger Station
15624 Highway 49
Camptonville, CA 95922-9797
(916) 288-3231

Notes on the trail: To do this ride as a clockwise loop: pedal west out of Downieville by following CA 49 to Saddleback Road, a dirt road, reached in about a mile or so. Go north, climbing up Saddleback Road toward the fire lookout, reached in about 8 miles near a five-way intersection. Just before reaching the lookout, bypass Telegraph Mine, a working gold mine. The view is spectacular from the lookout, which sits at 6,690 feet. Fill your bottles at the spring located just a few hundred yards up the lookout road on the left. (Point-to-point riders: here is where you could park your shuttle car and begin pedaling the loop clockwise. In fact, depending on the ability of your vehicle, you can park farther up this stretch, even all the way up to the trailhead of Chimney Rock Trail.)

RIDE 35 · Chimney Rock Trail

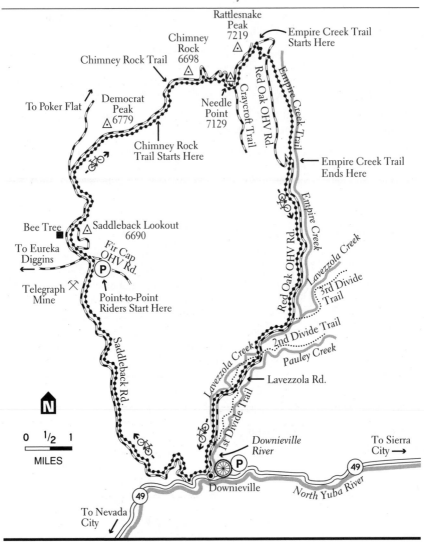

Continue pedaling through the intersection and past the Saddleback Lookout. Immediately after, on your left, there's a great view of Mt. Lassen at the Bee Tree. From the Bee Tree, the road starts to descend for a bit. Stay on this main road keeping to the right at the first two intersections. Left turns at either will take you down to Poker Flat. About 2 miles from the lookout road, bear right, bypassing the Poker Flat OHV Trail. Continue climbing the ridge, and at a little over 12 miles, pass Democrat Peak on the left. This is where the road gets steep. Gear down and prepare for three short, steep climbs. The road then descends steeply toward the Chimney Rock Trailhead, which you reach at roughly 12.5 miles.

Chimney Rock Trail is a technical trail characterized by rocks and loose sand. It climbs up and out of the trees and switches back seven times on its way up the mountain. You might have to walk and push your bike in some spots. About 0.2 mile beyond the switchbacks, the trail pops out at an incredible vista spot. Continuing on the trail, views of interesting rock outcroppings start to appear, including Chimney Rock, reached at about 14.5 miles. The view here is expansive, a 360-degree vista. Chimney Rock, sitting at elevation 6,700 feet on the left of the trail, is a massive vertically perched chunk of volcanic rock. It's at least 15 feet in diameter at its base and stretches skyward for approximately 25 feet. From here, the trail descends a bit through the forest and then starts to climb again toward Needle Point. There are five switchbacks up this face that are quite challenging to get through. The trail wraps around the southeast side of Needle Point and ducks into the trees. Immediately before reaching the trees, Craycroft Ridge OHV Trail intersects on the right at about 16 miles. Bypass Craycroft and continue past Rattlesnake Peak. Stay left and keep heading toward Empire Creek Trail, pedaling through an open valley amid panoramic views of the surrounding landscape.

At a little over 17 miles, Empire Creek Trail intersects on the right. Hop onto Empire and hold on as the trail starts off with high-speed switchbacks. It's an extreme descent on single-track. (Mere mortals can avoid this section by hopping onto Red Oak OHV Trail, a fire road. Empire Creek Trail rejoins Red Oak OHV Trail in just under 3 miles.) A mile down, Empire Creek Trail crosses Red Oak OHV Road. Continue on the trail through a lush meadow, usually filled with yellow wildflowers during the spring and early summer. The surrounding forest is made up of magnificent old-growth timber. After a few miles, a little shy of 21 miles, the trail pops you out onto Red Oak Road again. Keep to the left and continue descending to Lavezzola Road. Follow Lavezzola all the way down into Downieville. Enjoy! Total distance is about 28 miles.

RIDE 36 · North Yuba River Trail

AT A GLANCE

Length/configuration: 16.6-mile loop, clockwise; single-track and pavement. (Out-and-back option: 17.6 miles, 8.8 miles each way on single-track only. Halls Ranch–Fiddle Creek option: loop added onto the out-and-back for a total of almost 30 miles; includes dirt roads.)

Aerobic difficulty: Moderate due to short ups and downs (Halls Ranch–Fiddle Creek option is for longer and more strenuous loop)

Technical difficulty: Intermediate; rocky and abrupt roller-coaster conditions, with Halls Ranch–Fiddle Creek option as a more challenging ride

Scenery: Great overhead views of the North Yuba River, especially of whitewater sections in May and June.

Special comments: The out-and-back option is entirely on single-track. Not recommended for beginners who are not yet comfortable with single-track riding. This ride can also be expanded into a bigger, advanced-level ride by adding the Halls Ranch and Fiddle Creek Trails.

One of the finest single-tracks open to bikes, the newly built North Yuba Trail is a simple trail to follow as there are no other trails intersecting it. This short loop is 16.6 miles round-trip, and the first 8.8 miles of it clings to a north-facing slope above the North Yuba River. The remaining 7.7 miles rides the sometimes narrow shoulder of paved CA 49. But you needn't ride the highway if you don't want to. If it's all single-track riding you want, you can easily make it so by returning in the reverse direction. Whatever the direction, the trail is a fun roller-coaster path, punctuated with some steep but short ascents and descents while weaving through a forest of dogwood, big-leaf maples, and mixed conifers. Adding even more spice to the sweet trail is its narrowness, scattered patches of loose rocks, and some serious drop-offs into the river. Throw in great views of the river with sections of gushing whitewater and you have one heck of a fun ride. For riders aching to pedal more miles and more technically challenging terrain, the Halls Ranch and Fiddle Creek Trails are just the ticket, measuring about 30 miles when it's all said and done.

General location: About 4 miles west of Downieville, paralleling the North Yuba River and CA 49; about 70 miles north of Auburn.

Elevation change: 400 feet; starting elevation 2,700 feet; high point 2,800 feet; low point 2,400 feet. Lots of ups and downs throughout single-track portion, followed by gradual ascent on pavement. Halls Ranch–Fiddle Creek option has 3,300 feet gain.

Season: Spring through fall.

Services: Many services available in Nevada City and Downieville; more in Auburn.

Hazards: If you take CA 49 to complete the loop, beware of fast traffic while riding a sometimes narrow shoulder of the pavement.

Rescue index: During the summer, the river attracts numerous water lovers, especially on weekends. In case of emergency, you may be within shouting distance for help. Otherwise, you should make your way to either end of the trail to find help at Rocky Rest Campground and CA 49 or in the tiny community of Goodyears Bar. The area through which the Halls Ranch–Fiddle Creek optional loop travels sees fewer trail users. You need to be self-reliant.

Land status: Tahoe National Forest.

Maps: USGS Goodyears Bar 7.5 minute series.

Finding the trail: The short loop, out-and-back, and optional Halls Ranch–Fiddle Creek loop all begin at the Goodyears Bar trailhead. All routing configurations can also be started from Rocky Rest Campground, about 7.7 miles downstream from Goodyears Bar off CA 49. This description begins at the Goodyears Bar trailhead: From Downieville, head west on CA 49 for about 4 miles to Mountain House Road (CR 300, the turn off to Goodyears Bar). Go left onto Mountain House and follow the paved road over Goodyears Creek and as it curves left over North Yuba River. Make a right at a stop sign at a **T** intersection, and go through the tiny community of Goodyears Bar. Continue for almost 0.25 mile to where the pavement ends and a wide dirt road begins. Go a few yards farther, keeping an eye out for the back of a

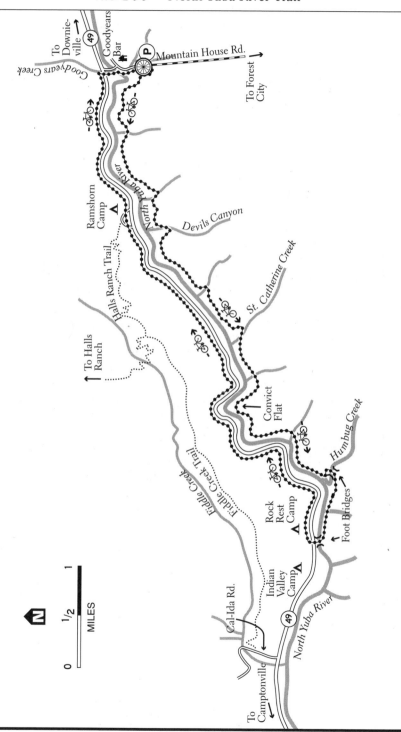

To Downieville

49

Goodyears Bar

P

Mountain House Rd.

Goodyears Creek

Goodyears Creek

To Forest City

Ramshorn Camp

North Yuba River

Devils Canyon

St. Catherine Creek

Halls Ranch Trail

To Halls Ranch

Convict Flat

Humbug Creek

Foot Bridges

Rock Rest Camp

Fiddle Creek Trail

Fiddle Creek

Cal-Ida Rd.

Indian Valley Camp

49

North Yuba River

To Camptonville

N

0   ½   1

MILES

brown sign that says North Yuba Trail on the front side, planted on the left (east) side of the road. The single-track multi-use trail is on the west side of the road, climbing steeply up the slope. Park in the small dirt pulloff on your left, next to the sign.

Sources of additional information:

Tahoe National Forest
Downieville Ranger District
North Yuba Ranger Station
15924 Hwy. 49
Camptonville, CA 95922-9707
(916) 288-3231

Notes on the trail: Pick up the trail on the west side of Mountain House Road, across from the dirt pulloff where your car is parked. The initial climb is steep but for a very short distance, and about 200 yards from the trailhead, you see a wooden sign declaring several distances: St. Catherine Creek in 3.5 miles and Rocky Rest Trailhead in 7.5 miles. (I confess that when I rode this trail, my trusty cyclometer clocked different mileages than what the sign indicated. From Goodyears Bar trail- head, I reached St. Catherine Creek in 4.6 miles (not 3.5) and the Rocky Rest Trailhead in 8.8 miles (not 7.5). If you ride with a cyclometer, I invite you to tell me your mile readings.)

Whatever the mileage, in less than a mile, the trail begins paralleling the river, al- ways on your right as you cruise downstream to Rocky Rest Campground. Although the trail is nearly at water level in some places, it is generally 100 to 200 yards above the river, giving you splendid views of some of the river's whitewater action. The trail crosses several creeks along the way, two of which use well-made wooden footbridges, while the others are generally tiny, possibly dry, depending on the time of year. On a hot day, look for enticing swimming holes to cool your jets. Expect to do a fair bit of steep but brief ups and downs over rocky and sometimes loose terrain. Since the trail is narrow, just wide enough for one cyclist (or hiker), stay alert for oncoming traffic.

When you reach Rocky Rest trailhead, you have three choices. One, you can re- turn to your car by retracing your path on North Yuba Trail. Two, you can return via paved CA 49. Three, you can add the Halls Ranch–Fiddle Creek Trails to create a loop before hopping back on North Yuba Trail at Rocky Rest camp trailhead and re- tracing your path back to the Goodyears Bar trailhead.

For the second and third options, follow the trail through a huge bridge that spans across North Yuba River. Pedal through the campground to CA 49. Make a right onto CA 49 and ride the sometimes generous shoulder. You now begin regaining the elevation you lost on North Yuba Trail. The ascent is gradual, and at about 14 miles from Goodyears Bar, Halls Ranch Trail leads off to the north on the other side of CA 49. (Riders opting for the third option, this is where you leave CA 49 and skip to the next paragraph.) At 15.7 miles, you reach the intersection of Mountain House Road on your right. Turn right here toward Goodyears Bar. Cruise over Goodyears Creek and continue following the road as it curves left, crossing over North Yuba River. In a few yards, now in a small residential community, you reach a T intersection con- trolled by a stop sign. Hang a right here, staying on Mountain House Road, and in less than a half mile, the pavement ends and the dirt road begins. You close the loop by pedaling a short distance to your car parked at the North Yuba Trail trailhead.

For the third option, proceed with the second option. At 14 miles, a little over 5 miles since hopping onto CA 49, Halls Ranch Trail leads off on your left on the other side of the road. Cautiously go across the road and follow the signs toward Halls Ranch. Climb through a forest of ponderosa pine and oak for about 2 miles to the intersection with Fiddle Creek Trail. At this junction, you've gained about 1,500 feet since leaving CA 49. Go left (west) onto Fiddle Creek Trail and enjoy a roller-coaster ride, mostly descending. Stay alert for rattlesnakes in the trail. Though the trail is not heavily enjoyed by other trail users, keep your radar on as you round blind curves. Continue cruising down Fiddle Creek Trail through the forest, and eventually the path twists and turns through tight curves before intersecting Cal-Ida Road. Go left onto Cal-Ida and follow it down to CA 49. Turn left onto CA 49 and head east for almost 2 miles to the Rocky Rest campground. Say good-bye to the highway as you turn into Rocky Rest. Make your way back to the footbridge over the river and pick up the now-familiar North Yuba Trail. Return to your car on North Yuba. Final mileage with this add-on is almost 30 miles.

RIDE 37 · Forest City's Pliocene–Sandusky Loop

AT A GLANCE

Length/configuration: 13-mile loop, counterclockwise; paved and dirt roads

Aerobic difficulty: Moderate due to elevation gain

Technical difficulty: Mild with an intensely intermediate stretch on Sandusky Creek Road (a nontechnical option bypasses this).

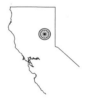

Scenery: Sweeping views of surrounding deep canyons and forested ridges; the jagged Sierra Buttes abruptly piercing the horizon in the distance; snow-patched mountaintops.

Special comments: Ruby Bluff overlook is a great place to camp, especially during summer meteor showers.

Compared to other trails in the Downieville district of Tahoe National Forest, Pliocene–Sandusky Loop, a 13-mile counterclockwise loop, is one of the few mildly technical rides around. Only 2 miles of the loop requires strong intermediate skills. Beginners can still enjoy this ride. They can bypass this intermediate section by taking a slightly longer option that finishes the loop via smooth, nontechnical dirt road. In both cases, the route is ridden counterclockwise and begins with a moderate climb on paved road to the highest point of the loop. The climbing is easily managed, and you can carry on a conversation with your riding buddies, catching up on all the latest news or making new acquaintances. All the climbing is on pavement and after that, it's all downhill on dirt roads through the pine and cedar forest. Along the way, a hidden side trail leads out to the Ruby Bluffs overlook, a stunning vertical face of a mountainside on the other side of a vast, deep canyon. The last part of the loop takes you through a different ecosystem, down a cool and lush ravine over several tiny creeks and through bushy, dense forest. Might you find gold here? Who knows—keep your eyes open.

The short life of the mining town known as Forest, now called Forest City, was directly linked to the lure of gold believed to be buried in the surrounding mountains. In 1852, the town was born near Oregon Creek when gold was discovered in the areas downstream. Riches were enormous and in two years, the population swelled to over 1,000. The mining frenzy was under way, seducing hopeful millionaires and merchants alike. Businesses were established to offer provisions: clothing, meat, blacksmith services, hotels, and, of course, saloons and brothels. Numerous fires and the dwindling vein of gold drove Forest to the brink of death. Then, in the early 1870s, some very smart miners reasoned that, given the nature of the drainage in the region, a "lost" river channel had to have existed somewhere nearby. Sure enough, their conjecture was right on the money. The river was found running under the bluffs of Bald Mountain. In 1872, the Bald Mountain Mine company was established, and the town was brought back to life, based on what turned out to be one of the richest drift mines in the state. The prosperity lasted for 15 years, reportedly totaling in the millions of dollars. Eventually, depleted of gold, the mine closed, and the town shrank.

Today, there's another kind of gold in "them thar hills." There's something potentially big happening in Forest City and the time couldn't be more ripe, especially with the dire need to lessen recreational impact on the trails around nearby Downieville. The U.S. Forest Service, the government agency that basically owns Forest City and its surrounding land, was approached by a handful of bike enthusiasts with the hopes of opening miles of old pack trails to biking. That was in the early 1990s. Now, what started off as a handful of dreamers has grown into a larger group of seriously dedicated people from all over California, determined to build their "field of dreams." Organized as the Forest City Trail Council (FCTC), their goal is to revitalize the area and make it a premier mountain bike–friendly area. To date, most, if not all, of the old, historic houses and structures in Forest City have been leased from the Forest Service by private individuals, many of whom are avid cyclists. Major renovation is slowly happening to many of the structures, and eventually Forest City will come back to life with full-time residents. Part of the overall plan is to establish small businesses that cater to recreation and, hopefully, will include eateries, lodging, and maybe even a bike shop.

A lot still needs to happen. Working with government agencies, celebrities, local residents, and enthusiastic out-of-towners, trying to keep everyone happy is a monumental task in itself. Though there have been setbacks and a lot of frustrations along the way, the movement is going forward and will ultimately benefit nearly everyone in the surrounding communities. It is hoped that new trails in the Forest City area will attract riders from the nearby Downieville and Lake Tahoe regions, thereby lessening trail impact in those areas. The income-generating potential of this sport called mountain biking has, up until now, been lightly tapped by the local communities. In a time when general sentiment is to protect and preserve our forests, what replaces the income these towns lose from diminishing logging and mining operations? Though mountain biking may never compare to the boom that gold mining did in the past, it is using the forest and land respectfully. That alone is a gold mine for all of us.

But to become a draw for bikers, plenty of great trails are needed. The FCTC have long realized that the land surrounding Forest City is rich with miles of old pack trails, long since abandoned after the gold in the local mines played out. After years of no use, trails have become overgrown to the point of disappearing and becoming one with the forest again. Working in conjunction with the Forest Service, FCTC is taking the lead in clearing and rebuilding miles of pack trails into world-class bike trails. A number of

RIDE 37 · Forest City's Pliocene–Sandusky Loop

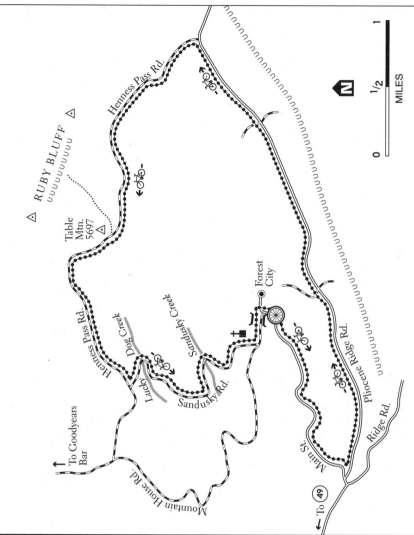

trails have been "rediscovered" by reconnaissance volunteers armed with topo maps. They assessed the kind and amount of work needed, addressing such issues as drainage and erosion control, creek crossings and trail bridges needed, and removing fallen trees and brush. And that's just to reopen existing trails, not blazing new trails. Trail-building is a slow and arduous job, and a weekend of volunteer work parties in June 1999 produced only a few miles of rideable trails. It goes without saying that the more people help, the faster the trails will open for all of us to enjoy. The Pliocene–Sandusky Loop presented here is just a taste of what can be mined around Forest City, and there's more, just waiting for you to help uncover it. For more information about volunteering, contact FCTC, listed below in "Sources of additional information."

General location: About 66 miles north of I-80, between Auburn and Downieville off CA 49, about 40 miles north of Nevada City.

Elevation change: 1,070 feet; starting elevation and low point 4,700 feet; high point 5,770 feet. Generally one gradual climb followed by easy descent over somewhat rough terrain.

Season: Late spring to mid-autumn.

Services: Pay phone in the town of Forest City. Food and gas in the tiny community of North San Juan. All other services in Nevada City and Downieville. As of 1998, long-range plans are under way to rebuild Forest City into a mountain biking community, complete with lodging, restaurants, and other amenities.

Hazards: Pliocene Ridge and Mountain House Roads are somewhat well traveled, so watch out for traffic when pedaling them. Avoid getting caught in a lightning storm while riding on exposed Pliocene Ridge Road and at Ruby Bluffs overlook. Deer hunting season begins with in mid-August, with rifles permitted from mid-September through early November. Riders are advised to wear brightly colored clothing at this time—or ride somewhere else where hunting is not allowed.

Rescue index: Because this trail is not well known, at least for now, you need to be self-reliant. For emergency situations, you may be able to flag down an occasional passing motorist on Pliocene Ridge or Mountain House Roads. In Forest City, there is a pay phone and a handful of residences. Medical clinic and other emergency services can be found in Downieville, about 16 miles away via Mountain House Road.

Land status: Tahoe National Forest.

Maps: USGS Pike, Alleghany, Downieville, and Goodyears Bar 7.5 minute series.

Finding the trail: From I-80 at Auburn, Forest City is about 66 miles north. Take CA 49 north out of Auburn. Drive through Grass Valley, Nevada City, and North San Juan (the last chance for food and gas) and after 48 miles on CA 49, turn right onto Ridge Road toward Pike and Alleghany. Stay on Ridge for about 14 miles until you see a sign for Forest City indicating another paved road going left down a canyon. Turn left here and descend into the canyon, and after approximately 4 miles, the road leads you into tiny Forest City. Park in the dirt lot next to a vehicle bridge at the intersection of Main Street and Mountain House Road, a wide dirt road.

Sources of additional information:

Tahoe National Forest
Downieville Ranger District
North Yuba Ranger Station
15924 Hwy. 49
Camptonville, CA 95922-9707
(916) 288-3231

Forest City Trail Council
Zach Anderson
P.O. Box 1202
Cedar Ridge, CA 95924
(530) 274-2388
zachi@netshel.net

Notes on the trail: Climbing on pavement is much easier than rock-strewn, rugged terrain. Conversely, riding down pavement is not nearly as fun, challenging, or as exhilarating as flying over rocks and ruts, whooping all the way down through the forest. That said, this ride is described in the counterclockwise direction, so that all 1,070 feet of climbing is done on pavement and the subsequent loss is on rugged dirt terrain. If you want more of an aerobic challenge, ride it clockwise, climbing up the rocky portion.

At about 4,700 feet elevation, Forest City sits in a canyon carved by Oregon Creek. Begin pedaling west following paved Main Street out of town. The quiet road curves left to the southwest as you begin climbing immediately toward Pliocene Ridge and Ridge Roads. Bypass all dirt trails shooting off the pavement. The road climbs moderately, gaining approximately 235 feet in 1.5 miles to the top of the ridge. Once on the ridge, just before Ridge Road, turn left onto paved Pliocene Road, which begins directly across from the County Dump entrance. If you reach Ridge Road, you've gone a few yards too far.

Though there isn't much of a shoulder on Pliocene Road, it sees only occasional traffic. Still, stay alert for vehicles. The road climbs gradually and the higher you go, the more sweeping the view becomes of the North San Juan Ridge off a short distance on your right. At about 4 miles, the road steepens and rewards you with a virtually unobstructed panorama to the south. You see the dramatically jagged Sierra Buttes, jutting straight up into the sky and possibly with lingering snow still sitting in its crevices. Just beyond the near ridge, Castle Peak and the high mountain ranges that surround Donner Pass can be seen.

At about 4.8 miles, bypass a dirt road coming up the hill that intersects Pliocene Road on your left. (It's a road that leads steeply and directly down to Forest City.) Pliocene levels and then climbs steeply again up the last hill. At about 5.7 miles, elevation about 5,700 feet, you reach the intersection of Henness Pass Road, a wide dirt and gravel road taking off on your left. Henness Pass is unsigned so look for the obvious landmark—a cattle chute—sitting at this junction. Take a breather and enjoy the view. The climbing is now finished and you've earned your reward: an exhilarating, slightly intermediate technical descent back down to Forest City through the forest, with a short excursion to the spectacular Ruby Bluffs overlook.

Turn left onto Henness Pass Road. It begins as a somewhat level two-car-width road, narrowing as it descends through the forest of conifer trees and low manzanita bushes. Trail conditions consist of packed dirt and gravel, occasionally strewn with loose rough rock, punctuated with semi-buried boulders and rain ruts. Bypass all lesser dirt roads leading off your trail until about 6.5 miles, at which point you reach an intersection where the main, wide road curves abruptly to the right and a narrow dirt road continues straight ahead. Stay straight, taking the narrow road. The main road curving right is gated closed in the distance. (The road serves privately owned and operated Ruby Mine. Sorry, no through access is available.)

Now on the narrower dirt road—still Henness Pass Road—continue the gradual downhill run as it traverses the southwestern slope of Table Mountain. Bypass lesser trails that intersect it. At about 7.3 miles, (less than a mile since the wider Ruby Mine Road), look for a lesser trail coming in behind your right shoulder. From Henness Pass Road, you can see that the right-hand trail runs through a small forested area devoid of underbrush. There's a stone fire ring behind one of the trees, evidence that this small clearing is a popular camping site. This is the beginning of a short 0.2-mile trail that leads to a cliff overlooking Ruby Bluffs and the surrounding northern mountain ranges. Leave the main dirt road and follow the faint single-track trail through the trees. Look for cairns that biking girlfriend Laura Anderson and I built along the way. The trail becomes less defined and the riding a bit more technical as you come into a small clearing completely strewn with loose chunks of rocks, ranging in size from golf ball to basketball, as well as shale rock varying from small saucer to huge dinner plate size. Check out the ground and you see a different sort of cairn fashioned into a 15-foot-wide Star of David. Follow more cairns as the trail weaves you through the

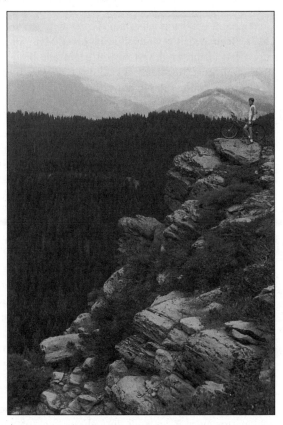

Laura soaks in the view
from Ruby Bluffs
Overlook.

manzanita bushes. In a few yards, at elevation 5,500 feet, you reach the overlook, a clearing at the edge of a cliff adjacent to impressive rock outcroppings. The cliff faces north, giving you a far-reaching view of the North Yuba River canyon with Ruby Bluff towering overhead on the other side. On clear days, a glimpse of the coastal ranges to the west can be had. Toward the east, the Downieville fire lookout is visible as well as the Sierra Buttes. Imagine watching a summer meteor shower up here. (Nowadays, powerful handlebar lights are available for night riders.) And what a great spot for a break or a picnic! When you're finished admiring the scenery, retrace the narrow trail back to Henness Pass Road and make a right onto it.

Continue the gradual downhill run. In almost 2 miles, keep an eye out for a small clearing sitting at the bottom of a gentle descent with a lesser road leading off on your left. This narrow dirt road on the left is Sandusky Creek Road, and because it's not signed, look for an isolated pair of pine trees growing at this intersection. At this point, you've pedaled about 10.6 miles since leaving Forest City. Sandusky is a 2-mile rugged unmaintained jeep trail, strewn with loose rocks and boulders ranging in size from golf ball to beach ball, spiced with rocky runoff ruts and tiny creek crossings. Winter storms have turned stretches of the jeep road into a narrow and fun obstacle course. Strong intermediate-level technical skills are required, although walking works just fine. The environment in which Sandusky travels is quite a bit different than what you found on Henness Pass Road. Sandusky gradually drops, following a cool ravine into which numerous tiny creeks drain. The abundance of so much moisture results in lush, thick vegetation made up of aromatic bear clover shrubs and fragrant dogwood, cedar, oak, and conifer trees, to name a few species. So, from Henness Pass Road, hang a left onto Sandusky Creek Road and put your technical skills to the test. Although the road may appear to peter out as it narrows and resembles a single-track bordered by overgrown bushes, the wide road does reappear.

Option to bypass Sandusky Creek Road: Stay on mildly technical Henness Pass Road, continuing past the pair of pine trees at the Sandusky Creek Road junction. In about a half mile, you reach Mountain House Road, a smooth, wide dirt road. Make a left onto Mountain House and follow it for almost 2.5 miles all the way back into Forest City. Expect to do some moderate climbing, made easier with short stretches of flats and descents. Though Mountain House sees only occasional traffic, stay alert for vehicles.

After descending about 210 feet on Sandusky Creek Road, you reach Mountain House Road, a wide, well-traveled dirt road. Turn left here and in a few yards, you come to the Forest City Cemetery. It's an historic cemetery worthy of a visit. Continue down Mountain House and in a short stretch, cross over Oregon Creek on a well-made vehicle bridge and enter Forest City. You finish the ride by closing the loop here at approximately 13 miles.

OTHER AREA RIDES

FEATHER FALLS OUT-AND-BACK: Located about 23 miles east of Oroville, in Plumas National Forest, this 7-mile out-and-back (3.5 miles each way) follows a single-track trail to the Feather Falls Overlook. Expect a significant amount of climbing and some technical terrain. The reward, however, is a spectacular view of the falls, the sixth highest in the nation. The most dramatic time to view the falls is in the spring, when runoff is heavy. You can extend the ride by adding 4 miles of pavement at the beginning (2 miles each way). Keep your speed in check at all times, as the trail is immensely popular with bikers and hikers.

Finding the trail: The town of Oroville is located about 70 miles north of Sacramento off CA 70. From Oroville, head east on CA 162 for about 7 miles to Forbestown Road. Go right onto Forbestown for approximately 6 miles, then turn left onto Lumpkin Road toward the town of Feather Falls. Park in town and pedal back on Lumpkin for a short distance to the outskirts of town. Watch for a sign indicating a dirt road to Feather Falls on the north side of the road. Follow this dirt road; it soon turns into a single-track and eventually ends at the overlook. Return the way you came.

Maps: USGS Brush Creek and Forbestown 7.5 minute series.

For more information, contact:
Plumas National Forest
Feather River Ranger District
875 Mitchell Ave.
Oroville, CA 95965-4699
(916) 534-6500

NEW MELONES LAKE—GLORY HOLE RECREATION AREA: New Melones Lake at Glory Hole Recreation Area: Admittedly, there are far more challenging and scenic trails in the Sierras, but this one offers a quick half-day or nearly full-day getaway for cyclists who live in the flatlands of the San Joaquin Valley. Over 12 miles of trails are open to bikes, most of which are suited for cyclists with intermediate-level technical skills. Numerous trails meander along the shoreline and cross paved access roads, which means you can configure your own route, making it as long or short, as easy or difficult as you like. The most challenging section reportedly is the Tower Trail, where there is some steep climbing and tight switchbacks involved.

Finding the trail: Glory Hole Rec Area is about 55 miles east of Stockton, just west of the town of Sonora. From Stockton, travel east on CA 4 toward Angels Camp. Turn right onto CA 49 and proceed through Angels Camp for about 12 miles. Look for the Glory Hole access road on your right. Go right and proceed to the entrance

of the recreation area. Park in any designated lot, and just start pedaling any configuration you wish.

Map: Available at the entrance station.

For more information, contact:

>   Bureau of Reclamation
>   New Melones Lake—Glory Hole Recreation Area
>   6850 Studhorse Flat Rd.
>   Sonora, CA 95370
>   (209) 536-9094

BRICEBERG LOOPS: (Thanks to Yosemite Bug Hostel Lodge & Campground for
providing info about this ride.) As you probably know, national parks like Yosemite are
off-limits to mountain bikes. The bike routes located near the town of Briceberg (a little over 20 miles from the main west entrance of Yosemite) is the closest you'll get to
riding off-road in this crown jewel of national parks. Reportedly, this ride measures between 19 and 33 miles round-trip, depending on which trails you follow. Though the
routes are made up of dirt roads and some pavement, moderate bike-handling skills are
recommended. Plenty of steep climbs between 1,250 to 3,550 feet elevation means
strong endurance is required. But, oh, the rewards of your efforts: Riding counterclockwise along Merced River gives you terrific views of Yosemite landmarks, namely
El Capitan, Half Dome, and Cloud's Rest, as well as the Merced River Valley.

Finding the trail: From Merced, follow CA 140 east through the towns of Mariposa
and Midpines, toward the main Yosemite entrance at Arch Way Ranger Station.
About 50 miles from Merced, where CA 140 meets the Merced River, is Briceberg.
Park in this vicinity. Begin your ride by pedaling over the Briceberg Suspension
Bridge on Bull Creek Road (also known as Briceberg Road). Bear right and grind up
the hill toward Burma Grade, which is reached in about 5 miles. Leave Bull Creek
Road and follow another dirt road on a rolling plateau riding due east by northeast
toward Jenkins Hill for about 7 miles. Along this stretch, be sure to check out several
side roads that lead off on the right—they offer views of those Yosemite landmarks.
The rest of the route loops around counterclockwise, connecting to Bonnell Gulch
Road, past Black Mountain and Halls Gulch before reaching Burma Grade again.

Maps: USGS Felicana Mountain and Kinsley 7.5 minute series.

For more information, contact:

>   Yosemite Bug Hostel Lodge &
>   Campground
>   6979 Highway 140
>   P.O. Box 81
>   Midpines, CA 95345
>   (209) 966-6666
>   www.yosemitebug.com

Visit the Bug for routing directions
and maps. They have the scoop on
other nearby bike trails, including
single-tracks, and biking in the winter. Check out their very informative
Web site.

Sierra National Forest
1600 Tollhouse Rd.
Clovis, CA 93611
(209) 297-0706

Stanislaus National Forest
19777 Greenley Rd.
Sonora, CA 95370
(209) 532-3671

Mariposa Ranger Station
(209) 966-3638

BEAR TRAP BASIN AND JELMINI BASIN LOOPS: This ride is located in the Calaveras Ranger District of Stanislaus National Forest, just south of the Mokelumne Wilderness. Bear Trap clocks in at 8 miles, and Jelmini Basin is 17 miles. Though each loop has its own starting point, a 1-mile dirt road connects the two loops, and hearty riders may want to tackle both rides as one outing. Both are suited for riders with intermediate-level technical skills on a combination of dirt roads, four-wheel-drive jeep roads, and some single-tracks. Strong endurance is required since the ride takes place between 6,800 and 8,100 feet, roughly. Views from the ridge tops are expansive, and the downhills are long and demanding, running through aspen groves and peaceful meadows. Views of the Mokelumne Wilderness are spectacular as are the lovely meadows surrounded by quaking aspen trees.

Finding the trail: From Stockton, follow CA 4 east into the mountains through Angels Camp and Arnold. Continue about 14 miles past Calaveras Big Trees State Park to the Cabbage Patch Maintenance Station, about 9 miles west of the town of Bear Valley. For the Jelmini Basin Loop, watch for FS 7N09 leading off on the north side of CA 4 (your left) near Cabbage Patch. You can park in the vicinity of this junction or head up FS 7N09 for a short distance. Limited parking alongside the road is available at both starting points. For the Bear Trap Basin Loop, continue past Cabbage Patch toward Bear Valley. Just before Bear Valley, still on CA 4, on the outskirts of town, look for Corral Hollow Road (a four-wheel-drive jeep road, FS 7N35). Plenty of parking is available at this trailhead. Begin pedaling by following the dirt road on the northwest side of CA 4, along Corral Gulch toward Corral Hollow.

Maps: USGS Tamarack and Calaveras Dome 7.5 minute series.

For more information, contact:

Stanislaus National Forest
19777 Greenley Rd.
Sonora, CA 95370
(209) 532-3671

SQUAW/SKY HARBOR RIDE: This gnarly ride is located at the eastern end of Millerton Lake, where the San Joaquin River empties, and is actually made up of two routes: the popular Squaw Leap Loop (2.5 miles) and the Squaw–Sky Harbor Out-and-Back (19 miles one way, 38 miles round-trip). Combine the two, and you have an all-day ride suited for expertly skilled riders with superhuman endurance. Squaw Leap leads over rolling hills dotted with chaparral, manzanita, oak, and pine trees. Rugged Sky Harbor trail offers spectacular views of the river gorge, whitewater, and granite cliffs. On both trails, expect some short, steep climbs and technically rocky sections. Bring plenty of food and water, allow plenty of time, avoid riding in the middle of summer, and don't ride alone.

Finding the trail: From Fresno, drive east on CA 168 (Shaw Avenue) to Prather. Continue through Prather for a short distance and then turn left (north) onto Auberry Road and go through Auberry to New Auberry. Once in New Auberry, make a left (west) onto Powerhouse Road, then a left onto Smalley Road. Smalley drops down into the river gorge and the Squaw Leap campground. Park here. The single-track Squaw Leap trail is signed and eventually leads you over the river on a bridge. The Sky Harbor trail, however, runs west along the south side of the river.

Maps: USGS Topo maps do not show the entire route. Instead, visit either Oakhurst Cycling Center or Tri-Sport Unlimited for a map, trail-finding advice, and tips on finding other trails in the area.

For more information, contact:

Oakhurst Cycling Center
39993 Highway 41
Oakhurst, CA 93644-9575
(209) 642-4606

Tri-Sport Unlimited
132 W. Nees
Fresno, CA 93711
(559) 432-0800

Bureau of Land Management
Folsom Resource Area
63 Natoma St.
Folsom, CA 95630
(916) 985-4474

Millerton Lake State Recreation
Area
San Joaquin District
5290 Millerton Rd.
Friant, CA 93626
(559) 822-2332

SOME LOCAL BICYCLE SHOPS & ORGANIZATIONS

Yuba Expeditions
P.O. Box 750
Nevada City, CA 95959
(530) 265-8779

Forest City Trail Council
Zach Anderson
P.O. Box 1202
Cedar Ridge, CA 95924
(530) 274-2388
zachi@netshel.net

Sports Fever
Pine Creek Shopping Center
Grass Valley, CA 95945
(530) 477-8006

Samurai Mountain Bikes
10028 Joerschke Drive
Grass Valley, CA 95945
(916) 477-0858

Tour of Nevada City Bicycle Shop
457 Sacramento St.
Nevada City, CA 95959
(530) 265-2187

Performance Bike Shop
5271 Sunrise Blvd.
Fair Oaks, CA 95628
(916) 961-1488

Rest Stop Bicycle Accessories
3230 Folsom Blvd.
Sacramento, CA 95816
(916) 453-1870

Oakhurst Cycling Center
39993 Highway 41
Oakhurst, CA 93644-9575
(209) 642-4606

Tri-Sport Unlimited
132 W. Nees
Fresno, CA 93711
(559) 432-0800

AROUND LAKE TAHOE

Brilliantly blue-green Lake Tahoe sits at about 6,200 feet, exactly on the California-Nevada stateline. Surrounded by tall mountain ranges, this mirror-like body of water is the largest alpine lake in the Western United States, drained only by the Truckee River. Volcanic activity and shifting earth created a kind of bowl, bounded by the Sierra Nevada mountains in the west and the Carson Range in the east. Plenty of snow melt and rain drained into the basin, forming the lake. To this day, Lake Tahoe's water quality is so incredibly pure, visibility is about 70 feet (and it used to be deeper). Measuring about 22 miles long, 12 miles wide, and over 72 miles of shoreline, the lake's average depth is 990 feet with the deepest point dropping to roughly 1,640 feet. On land, the lake is bordered by three national forests and a state park. The rest is private property.

Today, ironically, the lake's beauty maybe too much of a good thing. As one of the state's most popular recreation areas during the winter and summer, a by-product of great local concern is the increased air pollution, traffic, and construction projects — all of which aversely impacts the lake. Easy access by Interstate 80 to the north shore and CA 50 to the south shore only exacerbate the situation. Formulating a strategy to save Lake Tahoe was no easy task and you can imagine the kinds of battles that are still being fought between environmentalists and land developers. As recently as the late 1980s, a 20-year master plan was finally adopted, severely restricting new development. Many public and private agencies have joined forces in the continuing effort to preserve Lake Tahoe and to educate the public. One such group is the Tahoe Rim Trail Association, a non-profit volunteer organization that has been working long and hard to establish a 150-mile trail encircling the lake. Over 90% complete, the Tahoe Rim Trail (TRT), is a gem of a single-track trail, about half of which is open to bikes. There was a time when many more miles of the TRT were off-limits to us cyclists. Hats off to them for recognizing our sport as an acceptable, non-polluting form of recreation. We owe our thanks to the many dedicated two-wheelers who have participated in trail workdays and at the meetings—they give us all a good name. While the TRT is more suited to intermediate or better riders, a wide variety of other trails and roads suitable for everyone including beginners and youngsters can be found on both sides of the lake, in California and Nevada.

RIDE 38 · Hole-In-The-Ground Trail

AT A GLANCE

Length/configuration: 12.9-mile point-to-point; single-tracks and dirt jeep roads. (Loop option: add 3.7 miles of pavement to make this a 16.6-mile loop, counterclockwise.)

Aerobic difficulty: Moderately strenuous due to climbing and distance

Technical difficulty: Intermediate due to rugged and narrow single-tracks; some short sections are advanced due to steepness and boulder fields

Scenery: Spectacular view of Castle Peak and Donner Summit from an exhilaratingly narrow ridge.

Special comments: Nine miles of awesome single-track. Strong, advanced beginners can do this ride, but be sure to allow plenty of time for walking through difficult sections.

Here's a fairly new trail that opened in mid-1997, and its awesomeness is spreading the word faster than your fastest downhill run. Of the 12.9 miles that make up this point-to-point ride, 10 miles of it is on intermediately technical single-track with some advanced sections thrown in to keep you on your toes. The elevation gain is not exhausting, thanks to the variety of ups and downs throughout the route. And variety is what makes this trail a delight: twisting and turning, weaving past conifer forests and huge boulders, and ascending and descending steep terrain through tight and wide switchbacks. In August, you might even ride through tiny patches of snow, slowly melting in the shade of a boulder. You certainly won't get bored with this trail. Don't want to bother setting up shuttle cars for this fabulous point-to-point ride? Not a problem. It's a piece of cake to turn the ride into a 16.6-mile loop by tacking on a 3.7-mile stretch at the end. This connector stretch uses Donner Pass Road and a dirt road which cuts through the Boreal Ridge Ski Resort parking lot.

Both versions of the route are ridden counterclockwise. The first mile is a gradual uphill—a good warm-up. The following half mile has you pumping up 740 feet to a ridge line, through forests of mixed conifers via tight switchbacks. Ultimately, you top 8,040 feet. If you're not accustomed to the higher elevation, this is sure to get your heart thumping. But once you reach the top of the ridge, you're rewarded with spectacular views of Castle Peak, especially glorious when set against a brilliant blue sky and the wildflowers are in full bloom. As you ride down the narrow ridge through more switchbacks, you drop 540 feet in less than 3 miles into a canyon, weaving through boulder fields along the way. Eventually, you cross Lower Castle Creek and begin climbing to the next ridge where you enjoy a gradual descent toward Lower Lola Montez Lake. From there, it's more downhill fun on single-track, spiced with a few short rises. The trail eventually widens into an easy jeep road. And just when you thought you would fall asleep on this easy stretch, near the end of this great dirt ride, you're challenged yet again with several short single-track trails that

RIDE 38 · Hole-In-The-Ground Trail

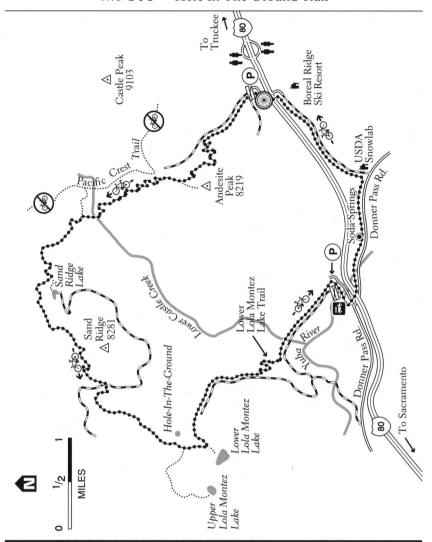

are steep and technically advanced before finishing the ride. Not up for this final technical stretch? No problem. There's an easy way down to the finishing point.

Many thanks to David Schotzko of Truckee for taking us on this outstanding ride. It turns out to be my favorite! —L.A.

General location: Near North Lake Tahoe, 7.5 miles west of Truckee, immediately off I-80, near Donner Summit.

Elevation change: 1,600 feet; starting elevation 7,280 feet; high point 8,040 feet; low point 6,440 feet. Initial long climb up to ridge, then drops into creek drainage, followed by climb out; lots of ups and downs throughout.

Season: Late spring to mid-autumn.

Services: None on the trail. Water taken from creeks and lakes needs to be treated. Water and rest rooms are located at the rest stop just east of the starting point on I-80. Very limited services in Soda Springs, near the end of the dirt route. Most services in Truckee, 7.5 miles east of the starting point.

Hazards: Stay alert for occasional vehicular traffic on the dirt road near the end of the ride. If you're tackling this route as a loop, watch out for considerable traffic on the paved roads as you cross I-80 twice via an overpass and underpass. The water level of Lower Castle Creek near the end of the ride is known to rise in the afternoon, though still passable, albeit a wet crossing.

Rescue index: While your chance of finding other trail users who might be of help is improving with the trail's growing popularity, the single-track nature of the trail still makes this a fairly remote area. The few homes near the end may provide assistance, but generally, in case of an emergency, you should make your way down to I-80. There's also a fire station a few yards from the ending trailhead on Sherrit Lane at the Soda Springs exit off I-80.

Land status: Tahoe National Forest.

Maps: *Hole-In-The-Ground Trail,* published by Sowarwe-Werher, P.O. Box 17, Weimar, CA 95736; USGS Soda Springs, Norden, Webber Peak 7.5 minute series.

Finding the trail: The entire ride is immediately on the north side of I-80. From Truckee or Sacramento, travel west or east respectively on I-80 to the Castle Peak exit, about 7.5 miles west of Truckee, across the freeway from Boreal Ridge Ski Resort. Take the exit and make your way to the north side of I-80. The paved road curves to the right and at about 0.1 mile, the pavement ends at a metal gate and a dirt road begins. Park just before the gate, on the side of the road. Be sure you're not blocking the gate from vehicle access. Begin pedaling from here.

To set up the end shuttle, take the Soda Springs exit, located 3.4 miles west of the Castle Peak exit on I-80. Make your way to the north side of the freeway and take the first right onto Sherrit Lane. Now heading northeast, go past the fire station to the Lower Lola Montez Lake trailhead, about 0.3 mile from the right turn. Park in the small dirt pulloff.

Sources of additional information:

Tahoe National Forest
Truckee Ranger District
10342 Hwy 89 North
Truckee, CA 96161
(916) 587-3558

Tahoe National Forest
   Headquarters
P.O. Box 6001
Nevada City, CA 95959
(916) 265-4531

Notes on the trail: This exceptional ride is fairly easy to follow. From the Castle Peak exit trailhead, begin by pedaling north through the metal gate up the dirt road. The road is about the width of a car and begins by gently ascending hard-pack dirt, punctuated by loose and semi-buried rocks and boulders. The terrain is mildly rugged and easy to ride. In the blink of an eye, you immediately reach a fork and there's a cross-country ski sign posted on one of the trees. Take the right fork, a narrow jeep road, and continue heading due north. At 0.5 mile, bypass another jeep road coming in on the right. The terrain steepens slightly, eased by a few level spots.

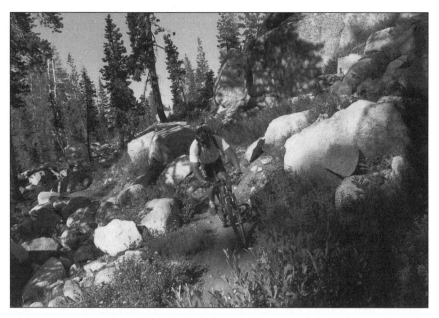

Agile David deftly maneuvers through the boulder fields on what is arguably the best single-track in the North Tahoe area.

One mile into the ride, you reach the junction of the Hole-In-The-Ground Trail, as marked by a prominent sign, leading off to the left. Say good-bye to the jeep road and hello to this fun and intermediately challenging single-track trail. You'll be following it for the next 9.1 miles. The adventure begins with a half-mile climb over very steep terrain to the first ridge traversing through a forest of mixed conifer trees. Never fear, switchbacks make the going manageable for mortals. The turns are tight and the trail may be loose with some rocks and soft dirt, but all in all, it's a good challenge to grind up the switchbacks without dabbing a foot. Along the way, you may see cinderblocks laid in the trail by hardworking, dedicated folks in an effort to stabilize and check erosion. Give a vocal "thanks a lot" to their efforts and consider volunteering on trail-maintenance days in the immediate future. As you continue up to the ridge, exhilarating views of Castle Peak, sitting at 9,103 feet, begin to emerge on your right, across another canyon. But keep an eye on the trail for it skirts a few short stretches of steep drop-offs. At approximately 2.4 miles, you reach the high point of the ride at the top of the ridge, elevation 8,040 feet. You're practically nose-to-nose with Castle Peak now. The view here is almost 360-degrees with Squaw Valley and Donner Pass toward the southeast. Take a moment and enjoy the view before dropping down to the other side of the ridge.

The gradual descent into the canyon is thrilling as you follow the narrow single-track over the equally narrow and wide-open ridge, sort of like riding a huge razor's edge. You'll feel as if you're liable to fall off the mountain if you don't keep your eye on the trail, which is tough to do since the scenery is so spectacular. The trail drops 540 feet in less than 3 miles via more switchbacks, threading you past boulders and trees, and cruising up and down fun, little dips. The terrain is intermediately challenging and strong beginners with the right attitude, including knowing when to dismount and walk, can enjoy this stretch. Cross Lower Castle Creek at 4 miles, approximate elevation 7,550 feet. You can keep your feet dry with fancy footwork as you portage your bike over the boulders.

After the creek, begin climbing up the other side of the canyon. About 0.3 mile from the creek, you reach the junction of a trail leading off on your right to the Pacific Crest Trail (PCT). Bypass it (no bikes allowed on the PCT), staying on your single-track, bearing left toward Sand Ridge Lake. Level stretches in the trail offer respite as you weave through fields of huge boulders. At 5.5 miles from the starting point, a trail to Sand Ridge Lake peels off on your left. (If you're looking for a great spot for a lunch break, check out the lake on this short side trip, distance 0.25 mile.) Continue past the Sand Ridge Lake trail, basically heading west and still climbing through more boulder fields. Just under 6 miles, you cross a tiny creek.

At about 6.3 miles, you reach the second highest point of the ride at approximately 7,800 feet. In 0.2 mile farther, bypass an unsigned logging road crossing your path. From this point, the trail is mostly a gentle and fun downhill cruise, meandering through the shady forest, dodging boulders along the way. You can pick up some speed here if you've got the hankering, popping up out of the tiny dips (more like wide and smooth-edged potholes) in the trail here and there. Stay on the main single-track, ignoring other intersecting trails. The terrain eventually becomes less boulder-strewn, and at 8.7 miles, a wood and gravel-filled footpath leads you through a small, marshy area. After weaving past a few more boulder patches, ride another wood-gravel footpath over another short, marshy stretch. Cross a tiny creek (which may be dry late in the summer), and skirt a wide-open meadow on your left.

At 9.7 miles, the small trail to Lower Lola Montez Lake takes off on your right. The lake is reached in 1.25 miles, and bikes are allowed on this side trail. (Warning: Voracious mosquitoes reside at the lake, so either bring repellent or keep moving!) If you visit the lake, retrace your path back to this intersection and resume your southerly descent on the main single-track. Before you know it, the trail widens into a dirt road, at 10 miles. You're now entering private property territory and posted signs ask that you stay on the road.

As you descend this mostly nontechnical stretch, keep an eye peeled for a narrow trail leading off on your left—it's easy to miss if you're bombing down the jeep road. That trail is signed Lower Lola Montez Trail, and it connects the previous lake trail with the trailhead at Soda Springs, your ultimate destination. (If you're riding this trail as a point-to-point, that Soda Springs trailhead is, hopefully, where you have left your end-shuttle car.) As promised, this left-hand trail is the half-mile descent that's suited for technically advanced riders due to extreme steepness, loose dirt and rock conditions, and twisty, narrow turns—all the ingredients that make controlling your speed and maintaining traction an extreme challenge. Of course, walking will get you down the trail, albeit not as much fun. This 0.5 mile hairy stretch soon rejoins the easy dirt road you've just been descending. (The easy option is to bypass this single-track trail and stay right on the wide dirt road. This option will add about a mile to the overall ride. Here's what you do: continue following the easy road and at almost a mile, cruise past another dirt road which leads off on the right. Bear left here and in almost 0.5 mile farther, your road is rejoined by the advanced single-track trail which you originally bypassed.)

The advanced trail rejoins the easy dirt road at mile 11.7. Go left onto the wide dirt road and pedal over several small hills. In just over 0.2 mile, cross Lower Castle Creek. The creek can be wide, but if the water is not too high, technically skilled riders can plow right through it. The creekbed is actually stabilized by a wire mesh blanket, so be careful as you ride over it. Bypass all lesser dirt roads (they're likely to be private dirt driveways) and power up and down several short hills. Watch for a narrow trail leading off on your left, at about 12.7 miles, simply signed "Trail." Hop onto this trail and climb over a steep but short rise, popping out of the forest and bushes at the end of the trail. Point-to-point riders: this is where your end-shuttle car is waiting. Loop riders: Follow the pavement down for about 0.3 mile, curving to the right and past the fire station. At the intersection, turn left onto Donner Pass Road and go over I-80 to its south side. Stay on Donner Pass Road, heading east toward Soda Springs. At about 1.3 miles from the overpass, go left at the USDA Snow Lab onto a dirt road. Follow the dirt road as it begins paralleling I-80 and climbs toward Boreal Ridge Ski Resort. Go through the resort parking lot and exit it via a paved road. Carry on to the north side of I-80 via an underpass. Follow the pavement as it curves right and in about 0.1 mile, you reach the starting point and your parked car, closing the loop in 16.6 miles.

RIDE 39 · Sardine Valley Loop

AT A GLANCE

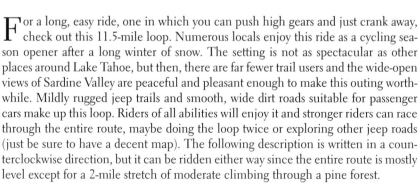

Length/configuration: 11.5-mile loop; double-track and dirt roads

Aerobic difficulty: Easy due to mostly flat riding

Technical difficulty: Mildly technical

Scenery: Wide-open views of Sardine Valley and Sardine Peak

Special comments: One of the few fairly level rides near mountainous Lake Tahoe. Great first-ride-of-the-season route. The best part of the loop is suitable for youngsters and kid-trailers.

For a long, easy ride, one in which you can push high gears and just crank away, check out this 11.5-mile loop. Numerous locals enjoy this ride as a cycling season opener after a long winter of snow. The setting is not as spectacular as other places around Lake Tahoe, but then, there are far fewer trail users and the wide-open views of Sardine Valley are peaceful and pleasant enough to make this outing worthwhile. Mildly rugged jeep trails and smooth, wide dirt roads suitable for passenger cars make up this loop. Riders of all abilities will enjoy it and stronger riders can race through the entire route, maybe doing the loop twice or exploring other jeep roads (just be sure to have a decent map). The following description is written in a counterclockwise direction, but it can be ridden either way since the entire route is mostly level except for a 2-mile stretch of moderate climbing through a pine forest.

The first 4.7 miles of the counterclockwise direction is free of vehicles, which makes it a great starting point for an out-and-back ride for freewheeling youngsters and kid-trailers—just turn around when the kiddies are good and tired. Riding this portion of the loop lets you avoid Smithneck Road, a dirt road with occasional car and truck traffic. Most of the loop is suitable for towing kids in a trailer (the 2-mile

RIDE 39 · Sardine Valley Loop

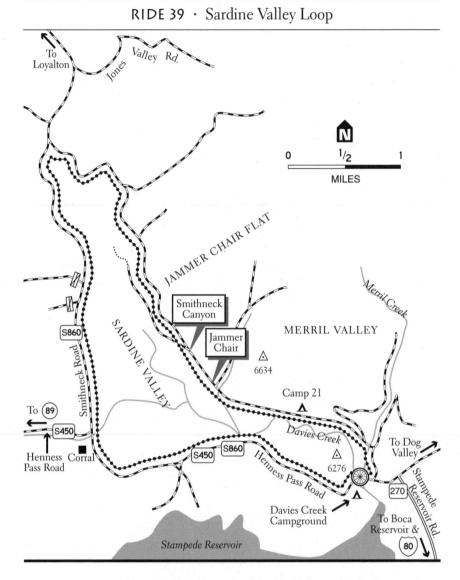

moderate stretch between the Smithneck Canyon Trail turn-off to Jones Valley Road is the exception). Thanks goes to Julie Maurer of Northstar-at-Tahoe for suggesting this ride. —L.A.

General location: About 11 miles north of I-80, north of Lake Tahoe, in California near the Nevada state line.

Elevation change: 300 feet; starting elevation and low point 6,000 feet; high point 6,300 feet. Mostly flat with a short section of moderate climbing.

Season: Mid-spring to mid-autumn.

Services: None on the trail. Piped water, pit toilets, and campsites at developed Logger Campground, located on the south side of Stampede Reservoir. Davies Creek campground, a less developed site, has a pit toilet but no water. All services available in Truckee.

Hazards: Occasional vehicular traffic on Smithneck, Jones Valley, and Henness Pass Roads.

Rescue index: The first 4.7-mile stretch is much less traveled; don't expect to encounter other trail users on this stretch. So, in case of emergency, make your way to occasionally traveled Smithneck Road or Henness Pass Road where you might be able to flag down a passing motorist. During the summer, you can find help at Logger Campground, located on the south side of Stampede Reservoir, about 2.5 miles south of Davies Campground.

Land status: Tahoe National Forest.

Maps: USGS Dog Valley and Sardine Valley 7.5 minute series.

Finding the trail: Take the Hirschdale Road exit off I-80, located about 7 miles east of Truckee. Make your way to the north side of the freeway where Hirschdale becomes Stampede Dam Road, County Road 270. About 10.5 miles from I-80, pass Boca Reservoir and then Stampede Reservoir, the pavement of CR 270 ends at a T intersection with Henness Pass Road, a dirt road that's also referred to as CR S860. Turn left onto Henness Pass, go over several little wooden bridges and then make a left into the Davies Campground, about a mile from the intersection. Park here.

Sources of additional information:

Tahoe National Forest
Truckee Ranger District
10342 Hwy 89 North
Truckee, CA 96161
(916) 587-3558

Tahoe National Forest
Headquarters
P.O. Box 6001
Nevada City, CA 95959
(916) 265-4531

Notes on the trail: Signed intersections, a couple of landmarks, and the obvious landscape of Sardine Valley make this route fairly easy to follow. Begin your counterclockwise loop by pedaling out of Davies Campground, going right on Henness Pass Road and crossing the two wooden bridges on which you initially drove over. In a few yards, a sign at this junction indicates the left trail leads to Camp 21, Murril Valley, and Jammer Chair. Hang a left onto the dirt jeep road masquerading as a double-track. Go through a cattle gate, leaving the gate open or closed, depending on how you found it. You may be tempted to ride past the gate as the barb-wire fencing is shabby with portions laying on the ground—just be careful not to puncture your tire!

The trail begins curving to the northwest, threading through the mixed conifer forest. At 0.5 mile, you reach a fork. Take the left fork, which leads directly across Murril Creek. This is a wet crossing, though the creek is tiny and most riders can plow right through it. In a few yards, another fork appears and the right fork is signed to Murril Valley. Ignore it, staying on the left trail. You soon begin edging the forest on your right while skirting the eastern side of Sardine Valley on your left. The trail now runs basically north by northwest, and for the next several miles, it parallels a power line that crisscrosses the road overhead. Get yourself into high gear and enjoy cruising the mildly rugged terrain. The trail is virtually flat, accented with a few semi-buried rocks and boulders to keep you awake.

Bypass lesser trails that lead away from your road. Basically, you should be skirting the forest and valley simultaneously while the power line roughly parallels your road. At 1.3 miles, the power line creeps away from your road, though still visible about 50 to 100 yards on your right through the forest. A barb-wire fence begins paralleling your road on the left. Beyond the fence is the valley, spreading out down a gentle slope. Continue heading northwest and at about 2.1 miles, you cross a tiny, perhaps dry creek. Immediately after the creek, a signed trail to Jammer Chair Flat takes off on your right. Bypass it, (although adventurous riders might enjoy exploring it). The trail becomes slightly more bumpy, still paralleling the fence on your left. At 2.8 miles, you reach a fork with a signed trail that leads to Smithneck Canyon off on your right. Hang a right here and begin a gentle climb, now deeply within the forest and still heading north by northwest. Cross under a power line at about 4.2 miles and a few yards farther, another trail to Jammer Chair Flat crosses your trail. Ignore Jammer Chair and continue the easy climb, following your trail as it curves to the west. At about 4.7 miles, bear left onto an obvious, well-traveled, narrow dirt road heading west. The forest visually insulates you from the valley momentarily. Soon, a great view of the valley emerges. The ride is smooth and easy, and the fragrance of the forest makes you glad to be here.

Your road intersects Smithneck Road, CR S860, at about 5.5 miles. Make a sharp left turn onto Smithneck, a well-traveled dirt and gravel road, and head south. The terrain is smooth and hard-packed and you're likely to encounter several cars or trucks on this road. For the next 6 miles back to Davies Campground, it's the perfect road for cranking in high gear. Be alert for a cattle guard crossing at about 6.7 miles. At 8.5 miles, go through a well-signed T intersection, ignoring Henness Pass Road (CR S450) running west toward CA 49. Stay on CR S450 (which becomes eastbound Henness Pass Road) as it reaches the southern edge of the valley. The road curves left (east) and you reach a signed triangular intersection at 11.2 miles. Bear left, following the road toward Stampede Reservoir, Hope Valley, and Dog Valley and in a short distance, turn right into Davies Campground, closing the loop at 11.5 miles.

RIDE 40 · Backside Loop at Northstar

AT A GLANCE

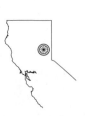

Length/configuration: 8.4-mile loop, clockwise; maintained fire roads and single-tracks

Aerobic difficulty: Easy with a few tougher short stretches

Technical difficulty: Mildly technical with a few brief intermediate sections

Scenery: Forest of mixed conifers. Views of nearby mountain ridges and Truckee River far below.

Special comments: Suitable for freewheeling children and alley cat riders (those contraptions made up of kid-sized seat, pedals and a wheel, and attaches to the back end of an adult bike). Helmets mandatory.

RIDE 40 · Backside Loop at Northstar

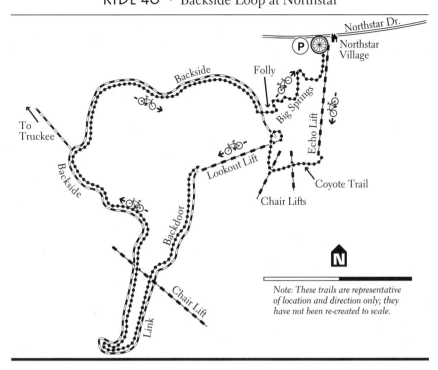

Note: These trails are representative of location and direction only; they have not been re-created to scale.

Anyone who's ever enjoyed downhill skiing at a resort knows how the whole system of chair lifts and trails generally work. The network of trails are well-marked in the field as well as on the resort's complimentary map. Lifts and trails are laid to minimize uphill exertion. In the summer, the experience at a ski resort–turned–mountain bike park is not much different although you'll need to pay attention to trails near the resort's boundaries. Without snow cover, other paths from outside the boundary that connect to a park's trail are exposed. Even with signs, it's easy to inadvertently follow a trail that leads you out of the park to somewhere you hadn't intended. Then, more than likely, you'll have to climb up a hill or ride pavement to where you should be. Having said that, make sure you pick up a complimentary map at any of the lift stations before enjoying the park. Inside the resort boundary though, it's pretty darn hard to get lost because all resort-maintained trails lead back down to the lifts or the main lodge. Emergency phones are fairly accessible at key locations, as are food joints with blaring music and civilized restrooms. Not exactly a raw and pristine outdoor experience but folks still manage to have a great time.

Of all the routes at Northstar-at-Tahoe bike park, this one is the most undeveloped in that you see fewer people and only a couple of lift lines overhead. Basically, this 8.4-mile point-to-point ride is mostly a mildly technical descent with a couple of brief, barely intermediate spots. Loose rocks scattered here and there and mostly hard-packed dirt add a bit of variety as you cruise this remote section of the bike park.

The route skirts the densely forested western edge of the bike park boundary. Peer through the forest of swaying tall pine trees and you have a view of the town of Truckee, the I-80 corridor and the Truckee River. Other than an occasional logging truck, this is the closest you come to a truly out-in-the-woods experience at Northstar. Make sure to bring a map with you as there are several trails that lead away from the park and down into Truckee. While those trails to Truckee are outstanding, aerobically challenging rides, you'll either have to ride back on pavement (ugh!) to your car at the Village or retrace your dirt path, climbing back up to the Northstar boundary. But then, that defeats the purpose of buying a lift ticket, doesn't it?

General location: Northstar-at-Tahoe Mountain Bike Park, between Truckee and the north shore of Lake Tahoe.

Elevation change: 1,350 feet gain via chair lifts, 1,350 feet loss while biking maintained trails.

Season: Weather permitting, the mountain bike park is open daily from mid-June to Labor Day, and thereafter, weekends only to about the second weekend in October, weather permitting.

Services: Northstar-at-Tahoe is practically a full-service resort. Lift ticket prices are about $16–21 for adults and $10–14 for children. (Biking the trails is free, using the lifts aren't.) Bike rentals are available from about $10–25. There's no grocery store but there is a deli/cafe, restaurant, rest rooms, and pay phones in the Village, the main access point to the bike park. Minor bike repairs can also be had at Northsport in the Village. Limited services may be offered at the Mid Mountain Day Lodge, including emergency phone and pay phone. Generally two lifts service the bike park: Echo and Lookout, and occasionally Vista Express. Lodging available on-site; for reservations, call (800) GO-NORTH (466-6784). The Tahoe Fat Tire Festival is usually held at Northstar in July. They also offer guided bike tours, dirt camps, and a BMX course for kids. Many other nonbike activities such as rope and wall climbing, horseback riding, golf, orienteering, and hiking are offered.

Hazards: Occasional logging trucks on the southwest edge of this loop.

Rescue index: Most of this loop is somewhat remote being the farthest route from the more well-used popular trails and lifts around the main and mid-mountain lodges. You might have to wait a long time before another biker or logger comes along. Emergency phones and first aid available at the top and bottom of Echo, Lookout, and Vista Express lifts, and at the Mid Mountain Day Lodge, and the Mountain Adventure Shop in the Village.

Land status: Northstar-at-Tahoe, a mountain bike park and skiing resort in Tahoe National Forest.

Maps: *Northstar-at-Tahoe Mountain Bike Park*, distributed in the Village and at each lift.

Finding the trail: Northstar-at-Tahoe is located halfway between I-80 and Kings Beach on the north side of Lake Tahoe. From I-80 in Truckee, go south on CA 267 for about 6 miles. Look for the Northstar-at-Tahoe signs and entry way and turn right (west) onto Northstar Drive and into the resort. Continue on Northstar Drive for about 2 miles to Northstar Village, the main access point to the bike park. (Incidentally, the Lodging Reservations offices are in the building located exactly at the intersection of CA 267 and Northstar Drive.)

Sources of additional information:

Northstar-at-Tahoe Resort
Highway 267 & Northstar Drive
P.O. Box 129
Truckee, CA 96160
(530) 562-2268; (530) 562-1010
Lodging: (800) GO-NORTH (466
    6784)
www.skinorthstar.com

Tahoe National Forest
Truckee Ranger District
10342 Hwy 89 North
Truckee, CA 96161
(916) 587-3558

Notes on the trail: From the Village, take Echo chair lift to its end. Trail signs welcome you at the top of the lift. Follow Coyote Trail, a 0.7-mile single-track connector trail to Lookout Lift, basically to the right as you unload from Echo. Hop onto Lookout Lift. At the top of Lookout, follow the sign to Backdoor Trail.

Backdoor Trail is an infrequently used narrow dirt road that's more like a double-track trail. After an initial short, easy climb, it basically descends as it winds through a mixed conifer forest on a remote slope of a mountain. Measuring from the top of Lookout, follow Backdoor to its junction with Sprocket at 0.5 mile. Stay right, continuing on Backdoor and at 1 mile, it runs into Link Trail, Road 701. Go left onto Link and begin a gradual climb interspersed with level stretches. To keep you awake, the trail becomes a bit more technical with semi-buried boulders and loose rocks — a fun, somewhat bumpy ride.

After cruising up and down through a small clearing, you reach the intersection of Link and Fibreboard Freeway, (Road 100), a wide dirt road. You're now at the western boundary of the bike park. If you were to follow Fibreboard (Road 100) on the soft right, you would eventually wind up in Truckee, 12.1 miles away. A left onto Fibreboard leads you toward Watson Lake and the other side of the Northstar Resort. Instead, make a hard right onto Backside Trail (Road 700) and begin gently descending. Backside Trail is not signed here. You may encounter a logging truck or two in this vicinity. Bypass other trails and dirt roads taking off from your trail. The path you want is usually signed by a mountain bike symbol. At 2.2 miles, go through a metal gate. A sign identifying Backside finally appears at 2.8 miles, at the junction with another wide trail. Stay on Backside, going straight and bearing left. Go underneath a quad chair lift at about 3 miles — an obvious clue that you're still within the bike park. Views of Truckee, the I-80 corridor and the Truckee River emerge through the trees. Continue on the main dirt road, still gradually descending.

At 4.4 miles, you reach a fork and Backside changes from Road 700 to Road 900 here. (If you were to continue following Road 700, you would reach Truckee in 6.1 miles.) Take the right fork, signed Backside, Road 900 and follow it up a gentle climb, still within view of the Truckee River area. Coming in on your right, at 6.3 miles is the bottom of Boondock Trail, a slightly more technically difficult trail. (If you're aching for tougher terrain, check out this trail out later.)

Stay on Road 900, going through a metal gate at about 6.7 miles. The trail immediately leads you through a kind of storage yard of old lift parts and maintenance parts. Fortunately, this unsightly stretch is very short and in less than 0.2 mile, intersects Folly and Shakedown Trails. Hang a left onto Folly and descend, bypassing other lesser trails. Folly becomes slightly more technical with some scattered loose rocks, ranging from baseball to basketball size. At just over 7 miles, Folly ends at Big Springs Trail.

Go left onto Big Springs. (A right here will take you to Lookout Lift.) Pass a water tank at 7.5 miles and in a few yards, the trail dumps you down onto pavement and you reach the end of the Northstar Trail System. Watch out for occasional vehicular traffic here. Continue straight on the pavement and in a few yards, unsigned Big Springs single-track trail peels off on the right, through the forest and bushes.

Hop onto the single-track and begin a moderately technical section, thanks to loose and semi-buried rocks and potholes. Enjoy a few yards of maneuvering because it quickly becomes less technical and starts a fun little up and down cruise. Go under an inoperative lift line and at 8 miles, the trail dumps you out onto pavement again, next to a small condominium complex. Continue left on the pavement toward the housing units and in a few yards, Big Springs single-track resumes, taking off on your right. Hop onto Big Springs and it soon intersects Creekside Trail, a wide, somewhat bumpy dirt road running left and right. Follow Creekside past some more condos, basically following the inoperative gondola line down to the Village. At 8.3 miles, go under Echo Lift and reach the end of the route at the Village. Make your way through the Village for a break or hop back on Echo Lift for another run.

RIDE 41 · TRT–Cinder Cone Loop

AT A GLANCE

Length/configuration: 11.9-mile loop, counterclockwise; jeep roads and single-tracks

Aerobic difficulty: Moderately strenuous due to long stretches of rugged terrain and elevation gain

Technical difficulty: Intermediate overall. The first 5.5 miles is mildly technical, smooth trails and dirt roads; the rest is mostly intermediate with an intensely advanced section over steep and loose trail conditions.

Scenery: No great views of Lake Tahoe, but then, spending a few hours in the woods and riding the Tahoe Rim Trail, a premier single-track, makes it a worthy ride.

Special comments: Strong beginners can ride the first 5.5 miles as an out-and-back. Easier trails can be found in Burton Creek State Park, also accessible from this parking area. Also referred to as the Rim Trail and the TRT, portions of the 150-mile Tahoe Rim Trail are off-limits to bikes. Sections described in this ride permit bikes. Please obey all posted signs.

This 11.9-mile loop saves the toughest section for the end and it's guaranteed to test your mettle. The loop is best ridden counterclockwise, which means you tackle the thrilling and toughest section going downhill. About a third of the ride is on dirt road; the rest is single-track. The first 6.3 miles is a mix of mildly and intermediately technical terrain, cruising on single-track and dirt roads, including the Tahoe Rim Trail (TRT). After that, the next mile becomes more technically challenging thanks to rocky terrain. Near the end, a half-mile section of easy riding offers respite and then POW! The seriously advanced section hits, dropping about

RIDE 41 · TRT–Cinder Cone Loop

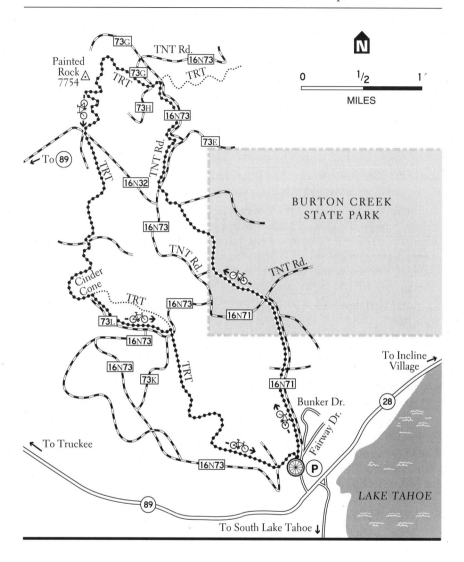

1,000 feet in less than 4 miles via rocky and loose dirt terrain. Most riders can enjoy the first 6.3 miles because a bail-out option exists. In fact, the area is a network of jeep roads and single-tracks, and less challenging configurations can be enjoyed. A portion near the beginning of the loop runs into Burton Creek State Park, giving you access to easier trails on which bikes are allowed.

A geological wonder on this loop is a short section referred to as Cinder Cone, the result of volcanic action eons ago. Here, the Tahoe Rim Trail is peppered with schist, a shale-like rock that produces a unique musical crunch underneath your wheels, like the sound of breaking glass. Schist is a rock with different minerals that easily split into thin layers. Less musical but still interesting is the feldspar covering another short section of the TRT near Cinder Cone. It's a kind of white lava-rock that has undergone metamorphosis, combining white minerals into a grey substructure. See, you can learn a bit of geology while enjoying the ride.

General location: North shore of Lake Tahoe, beginning in Tahoe City.

Elevation change: 1,330 feet; starting elevation and low point 6,320 feet; high point 7,650 feet. Easy climbs interspersed with flat stretches, followed by a rugged, technically steep downhill section.

Season: Late spring to mid-autumn.

Services: Rest room and water is available at the trailhead in the Fairway Community Center, generally open throughout most of the day and into the early evening. There are no services on the route. All services available in Tahoe City and Truckee.

Hazards: Watch out for oncoming hikers and bikers on the single-tracks. Dirt roads see very little vehicular traffic but stay alert just in case.

Rescue index: This area is a maze of trails and jeep roads. Portions of the route follow the popular TNT Road (Tahoe-to-Truckee bike route), which is well-traveled during the weekends. Chances are fair that you meet another trail user who may be of help during an emergency. Otherwise, you should make your way back to the trailhead where you can find help at the Fairway Community Center and surrounding residential neighborhood.

Land status: Tahoe National Forest, Lake Tahoe Basin Management, Burton Creek State Park.

Maps: *Burton Creek–Lake Tahoe Area Recreation Map*, published by Solstice Adventures, (916) 582-1836. (Its depiction of the Tahoe Rim Trail is slightly inaccurate. Nevertheless, the map is still very useful.) *Recreation Map of Lake Tahoe*, published by Tom Harrison Maps, 2 Falmouth Cove, San Rafael, CA 94901, (800) 265-9090, www.tomharrisonmaps.com. (Not all trails and jeep roads which appear on the map are labeled. Nevertheless, the map is still very useful.) USGS Tahoe City 7.5 minute series.

Finding the trail: From CA 28 in Tahoe City, go north on Fairway Drive for less than 0.25 mile to the Fairway Community Center. Park here, across the road from the Tahoe Rim Trail trailhead.

Sources of additional information:

Tahoe National Forest
631 Coyote Street
P.O. Box 6003
Nevada City, CA 95959
(916) 265-4531

U.S. Forest Service
Lake Tahoe Basin Management Unit
870 Emerald Bay Rd.

South Lake Tahoe, CA 96150
(916) 573-2600

Tahoe Rim Trail Association
P.O. Box 4647
Stateline, Nevada 89449
(775) 588-0686
TahoeRim@aol.com
www.tahoerimtrail.org

Notes on the trail: The first half of this counterclockwise loop goes up a dirt road to the Tahoe Rim Trail (TRT). The loop ends here, coming out on the TRT. Facing the TRT trailhead across from the Fairway Community Center, begin your adven-

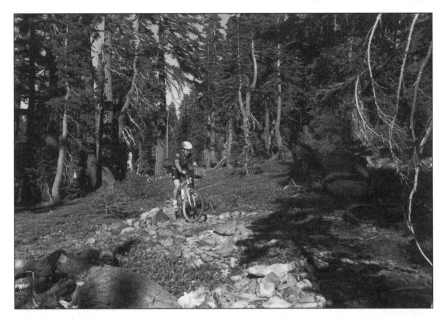

Here, Bruce rides over some schist, shale-like rock which sounds like breaking glass when crushed.

ture by pedaling right (north) on Fairway Drive, away from CA 28 and Lake Tahoe. In a few yards, Bunker Drive, another paved residential street, peels off of Fairway on your left. Follow Bunker up a gradual hill and in a few more yards, veer left toward the "Fire Protection" dirt road next to a home at 836 Bunker Drive. Leaving the pavement, the rough jeep road begins climbing through a quiet forest of conifers and deciduous trees. The trail and grade varies from hard-packed and loose dirt, and gentle to steep, interspersed with welcomed, brief level stretches.

A mile into the ride, bypass a trail leading off on your right and a few yards farther, you see a trail marker indicating that the trail you're riding is 16N71 (although several of the numbers were beginning to peel off when I last saw it). Cross into state park boundary, as indicated by a sign. A bit farther and another sign, planted next to a dirt road, states that you're in Burton Creek State Park. Stay on 16N71 and continue the gradual climb. At 1.5 miles, a short stretch becomes slightly more technically challenging due to semi-buried rocks and boulders in the trail. Once through this rocky section, you reach a sort of four-way intersection with a dirt road running both soft left and hard right, and a single-track going straight, (actually, a very soft right). (This unsigned dirt road is the TNT Road, short for Tahoe-to-Truckee—a dirt road that dumps you into Truckee. It's a popular out-and-back or point-to-point, depending on the endurance of the rider.) Follow the single-track and in about 2 miles, you reach a fork with a wide single-track peeling off on your left. There's a sign in the opposite direction stating "No Motor Vehicles." Stay right on your single-track trail which is really an overgrown double-track. At this point, you leave the state park and cross back into national forest land. The forest opens into a small, bushy clearing. The trail is mildly technical, fairly level, and occasional boulders and rocks make the riding fast and fun. (If you turn left onto the dirt TNT road back at that four-way intersection, you'll pedal about 2 miles before rejoining the described route. I recommend staying on the single-track though—the riding is more fun than the wide, dirt road.)

At 2.8 miles, go past a trail coming in on your right, staying left on the single-track. Go through a small meadow and cross a tiny creek (which may be dry, depending on the time of year). Your trail intersects the unsigned wide, TNT Road again at about 2.9 miles. The road is a combination of dirt and gravel, and is basically smooth riding, especially if it has been graded recently. Hang a right onto the TNT Road and begin a moderate climb.

At almost 3.5 miles, you reach a junction with another road leading off on the right, signed 73E. Still climbing toward the ridge, keep an eye peeled for the Tahoe Rim Trail crossing the dirt road you're on. It's a narrow single-track indicated by a single wooden post decorated with the small TRT crest symbol. You reach the TRT at about 4.2 miles. (If you reach a junction with a left-hand road signed 16G, you've gone too far. Backtrack about 0.2 mile to the TRT.) Hang a left onto the TRT, heading basically west. From this point, the route becomes more technically challenging and anyone who's not comfortable with their technical skills may want to turn around here. Attitude is everything! Strong beginners with the right frame of mind may enjoy the first several miles of the TRT to mile 6.3, at which point there is a bail-out option.

Follow the TRT as it gradually climbs and in less than 0.5 miles, you reach the top of the ridge at approximately 7,650 feet. The trail is mildly technical with loose dirt and a few boulders. (If you have time, leave your bike on the trail and explore Painted Rock by hiking up its peak at 7,754 feet.) Cruise along the top of the ridge here, curving south, and at about 5.4 miles, you catch a glimpse of Lake Tahoe through the trees. From here the single-track TRT begins a fun, easy descent, becoming slightly more technical with semi-buried boulders, exposed tree roots, and abrupt dips. At 6.3 miles, the trail intersects an unsigned jeep road. (This is the bail-out option. According to the map published by Solstice Adventures, this road is 16N32. Hang a left here and in about 0.8 mile, it will intersect the TNT Road just south of where you originally joined it back at 2.9 miles. Riders who take this option can then retrace their path back to their car at the Fairway Community Center.) Advanced riders up for the challenge, go left onto the dirt road and in a few yards, hang a right onto the TRT, heading south. The trail begins to climb, becoming steeper and rockier, and depending on your skill level, you may have to dismount and walk in a few places. You're now heading into a geologic area greatly influenced by volcanic action eons ago. Covering the trail are small chunks of feldspar, a kind of white lava-rock. As you continue on, you catch a glimpse of Lake Tahoe and the trail becomes even more challenging with huge boulders.

At 7.3 miles, the TRT intersects a jeep road. Go right onto the road and in a few yards, the TRT peels off on the left. Follow the TRT and the trail leads you to the top of the saddle through a grassy clearing toward the Cinder Cone, another result of ancient volcanic action. Soon, your tires begin rolling over schist strewn on the trail, producing an distinctive sound like breaking glass. It's an interesting but short stretch, less than 0.5 mile. The trail remains rocky and technically challenging as it meanders through the woods.

At about 8.6 miles, the TRT intersects jeep road 73L (it's unsigned here but in less than a mile, you find a sign identifying it as such). Expert riders who love tackling humongous boulder fields may enjoy staying on the TRT for this stretch. We attempted this stretch but aborted our efforts since we lost the trail among the boulders and ended up portaging our bikes. So, hang a right here, leaving the TRT for the time being. Follow the dirt road and at almost 9 miles, you reached an intersection with another unsigned jeep road, which according to the Solstice map, is probably 16N73. The road which you've been riding, however, is signed here as 73L. Stay on the road you've been following and in about 0.2 mile, at 9.2 miles from the Community Center, intersect another jeep road on your right, signed 73K. A few yards straight ahead is the TRT crossing your road.

Go right onto the TRT, and begin the final stretch back to your car. Hang on. Here comes that intensely technical section. Your tire crunches over more schist. The trail narrows, bounded on both sides by tall bushes, and begins descending over increasingly steeper and intensely rocky terrain. Maintaining traction is more challenging due to sections of loose dirt and steepness. Fortunately, walking is an option. At 11.3 miles, the TRT intersects a rugged unsigned jeep road, running both left and right. According to the map, this is 16N73. Bypass this road, staying on the TRT, still plunging downward. At 11.9 miles, you close the loop and the TRT literally dumps you out onto Fairway Drive, across from the Community Center, next to your parked car. Congratulate yourself for having made it down this last stretch of the TRT, even if you walked parts of it.

SKI RESORTS BECOME MOUNTAIN BIKE PARKS IN THE SUMMER

An economical and logical trend for the past 6-plus years is ski resorts becoming mountain bike parks in the summer. And no where else but in the Lake Tahoe region will you find the biggest concentration of such chameleon resorts. Purists may call riding at a maintained park not real mountain biking but there's no denying the popularity of the concept. Summer attendance at Mammoth Mountain Bike Park has now outpaced skiers in the winter and that translates to more year-round employment and a happy community. Besides, why let precious land sit unappreciated in the summer? The operating season for the parks are typically June through Labor Day, and then on weekends to the end of September, depending on weather conditions. So, if biking in tame environments is your cup of tea, then check out these other Ski/Bike resorts.

EAGLE MOUNTAIN CROSS-COUNTRY SKI AREA AND MOUNTAIN BIKE PARK: A cross-country ski area in the winter, Eagle Mountain offers over 31 miles of marked roads, and that's not counting the myriad of single-track trails available. Not serviced by lifts, more serious riders looking for a great day of exertion on the trail and equally great amenities off the trail, will enjoy this park. Aerobic and technical challenges ranging from easy to very strenuous, and nontechnical to expert, respectively, are offered. Elevation ranging from 5,800 to 6,600 feet, which is considerably lower than the other Tahoe resorts, means the riding season is slightly longer.

General location: Just on the south side of I-80, halfway between Auburn and Truckee. Take the Yuba Gap exit off I-80 and head south.

Services: Trail pass costs range from about $8–15. Amenities include a day lodge with snacks and gourmet food service, bike rental, showers, rest rooms, and tent cabins. Fun events are offered, including moonlight dinner rides, mountain bike snow races in the winter, riding instruction classes, guided tours, children's obstacle course, and climbing wall. If you're interested in biking classes, other activities can be combined, such as kayaking and climbing. Wearing a helmet is mandatory.

For additional information: Call (800) 391-2254 or (530) 389-8033 or visit www. eaglemtnresort.com

DONNER SKI RANCH MOUNTAIN BIKE PARK: Not a huge park, Donner's 30-plus miles of trails include single-tracks serviced by one chair lift. Routes for riders of all abilities are offered. One of its more popular events is the annual Rage'n at the Ranch, a NORBA-sanctioned race series.

General location: Almost 11 miles west of Truckee, just on the south side of I-80. Take the Soda Springs/Norden exit (the same exit as the end-shuttle location for the Hole-In-The-Ground Ride).

Services: Lift price ranges from $4–8. Amenities include food and drink services, rest rooms, bike rentals, and cycling clinics. Helmet mandatory.

For additional information: 19320 Donner Pass Road, Norden, CA 95724; (530) 426-3635

SQUAW VALLEY BIKE PARK: Most of the dirt roads and single-tracks that form the network of trails throughout Squaw Valley will delight strong riders with technical skills ranging from intermediate to advanced. Few routes are suited for beginners. The terrain is generally rocky and without tree cover. The elevation ranges from 6,200 to 8,200 feet, which means long or short runs can be had—especially thrilling for those of you who like intense vertical drops.

General location: Northwest of Lake Tahoe, between Truckee and Tahoe City, on the west side of CA 89.

Services: Only one cable car services the entire park and its cost ranges from $20–28. Amenities include food services, bike rentals, rest rooms, lodging, and a sport shop offering clothing and accessories.

For additional information: P.O. Box 2007, Olympic Valley, CA 96146; (800) 545-4350; (530) 583-5585; www.squaw.com

KIRKWOOD RESORT: Kirkwood is the highest of all the resorts in the Tahoe area, sitting atop Carson Pass at 9,000-plus feet. The views are exceptionally spectacular here, with it fields of wildflowers and distant volcanic landscape. Technically, its network of dirt roads and single-tracks are mostly intermediately rated, about 55%. Of the rest, 25% are rated mild (perfect for beginners) and 20% advanced/expert.

General location: Basically south of Lake Tahoe, near the intersection of CA 89 and CA 88.

Services: Two lifts service the park and cost about $15 for adults and $8 for children. To access the trails without the lift service, the fee is about $4. Season individual and family passes are offered as well as groups rates. Amenities include many food service establishments, a grocery store, bike rentals, sport clothing and accessories shop, and lodging. A variety of activities such as bike lessons and races, guided tours, horseback riding, a climbing wall, rock climbing, and tennis are also offered.

For additional information: P.O. Box 1, Kirkwood, CA 95646; (209) 258-7283; (209) 258-6000; (209) 258-3000

NORTH TAHOE REGIONAL PARK: This park is not like the other resorts listed here. It's just a small local park with a smattering of nice trails, managed by the North Tahoe Public Utility District. But don't let the smallness or manager fool you. You can expand your ride by connecting to any number of dirt roads that lead into Northstar-at-Tahoe, bikes-allowed portions of the Tahoe Rim Trail, even the Truckee-To-Tahoe Ride. But, in this park alone, the terrain is suitable for riders of all abilities, from easy to strenuous aerobically, and mild to advanced technically. There's even a mile-long paved easy trail.

General location: On the north shore of Lake Tahoe, on the northern edge of the town of Tahoe Vista, near the intersection of CA 28 and CA 267.

Services: Using the park is free but parking is about $2 per car. There are no resort-style services here. But you will find water, rest rooms, a mountain bike race track, softball field, a playground, and picnic areas. Limited services found in Tahoe Vista and Kings Beach. Complete services available in Tahoe City and Truckee.

For additional information: (530) 546-5043

MAMMOTH MOUNTAIN BIKE PARK

For additional information: P.O. Box 24, Mammoth Lakes, CA 93546; (888) 4-MAMMOTH; (619) 934-2581. (See the trail descriptions in the next chapter.)

RIDE 42 · TRT–WST–Paige Meadows Point-to-Point

AT A GLANCE

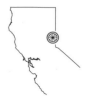

Length/configuration: 31.9- to 33.7-mile point-to-point, (depending on where you park your end-shuttle car); fire roads, single- and double-tracks, and paved bike path

Aerobic difficulty: Very strenuous due to distance and some climbing

Technical difficulty: Intermediate to advanced; occasional spots of very rugged terrain

Scenery: Thick forests on ancient volcanic terrain; open meadows; postcard views of Lake Tahoe; awesome views of Squaw Valley, the Truckee River canyon, and peaks in distant Granite Chief Wilderness

RIDE 42 · TRT–WST–Paige Meadows Point-to-Point

Special comments: Available are several bail-out options which shorten the ride considerably. Arranging two shuttle vehicles required. Shuttle services conveniently offered by CyclePaths for a nominal fee. Also referred to as the Rim Trail and the TRT, portions of the 150-mile Tahoe Rim Trail are off-limits to bikes. Sections described in this ride and elsewhere in this chapter permit bikes. Please obey all posted signs.

Seekers of epic rides . . . check this one out! This route makes use of a recently opened (1998) portion of the fabulous Tahoe Rim Trail west of Brockway Summit on the northwest shore of Lake Tahoe. Greg Forsyth, owner of CyclePaths

Mountain Bike Adventures was instrumental in helping me put this ride on paper. As one of the first guided mountain bike touring companies, he and his staff scouted the trails, piecing together this route to create a challenging, advance-level 33.7-mile point-to-point ride. How to arrange a shuttle car if you and your buddies have only one car among you? Not a problem. You, your buddies, bikes, and gear can catch a lift to the trailhead from CyclePaths for a nominal fee.

Not sure if this ride is worth the hassle of setting up a shuttle? Trust me. It's worth the effort and the bucks. Consider this: You'll begin this ride at 7,200 feet near Brockway Summit on the Tahoe Rim Trail and head west towards Watson Lake and Painted Rock—the high point of the ride. This section is a combination of mostly awesome single-track and some dirt roads, weaving through thick forests, down slopes, and on ridges for 15 miles before its junction with the Western States Trail (WST). Six-acre Watson Lake is unique in that it is the only lake in the Sierras around Lake Tahoe that lies entirely on volcanic bedrock. All other lakes in this area sit on either granite or metamorphic bedrock, having been formed by the scooping action of glaciers. In the spring, wildflowers line the banks of the Watson Lake and it's a lovely spot to take a short break. And immediately before you reach the WST, you get to test your bike handling skills on "The Wall," an incredibly steep and rugged descent of about a quarter of a mile on 13%-plus grade. (Just be glad you don't have to ride up it.) WST then drops down to CA 89 via a series of hairpin turns on single-track, losing 720 feet in less than a mile. Whew! Then, you get a bit of a reprieve as you ride the paved bike path for a short spin before tackling 14.7 miles more of dirt roads and single-track in the vicinity of Alpine Meadows and Paige Meadows. The dirt portion of the route basically ends near Granlibakken ski area, just south of Tahoe City, where you can leave your end-shuttle car. If you leave your car at CyclePaths, then the last 1.8 miles of your epic journey leisurely follows the West Shore Bike Path, leading past several tempting watering holes. By this point, you should just give in to the temptation—you will have earned it!

General location: Northwest shore of Lake Tahoe.

Elevation change: 1,400 feet; starting elevation 7,200 feet; high point 7,700 feet; low point 6,200 feet to 6,300 feet (depending on where you leave your end-shuttle car). The route generally descends but there are numerous ups and downs along the way.

Season: June through October, or until the first snow falls.

Services: Many eateries, watering holes, small food stores, lodging, phones, rest rooms (please patronize the merchant), and gas stations located along the West Shore Bike Path between Tahoe City and CyclePaths bike shop as well as around the Y (CA 89 and CA 28 intersection) in Tahoe City. CyclePaths is a well-equipped, full-service bike shop and mountain bike tour operator. They also offer shuttle services to many of the areas trailheads, including this epic ride. The Fire Sign Café, next door to the bike shop, offers outstanding breakfast and lunch. Campgrounds available along the western shore of Lake Tahoe. All other services in Tahoe City and Truckee.

Hazards: Be aware that the narrow single-track portions of this route are open to bikers and hikers going in either direction. When riding all bike paths, stay alert for vehicles crossing the paved trail. The bike path is a multi-use trail so expect to share the path with other bikers, pedestrians, joggers, and skaters. Please respect private property by staying on roads, especially when riding through residential areas. Be alert for occasionally seen mountain lions and bears.

Rescue index: Some—but not all—portions of this route are well traveled. If you ride during the weekday, you may not encounter any other trail users. For that reason, you need be self-reliant. Instead of waiting for help during an emergency, you should make your way down to a main highway where you can either flag down a passing motorist or find a phone at many roadside businesses. Fibreboard Freeway, a dirt road (Forest Service 16N73), closely parallels the first 12 miles of the TRT and at 11.1 miles, near Painted Rock, it offers a fast and easy shortcut into Tahoe City.

Land status: Tahoe National Forest and some private property with public access roads.

Maps: Though several recreational maps of Lake Tahoe including USGS topographical maps are available, none show the trails and roads of this route accurately or completely. As of the end of 1999, the only map that displayed the entire route was the one custom-made by CyclePaths and it's available for a pittance at their store or from their Web site.

Finding the trail: The trailhead is near Brockway Summit, just on the west side of CA 267. To set up your two-car shuttle, park your end vehicle in Tahoe City in the small dirt parking area along the west side of CA 89 about 0.2 mile south of the Y (CA 89 and CA 28 intersection). To reach the starting point of the ride, leave this parking area by driving north on CA 89 and immediately go right onto CA 28. Follow CA 28 for about 9.5 miles and then turn left onto CA 267. Now driving north with the lake behind you, go about 3 miles towards Brockway Summit. Keep your eyes peeled to your left for a sign identifying the paved beginning of Fibreboard Freeway (FS 16N73—it becomes chipped gravel and then dirt about 3 miles in). The Tahoe Rim Trail (signed by tiny TRT blue crest markers) crosses Fibreboard in several places. Turn onto Fibreboard heading west and immediately bypass the first TRT crossing within a few yards from CA 267. Continue for just over a mile more—about 2 miles total from CA 267—to the next TRT junction. Park here, pulling well off the road, and begin pedaling.

Sources of additional information:

Tahoe National Forest
Truckee Ranger District
10342 Hwy 89 North
Truckee, CA 96161
(530) 587-3558

Tahoe Rim Trail Association
P.O. Box 4647
Stateline, Nevada 89449
(775) 588-0686
TahoeRim@aol.com

CyclePaths Mountain Bike
  Adventures
1785 Westlake Blvd.
P.O. Box 887
Tahoe City, CA 96145
(800) 780-BIKE or (530) 581-1171
www.cyclepaths.com

Notes on the trail: Begin your epic ride by hopping on the Tahoe Rim Trail on the south side of the road (Lake Tahoe side) and head west by southwest. The single-track begins with a gradual descent, mixed with a few short boulder drops. For the first 3 to 4 miles, expect a slew of twists and turns in the TRT as it leads you down the Watson Creek drainage. The forest is thick through this section and open views of Lake Tahoe, an obvious landmark from which to orient yourself, don't exist. Keep following the TRT and at 2.8 miles from the starting point, go across a dirt road. Continue on the TRT as it climbs steadily back up the ridge. Cross another dirt road at 4.1 miles and cruise through a meadow. To the right off in the near distance is the dirt road Fibreboard Freeway (FS 16N73), closely paralleling your trail. When the trail splits at 5.8 miles, stay right (the left dead ends at Fibreboard in less than a mile). Watch for a TRT marker on the left. Bear left and at about 5.9 miles, you reach Watson Lake. Stay on the TRT, veering left twice and almost immediately, at 6.1 miles, look for the TRT, now a narrow single-track, splitting off on the left. Just after this left curve, you should pass a "No Motor Vehicles" and a TRT marker. This is an easy turn to miss so keep a your eyes peeled!

Still following the TRT, you soon reach a four-way intersection with other single-tracks at 6.3 miles; continue straight. Take a peek through the trees on your left and you'll have a filtered view of Lake Tahoe. Don't fret for in a short distance, past large boulders on your right, great postcard views of the lake emerge around 6.7 miles. In 0.3 mile farther, the TRT runs through "The Rockgarden" for several hundred yards and you might want to walk your bike. The trail's technical nature soon mellows out, regaining its sweet, rideable character again.

Continue following the TRT and at 8.6 miles, veer right and begin an uphill push. In just 0.1 mile further, just after you pass through two, low, wooden pillars that mark your single-track, immediately turn right onto a dirt road. Follow the road and at 10.3 miles, watch for a sharp left turn onto the single-track TRT again, identified by both TRT and American Discovery Trail markers. Now back on the TRT, your trail crosses Fibreboard Freeway (FS 16N73) at 11.1 miles. Bail-out Option #1: Ride too difficult or running out of time? Hang a left onto Fibreboard, a dirt road, and follow it all the way down into Tahoe City, a distance of about 6.5 miles.] Assuming you skip the bail-out option, continue following the TRT and begin a steady climb up to Painted Rock. There, you have awesome views of Squaw Valley and the Truckee River canyon.

Enjoy the next 2 miles cruising over the volcanic terrain which the TRT traverses. After that, get ready to lose some elevation like there's no tomorrow. When you hit 13 miles, turn left at a junction with a jeep road and say good-bye to the TRT. Now on the dirt road, go through a green gate and begin heading down "The Wall." As its name implies, it's extremely steep. Walk or let 'er rip for the next half-mile down but don't blow straight through an intersection at 13.6 miles. Here, instead of going straight, turn left. The trail's steepness mellows slightly. At 13.9 miles, bear right at a Y intersection and continue descending. Enjoy your downhill run but at 14.7 miles, keep an eye out for a small, brown sign marking a single-track trail on your right. It's the Western States Trail (WST) and at this point, make a sharp right turn onto it and continue descending. For the next 0.3 mile, the WST leads you through small creeks. After you go across a creek on a series of wooden planks at 15 miles, get ready: Another thrillingly steep downhill section begins. This time, a series of hairpin turns help you negotiate the descent. Still, exercise caution. At 15.3 miles, continue straight through a four-way intersection with a fire road, staying on the WST. A short distance further at 15.6 miles, veer right at a Y intersection and go underneath the CA 89 bridge. You survived the drop!

Now on the west side of CA 89, hop on the Truckee River Bike Path and head upriver (south) to Alpine Meadows Road which you reach at 16.4 miles. [Bail-Out Option #2: Stay on the bike path and follow it 3 miles into Tahoe City. Carefully make your way through the Y intersection and turn right to continue on the bike path along CA 89 back to where your car is parked, either 0.2 mile south in the dirt pulloff or almost 2 miles further at CyclePaths.] Assuming you skip this bail-out, turn right onto Alpine Meadows Road and begin a gradual climb up the paved vehicle road towards the Alpine Meadows ski area. After a quick 0.1 mile, hang a left onto Snow Crest Road, another paved road. Continue straight on Snow Crest, pass the condos, and at 17.2 miles, bear left onto a dirt road with a green gate. A few yards farther, at a **T** intersection, continue going uphill on a single-track. The trail gives you a short breather as it levels out at 18 miles. Enjoy it while you can because before you know it, at 18.3 miles, a steep climb begins. At this point, bear right to continue on the main trail and bypass the north end of Drunken Bear Trail, a narrow single-track which peels off on the left. A short distance further, at 19.9 miles, your trail crests at a fork with another trail on the right which leads uphill to Scott Peak and the ski lifts of Alpine Meadows; stay straight bearing left.

You're now approaching the Paige Meadows area, the site of many popular and moderate bike trails. (See the next ride description for more riding options.) At 20.6 miles, veer left at a **Y** intersection and follow the single-track trail through two, short, wooden posts. Stay straight on the main trail, ignoring narrow single-tracks on the right. (Those trails lead into a soggy portion of the Meadows and since this is ecologically sensitive area, please stay out!) You reach another **Y** intersection at 21.8 miles; stay left. A few yards further, the narrow trail coming in on your left is the south end of Drunken Bear Trail; bypass it. In another 8.1 miles, at 30 miles, cross a swale and climb a brief hill. Almost immediately at 30.1 miles, turn left at a **T** intersection and then continue straight along the main trail as it descends. Bypass trails leading off on your right (they lead into a residential subdivision). At 31.3 miles, veer right at a **Y** intersection and stay on the main trail. Finally, at 31.9 miles, watch out for a green gate. Go around the gate by bearing right and continue to follow the dirt and gravel road about 100 feet to where paved Rawhide Drive begins at its intersection with Bonanza Drive. Now within a residential neighborhood, continue straight on Rawhide for a few blocks and then right onto Granlibakken Road. Go three blocks to the paved bike path. If your car is parked at the dirt pulloff near the **Y** (CA 89 and CA 28 intersection), turn left onto the bike path and pedal about 0.2 mile back to your end-shuttle car. If your car is at CyclePaths, go right and follow the bike path for 1.8 miles.

RIDE 43 · Paige Meadows Ride

AT A GLANCE

Length/configuration: 12-mile double loop (small counterclockwise loop inside a bigger clockwise loop); paved and dirt roads, single- and double-tracks, and paved bike path. Several options to shorten the route available.

Aerobic difficulty: Easy to moderate; some easy climbing

Technical difficulty: Mild; single-tracks with a few rugged sections

Scenery: Peaks in the Granite Chief Wilderness; conifer forests; riding the bike path along the edge of Lake Tahoe. Display of a wide variety of wildflowers in the meadows during the spring is outstanding.

RIDE 43 · Paige Meadows Ride

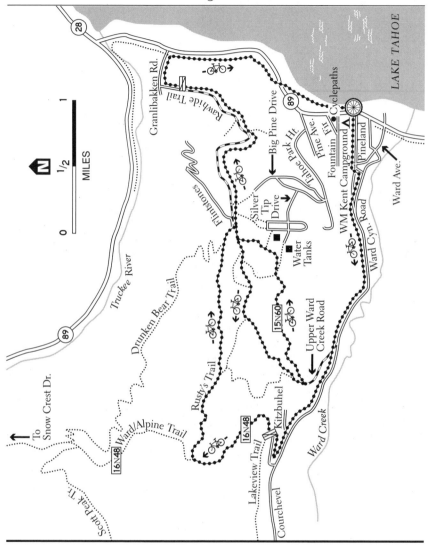

Special comments: Can also be ridden as a single, short loop, or a point-to-point requiring a shuttle car. Shuttle services are conveniently offered by CyclePaths. Advanced riders can access Drunken Bear Trail for a much longer loop ride.

If you're a strong beginner seeking more thrilling rides than the nearby paved bike path, you'll be glad to know you can find mild to intermediate technical single-track trails in the popular Paige Meadows area. The Meadows is actually a group of several open fields nestled on the top of a hill. Getting there entails some moderate climbing but beginners with good endurance are likely to find this suggested route worthy of their efforts. Even though these trails link to a wide-ranging network of outstanding trails, Paige Meadows by itself is a favorite area among riders of all abilities statewide, thanks to miles of sweet single-tracks that run through thick evergreen forests and open meadows. Stronger and more technically skilled riders can access several other trails that connect to this ride and create a much longer, more technically challenging adventure. The configuration of the loop described below clocks in at almost 12 miles, using about 3.5 miles of paved roads, 6.5 miles single- and double-tracks, and 2 miles on the paved West Shore Bike Path. The climbs are easy to moderate, ascending a respectable 1,000 feet to the high point of about 7,240 feet. The views of the peaks in nearby Granite Chief Wilderness from the open meadows are gloriously breathtaking and in late spring, the meadows are adorned with a wide variety of wildflowers. For those of you who are low on stamina or unaccustomed to the higher altitude, you can enjoy this area as a point-to-point ride with a two-car shuttle arrangement. This option shortens the ride by eliminating 3 miles of moderate climbing up Ward Canyon Road, a well-traveled, paved residential road.

Years ago, jeep-driving yahoos made Paige Meadows a favorite playground, crisscrossing the meadows and leaving a mess of tracks behind. Today, the roar and the stench of the gas-guzzling shedders are replaced by mountain bikers and hikers. So, when you're pedaling here, don't be surprised to find some trails not depicted on maps. If you're unsure of your trail-finding skills, not to worry. You're never too far from civilization. You won't be grinding up anything terrifically steep, long, and rugged (if you do, you're way off the route). Generally, when in doubt, follow the more well-traveled trail. Lesser trails may lead into marshy areas. Please obey all posted trail closures and stay on the trail. Don't bushwhack through the ecologically sensitive terrain and avoid riding when trails are muddy.

Want to ride Paige Meadows as a point-to-point but only have one car between you and your riding buddies? Not a problem. CyclePaths Mountain Bike Adventures, a full-service bike shop offers more than mountain bike hard- and soft-goods—they run a convenient, reasonably priced shuttle service to many trailheads around Lake Tahoe, including this one. CyclePaths is one of the first mountain bike touring companies in the region. They offer a delectable menu of guided and self-guided tours for riders of all abilities. From their economical "Blue Plate Special" (ride your own bike, schlep your own gear, and just follow the CyclePaths trail guide) to "The Whole Enchilada" (a demo bike, van support, and great food, in addition to a trail guide). Located just north of the intersection of CA 89 and Ward Canyon Road, you'll either drive or pedal past them, or park there for this ride. Sincere thanks to Greg Forsyth, owner of CyclePaths for his trail notes on Paige Meadows, an area he considers his "backyard." He and his staff often sponsor trail maintenance days and work with the Forest Service in protecting and promoting the wise use of the surrounding natural resources which are key to making Lake Tahoe one of the crown jewels of California.

General location: Northwest shore of Lake Tahoe.

Elevation change: 1,000 feet; starting elevation and low point 6,240 feet; high point 7,240 feet. Most of the climbing is on Ward Canyon Road; thereafter, some ups and downs through the meadows, followed by a long, gradual descent into Tahoe City.

Season: June through October, or until the first snow falls.

Services: Located at the starting point of this ride is CyclePaths, a well-equipped, full-service bike shop which also offers shuttle service and an array of guided mountain bike tours. Many eateries, watering holes, small food stores, lodging, phones, rest rooms (please patronize the merchant), and gas stations are located along CA 89 between Tahoe City and CyclePaths. The Fire Sign Café, located next door to the bike shop, offers outstanding breakfast and lunch. William Kent Campground, less than a half mile further south on CA 89, has water and rest rooms, and if you're planning to ride for several days, makes a splendid base camp. All other services in Tahoe City and Truckee.

Hazards: Watch out for motorists as you ride up well-traveled Ward Canyon Road which serves the residential subdivision near the dirt trailhead. When riding West Shore Bike Path along CA 89, stay alert for vehicles crossing the paved trail. The bike path is a multi-use trail so expect to share the path with other bikers, pedestrians, joggers, and skaters. Please respect private property by staying on roads, especially when riding through residential areas. Be alert for occasionally seen mountain lions and bears.

Rescue index: During the popular summer months, you're likely to meet other persons on the trails who may be of help. Other times of the year, you may not see a soul, in which case, be prepared to make your way down to the bike path in order to phone for help. The south and southeast edge of Paige Meadows borders several residential subdivisions, so you're never too far from civilization.

Land status: Tahoe National Forest and some private property with public access roads.

Maps: Several maps of the area are available in a few local bike shops. Note however, that Paige Meadows is an area crisscrossed by many minor trails and dirt roads, and some trails may be closed to allow certain areas to recover from overuse. For that reason, maps you find of the area may not be current, accurate, or show all trails and roads. CyclePaths has a custom map and it's available for a pittance.

Finding the trail: From Truckee, drive south on CA 89 to Tahoe City. When you reach the Y in Tahoe City (intersection of CA 89 and CA 28), go right/south on CA 89 (Westlake Boulevard) for about 2 miles. On your right, watch for CyclePaths (1785 Westlake Blvd.), just after Fir Street and before William Kent Campground and Pineland Drive. Park in this vicinity and begin pedaling from here. You can also park and begin from the campground too.

Sources of additional information:

Tahoe National Forest
Truckee Ranger District
10342 Hwy 89 North
Truckee, CA 96161
(530) 587-3558

William Kent Campground
(On CA 89 just south of CyclePaths)
(530) 573-2600 or (530) 544-5994

CyclePaths Mountain Bike
   Adventures
1785 Westlake Blvd.
P.O. Box 887
Tahoe City, CA 96145
(800) 780-BIKE or (530) 581-1171
www.cyclepaths.com

Notes on the trail: From CyclePaths (or the William Kent Campground), pedal south on the bike path for less than a half mile to Pineland Drive. Watch for a two-post wooden sign declaring "Pineland." Go right onto Pineland. Proceed west for a short distance, about 0.4 mile, and then turn left onto Twin Peaks Road, following the sign to Ward Valley. Twin Peaks soon runs into Ward Canyon Road, also called Ward

Creek Boulevard and farther west, becomes Courchevel Road. Go right on Ward Canyon Road, gradually climbing away from Lake Tahoe. Continue past Upper Ward Creek Road (a dirt road on your right) and later past Kitzbuhel Road. You're in a residential subdivision now and Ward Canyon Road becomes Courchevel Road. Almost 3 miles from CyclePaths, turn right onto Chamonix Road and begin riding uphill, due northeast to the end of the pavement and a gate.

Get ready—here comes the dirt! And don't expect to see any trail-markers because the trails are basically unsigned. Trail names used here are unofficial monikers used by locals. Go through the gate and take the single-track trail to the right of the gate. (The following mileages use the gate at the end of Chamonix as the beginning measuring point.) In about 100 yards, the trail becomes a double-track. In less than a mile, keep your eyes peeled for two, short, wooden posts marking the beginning of a single-track trail leading off on your right. Turn right onto this single-track, which is the beginning of unsigned Rusty's Trail. (Incidentally, the double-track which continues straight bearing left is the Ward/Alpine Trail, FS 16N48. It leads to the Scott Peak Trail and is where the finishing end of the epic TRT–Western States Ride comes in; it's also described in the next chapter.) From the two wooden posts, for the next 1.5 miles or so, stay straight, and bypass trails on your right (they lead into the marshy area of Paige Meadows). Along the way, at approximately 2 miles from the Chamonix gate, stay straight, bypassing a minor trail on the right. In a few yards, your trail reaches a junction with Drunken Bear Trail on your left; ignore it. (Drunken Bear is partially blocked by several cut logs. If you're an advanced rider looking for a technical challenge, this route is for you. Note, however, that the suggested direction is to begin riding from its other end near Alpine Meadows, finishing here.) Continue on Rusty's Trail and soon, make a hard right turn instead of going straight onto Flintstones Trails. (Don't miss this turn! If you begin a loose, technical descent, you've just missed it.) Proceed across a small creek and climb a steep little hill and at the top, at 2.3 miles from Chamonix, you reach a **T** intersection with Rawhide Trail, an old jeep road that looks more like a wide single-track. This is the beginning of the smaller loop which follows single-track trails through Paige Meadows. (First bail-out option: For those of you who want to shorten the ride, you can forego the smaller loop by taking the wide single-track to the left. This will eliminate almost 3 miles.)

To pedal the smaller loop through the meadows, go right for a few yards and then stay straight on the main trail, still within the forest. Ignore a left trail which leads uphill. About 200 yards further at 2.5 miles, bear left at another fork. Ride to 0.2 mile and turn left onto a narrow single-track; do not go through the low, wooden pillars. In a short ways, you emerge from the forest. The meadow is a bit marshy here but not to worry. Pavers and a man-made elevated path protect the wet ground as it leads you through the first meadow, basically due west. At the edge of the meadow, go through a quick 100 yards of forest and then begin crossing the second meadow to a **Y** intersection. Head straight, bearing left and continue on the main trail, making no turns onto lesser trails. Eventually, ride through three, short, wooden posts as you enter another section of forest, still heading west on the single-track. Proceed down a slight descent, following the curvy trail until it pops you out onto a jeep road. Hang a left onto the jeep road and carry on for about 100 yards to the next fork. Bear left at the fork and enjoy very brief ups and downs as you roll along through the woods. Ignore any single-tracks leading off on your left until you reach the top of the hill, at which point turn left. (Second bail-out option: The dirt trail on the right eventually runs into Silver Tip Drive and a residential subdivision. You can reach CA 89 and the bike path by making your way through the neighborhood via paved roads.) The single-track trail winds down a narrow, steep stretch for about 0.25 mile and beginners may want to walk this somewhat technical section. You soon close the smaller loop by reaching a familiar intersection. Bear right and retrace your path back to the first bail-out opportunity at Rawhide Trail as described earlier. This time, turn right onto Rawhide.

Whether you bailed out early or rode the small loop, continue on Rawhide, a well-defined jeep road masquerading as a single-track and bypass other trails leading off on your right (they lead into a residential subdivision). When you reach a **Y** intersection at 6.4 miles, bear right and continue down on the main trail. Watch out for a green gate at 6.8 miles. Go around the right side of the gate and follow the gravel road about a 100 yards farther to where paved Rawhide Drive begins at its intersection with Bonanza Drive. Now within a residential neighborhood, continue straight on Rawhide for a few blocks and then right onto Granlibakken Road. Go 3 blocks and turn right onto the paved bike path and follow it for almost 2 miles back to your car parked at either CyclePaths or William Kent Campground.

RIDE 44 · Tahoe City Bike Paths

AT A GLANCE

Length/configuration: 3 sections of closely linked paved bike paths: 21.4-mile out-and-back (10.7 miles each way); 9-mile out-and-back (4.5 miles each way); 5 mile out-and-back (2.5 miles each way)

Aerobic difficulty: Easy

Technical difficulty: Not technical, though all riders should be comfortable sharing the path with a variety of trail users, including rollerbladers and walkers with baby-strollers or a dog or two.

Scenery: Varies from forests of mixed conifers, water-level views of Lake Tahoe, and scenic Truckee River

Special comments: The path is heavily used by riders of all ages and abilities. Numerous dirt bike trails of varying aerobic and technical levels can be accessed off these bikeways.

Located in the region west and northwest of Lake Tahoe are three popular paved bike paths: West Shore Bike Path, Truckee River Recreation Trail, and Dollar Point Trail. They're sometimes collectively called the Tahoe City Bike Paths because they all radiate from the intersection of CA 28 and CA 89 in the bustling community of Tahoe City. And believe me, this is a busy intersection. During the summer, it's a zoo of insane traffic and pedestrians, with cars crossing the bike path as they pull in and out of parking lots. Bumper-to-bumper traffic is a common occurrence. If you have youngsters riding with you, I suggest that you avoid pedaling through this intersection. Fortunately, several of the paved trails offer great riding without dealing with this mess.

The West Shore Bike Path generally refers to the section between Tahoe City to Sugar Pine Point State Park, running 10.7 miles (21.4 miles total as an out-and-back), paralleling CA 89 and the western shore of Lake Tahoe for its entire length. The path is generally flat, cruising through pine forests, occasionally skirting sparkling blue

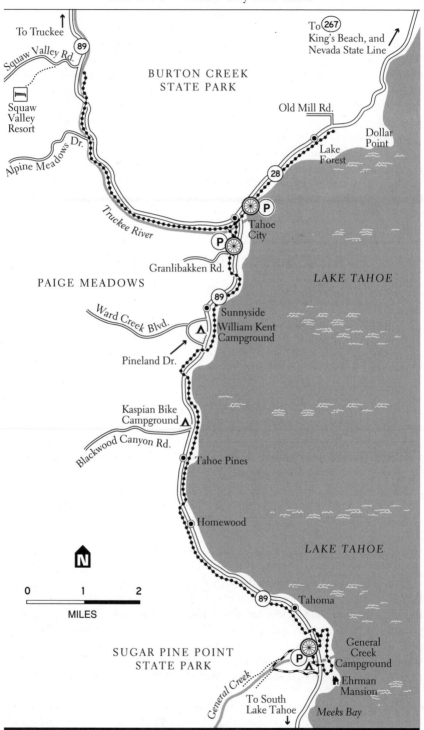

To Truckee

Squaw Valley Rd.

89

Squaw Valley Resort

Alpine Meadows Dr.

BURTON CREEK STATE PARK

To 267
King's Beach, and Nevada State Line

Old Mill Rd.

Dollar Point

Lake Forest

28

Truckee River

Tahoe City

P

P

Granlibakken Rd.

LAKE TAHOE

PAIGE MEADOWS

89

Ward Creek Blvd.

Sunnyside
William Kent Campground

Pineland Dr.

Kaspian Bike Campground

Blackwood Canyon Rd.

Tahoe Pines

Homewood

LAKE TAHOE

N

0   1   2
MILES

89

Tahoma

SUGAR PINE POINT STATE PARK

General Creek

To South Lake Tahoe

P

General Creek Campground

Ehrman Mansion

Meeks Bay

Lake Tahoe, and passing cozy homes and extravagant estates. Picnic tables and beaches along the way invite you to linger over lunch or snack. Quaint cafés along the path offer refreshments. You can even take a long break in any of the decent restaurants found along the path (bring a bike lock). West Shore Bike Path is mostly Class 1, crossing CA 89 several times, with occasional few yards of Class 2 and an almost one-mile stretch of Class 3. (Class 1 is a paved path that's physically separated from a vehicle road. Class 2 is a bike lane sharing the shoulder of a road. Class 3 is basically the same as the road, with or without a shoulder.) Despite crossing CA 89 several times, West Shore Bike Path is a great route for young families. Accessible at almost anyplace along its north-south route, the longest uninterrupted stretch is at either Sugar Pine Point State Park or the parking area just south of the insane CA 89 and CA 28 intersection in Tahoe City.

The scenic Truckee River Recreation Trail leads northwest out of Tahoe City, sandwiched between the Truckee River and CA 28. A Class 1 bikeway, it's an extremely slight downhill cruise away from Tahoe City, running 4.5 miles one way past Alpine Meadows to Midway Bridge (9 miles out-and-back, round-trip). This path is arguably the most frequently used path, popular with bikers of all abilities (it connects with other known bike trails). Rollerbladers, pedestrians, and water-recreationists accessing the river use it too. Indeed, during the summer, the river is virtually a freeway of rafters, floating, laughing, and screaming down the river. The bike path can get congested, particularly near Tahoe City.

The Dollar Point Trail is a 2.5-mile stretch running northeast out of Tahoe City, paralleling CA 28. It's mostly flat except for the last 0.5 mile which is a gentle climb up to Dollar Point. Along the way, the path leads past Lake Forest Beach, campgrounds, athletic playgrounds, picnic areas, restaurants, and retail shops, including several bike stores. Locals use this path to access a great network of mountain biking trails in the Lakeview Cross-Country Ski Area and Burton Creek State Park, about a half mile north of CA 28. Beginning about 0.5 mile east of the insane intersection, the path actually starts at the Safeway parking lot and is mostly a Class 1 bikeway, with occasional sections of Class 2 and 3. Of the three bike paths mentioned here, this is the least scenic and the busiest, due to lots of businesses bordering the path and numerous vehicle road crossings. If you have freewheeling kids with you, my first recommendation is West Shore Bike Path from its southern trailhead in Sugar Pine Point State Park. (Also found in this state park is Ride 45, another family favorite.) Second recommendation is the Truckee River Recreation Path.

General location: Mostly along the west and northwest shore of Lake Tahoe, near Tahoe City and Sugar Pine Point State Park.

Elevation change: Virtually none.

Season: Spring though fall.

Services: Many cafés, restaurants, delis, and other conveniences can be found in the numerous towns along the bike path. Major services available in Tahoe City, Truckee and South Lake Tahoe. Sugar Pine Point State Park offers General Creek Campground, one of the best camping sites in the entire Lake Tahoe area, with hot showers and a splendid setting.

Hazards: On the West Shore Bike Path, a brief stretch uses the shoulder of heavily traveled CA 89 (class 2), especially busy on summer weekends. Generally well marked with a wide shoulder, freewheeling kiddies will require constant attention on these sections. The bike route through the town of Homewood is Class 3, using quiet residential roads. On the Truckee River Bike Path, watch out for other trail users, especially on summer weekends. On the Dollar Point section, be alert for cars crossing the bike path.

Rescue index: Assistance from other trail users and passing motorists is generally available, especially during the summer. Plenty of businesses line the path and you're sure to find one who'll let you use their phone.

Land status: Tahoe National Forest and Eldorado National Forest.

Maps: *Recreation Map of Lake Tahoe*, published by Tom Harrison Maps, 2 Falmouth Cove, San Rafael, CA 94901, (800) 265-9090, www.tomharrisonmaps.com. *North Lake Tahoe Basin Recreation Topo Map*, published by Fine Edge Productions.

Finding the trail: The West Shore Bike Path can be accessed by parking in Tahoe City or at Sugar Pine Point State Park. In Tahoe City, park in the small dirt parking area along the west side of CA 89 about 0.25 mile south of its intersection with CA 28. At Sugar Pine Point State Park (10.7 miles south of this intersection on CA 89), park in the General Creek campground day-use parking area (small fee required) or in the Ehrman Mansion historic site across CA 89. You can also access the bike path at many points in between along CA 89. To reach Tahoe City from I-80, drive south by southwest on CA 89, reaching Tahoe City in about 13.5 miles. Turn left onto CA 89, cross the Truckee River, and continue a short distance to the parking area on the west side of the road, or continue south to Sugar Pine Point State Park. If you're driving from the east shore of the lake, go west on CA 28 past CA 267 and Kings Beach. Continue about 9.5 miles from the CA 267 intersection and turn left onto CA 89. Cross the Truckee River and in a few yards, pull into the parking area on the right (or continue 10.7 miles farther to Sugar Pine Point.) If you're coming from South Lake Tahoe, go north on CA 89 for about 18 miles to Sugar Pine Point or continue 10.7 miles farther to the parking area in Tahoe City.

To access the Truckee River Recreation Trail, you can park in the small dirt lot described above but that means you'll have to make your way through the insane CA 89 and CA 28 intersection. Otherwise, you might find legal parking off CA 89 along the Truckee River Recreation Trail, just prior to intersecting CA 28. Also, parking in any of the pulloffs of CA 89 is permitted—just park completely off the pavement.

To access the Dollar Point Trail, you can avoid pedaling through the insane intersection by parking in a legal spot along CA 28, near the Safeway store.

Sources of additional information:

Cyclepaths Mountain Bike
  Adventures
1785 Westlake Blvd.
P.O. Box 887
Tahoe City, CA 96145
(800) 780-BIKE or (530) 581-1171
www.cyclepaths.com
The West Shore Bike Path runs past it. Service and retail sales of bicycles and accessories. They also offer guided backcountry tours for all skill levels and of varying lengths.

Olympic Bike Shop
620 N. Lake Blvd.
Tahoe City, CA 96145
(916) 581-2500
The Dollar Point Trail runs past it. Service and retail sales of bicycles and accessories as well as rentals. Great staff.

Eldorado National Forest
3070 Camino Heights Dr.
Camino, CA 95709
(916) 622-5062

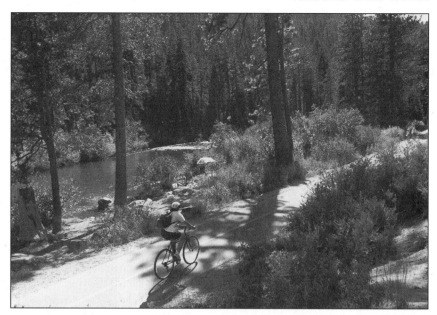

Skirting the river for most of its northwest direction, the Truckee River Recreation Trail is popular with bikers, as well as rafters and sunbathers seeking easy access to the water.

Tahoe National Forest
631 Coyote St.
P.O. Box 6003
Nevada City, CA 95959
(916) 265-4531

Notes on the trail: There's not much to the Truckee River Recreation Trail other than it being an outstanding, scenic Class 1 bikeway that flows as pleasantly as the river it follows. The setting is beautiful, if you ignore busy CA 89. You can access the river in many spots along the way. Unlike the other two bikeways, there are no cafés or other eateries on the route, but there are pit toilets.

The West Shore Bike Path, on the other hand, offers lots of sites of interest. Before hopping on your bike, consider bringing a bike lock and some form of money—lots of eateries and shops line the path. I recommend starting from Sugar Pine Point State Park. Here are a few of those nuggets, as described riding south to north from Sugar Pine Point to Tahoe City. From General Creek campground in the state park, pedal east toward CA 89, hop onto the bike path, northbound, and immediately, though cautiously, follow the path as it crosses CA 89, putting you on the lake side of the busy road. Look for an interpretative path (paved). This side path gives a short and interesting history lesson of the flora and fauna of the immediate terrain. Also worth checking out is the Ehrman Mansion. Owned by San Francisco businessman I.W. Hellman in 1897, it's an example of fine opulent summer homes that colored the shoreline in the early 1900s. Acquired by the state park in 1965, the house and its nearby Nature Center (also on the estate) is open to the public during the summer.

Hop back on the main bike path and continue north with the lake off on your right in the distance. In a few yards, the paved path crosses over to the west side of

CA 89. Cruise through the quiet town of Tahoma at about 1.5 miles. At about 2.6 miles, coming in on your left is McKinney-Rubicon Springs Road which leads to Ellis and Barker Peaks via several popular dirt mountain bike trails. Continue north on the paved bike path and when you reach the quiet town of Homewood at about 3.5 miles, the bike path becomes residential streets (Class 2 and 3). Make your way through the neighborhood, following bike route signs along the way, sometimes sharing the road and sometimes in a designated bike lane. Leave Homewood and in less than a mile, the path cruises through Tahoe Pines and crosses CA 89 again. Keep an eye out for the impressive but understated estate, "Fleur du Lac," built in 1937 by industrialist Henry J. Kaiser. It was the location for a scene in the movie "The Godfather II." (Sorry, it's not open to the public.) Continuing on, just after 6 miles from Sugar Pine Point State Park, you begin skirting the water's edge of Lake Tahoe. Picnic tables and pit toilets can be found along this stretch. On your left, leading west is Blackwood Canyon Road which leads to other mountain bike trails. Staying on the bike path, continue north and at about 7.7 miles, the trail leads you across CA 89 to the west side. The bikeway shares the road with cars but in a short distance, it becomes a separate bike path again. At almost 9 miles, in Sunnyside, Ward Creek Road takes off on your left, leading to Paige Meadows and fine dirt mountain bike trails (see Ride 43). Continuing on, the bike path leads you across CA 89 several more times and at just over 10.5 miles, you reach Tahoe City where the Class 1 paved path ends, next to the parking area.

From here, you can turn around and head back the way you came or continue on to the Truckee River Recreation Trail. To pick up that path, make your way through the busy intersection (CA 89 and CA 28), crossing over the Truckee River and watching out for automobile and pedestrian traffic. Follow CA 89 due northwest, looking for the Truckee River Recreation Trail on your left, next to the river. The bike path runs about 4.5 miles, ending at Midway Bridge near Squaw Valley Road. At this point, you can turn left into Squaw Valley and pick up another paved bike path (actually, it's more like a sidewalk) and ride a couple of miles to the resort area. Incidentally, Squaw Valley operates a mountain biking park during the summer, complete with lift service, hotel, eateries, and other conveniences; (800) 545-4350. Otherwise, turn around and return the way you came.

RIDE 45 · General Creek Easy Loop

AT A GLANCE

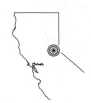

Length/configuration: 5.7-mile loop, counterclockwise; double-track and paved bike path

Aerobic difficulty: Easy

Technical difficulty: Not technical

Scenery: Gently rolling terrain paralleling General Creek. The route includes a stretch through the Ehrman Mansion grounds and an interpretive paved path.

Special comments: This is a perfect loop for young families. For a longer, full day of easy riding, consider adding the West Shore Bike Path out-and-back as well as the Truckee River Recreation Trail, for a total round-trip over 20 miles (see Ride 44).

Perfect for families with freewheeling youngsters or kid-trailers, the General Creek campground loop is easy, short and, (dare I say?) educational. As the name implies, the loop begins right smack in the middle of the campground. This 5.7-mile dirt loop is mostly free of vehicular traffic, cruising through the forest along-side General Creek. Included on the loop is an interpretive path on which bikes are allowed. A visit to the Ehrman Mansion is a must, if only to see how the rich lived in the early 1900s. An opulent summer home built in the rustic architectural style of Tahoe, the California State Park System acquired the Mansion in 1965 and it's now opened to the public for viewing. It's gorgeous interior is worth a visit, even if the kiddies find it boring. But the Nature Center adjacent to the Mansion is sure to pique their attention. There, they might learn something about the local environment through exhibits and hands-on displays. They might even be fascinated by the Washoe Indian myth about Water Babies—small grey creatures living in the lakes and streams—and how they created the area's many lakes. The area which Sugar Pine Point State Park now occupies was once the summer home for generations of Washoe Indians. In fact, bedrock mortars and grinding rocks just offshore from the Ehrman Mansion are still visible.

General Creek Camp, located in Sugar Pine Point State Park, is one of the finest—and most popular—maintained campgrounds in the Lake Tahoe vicinity. Shaded by dense forests of pine, fir, aspen, and juniper, Sugar Pine Point is a great place to set up a budget-conscious base camp for riders planning to partake of the region's many fine bike trails and other outdoor amenities. Facilities here at the camp include two of the most important ones of all: hot showers and rest rooms. If you want to camp here, reservations are strongly advised for summertime dates. (See "Sources of additional information" below for making reservations.) Though there are 175 campsites, the camp fills rapidly in the summer.

General location: 10 miles south of Tahoe City, on the west shore of Lake Tahoe.

Elevation change: Negligible change; mostly at 6,200 feet.

Season: Spring through fall.

Services: Water, rest rooms, picnic tables, and campsites available at General Creek campground within the park. Open year-round, hot showers available in the summer. Small grocery stores, cafes, and eateries nearby, north of the park entrance on CA 89. All other major services in Tahoe City and South Lake Tahoe.

Hazards: Watch for automobile traffic when crossing CA 89.

Rescue index: This route is popular with other trail users, especially in the summer, making your chances of find help very good. Otherwise, make your way back to the campground or CA 89 to find someone who can be of help.

Land status: Sugar Pine Point State Park.

Maps: *Recreation Map of Lake Tahoe*, published by Tom Harrison Maps, 2 Falmouth Cove, San Rafael, CA 94901, (800) 265-9090, www.tomharrisonmaps.com. *North Lake Tahoe Basin Recreation Topo Map*, published by Fine Edge Productions.

RIDE 45 · General Creek Easy Loop

Finding the trail: From Tahoe City, travel south on CA 89 for almost 11 miles to Sugar Pine Point State Park. Turn right into the park and park in the day-use parking area (fee required), or continue less than a half mile farther and turn left into the Ehrman Mansion estate where you may find free but limited parking. In any case, to access the trailhead, begin by pedaling west through the campground via the paved roads, heading for campsites 149 and 150. (The single-track trails which weave through the campground are hiking-only). The beginning of General Creek Easy Loop (also signed as Red Loop) is found between these two campsites.

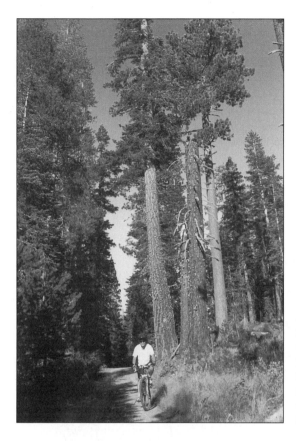

A short and sweet route amid graceful evergreens, this ride is perfect for novices and children, while more skilled riders have a chance to explore narrow, twisty single-track.

Sources of additional information:

Sugar Pine Point State Park
P.O. Box 266
Tahoma, CA 96142
(530) 525-7982
Campground reservations: (800) 444-7275

Notes on the trail: This loop is described in a counterclockwise direction, though you can easily ride it in reverse. Having found the dirt trail between campsites 149 and 150, follow it due west. The route quickly leads you into a clearing surrounded by mixed conifer trees with General Creek off in the distance on your left. In less than a half mile from campsite 149, a wide single-track trail cruises past a dirt road taking off on your left. That road crosses the creek on a well-made steel and wooden bridge, and connects to the south side of the loop. Bypass that road, continuing straight on the north side of the creek. At 1.6 miles from campsite 149, you reach a signed junction with a trail peeling off on your left toward the creek. Hang a left here and make your way over the creek via a bridge and boardwalk.

(If you stay straight instead of crossing the creek here, you'll find the trail narrows as it weaves through the pine and aspen forest, and the terrain becomes slightly more technical thanks to small rocks, boulders and exposed tree roots. Beginners wanting to hone their single-track riding skills will enjoy this trail—up to a point. The slightly challenging terrain goes about 2.5 miles, gradually gaining elevation as it runs through steep but short dips. Eventually, the riding becomes less enjoyable because the fallen trees and rugged dips in the twisting trail require you to dismount and walk a couple of steps. Following the trail becomes a bike 'n' hike affair and not much fun after a while. Still, the forest is gorgeous, fragrant, and serene, and if you're up for the adventure, go for it. You can always turn around when you've had enough.)

Instead of continuing straight ahead, turn left here and cross the creek via a bridge and boardwalk. Once on the other side of General Creek, the route loops back toward the east. The creek is still on your left and the single-track remains relatively easy as you cruise alongside the creek through the pine forest. Pedal about 1.2 miles and you reach a dirt road leading off on your left which runs over the creek via the first bridge you encountered at the very beginning of the ride. (Taking this bridge road will return you to the campground in approximately 0.5 mile.) Bypass the bridge road, following the trail straight ahead as it becomes wider and more like a smooth jeep road. In about a mile from this last bridge, the trail intersects CA 89, near the entrance to the Ehrman Mansion. Cautiously cross CA 89, bypass the paved bike path that runs alongside the road, and continue straight into the grounds of the historic mansion. In the summer, the mansion and the nearby Nature Center is open for visitors. Here's your chance to check out the interior of one of Tahoe's most elegantly rustic old estates.

When you're ready to continue the ride, look for a paved interpretive path leading due north through the trees and bushes (not the bikeway next to CA 89). This short one-mile path is a worthwhile ride just to read the interesting signs which describe the local vegetation and the Washoe Indian myth of the water babies. The interpretive path ends when it intersects the original bike path at CA 89. Follow the bike path as it crosses to the west side of CA 89. In a few yards, a dirt single-track trail peels off on the left at a signboard indicating the site of the old Bellevue Hotel. Stay left, following the paved path as it leads you back into the campground and to your parked car (or camp). Total mileage of the loop, including the side trip through the Ehrman Mansion grounds and interpretative path is about 5.7 miles.

RIDE 46 · Fallen Leaf Lake Easy Loop

AT A GLANCE

Length/configuration: 5.4-mile loop, clockwise; single-track, jeep and paved roads, and paved bike path

Aerobic difficulty: Easy due to flatness and length

Technical difficulty: Mildly technical

Scenery: Dense forest of aspen, lodgepole pine, and spruce trees, paralleling the northern edge of Fallen Leaf Lake and Taylor Creek. Especially lovely during the fall when the aspens turn fiery yellow-orange.

Special comments: A great add-on to the Angora Lakes Out-and-Back, which uses the same starting point. Well-suited for youngsters and beginners.

Fallen Leaf Lake is like a miniature Lake Tahoe sitting at approximately 6,370 feet elevation. The water is sparkling sapphire blue and mostly clear. Its deepest point is about 430 feet. Most of its southern shoreline is lined with gorgeous homes. The north shore, however, is free of homes, forming the densely forested backyard, so to speak, of Fallen Leaf campground. Numerous trails crisscross this small, wooded area and most of them are not marked. You really can't get lost because the entire area is basically enclosed by obvious landmarks: the lake's northern edge, Cathedral Road, Fallen Leaf Lake Road, and CA 89. The trails are aerobically easy thanks to its relative flatness. Other than a few semi-buried boulders, a storm-downed tree or two, and some tiny patches of sand, the trail is mostly mildly technical. The 5.4-mile clockwise loop described here is composed of 3.1 miles of easy single-tracks and 2.3 miles of combined paved, quiet car roads, and bike path. For more mileage, consider adding the Angora Lakes Out-and-Back (Ride 47), which begins at the same parking lot.

General location: About 3.5 miles northwest of South Lake Tahoe, at the southern end of Lake Tahoe.

Elevation change: Negligible change; mostly at 6,400 feet.

Season: Spring through fall.

Services: Fallen Leaf Campground is adjacent to Fallen Leaf Lake. Limited services are available at Camp Richardson, a privately owned and operated motor campground. A small bike rental shop is located at Camp Richardson. All other services can be found in South Lake Tahoe.

Hazards: Some car traffic on Cathedral and Fallen Leaf Lake Roads, especially during the summer. CA 89 is busy and extreme caution is required when crossing it. If you're accustomed to wearing eye protection when riding, consider clear or yellow glasses as the single-track portion of this loop is through dense, dark forest. Expect to share the trail with hikers and other bikers, especially during the popular summer months.

Rescue index: The single-track is frequently used by walkers and other cyclists, and Fallen Leaf campground is generally staffed. So, you shouldn't have any trouble finding someone who may be of help. Because Cathedral Road and Fallen Leaf Lake Road are major access roads to the gorgeous homes located on the southern end of Fallen Leaf Lake, passing motorists may be able to assist in an emergency.

Land status: El Dorado National Forest, Lake Tahoe Basin Management Unit.

Maps: *Recreation Map of Lake Tahoe*, published by Tom Harrison Maps, 2 Falmouth Cove, San Rafael, CA 94901, (800) 265-9090, www.tomharrisonmaps.com.

Finding the trail: From the Y (intersection of US 50 and CA 89) in South Lake Tahoe, travel north on CA 89 for 3.2 miles, going past Camp Richardson. Turn left (due south) onto Fallen Leaf Road which is directly opposite the entrance of Tallac Historic Site. Continue toward Fallen Leaf Lake and go past the campground entrance at 1.5 miles. About 0.25 mile farther, look for the Fallen Leaf Lake trailhead sign adjacent to a small dirt parking area. Park and begin your ride here.

Sources of additional information:

U.S. Forest Service—Lake Tahoe Basin Management Unit
870 Emerald Bay Rd.
South Lake Tahoe, CA 96150
(916) 573-2600; (916) 573-2674

Notes on the trail: From the dirt parking area adjacent to Fallen Leaf Lake trail-head, begin by pedaling the single-track trail, heading south by southwest through the forest toward the lake. Beginners may want to walk the first 0.3 mile as the terrain is a bit rocky leading up and over a berm. When you reach the water's edge, the trail levels and intersects another trail going both left and right; turn right. (Go left if you'd like, for that trail will loop you back to this vicinity in a few yards.) Follow the single-track and re-enter the cover of the shady forest. In less than a few yards, intersect a wide gravel road and go right onto it for a few yards. Pick up the single-track again leading off on the left. The trail continues to weave through the forest, about 50 yards from the shoreline. As you follow the edge of the lake, at about 1.1 miles, you come to a spillway with a wooden bridge across the mouth of Taylor Creek. Dismount and walk through the narrow bridge.

With the lake still on your left, continue following the narrow trail through the forest, heading south. At about 1.7 miles, you reach a rustic tiny building and next to it, near the lake edge, is the foundation of what use to be a house, the obvious evidence being its the stone fireplace. Though a narrow trail meanders off through the trees and bushes, it eventually peters out in a few yards. Don't follow that trail. Instead, at this foundation, take the dirt road leading off on your right, away from the lake. In a few minutes, you reach the intersection with paved Cathedral Road. There's a sign here indicating that the dirt road you've just ridden is 1304c.

Turn right onto Cathedral Road and follow it for about a half mile, at which point you see a dirt road leading off on your right. It's signed 1304b and gated. Take this dirt road and go around the gate. The path varies from a wide single-track to a double-track to a narrow jeep road. You're now deep in the forest again, weaving through aspen, spruce, and lodgepole pine trees. At about 2.8 miles, begin paralleling Taylor Creek on your right, sometimes riding alongside it, other times a few yards away. Watch out for water bars in the trail. Go past a green metal cylindrical structure in the creek sitting about 7 feet tall.

When you come to a huge granite boulder sitting right smack in the middle of your trail, you've pedaled about 3.3 miles. Straight ahead, surrounded by a small grove of aspens, is a towering but dead lodgepole pine tree. The trail has now become a narrow double-track jeep road. A few yards beyond the boulder is a walking trail leading off on the right. It leads to an interpretive sign and popular swimming hole alongside Taylor Creek. Check it out: the Forest Service has placed large logs in the creek bed to help flowing water carve out sheltered pools, providing a cozy home for the native fish.

Next to the interpretive sign is a narrow single-track trail; don't follow it, because it dead ends after a few yards. Back in the saddle, retrace your path back to the main trail and continue the direction in which you were headed. In a few yards, at about 3.6 miles, you reach paved Cathedral Road again. Hang a right here, riding due north, and enjoy a sweet, gradual descent, passing pine, and fat and thin aspen trees along the way. Continue past a green gate and the California Snow Park (a paved parking lot). In a little over 4 miles, Cathedral intersects CA 89. Go across CA 89 (watch for cars) and immediately go right on the Pope Baldwin Bike Path. At 4.6 miles, directly across CA 89 from Tallac Historic Site is Fallen Leaf Lake Road. Go right across CA 89 and follow Fallen Leaf Lake Road for just under a mile to reach your parked car, closing the loop in about 5.4 miles.

RIDE 47 · Angora Lakes Out-and-Back

AT A GLANCE

Length/configuration: 8.5-mile out-and-back (4.25 miles each way); wide dirt road with some stretches of pavement

Aerobic difficulty: Moderate especially if you're not ac-climated to the higher elevation

Technical difficulty: Nontechnical except for a few small sandy patches

Scenery: Surrounded by mixed forests of pine and aspen. Splendid views of Lake Tahoe and Fallen Leaf as well as Upper Truckee River Valley from the ridgetop.

Special comments: Suitable for strong youngsters. Tow a kid-trailer if you want a workout. The ride can be shortened and the climbing dimin-ished by driving up the ridge to one of several alternate starting points. Aspen leaves turn fiery red, yellow, and orange during the fall. A quaint snack bar and beach resort at the lake is a fun place to hang out with the kiddies. This ride can be combined with the Fallen Leaf Lake Easy Loop for a longer ride (Ride 46).

Lying side by side at 7,440 feet are two little pristine lakes—Lower Angora and Upper Angora. Together they're referred to as Angora Lakes and they sit within a carved bowl of towering granite cliffs. The smooth, wide dirt road leading up to the lakes climbs steadily, traversing up a ridge, gaining 1,040 feet in 4.25 miles. Once on the ridge, splendid views emerge, Fallen Leaf Lake and Lake Tahoe on the right and the narrow Upper Truckee River valley and the US 50 corridor on the left. The return trip is an exhilarating downhill flight—all the way—for a total round-trip of 8.5 miles.

If you're looking to get away from everyone and civilization, this isn't the route. But, if you're looking for an easy-to-follow, nontechnical, short, and moderate work-out with homemade, ice-cold lemonade as a reward on a hot day, this is the ride for you. Include freewheeling youngsters and/or a kid trailer, and you'll have one heck of a workout, in which you'll also be entitled to an ice cream bar. That's right! At the far end of this out-and-back ride is a quaint resort, complete with cute cabins, a snack bar, and a beach on which to relax and soak in the sun. (Bring a bathing suit if you want to take a dip in the typically ice cold lake.) Since it's accessible by cars, it's a popular spot, especially during the summer. Fortunately, the road is mostly wide and the traffic slow enough making the route fairly safe for kids. To shorten the ride for

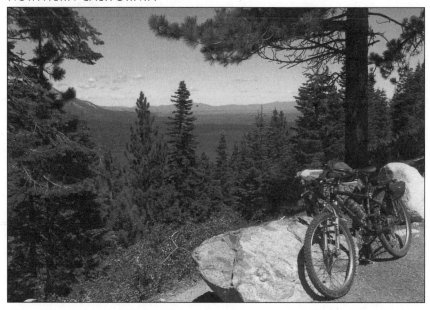

A view of Emerald Lake from a small clearing at Angora Lookout.

youngsters, you can certainly drive part way up the dirt road, parking at one of several spots, depending on the amount of mileage and climbing you want to eliminate. To lengthen the ride, consider adding the Fallen Leaf Lake Easy Loop (Ride 46), which is accessed from the same trailhead as this ride.

General location: About 3.5 miles northwest of South Lake Tahoe, at the southern end of Lake Tahoe.

Elevation change: 1,000 feet; starting elevation and low point 6,400 feet; high point 7,400 feet. One long, moderate climb with short level stretch in the middle; return is downhill coasting.

Season: Spring through fall.

Services: Water, snacks, rest rooms, bike locks, phone, rowboat rentals, and lodging available at the Angora Lakes Resort during the summer months. Developed campground adjacent to Fallen Leaf Lake. Limited services available at Camp Richardson, including a small bike rental shop. All other services can be found in South Lake Tahoe.

Hazards: Some car traffic, especially during the summer.

Rescue index: Since the road is the only road leading to the resort, you're sure to encounter motorists and other riders who may be of assistance.

Land status: El Dorado National Forest, Lake Tahoe Basin Management Unit.

Maps: *Recreation Map of Lake Tahoe*, published by Tom Harrison Maps, 2 Falmouth Cove, San Rafael, CA 94901, (800) 265-9090, www.tomharrisonmaps.com. *South Lake Tahoe Basin Recreation Topo Map*, published by Fine Edge Productions.

Finding the trail: From the Y (intersection of US 50 and CA 89) in South Lake Tahoe, travel north on CA 89 for 3.2 miles, going past Camp Richardson. Turn left (due south) onto Fallen Leaf Road which is directly opposite the entrance of Tallac

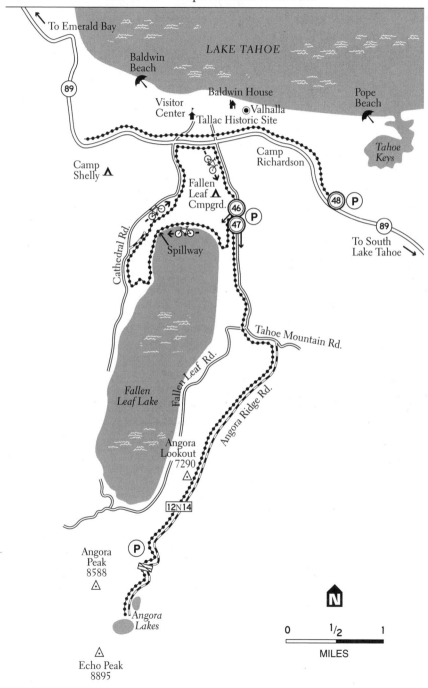

Historic Site. Continue toward Fallen Leaf Lake and go past the campground entrance at 1.5 miles. About 0.25 mile farther, look for the Fallen Leaf Lake trailhead sign adjacent to a small dirt parking area. Park and begin your ride here. If you wish to shorten the ride to Angora Lakes, there are several places at which to park: Continue on Fallen Leaf Lake Road past the trailhead and in about 0.2 mile, turn left (due southeast) onto Tahoe Mountain Road. Follow it for about 0.4 mile to the intersection of a dirt road leading off on your right, signed 12N14 (also known as 1214 and Angora Ridge Road). There's a small pulloff at this intersection and you can park here. From here, your distance to Upper Angora Lake is about 3.7 miles. If you want to shorten the ride further, especially if you have youngsters in tow, turn right onto the dirt road and continue up for about 1.8 miles at which point you reach the Angora Lookout (a tiny white structure) sitting next to a generous pulloff. Parking here means the distance to Angora Lakes is about 1.9 miles. If you still want to shorten the ride even more, continue a mile more to the end of the road and into a parking lot. Parking here shortens the ride considerably to about 0.9 mile to the upper lake.

Sources of additional information:

U.S. Forest Service
Lake Tahoe Basin Management Unit
870 Emerald Bay Rd.
South Lake Tahoe, CA 96150
(530) 573-2600; (530) 573-2674

Angora Lakes Resort
Angora Ridge Rd.
South Lake Tahoe, CA 96158
(530) 541-2092; (530) 577-3593

Notes on the trail: From the Fallen Leaf Lake trailhead near the campground, begin pedaling due south on the paved road. At about 0.2 mile, turn left onto paved Tahoe Mountain Road and begin gaining a bit of elevation. In less than 0.5 mile, you reach the intersection with dirt road 12N14 leading off on your right, also known as 1214 and Angora Ridge Road. Make the right here and follow the dirt road as it begins climbing gradually. Stay to the right of the road as this is a popular route for vehicles driving up to Angora Lakes.

The route is mostly dirt with occasional stretches of broken pavement. As you steadily grind your way up to the ridge, enjoy the slowly emerging view of the Fallen Leaf Lake and Lake Tahoe, visible through the pine and aspen forest on your right. When you reach the Angora Lookout (a tiny white structure) at 2.4 miles, the views of the lakes and the Upper Truckee River valley to the right and left of you, respectively, is commanding.

Continue ascending the ridge and at about 3.4 miles, the road ends in a parking lot. Make your way to the far end of the parking lot, toward a gate that typically closes off a jeep road. Go around the gate and begin a somewhat steeper climb. The terrain becomes slightly more technical, thanks to some sandy patches and semi-buried small boulders.

In just over 0.5 mile, the jeep road leads you past Lower Angora Lake, visible on your left through the pine forest. A bit farther and you begin to see Upper Angora Lake. At 4.25 miles, you reach the resort area, next to the lake's edge. Lock up your bike here (locks and rack provided) and treat yourself to a refreshment. Kiddies will probably want to splash their hands and toes in the icy lake water. When you've had enough, turn around and enjoy a 4.25 mile downhill run back to your car at the trailhead near the campground, clocking in at almost 8.5 miles round-trip. Watch out for traffic on the way down.

RIDE 48 · Pope Baldwin Bike Path

AT A GLANCE

Length/configuration: 7.8-mile out-and-back (3.9 miles each way); paved bike path

Aerobic difficulty: Easy

Technical difficulty: Not technical

Scenery: Path through pine forests, running past several splendid beaches and three of the region's finest old estates

Special comments: Suitable for young children, including kid trailers. Adult riders (and older, stronger kids) can add more mileage by including the Fallen Leaf–Taylor Creek Loop. For a moderately aerobic, nontechnical ride, the Angora Lakes Out-and-Back ride is easily accessed from the bike path.

This is a great route to take the kiddies. Though it's only 3.9 miles of paved bike path, riding the entire route as an out-and-back makes the effort an easy 7.8-mile round-trip journey through a lovely pine and aspen forest. Add to that a picnic stop at Pope or Baldwin Beach, Camp Richardson, or Tallac Historic Site, throw in a short hike and visit several fancy estates and you have a nice outing. And this isn't a bike route that shares the shoulder of an automobile road—it's completely separated. The path is sandwiched between CA 89 and the southwest shoreline of Lake Tahoe. Except for several minor roads crossing the path, you needn't worry about cars. The route runs basically north to south and can be conveniently accessed at many points. Pack a picnic or pick up goodies at the Camp Richardson deli—there are lots of great lunch spots available, either on the beach, at Camp Richardson, or on the splendid grounds of Tallac Historic Site.

Adults will find this an enjoyable outing because it gives them a chance to visit historic sites. Here, the history of Lucky Baldwin and his "greatest casino in America" added color to this luxuriously rustic playground of the rich and famous, circa 1890s. The bike path gives you an option to ride through the historic grounds, taking you past three magnificent old residences on the banks of Lake Tahoe: the Valhalla, Pope, and Baldwin Estates. Park your bike and stroll through the beautifully maintained grounds and gardens. A visit to the Tallac Museum (housed in the Baldwin Estate) is well worth the detour. During the summer, special events are held, including Great Gatsby Days, Wa She Shu Way, and Wa She Shu it Deh (both of which celebrate the culture of the Washoe Indians who inhabited the region long before Lucky and his party animals invaded), concerts, and children's programs. And the Taylor Creek Visitor Center, located just north of Tallac Historic Site, offers its own set of special events, too. If you're looking for a great bicycle outing with some mileage and lots of variety to keep yourself and the kids entertained, this route is a winner.

General location: Located on the southwestern edge of Lake Tahoe paralleling CA 89, just west of South Lake Tahoe.

Elevation change: Negligible change; mostly at 6,220 feet.

Season: Spring through fall.

Services: Camp Richardson, which the path runs through, is a privately owned and operated motor campground. Nearby is a bike rental shop, an ice cream parlor, a restaurant, and grassy picnic spots. Pope and Baldwin Beaches are accessible from the path. Paved parking is available at Tallac Historic Site (fee may be required) and Taylor Creek Visitor Center (free). All other services available in South Lake Tahoe.

Hazards: Watch out for other trail users, especially during the summer. Though the paved path is about 10 feet wide, it is a popular route, frequently used by rollerbladers, fast bikers, joggers, and walkers, as well as four-wheel bicycle carriages. There are five places where a vehicle road crosses the bike path and extreme caution is required here, especially if you're accompanied by freewheeling kids. Bringing and using a bike lock is recommended so that you can enjoy visiting the estates, museum, and beaches.

Rescue index: Lots of trail users and plenty of nearby places of business means your chance of finding help is great.

Land status: Lake Tahoe Basin Management Unit (a part of the USDA Forest Service).

Maps: General map printed in many free tourist publications found at visitor centers and places of businesses in nearly all communities around Lake Tahoe.

Finding the trail: You can access the bike path from seven locations, though parking anywhere alongside CA 89 is permitted, unless posted otherwise. (Park well off the pavement.) From the Y (intersection of CA 89 and US 50) in South Lake Tahoe, travel north on CA 89 for about 1.5 miles. The paved bike path begins abruptly on the right side (east) of the road, across from a gated forest road. Next to the trailhead, on both sides of the road, are small dirt pulloffs, suitable for parking your car. Or, you can continue almost 0.8 mile farther north on CA 89 to Pope Beach where you turn right, crossing the bike path, and park in the lot (small fee charged). Or continue 0.3 mile past Pope Beach and park at Camp Richardson, a little community composed of a bike rental shop, deli and other tourist conveniences. Or continue 0.9 mile more and turn right into the Tallac Historic Site parking lot. Or continue a few yards farther, still on CA 89 and turn right into the Taylor Creek Visitor Center parking lot. Or continue 1.1 miles farther north on CA 89 and turn right to Baldwin Beach parking lot (a small fee charged). In 0.8 mile past Baldwin Beach, you reach the northern end of the bike path with a parking lot on the left side (west) of CA 89.

Sources of additional information:

U.S. Forest Service
Lake Tahoe Basin Management Unit
870 Emerald Bay Rd.
South Lake Tahoe, CA 96150
(916) 573-2600; (916) 573-2674

Taylor Creek Visitor Center
(adjacent to Tallac Historic Site)

Summer hours: 8:00 a.m.–5:30 p.m.
(916) 573-2674

Tallac Historic Site Museum
Summer hours: 10:00 a.m.–
    4:00 p.m.
(916) 541-5227

Notes on the trail: You don't really need a map to follow the route and you can't get lost since the bike path parallels CA 89 for its entire 3.9-mile length. The hardest part is deciding where to park to access the trail and where to picnic. Starting at either the north or south end at least gives you the longest stretch of riding before turning around.

RIDE 49 · Burnside Lake Out-and-Back

AT A GLANCE

Length/configuration: 11.4 miles round-trip (5.7 miles each way); dirt road

Aerobic difficulty: Moderate elevation gain; can be moderately strenuous if you're not acclimated to the higher elevation

Technical difficulty: Not technical since the road is smooth and wide

Scenery: A tiny, undeveloped and peaceful blue lake sitting in a forest of mixed conifers. Carson Ridge rises over the lake to over 10,000 feet. A side trip from the lake leads to an overlook area, offering dramatic views of Markleeville and the Mokelumne Wilderness beyond it.

Special comments: Suitable for strong young riders. Optional side trails offer more aerobic and technical challenge, including an experts-only single-track trail which leads from the lake down a rocky mountainside and into Grover Hot Springs.

For a no-brainer moderate workout that's far from the maddening crowd of South Lake Tahoe, this out-and-back ride up to Burnside Lake fits the bill. The basic route follows Burnside Lake Road, a wide, hard-packed dirt road that's not technical though small stretches may be accented with eyeball rattling washboard terrain, depending on the last time the surface was graded. It's 11.4 miles round-trip (5.7 miles each way) with opportunities to extend your mileage and seriously tax your cardiovascular system. If you're looking for a strenuous day, add an out-and-back climbing to Pickett Peak and/or Hawkins Peak.

The attraction of Burnside Lake, especially with local folks, is that it's a pristine, peaceful, tiny lake sitting at about 8,080 feet. Completely devoid of commercial development, it's a popular place for fishing and just plain relaxing on a sunny day. Beyond the lake is a single-track trail that overlooks Markleeville Peak, Mokelumne Wilderness, and Charity Valley where Grover Hot Springs lies. The overlook is worth the short out-and-back "bike 'n' hike." This overlook trail is an intermediately technical path and beginners may prefer hiking it after stashing their bike in the bushes. Reportedly, expertly skilled strong riders can actually reach Grover Hot Springs State Park by following a rocky trail skirting stretches of very steep, unnerving drop-offs. (Check out topographic maps and you'll agree that advance planning is highly recommended on this optional route. A shuttle-car arrangement is recommended.)

General location: About 12 miles southeast of South Lake Tahoe.

Elevation change: 1,080 feet; starting elevation and low point 7,000 feet; high point 8,080 feet. Easily sustained climb up with few flat stretches.

Season: Late spring through fall.

Services: None on the trail. Limited services in Crystal Springs Campground, and the towns of Markleeville and Woodfords. All services available in South Lake Tahoe.

Hazards: Hunting is permitted in the fall and if you must ride, wear brightly colored clothing such as the familiar blaze orange. The optional experts-only single-track trail leading to the Grover Hot Springs overlook area and beyond is narrow with treacherously deep drop-offs. The road to the lake sees occasional automobile traffic.

Rescue index: The route is the only road leading up to the lake. During the summer, the lake is a somewhat popular fishing and relaxing destination for local people. You may get lucky and find someone who may be of assistance. Otherwise, continue back down to your car at the well-traveled CA 88 and CA 89 intersection and flag down a passing motorist for help.

Land status: Toiyabe National Forest.

Maps: *South Lake Tahoe Basin Recreation Topo Map*, published by Fine Edge Productions; USGS Freel Peak, Carson Pass (and Markleeville for the expert-only portion) 7.5 minute series.

Finding the trail: From the Y in South Lake Tahoe (the intersection of US 50 and CA 89), travel south on CA 89 for 11.6 miles to its intersection with CA 88. Directly across CA 88 is a dirt road and a wide-open parking lot marked by a national forest informational signboard. The dirt road is Burnside Lake Road. Park here.

Sources of additional information:

Toiyabe National Forest
U. S. Forest Service, Headquarters
1200 Franklin Way
Sparks, NV 89431
(702) 331-6444

Grover Hot Springs State Park
P.O. Box 188
Markleeville, CA 96120
(916) 694-2248

Notes on the trail: This is an easy route to follow. Though unsigned, the main route is Burnside Lake Road, an obviously well-traveled, wide dirt road suitable for passenger vehicles. Other trails will intersect but stay on the main road, always heading south. Along the way, several small jeep roads leading off the main road offer you the chance to add a few more miles, albeit rated slightly more technical and aerobically taxing.

Begin by pedaling from the dirt parking area on the wide dirt road and head south from CA 88 and CA 89. Do not take the dirt road alongside CA 88 which is signed "Do Not Enter." In less than a mile after riding through an open area, you see a sign identifying your road as FS 019. Throughout the ride, the road surface is generally smooth and not technical except for long patches of washboard terrain—just like those annoying highway dots that keep you from falling asleep behind the wheel of your car. The road begins its steady march, gradually gaining elevation. Along the way, you pass aspen groves, and fragrant juniper bushes, pines, and spruce trees.

At 0.4 mile, bypass a lesser dirt road leading off on your left, staying on FS 019. At 0.9 mile, another dirt road shoots off on your right, going slightly downhill as the main road you're on continues straight ahead. This is worth noting because this offshoot road is also signed 019, at least it was the case when I last pedaled this route. Sound confusing? If the sign is still here, take a closer look and you'll see that the sign is missing another number. The big clue I noticed was that "019" was not centered on the signboard, which led me to conclude that another number (in this case, according to my map, the letter "g," designating "019g") had probably fallen off. In any case, bypass it, staying straight on the main road as it leads you past a metal gate.

RIDE 49 · Burnside Lake Out-and-Back

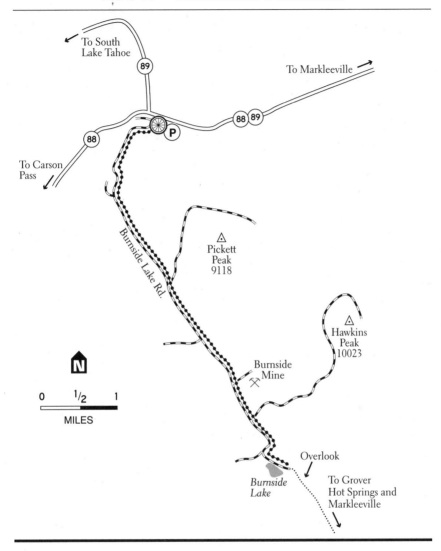

The climb steepens slightly in some stretches, especially where black asphalt patches have been placed on the road.

At nearly 2.9 miles, FS 053 peels off on your left. It's a lesser dirt road that leads up to Pickett Peak, a climb of over 1,400 feet. Continuing on FS 019 and the view of the granite face of Carson Ridge emerges on your right (west). It may still be patched with snow, clinging to its crevices. At about 3.6 miles, bypass signed FS 19h, an all-terrain road for motorbikes and jeeps taking off on your right. In less than 0.5 mile, the road crosses over a tiny creek and shortly thereafter, another lesser road leads off on your left. Continue past it to another little creek crossing. At 4.7 miles,

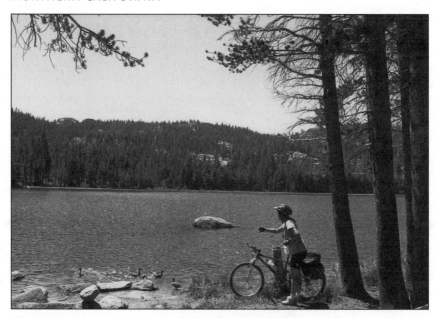

A peaceful, undeveloped alpine lake, mostly enjoyed by locals.

bypass another lesser road on your right. In a few yards, another road takes off on your left, signed "Dead End." (This is the road that leads to Hawkins Peak, elevation 10, 023 feet. It's worth exploring if you're up for the strenuous climb of about 1,400 feet in 3 to 4 miles.) Still following the main road, push on, bypassing yet another unsigned road on your right. After a couple of gentle turns, Burnside Lake comes into view. At 5.7 miles, you reach the eastern edge of the lake.

The Grover Hot Springs overlook is worth the extra 1-mile trek from the lake on a narrow single-track. The trail starts off easy but soon becomes more technical due to fallen trees, small boulders, and loose rocks in the trail, especially as you approach the point where the canyon opens up, revealing Markleeville and Grover Hot Springs far below. Beginners can bike and/or walk this short out-and-back stretch. To access the single-track trail, look for a humongous, lone-standing boulder sitting immediately next to the water's edge—it's marked by a faded white painted 11 and there's evidence of a campfire pit behind it. As you face south, looking at this boulder, turn directly left toward a small mound of rocks and boulder. The trail begins there, faintly leading over and around the boulders. After riding (or walking) up the mound, the trail levels and weaves through the shady forest, leading you over tiny creeks. Look for footbridges to keep your feet dry. Blazed trees help you stay on the trail. The understory becomes dense and the trail runs through a small marshy section. In a few yards, the terrain becomes strewn with huge boulders in between fewer mixed conifer trees. There may be storm-downed trees lying across the trail. At about a mile from the lake, you have a tremendous view looking into the valley below. The trail eventually begins to descend steeply through switchbacks and the terrain becomes a bit more rugged. Turn around and retrace your path back to the lake at any time.

From the overlook, expert riders can actually ride down to Grover Hot Springs where an end-shuttle should have been arranged prior to hitting the trail. The option is epic in portion and involves pedaling a loop on CA 89 and CA 88, two heavily traveled paved roads. If you decide to tackle this major loop, you need to be prepared with maps and food. More importantly, you should have expert technical skills as the descent from Burnside Lake to Grover is reportedly very rocky and steep, and the drop-offs are not for the faint of heart.

The return run back down to your car promises to be a nonstop, sweet and fast descent. Want more of a workout? Consider exploring any of the lesser roads that you bypassed along the way.

RIDE 50 · Genoa Road–TRT Loop

AT A GLANCE

Length/configuration: 16.2-mile loop (short loop: 8.6-mile loop), counterclockwise; jeep road and single-track

Aerobic difficulty: Strenuous, especially if you're not acclimated to the higher altitude. (Short loop: moderately strenuous.)

Technical difficulty: Advanced due to loose rocks, steepness and rough jeep roads. (Short loop: Intermediate with slightly less climbing.)

Scenery: Outstanding views of Lake Tahoe, especially from the Tahoe Rim Trail

Special comments: The loops can be ridden in any configuration, even as an out-and-back, turning around whenever you like. This route can be combined with The Flume–TRT Ride (Ride 51) for an epic outing. Also referred to as the Rim Trail and the TRT, portions of the 150-mile Tahoe Rim Trail are off-limits to bikes. Sections described in this ride permit bikes. Please obey all posted signs.

With the opening of the Tahoe Rim Trail to bikes, this already scenic ride on a rugged jeep road becomes even more spectacular with views of glorious Lake Tahoe throughout most of the ride. Throw in some twisty single-track through pine forested slopes spiced with dips and rises and you have a route that requires at least intermediate bike handling skills. Aerobically, even strong riders coming from the flatlands will find this route moderately strenuous. And there are mileage options, too. This 16.2-mile loop can be shorten to an 8.6-mile loop, a perfect bailout option if it's too arduous or technical, or if you have little time. But if you're a hard-core, highly skilled hammerhead aching for an all-day major epic adventure, consider combining this 16.2-mile loop with The Flume –TRT Ride via Spooner & Marlette Loop for a 40-plus-mile adventure—an incredible route that has you riding nearly the entire eastern length of Lake Tahoe. Strong beginners who are uncomfortable with narrow single-track riding can avoid the Tahoe Rim Trail by riding Genoa Peak Road, a wide rugged jeep road, as an out-and-back. Walking, of course, is always an option. Whatever configuration you choose and no matter how much effort you exert, this is classic Tahoe mountain biking.

General location: About 8 miles east of Stateline in South Lake Tahoe. The entire ride is in Nevada.

Elevation change: Starting elevation and low point 7,900 feet; high point 8,720 feet. First half climbs over uneven, rugged terrain of varying steepness. Second half descends through both gentle and abrupt dips. (Short loop: High point 8,400.)

Season: Early summer to late fall.

Services: None on the trail. All services in South Lake Tahoe and nearby communities, about 6 to 8 miles away.

Hazards: The TRT is a narrow single-track that sees lots of use so watch out for oncoming traffic by other bikers and hikers, especially during the last 5 miles leading back to the parking area. Genoa Peak Road is open to off-highway vehicles.

Rescue index: Since this is a popular biking and hiking route, especially on summer weekends, chances are good that you'll find other trail users who may be of assistance. During the week, late in the day, you can expect to meet local trail users who are out for an after-work ride or hike.

Land status: Lake Tahoe Basin Management Unit (a part of the USDA Forest Service).

Maps: *Recreation Map of Lake Tahoe,* published by Tom Harrison Maps, 2 Falmouth Cove, San Rafael, CA 94901, (800) 265-9090, www.tomharrisonmaps.com. USGS South Lake Tahoe and Glenbrook 7.5 minute series.

Finding the trail: Starting at the intersection of CA 89 and US 50 (also known as the Y) in South Lake Tahoe, head east on US 50 and into Nevada. Drive for about 5.9 miles, to the intersection with NV 207, Kingsbury Grade. Go right onto Kingsbury for 2.9 miles to North Benjamin Drive, then go left. Follow North Benjamin as it becomes Andria Drive. Stay on Andria until the pavement ends at a small dirt parking area, about 1.8 miles from Kingsbury. Park here. You immediately notice that the Tahoe Rim Trail and jeep road 13n80 run into this parking area. This loops begins on the jeep road, straight ahead, due north through the gate.

Sources of additional information:

U.S. Forest Service
Lake Tahoe Basin Management Unit
870 Emerald Bay Rd.
South Lake Tahoe, CA 96150
(916) 573-2600

Nevada State Parks
P.O. Box 8867
Incline Village, NV 89452
(702) 831-0494

Tahoe Rim Trail Association
P.O. Box 4647
Stateline, Nevada 89449
(775) 588-0686
TahoeRim@aol.com
www.tahoerimtrail.org

Notes on the trail: Begin by pedaling north through the gate, following the rough jeep road. Though it's not signed here, the jeep road is Forest Service Road 14N33 and is labeled as such on many topo maps. Throughout the loop, you're likely to see orange or aluminum-grey diamonds nailed high up on trees. They're cross-country skiing and snowmobiling markers and do not necessarily indicate the route being described here.

The first few yards of the ride is a rude welcome, subjecting you to a steep climb over rough and dusty terrain. If you're not accustomed to the altitude, don't be surprised to find yourself quickly gasping for air. Fortunately, the climb is short, leaving only the rugged road as your challenge. The climb mellows a bit and you soon begin enjoying the fresh mountain air. For the next half mile or so, bypass several other trails leading off of your main jeep road.

At about 0.9 miles, after a steep but short climb, the dirt road quickly descends into a small clearing surrounded by tall pine trees. There are lots of unsigned jeep and motorbike trails crisscrossing and radiating from the clearing and picking the correct path is not easy. As you descend the hill, look straight ahead, due west directly toward the lake. You see a trail leading away on the far side of the clearing almost directly straight ahead. This trail runs steeply up a berm, looking like a big launching pad to catch a lot of air. That's the continuation of the jeep road. Follow it and once over the berm, the road curves slightly north with the lake now on your left. Cruise downhill for about a half mile and go through a green gate.

At about 2 miles, amid views of the lake and the mouth of Emerald Bay on the far western shore, you reach a fork. There's an orange or aluminum-grey diamond and right-pointing arrow on a tree here. Take the right fork, following the arrow and gently descend. At about 3.7 miles, you reach another junction with a road leading off on your right; ignore it, staying straight. In a few yards, you come to the junction of another dirt road peeling off on the left, this time it's simply signed US Forest Route. Maps identify this as 14N33. (For those of you electing to do the shorter loop, this is your short cut. Turn left here and in 0.2 miles, turn left again, this time onto the signed Tahoe Rim Trail. The longer loop passes this point later at approximately 11 miles. From here, you reach the parking area in 4.8 miles, via a delightfully twisty, abruptly up and down single-track trail.)

Bypass the left road and in less than a mile, (4.5 miles from the start), you reach the intersection of the Genoa Peak Road leading off on your right. Looking for an expansive view of Lake Tahoe as well as Carson Valley to the east? Then tackle this half-mile road up to Genoa Peak sitting at 9,150 feet—a climb of about 480 feet over rugged and steep terrain. Otherwise, stay straight on the main road where the climb is more tame. At just over 5 miles, you reach the wide-open crest of a ridge near the top of South Camp Peak. The road levels as it leads around the southeast side of South Camp Peak. Look straight ahead down the jeep road through the trees and you can see Carson Valley lying below. Get ready: here comes a short but steep and rugged descent, losing almost 300 feet in less than 0.5 miles—guaranteed to challenge your bike-handling skills. The road soon mellows out, descending gradually through the forest until you reach the intersection with the Tahoe Rim Trail, roughly 2 miles from the open ridge near South Camp Peak (about 7.7 miles from the start).

Go left onto the TRT, a sweet single-track, and begin recovering the lost elevation. The trail loops back toward the south and after climbing just over 700 feet in almost 1.5 miles, you reach the high point of the loop on the western slope of South Camp Peak at approximately 8,720 feet. Take a breather and enjoy cruising the wide-open slope, taking in the views of magnificent Lake Tahoe and the surrounding mountain ridges. A little over 2 miles farther (3.7 miles from where you hopped onto the TRT and just over 11 miles from the start), you reach the intersection with FS 14N33, though it's not signed as such here. (This is the short cut that the shorter loop uses.) Continue across the road, staying on the TRT.

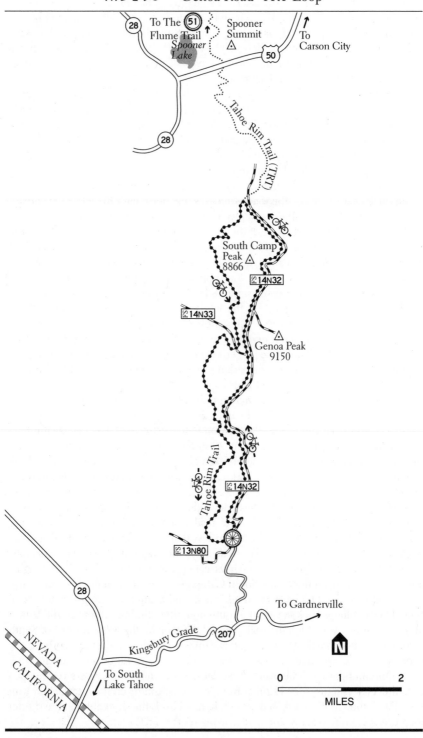

For the next 4.8 miles to the parking area, the TRT threads through forested slopes, traversing through numerous tiny ravines. Be alert for oncoming bikers and hikers, especially since the narrow trail is punctuated with twisty ups and downs, weaving around boulders and blind curves. Go through an intersection, staying on the TRT and in a short distance you reach the parking area. Total distance is about 16.2 miles. (The shorter loop is about 8.6 miles.)

RIDE 51 · The Flume–TRT Ride

AT A GLANCE

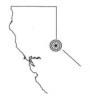

Length/configuration: 22-mile out-and-back with a loop, clockwise only; dirt roads, single- and double-tracks. (Options exist for shorter and longer rides.)

Aerobic difficulty: Very strenuous due to length, elevation gain, and altitude. (The first 9.2 miles is only moderately strenuous and can be ridden as an out-and-back.)

Technical difficulty: Intermediate due to narrow, exposed single-track riding along deep drop-offs and rough terrain particularly on the return half of the ride. (Options exist for advanced terrain.)

Scenery: Views of Lake Tahoe, Marlette Lake, and the Carson Valley. The Flume Trail portion skirts a mountainside that rises immediately up from the east shoreline of turquoise-blue Lake Tahoe.

Special comments: The stretch from the starting point at Spooner State Park to Marlette Lake where the Flume Trail actually begins, is suitable for strong beginners. The Flume Trail itself, however, is not recommended for beginners and other riders who are fearful of heights, especially while on narrow, exposed single-track trails that skirt deep drop-offs. Can be combined with the Genoa Road–TRT Loop (Ride 50).

Arguably the best mountain bike route in the west, the Flume Trail has been featured on postcards and in a gazillion bicycle publications. But, this ride's popularity almost contradicts the claim. During the summer, this loop is likened to a crowded freeway. But in early May or late October-November, when the hordes of vacationing crowds have left town, it's easy to understand why the Flume–TRT Ride is a strong contender for the title. This 22-mile ride has a lot to offer. Like gorgeous sweeping views of Lake Tahoe. Peaceful lakes where bald eagles soar from tree to tree. Thrilling single-track that clings precariously to a steep, exposed slope, bordered by deep drop-offs. Heart-pounding climbs through forests of aspens and conifers. Boulder fields and switchbacks. The terrain is well-suited for intermediate-level riders. If you have a hankering for an all-day outing that's exhilarating for the body and soul, this is the ride for you.

The first five miles of the ride from Spooner Lake to Marlette Lake climbs basically smooth dirt roads. From Marlette Lake, the next portion rides the famous Flume Trail, a single-track that desperately hugs the mountain slope as it twists and turns around boulders and blind curves. Portions of the trail may require you to portage your bike a couple yards. After riding the Flume to its northern terminus at Tunnel Creek Road, the next 4.5 miles partakes of the awesome Tahoe Rim Trail, a single-track that climbs up to the highest point of the ride and weaves through boulder fields hidden in the forest. (Also referred to as the Rim Trail and the TRT, portions of the 150-mile Tahoe Rim Trail are off-limits to bikes. Sections described in this ride and elsewhere in this chapter permit bikes. Please obey all posted signs.) The TRT then descends toward Marlette Lake where it intersects a dirt road and closes the loop. After that, it's a sweet descent back to Spooner Lake.

Up until 1997, the TRT in this area was originally deemed off-limits to mountain bikers by its primary creator, the Friends of the Tahoe Rim Trail, an all-volunteer, nonprofit organization which spearheads the 150-mile trail construction in conjunction with the U.S. Forest Service and the Nevada Division of State Parks. Signs prohibiting bikes were posted but the sheer beauty and joy of riding this gorgeous single-track trail didn't deter cyclists. Enforcing the no-bikes rule was nearly impossible. Add to that the fact that trail-maintenance days organized by the Friends sometimes attracted more bikers than hikers. And so, after a short trial period, this section of the TRT was officially opened to bikers. Prior to this, riders of the famous Spooner-to–the Flume Trail route either pedaled it as a 18.4 mile out-and-back (9.2 mile each way), or point-to-point with shuttle in the Sand Harbor vicinity. Moderately strong riders who didn't set up a shuttle car used to make a loop by riding back to their parked car via paved NV 28 for 9 miles (not a pleasant stretch due to heavy traffic and narrow shoulders). An option enjoyed by stronger riders was making an all-dirt loop via the steep jeep roads to the east of the Flume Trail, passing Red House and Hobart Creek Reservoir—a 23-plus-mile loop back to their parked car. Today, you can still ride any of these configurations, adding all the miles and adventures your climbing legs and lungs will allow. And now, with the opening of the TRT to bikes, more outstanding single-track riding is added to this already classic ride.

General location: East shore of Lake Tahoe.

Elevation change: 2,260 feet; starting elevation and low point 6,940 feet; high point 8,800 feet. Mixed terrain of flat stretches and ups and downs; moderately steep, sustained climb and a long coasting descent.

Season: Late spring to mid-fall, or until the first big winter snow storm hits. Autumn colors, golden after sunlight low on the horizon, and the lack of crowds make October and early November the ideal time to enjoy this ride.

Services: None on the trail. Water, rest room, and picnic tables at Spooner Lake State Park. A small parking fee required to park in the state park. All services in Incline Village or South Lake Tahoe.

Hazards: During the summer months, trail use by bikers and hikers is the heaviest. Passing other bikers and oncoming traffic requires extreme caution and alertness, especially while riding the Flume Trail, a narrow and twisty path with blind curves. If you decide to complete the loop via NV 28, be aware that the shoulder is narrow and the automobile traffic can be heavy at times. If you intend on riding the Flume Trail as a point-to-point, parking near Tunnel Creek Road is extremely limited and you may be force to park your end-shuttle at Sand Harbor, which means you'll be riding almost 2 miles on the narrow shoulders of NV 28.

Rescue index: Since this is a popular route in the summer, you're sure to find help from other trail users. In the off-season, though, you need to be self-reliant. (When

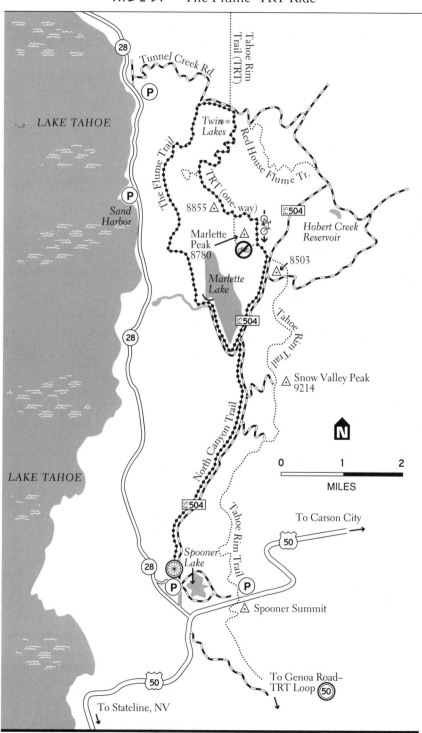

we rode this trail in mid-October, we didn't see a soul.) The northern end of the ride borders the Ponderosa Ranch (a tourist joint) as well as a few residential homes and you might be able to find help there. Your chances of flagging down a passing motorist on NV 28 are very good. During the summer, Spooner Lake State Park rangers frequently patrol the area.

Land status: Spooner Lake State Park, Lake Tahoe Nevada State Park, Lake Tahoe Basin Management Unit, and Toiyabe National Forest.

Maps: *Recreation Map of Lake Tahoe,* published by Tom Harrison Maps, 2 Falmouth Cove, San Rafael, CA 94901, (800) 265-9090, www.tomharrisonmaps.com. USGS Marlette Lake and Glenbrook 7.5 minute series.

Finding the trail: From Incline Village on the north shore of Lake Tahoe, follow NV 28 around to the east side of the lake. Drive 10 miles south on NV 28, passing Tunnel Creek Road at about 1.5 miles and Sand Harbor at 3.5 miles. You reach Spooner State Park at about 10 miles. Turn left into the park, pass the entrance pay booth, and park here. If you reach US 50, you've gone too far. For point-to-point shuttle riders, park your end-shuttle car alongside NV 28, just south of the Ponderosa Ranch, near Tunnel Creek Road (very limited parking on shoulder). A better place to park is at Sand Harbor picnic grounds (small fee required), about 2 miles south of Tunnel Creek Road on NV 28 (although bear in mind that you'll have to pedal the pavement and put up with the traffic). For the advanced option, park at Spooner Summit by continuing past the Spooner State Park entrance, turning left onto US 50 and in less than a mile, park at the summit where the Tahoe Rim Trail intersects the road.

Sources of additional information:

U.S. Forest Service
Lake Tahoe Basin Management Unit
870 Emerald Bay Rd.
South Lake Tahoe, CA 96150
(916) 573-2600

Nevada State Parks
P.O. Box 8867
Incline Village, NV 89452
(702) 831-0494

Tahoe Rim Trail Association
P.O. Box 4647
Stateline, Nevada 89449
(775) 588-0686
TahoeRim@aol.com
www.tahoerimtrail.org

Notes on the trail: Before you hit the trail, consider bringing a camera because the stretch along the Flume Trail is like no other! It really is that spectacular, especially on a sunny day.

From the Spooner Lake parking lot, begin pedaling north through the lot, descending a short dirt single-track trail to the beginning of North Canyon Trail. A big brown sign marks the trailhead along with mileages to various destinations. The North Canyon Trail starts off as a narrow, smooth, semi-packed dirt road and cruises through an open meadow, heading north toward Marlette Lake. As you leave the meadow, the gradual climb begins, taking you past stands of aspen, conifers, and deciduous trees. Stay on the main, well-traveled dirt road, bypassing other roads leading from it. At almost a mile from the trailhead, you reach a white metal gate and a Lake Tahoe–Nevada State Park bulletin board. Here, another jeep road peels off on the left. Continue past the bulletin board due north, ignoring the left road.

At about 2.7 miles, having climbed nearly 670 feet, you reach the signed intersection with a trail leading off on your right toward the North Canyon campground. Bypass it, staying on the main road and keep heading due north. The climb eventually steepens to about 9% grade. At about 3.7 miles, Snow Valley Peak Trail intersects your road. Continue straight, still climbing on North Canyon and in a few yards, you catch your first glimpse of Marlette Lake through the trees.

At just under 4 miles, after huffing and puffing up 1,175 feet since the start, the trail gives you a break and begins a short but welcome descent to the southern edge of the lake. You reach the lake at about 5 miles. North Canyon Trail ends at a sort of T intersection, across from the interpretive signs. Take a breather and check out these signboards planted next to the lake. From these signs, you'll learn that mining activity in the Virginia City region north of here motivated the construction of a 4.5-mile flume to transport much needed water. Today, not much of the flume remains along the now popular Flume Trail. Adding color to the local history is Jack Ferguson, the flumekeeper and lone resident at Marlette Lake who, in 1948–1953, built a 48-foot ocean-worthy vessel here, high in the Sierras. In 1957, the land was acquired by the Curtis Wright Corporation with intentions to use the lake as a missile test site. In 1963, the State of Nevada took over the land and eventually deemed it the crown jewel in its Lake Tahoe–Nevada State Park system.

After your educational break, hop back on your bike and begin the loop portion of the ride. The direction is clockwise. Follow the dirt road leading south from the signs to the dam and the Flume Trail. (The road coming in from the north is your return route.) The road you're following is level and follows the edge of the lake, heading south, then west. In less than 1.5 miles from the interpretive signs, you reach small Marlette Dam. The smooth road ends here and the Flume Trail begins. (Beginners who are unaccustomed to narrow single-tracks and steep drop-offs should turn around here.) Look for a signed single-track trail that descends over rocky terrain. Cross Marlette Creek. You may have to portage your bike along the water's edge to reach the beginning of the trail.

For the next 4.5 miles, the breath-taking Flume Trail weaves around boulders and skirts steep drop-offs, all the while cruising at a consistent 7,680 feet. The sweeping views of Lake Tahoe are truly spectacular and in some exposed sections, you feel as if you can dive right into the crystal blue lake. But stay alert: The trail is narrow, just barely enough room for two cyclists to pass, and the huge boulders combined with twisty turns often obscure oncoming traffic until you're nearly face-to-face. The Flume Trail can be ridden in both directions, while the following portion of the TRT is one-way.

At about 10 miles from the Spooner State Park, the Flume Trail ends, intersecting unsigned Tunnel Creek Road, a dirt road. (Here's where the options come into play: If you have arranged a shuttle car near here, turn left here toward Lake Tahoe. Follow Tunnel Creek Road as it descends over sometimes loose, sandy terrain, and through several wide switchbacks. In just over 3 miles, you approach the Ponderosa Ranch and intersect NV 28. If you've parked your end-shuttle at Sand Harbor, cautiously turn left onto NV 28 and pedal the shoulder for about 2 miles to your car. If your car is back at Spooner State Park, you can either pedal NV 28 for about 9 miles or hop on the TART bus which will stop at the state park. Look for the appropriate bus stop near the entrance to the Ponderosa Ranch, just north of Tunnel Creek Road on NV 28. Another option is to simply turn around and retrace your path.)

Intermediate and advanced riders, turn right onto Tunnel Creek Road and head east away from Lake Tahoe. The wide dirt road leads you underneath a power line,

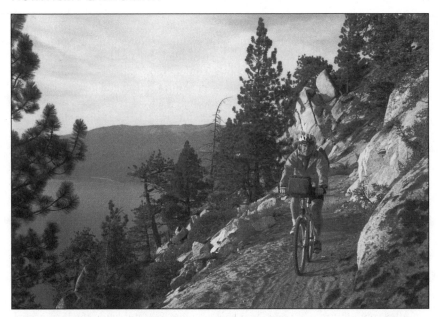

What puts a grin on Bruce's face? The stunning views of Lake Tahoe as seen from the Flume Trail, a level single-track just wide enough for one cyclist. And thanks to the time of year, he has the trail all to himself.

then up a short hill. Descend the fast but short hill and in less than 0.5 mile from the Flume Trail, go past the signed Tahoe Rim Trail which peels off on your left. A few yards farther, you reach another junction where the TRT leads off on your right. Hang a right onto the TRT, toward Twin Lakes and head south. From this point, the TRT is one-way for the next 5 miles. Get psyched because the very strenuous task of climbing almost 1,200 feet begins. The elevation gain may not sound like much but if you're not accustomed to the higher altitude, your ticker is sure to feel it on this return portion of the loop.

At this point here's an option for all you advanced riders: Stay on Tunnel Creek Road, bypassing the TRT about 0.5 miles farther to Red House Flume Trail. Make a right onto Red House Flume and follow the single-track due south and then southeast toward Red House and Hobart Creek Reservoir. This sweet, intermediate section rolls along on the ridge before intersecting a jeep road in about 2 miles at the Red House. Portage the dam and Red House Flume Trail becomes FS 186. After approximately 0.5 miles on 186, turn right onto FS 504 and follow it for almost 2 miles to its intersection with the TRT, just south of Marlette Peak. Advanced riders can go left onto the TRT and continue the technically challenging terrain, reaching Spooner Summit and US 50 in almost 8.5 miles. Or, if you've had enough of the tough terrain, stay on FS 186 and enjoy a fast and technically easy descent to Marlette Lake and North Canyon Trail, where you rejoin the ride description as follows.

Assuming you're a mere mortal like most of us intermediates, turn right onto the TRT and head south. The trail is level and wide but the condition is a bit sandy. Persevere. Walking through the somewhat deep but small patch of sand works just fine. Follow the signs to Twin Lakes, still on the TRT south trail. Stay on the dirt road (the TRT), bypassing other jeep roads as you skirt Lower and Upper Twin Lakes (actually, two tiny intermittent lakes that may resemble huge ponds in the summer). The trail narrows as it begins to steepen, becoming more technical with semi-buried boulders in the trail. For the next 2.4 miles, the TRT continues its unrelenting uphill march through several wide switchbacks. Some of the boulders planted in the trail are humongous, forcing most riders to portage every now and then.

At about 13.3 miles, you reach the Sand Harbor Overlook near Herlan Peak. You've ascended almost 900 feet in 2.8 miles since hopping onto the TRT from Tunnel Creek Road. When you reach this point, you can take a well-deserved break, knowing that most of the tough climbing is behind you. Check out the view of Sand Harbor and all of Lake Tahoe by walking to the top of the hill (the trail is fragile and a sign asks that you walk your bike). Back on the TRT, continue heading south and in less than a mile, there's another side trail peeling off toward Lake Tahoe, about 200 yards over a treeless mound. At the top of this mound, you have a virtually unobstructed view of the Lake Tahoe and Marlette Lake as well as the Carson Valley in the east. Wow! A view of two lakes for the price of one, and a valley to boot!

Continue on the TRT toward Marlette Peak. At approximately 14.5 miles, the trail forks. A sign directs bikers to the east side of Marlette Peak, hikers to the west, and also warns that violators will be fined $100. Honor the sign, taking the left fork and after 0.7 miles of weaving through a conifer forest, the split trail rejoins on the south side of Marlette Peak. At 15.6 miles, the TRT converges with a mess of other trails in a small clearing. Advanced riders can continue on the TRT toward Spooner Summit and US 50. The rest of us mortals take the well-traveled dirt road leading south and down the east side of Marlette Lake. Go silently and slowing here. Keep a sharp eye out, especially focusing on the top of snags (dead, bare but still standing trees)—you might get lucky and spot a bald eagle.

In just over a mile, at 16.7 miles from your start at Spooner State Park, you close the loop on the southeast side of Marlette, near the interpretive signs. From here, retrace your path on North Canyon Trail and enjoy an easy, 5-mile downhill cruise back to your car. The speed limit for bikes is 20 mph and rangers do patrol the area. But that's OK: Keeping the speed of your trusty two-wheel steed in check lets you prolong the aura of a truly great day of riding. Savor it as you float down this last run to your car.

RIDE 52 · TRT: Big Meadows to Kingsbury Grade

AT A GLANCE

Length/configuration: 27.5-mile point-to-point (or 41.5-mile loop, counterclockwise); mostly single-track with some dirt roads and paved roads (both well-traveled and abandoned roads)

Aerobic difficulty: Very strenuous due to distance, elevation and rugged terrain

Technical difficulty: Mostly strong intermediate with some very advanced sections; boulder staircases; narrow, exposed trail; good trail-finding skills required.

Scenery: Awesome. Gorgeous alpine meadows and lakes, wildflowers, terrific views of the Tahoe Basin including Lake Tahoe, Carson Valley, Great Basin, peaks of surrounding wilderness areas, glacier-carved canyons, and high mountain passes.

Special comments: Not recommended for beginners. This is an all-day affair. Shorter out-and-back rides from either ends of the Tahoe Rim Trail are possible. Occasional summer electrical thunderstorms . Several bail-out options exist that shorten the ride considerably but they're both intense, advanced-level trails.

G ot a jones for a big, all-day epic ride around the Tahoe Basin that's technically challenging as well as incredibly scenic? How does a 27.5-mile point-to-point with 22.5 miles of awesome single-track on the Tahoe Rim Trail at elevations close to the 10,000 feet sound? And from that altitude, think of the stunning vistas of far away peaks, lush alpine meadows dotted with wildflowers, deep glacial canyons and valleys, and windswept mountain passes. How about weaving up, down, or through gardens of monolithic granite boulders, thick stands of fragrant pine forests, spiced with occasional panoramic views of Lake Tahoe, and thrillingly exposed, cliff-hugging sections along a narrow ridge? Look no further: this ride is it. Also referred to as the Rim Trail and the TRT, portions of the 150-mile Tahoe Rim Trail are off-limits to bikes. Sections described in this ride and elsewhere in this chapter permit bikes. Please obey all posted signs. Of all the sections of the Tahoe Rim Trail system (TRT) open to bikes, this is the longest, continuous stretch of single-track.

Peter Underwood, one of the owners of Olympic Bike Shop, the oldest, most established dealer and repair service in the north shore area, brought this adventure to my attention. If you're staying around north Lake Tahoe, Peter claims it's worth the 45-minute drive down to the south shore because this is one of the best rides in the entire Tahoe Basin. But this is not for beginners or recreational riders with only basic technical skills or for the once-a-month cyclist. "We recommend this ride to those people looking for a big adventure and are not afraid of getting away from the roads in order to do a little reconnaissance with maps and route finding once in a while. They have to have good survival sense and good mechanical skills because there aren't any real quick bail-outs." He goes further to say "Definitely not a two PowerBar® ride. This is a giant deli sandwich kind of ride because you'll be burning lots of calories." That said, you'll need to bring plenty of long-burning energy food. As for water, you can do one of three solutions: lug enough water, which means gallons. Or take your chances and drink from a number of quality, ice cold alpine creeks and springs. "I've been drinking it for years and have not had any problems with it," declares Peter. Or, if you're tentative about that, bring along a backpacker's water filter system or those dreaded iodine pills.

Because this route leads to elevations and exposed ridges where electrical storms do occur, riders need to be constantly mindful of that potentially dangerous situation. Several bail-out trails exist that shorten the ride considerably but they're intensively technical and require advanced-level skills—not exactly a quick escape hatch. Regarding rain, you might get lucky and endure a momentary drizzle. However, hypothermia is a very real possibility and riding at high altitudes only increases the risk. Avoiding this life-threatening situation starts with proper clothing. Peter urges all cyclists to wear only synthetic garments. "No cotton!" You'll be perspiring heavily on this ride which means if you're sporting a cotton T-shirt or sweatshirt, it'll be soaking. Combine a cold, wet, clammy, heavy cotton shirt with fast, wind-chilling descents and you can quickly become hypothermic. So, no cotton anything, not even cotton socks. A waterproof windbreaker is worth carrying, even if the day is clear and hot. This route, after all, takes place around 10,000 feet, give or take.

Regarding the best time to ride, there's a small window of opportunity during the year in which to enjoy this adventure. Because the elevation and north-facing slopes and canyons hold snow well into the summer, this ride doesn't usually open up until August, maybe as early as July and into September, depending on the intensity of the preceding winter or the occurrence of Indian summer, respectively. Even if you're super-human, it's a good idea to start early in the day. Fall is not a good time to ride for most cyclists because there's not enough hours of daylight for the entire loop. But if you do ride in the fall, even with a shuttle arrangement, remember that the sun sets early and temperatures then drop quickly, so allow plenty of time, particularly for the slowest person in your group. Don't ride solo. (Carrying a cell phone doesn't qualify as a riding buddy. See the discussion about cell phones in the Introduction.) Be prepared in the event you must spend the night out on the trail—among other items, matches or a lighter can be a life-saver.

Several routing options are available. You can shorten this ride to a 22-mile point-to-point by eliminating a warm-up section on a partially abandoned paved road (South Upper Truckee Road). Both long and short point-to-point configurations require a two-car shuttle arrangement. If you're a bionic rider, you can hammer yourself by riding a 41.5-mile loop, which includes an 8-mile stretch on Pioneer Trail, a well-traveled paved road. Consider too, the idea of riding an out-and-back configuration from either end of the Rim Trail, turning around when you've had enough. Big Meadows Trailhead to Freel Pass is a 25.6-mile out-and-back (12.8 miles each way). Kingsbury Grade to Star Lake is about 17.6-mile out-and-back (8.8 miles each way).

In the event that mechanical problems, inclement weather, or an emergency force you to bail-out, two trails offer a shorter, albeit technically challenging way back down into South Lake Tahoe (Mr. Toad's Wild Ride/Saxon Creek Trail and Fountain Place Road). If your car is down at the junction of CA 50 and CA 89 (the suggested starting point of this description), you can reach it in record time by descending the narrow shoulder on busy CA 89, though you'll have to share the road with speeding motorists.

All that said, are you still up for the challenge? All your huffin' and puffin' and cussin' and discussin' is well-worth the effort, according to Peter. This ride quite possibly may surpass the grandeur of the famed Flume Trail on the east shore (Ride 51); at the very least, it will definitely have far fewer trail users. Sincere thanks to Peter and Olympic Bike Shop for contributing trail notes for this ride.

General location: South Lake Tahoe.

Elevation change: 3,860 feet; starting elevation 6,400 feet; high point 10,160 feet; low point 6,300 feet. Lots of ascents and descents throughout the Rim Trail.

Season: Late July to September, depending on the intensity of the previous winter and when the autumn's first snowstorm hits. Since this is easily an all-day ride for strong riders, this adventure requires an early start, especially in the fall.

Services: Limited parking near the KOA campground near the beginning of Old Luther Pass Road (also known as South Upper Truckee Road). At the Big Meadows trailhead, rest rooms and limited parking are available but water is not. Bring plenty of water. Though locals swear that the water from streams and springs found along the trail between Armstrong Pass and Star Lake is safe for drinking, do so at your own

RIDE 52 · TRT: Big Meadows to Kingsbury Grade

risk. If you're skeptical, bring a water filter or iodine for treating before consumption. All services can be found in greater South Lake Tahoe.

Hazards: If you're riding the entire loop, expect lots of vehicular traffic on well-traveled Kingsbury Grade, Pioneer Trail (a paved road), US 50, and also when crossing CA 89 at several places. Stay alert for on-coming traffic from other trail users on the narrow Tahoe Rim Trail. Most of the Rim Trail traverses a high ridge so be mindful of changes in the weather as electrical storms do occur. Dress appropriately in synthetics and be sure to bring a windbreaker. Be prepared for an unexpected night out in the woods.

Rescue index: The Tahoe Rim Trail stretch of this ride traverses through steep and remote territory. Though there are several challenging bail-out trails, (Mr. Toad's Wild Ride/Saxon Creek Trail and Fountain Place Road), the bulk of the Rim Trail is not easily accessible by emergency help. That said, you need to be self-reliant, which means know how to repair your bike, which also means know how to use appropriate tools. Do not ride solo. In case of a medical emergency, a buddy can go for help. Be prepared, however, for self-evacuation should inclement weather compromise you or your group's safety. If you're not too far from the Big Meadows Trailhead of the TRT, retreating to CA 89 in order to flag down a passing motorist for emergency help is a good option.

Land status: Eldorado National Forest, Toiyabe National Forest, Lake Tahoe Basin Management Unit.

Maps: *Recreation Map of Lake Tahoe,* published by Tom Harrison Maps, 2 Falmouth Cove, San Rafael, CA 94901, (800) 265-9090, www.tomharrisonmaps.com. *South Lake Tahoe Basin Recreation Topo Map,* published by Fine Edge Productions.

Finding the trail: From the Y in South Lake Tahoe (the intersection of US 50 and CA 89), travel south on US 50/CA 89 (they're one and the same along this stretch), going past the airport and the agricultural inspections station along the way. Proceed through the town of Meyers to the junction with CA 89 (also known as "New" Luther Pass Road). Continue past CA 89, staying on US 50 for a short distance and park in the vicinity of the KOA and Tahoe Pines Campgrounds. The ride begins on South Upper Truckee Road, (also known as "Old" Luther Pass Road), a lightly used paved residential road located between Tahoe Pines and KOA.

If you plan to ride this route as a point-to-point, leave your end-shuttle vehicle at either the parking lot next to the Heavenly Valley Stagecoach ski lift off NV 207 (Kingsbury Grade), somewhere along NV 207, or in Stateline (preferably next to one of those all-you-can-eat buffets in a casino—you'll be famished after this ride). To reach the Heavenly-Stagecoach parking lot from the California side: Starting at the intersection of the Y (CA 89 and US 50) in South Lake Tahoe, head northeast on US 50 and into Nevada, passing the casinos in Stateline along the way. About 5.9 miles from the Y, go right onto Kingsbury Grade (NV 207). Travel about 3 miles to Daggett Pass, going past North Benjamin Drive along the way. Keep an eye out for Tramway Drive on the south side of the road. Turn right onto Tramway, proceed through Jack Drive and towards the Stagecoach Lodge. Follow Tramway into Tahoe Village. Watch for a sign that reads "Ridge Tahoe Heavenly Stagecoach" which directs you to the parking lot next to the ski lift named Stagecoach. The Rim Trail is adjacent to the ski lift. Leave your end-shuttle here. From the Nevada side, follow Kingsbury Grade west towards California and Daggett Pass. After Daggett, turn left onto Tramway Drive and follow the directions described above.

Sources of additional information:

U.S. Forest Service
Lake Tahoe Basin Management Unit
870 Emerald Bay Rd.
South Lake Tahoe, CA 96150
(916) 573-2600; (916) 573-2674

Tahoe Rim Trail Association
P.O. Box 4647
Stateline, Nevada 89449
(775) 588-0686
TahoeRim@aol.com
www.tahoerimtrail.org

KOA Campground; (916) 577-3693. Tahoe Pines Campground & R.V. Park; (916) 577-1658

Two separate private campgrounds, located within a half mile of each other in South Lake Tahoe, at the junction of CA 50 and 89. Neither are especially lovely campgrounds, but hey, they offer hot showers and are, for the most part, at the beginning of this ride. That means if you plan to tackle the 41.5-mile loop, camping here gives you an early start—just roll out of your sleeping bag, climb into the saddle of your trusty two-wheel steed, and start pedaling.

Olympic Bike Shop
620 N. Lake Blvd.
Tahoe City, CA 96145
(530) 581-2500

In addition to sales, service, and being a great source for local bicycling information, Olympic offers an amazing selection of rentals, from basic, quality models to exotic, full-suspension bicycles.

Notes on the trail: From the KOA/Tahoe Pines campground area, hop onto South Upper Truckee Road (also known as "Old" Luther Pass Road), located between the two campgrounds and begin pedaling south. The next 4 to 5 miles follows this lightly-used paved road. Portions are closed to vehicles as it passes through a residential neighborhood and lovely old ranch. Sections lead through private property but through-access is allowed so long as you stay on the road. South Upper Truckee Road ascends moderately, giving you a good warm-up before tackling the rigorous Tahoe Rim Trail. At about 4.5 miles, the abandoned road you're savoring leads you across busy CA 89. Continue on the paved road (closed to vehicles) and in about a mile, after an approximate 900-foot gain from US 50, you reach the Big Meadows Trailhead of the Rim Trail parking area. (If you want to skip the warm-up on South Upper Truckee, you can park your car here at Big Meadows and immediately begin climbing difficult terrain on the TRT.)

Get ready. Here comes 22.5 miles of incredible single-track. The first 1.8 miles of the Rim Trail climbs and rolls, steadily gaining elevation on its way to the Grass Lake on-ramp (that is, another trail off CA 89 that accesses the TRT). Continue past the on-ramp heading basically east.

The next 2.5 miles or so to Tucker Flat will test your bike-handling ability. Along this stretch, the Rim Trail is spiced with staircases of granite boulders and some switchbacks, all while climbing over rugged terrain. It's more or less rideable, depending on your technical level. You reach Tucker Flat when you see a sign designating Saxon Creek Trail, more fondly known as Mr. Toad's Wild Ride leading off on your left. This is the first bail-out opportunity. Bear in mind that Mr. Toad's is indeed a wild ride, classified as advanced-level, very technical terrain.

From Tucker Flat, the next 4.7 miles climbs for about the first half—super-humans will be able to pedal it, the rest of us may have to walk a bit. Unique perspectives of Desolation and Mokelumne Wilderness Areas and Hope Valley temper the burning in your legs. On this stretch, one of the rewards for your efforts thus far comes in the way of Freel Meadows, a stunningly beautiful alpine meadow lying at almost 9,400 feet. Because the ground is almost always wet, the meadow stays green well into the fall, often accompanied by a dazzling display of wildflowers. Deep within the meadows is a very uniformly circular shaped warm spring, about 10 to 15 feet in diameter and graced by almost milk-blue water. The surrounding is inspiring, but before you can break out into song like Julie Andrews in *The Sound of Music*, bugs will likely chase you away or make a meal of you. You can probably out-pedal the pesky critters since the Rim Trail becomes quite rideable again.

The single-track continues its temper, rolling along as it gradually climbs to a little over 9,400 feet. Shortly after Freel Meadows, the trail creeps up a fairly narrow ridge, though you wouldn't know you're on such a precipitous spot unless you walked to the edge of the cliff. Along this stretch, there's an exceptional vista point of Hell Hole and the Tahoe Basin that is worth seeking. Watch for tire tracks that lead off the Rim Trail for about 10 to 15 feet. Hell Hole, sitting deep below the trail, is a beautiful glacial cirque (a steep hollow scoured by glaciers) that's graced by lush, green alpine meadows.

Here comes your next reward: a steep descent towards Armstrong Pass which sits at about 9,000 feet. When you reach a major intersection of trails, you're at Armstrong Pass. The single-track trail coming up on the left is Fountain Place Road. It's the second bail-out option and it drops into South Lake Tahoe. Keep this option in mind because if there's to be an electrical storm, it's likely to occur along this stretch of the Rim Trail. (Incidentally, starting from town, locals like to ride Fountain Place up to this point, then hang a right onto the Rim Trail and then descend Mr. Toad's for a gnarly loop—something else to keep in mind if you're looking for more technically challenging terrain, on another day, of course.)

The next stretch between Armstrong Pass and Freel Pass is about 3 miles and is probably the most difficult segment of the entire ride, due to the combination of climbing, high elevation, and loose sand under your wheels. In fact, Freel Peak is like a huge sand pile, peaking at 10,881 feet, which also makes it the highest peak in the entire Tahoe Basin. The Rim Trail zigzags at a fairly steep pitch, climbing up the southwestern flank of Freel, completely exposed to the sun and the elements. Take a breather and check out the landscape behind you. You can really get a sense of how far you've pedaled as you look south by southwest towards Luther Pass. Numerous crystal-clear springs and creeks run off the mountain amid a welcoming garden of wildflowers. This is a good place to refill your bottles and the ice cold, pure water up here is reportedly potable. Still, if you're apprehensive, treat it with a water filter or iodine tablets before consuming. At about 16 miles from your starting point at the bottom near the KOA, you finally reach Freel Pass, the high point of the ride at about 10,160 feet. The pass sits on a saddle between Freel Peak and Trimmer Peak (9,915 feet) in the northwest.

From Freel Pass to Star Lake, the Rim Trail leads you on a roller coaster ride for almost 2 miles, mostly descending through a glacial cirque and into the woods again. Water sources are available on this stretch to the lake and this is your last chance to refill your bottles. When you reach Star Lake, you are essentially 8.8 miles from Kingsbury Grade. Ringed by evergreen trees, this pristine blue, glacial lake is a terrific picnic spot and an exhilarating swimming hole on a hot summer day. Though this lovely lake is still recovering from years of abuse by off-road vehicles, it's worth taking time out to explore. When you're ready to leave Star Lake, you'll discover the Rim Trail is a bit difficult to find. The trail gets lost in the thicket as it crosses the outlet of the lake but keep looking—it's there, basically on the other side of the creek near the mouth of the lake.

From Star Lake, the trail continues its roller coaster attitude for about 3.5 miles towards Monument Pass. Though Monument Peak sits at 10,067 feet, you can breathe easy because you won't be climbing it. Instead, the Rim Trail leads you around, across, and slightly up the peak's eastern flank towards the pass. At Monument Pass, the trail leads you out of the Tahoe Basin and into the Great Basin. You begin to get glimpses of the Carson Valley below at approximately 4,600 feet, a difference of 4,400 feet. The views are terrific and lingering here is worth it. Welcome to Nevada: you cross the state line about a half mile from the pass.

The segment between Monument Pass (9,000 feet) and Kingsbury Grade (7,300 feet) is about 5.5 miles. You will ultimately lose roughly 1,700 feet in that distance. The Rim Trail begins descending towards Kingsbury, punctuated by plenty of rigorous ups and downs. The vista changes dramatically and you feel like you're hanging out over the Carson Valley. It's a strange sensation, as if you're about to fall into the valley at any moment. Your senses are tantalized further because the direction in which the Rim Trail descends might make you feel a bit discombobulated as it threads through switchbacks. It may seem like you're on the wrong trail, dropping down into the Carson Valley instead of continuing north. Fortunately, the Rim Trail makes a hard left at the base of the switchbacks and continues down toward Kingsbury.

Just enjoy the ride and let your senses be entertained. The trail leads you through two beautiful canyons carved by winter avalanches on the east slope of Monument Peak and East Peak. In fact, if you've ever skied the back bowls of Heavenly Valley, you may recognize the terrain along this stretch—the Rim Trail is the boundary for the ski resort. As you and the trail zigzag in and out of the wooded canyons above Carson Valley, the path seems to just fall off the mountain and into space at times. This illusion is especially magnified if you're riding behind another biker. Kind of like the feeling you get as a passenger on one of those little, zippy "Mighty Mouse" roller coasters, when the car you're riding approaches a tight turn except there doesn't seem to be anymore track and you think you're going to shoot off the end and into space. The trail is gorgeous, weaving through mature pine forests alongside very steep slopes. Some spots receive only brief sunshine, never really experiencing summer. If you're to see snow on this ride, this is usually the place, even well into August.

The Rim Trail drops you into Mott Canyon and eventually to the base of Heavenly's Mott Canyon chairlift. Welcome back to civilization. At this point, the Rim Trail follows a service road, which can be unpleasantly rough to pedal because tractors pulverize the dirt into moon dust. It's a bear to ride. Consider yourself lucky if a recent rainstorm settles the dust, making the trail condition behave itself. Follow this service road for less than a half mile and keep a sharp eye out for the Rim Trail peeling off on your right.

Hop onto the Rim Trail and follow it as it begins a wild, roller-coaster descent, punctuated by rocky staircases. Two extremes make up the technical condition of the trail along this stretch: incredibly smooth and very rideable to extremely challenging. It's an intense, steep downhill over big granite boulders and, by now, after 24-plus miles of rigorous riding at altitude, some of you may prefer to walk over the more difficult sections. By all means take a break, walk a bit, and "smell the roses." The huge boulders here are especially beautiful.

Finally, the Rim Trail dumps you out onto a ski run at Heavenly Valley near the Stagecoach lift. At this point, you're still high up on the mountain. Following the Rim Trail down to Kingsbury gets a bit convoluted due to the many service roads and ski runs that crisscross this stretch. As you make your way down, keep in mind that you want to descend into the Tahoe Basin towards the west and not the Carson Valley on the east. Of course, if you parked your end-shuttle vehicle at the bottom of the Stagecoach lift, following the chair's cables to the end of your epic journey is a piece of cake. If you left your end-shuttle in town or are planning to ride the entire loop, continue past the bottom of Stagecoach and follow the paved road down to Kingsbury Grade. Hang a left onto paved Kingsbury and enjoy a well-deserved downhill coast on the shoulder, being mindful of vehicles. Make your way to your end-car and give everyone in your group a congratulatory high-five for an incredible experience together.

For all you super-human loop riders: Close the loop by proceeding west (left) on Kingsbury and then turn left again (south) onto US 50. Head towards Stateline. Traffic can be insane here so stay alert. In almost a mile after re-entering California, watch for Pioneer Trail (a well-traveled paved road) veering off on your left, next to the Raley's Supermarket. Follow Pioneer for about 8 miles to US 50 and the town of Meyers. Hang a left onto a paved bike path (you won't have to cross US 50) and follow it south to the familiar junction of US 50 and CA 89. From there, make your way back to your car. Time to celebrate your epic adventure.

RIDE 53 · TRT: Big Meadows to Round Lake

AT A GLANCE

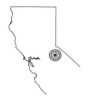

Length/configuration: 14.6-mile loop which includes two out-and-back spurs; mostly single-track and some abandoned pavement

Aerobic difficulty: Mostly moderately strenuous with some very strenuous sections; elevation contributes to the difficulty

Technical difficulty: Intermediate with a few advanced spots; stretches of both smooth and rocky terrain

Scenery: Alpine meadows, dazzling display of wildflowers in season, glacial lake basin, volcanic conglomerate, granite boulders, riparian environment of the Upper Truckee River and a rustic yet beautiful old cow camp.

Special comments: This portion of the TRT intersects with the Pacific Crest Trail on which bikes are not permitted. Also referred to as the Rim Trail and the TRT, portions of the 150-mile Tahoe Rim Trail are off-limits to bikes. Sections described in this ride permit bikes. Please obey all signs.

B ecause not everyone is capable of the previously described epic adventure, Peter Underwood of Olympic Bike Shop highly recommends this ride for cyclists who seek something easier but just as scenic. You'll find this 14.6-mile route the perfect alternative. Located across CA 89 from the previous ride, this moderately strenuous route is spiced with a few sections of very strenuous terrain, but, for the most part, is very rideable for bikers with intermediate-level technical skills. Though some brief sections are rocky and may force you to resort to the always effective bike-and-hike technique, your efforts will be rewarded with spectacular mountain scenery. Autumn is an especially magical time to enjoy this ride because the foliage on the aspens and other deciduous trees are brilliant golds, yellows, and reds, splashed across the landscape.

The route takes place between 6,500–8,500 feet elevation, and begins from the Big Meadows Trailhead and parking lot. This decidedly less challenging adventure is essentially a loop with two out-and-back segments. The first 4.8 miles follows the

RIDE 53 · TRT: Big Meadows to Round Lake

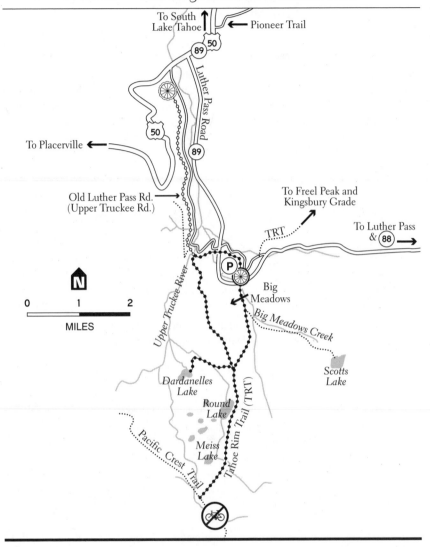

phenomenal Tahoe Rim Trail to the Pacific Crest Trail (PCT), leading you through Big Meadows, volcanic rock and granite boulder patches, peaceful aspen and evergreen forests, and past lovely Round Lake along the way. Since the PCT is off-limits to bikes, you have no choice but to turn around and retrace your path on the Rim Trail for almost 3 miles. Hopping onto Christmas Valley Trail then gives you the opportunity to check out Dardanelles Lake, another peaceful alpine lake at the end of a moderate 1.2-mile out-and-back stretch (2.4 miles round-trip). Following that pleasant side-trip, you'll then descend almost 3 miles on Christmas Valley Trail, before hopping onto an abandoned paved road that climbs easily back up to the Big Meadows Trailhead and parking lot.

Thanks goes to Peter of Olympic Bike Shop for furnishing the trail notes for this great ride. He and his staff can offer more trail suggestions for riders of all abilities. In addition to retail sales, this oldest, most well-stocked bike dealer on the north shore also provides repair service and rental bikes.

General location: South Lake Tahoe.

Elevation change: 1,920 feet; starting elevation 7,200 feet; high point 8,480 feet; low point 6,560 feet. Initial steep uphill stretch followed by shorter ups and downs.

Season: Late June through September or until the first snowstorm hits.

Services: At the Big Meadows trailhead, rest rooms and limited parking are available but water is not. Bring plenty of water or be prepared to treat any water you find on the route. All services can be found in greater South Lake Tahoe.

Hazards: CA 89 is a busy highway and extreme caution is necessary when crossing it at the beginning and end of the ride. Watch out for other trail users, especially along the Rim Trail leading up to Round Lake. Keep your speed in control at all times. Be prepared to dismount and step off the trail to allow hikers, equestrians, and other bikers to pass.

Rescue index: The Rim Trail from Big Meadows Trailhead to Round Lake is popular with hikers, especially on weekends. In case of an emergency, you may get lucky and meet other trail users of may be of help. Otherwise, your best course of action is to make your way back down to CA 89 where you can flag down a passing motorist. The nearest public phone is in the vicinity of the CA 89 and US 50 intersection.

Land status: Eldorado National Forest, Lake Tahoe Basin Management Unit.

Maps: *Recreation Map of Lake Tahoe*, published by Tom Harrison Maps, 2 Falmouth Cove, San Rafael, CA 94901, (800) 265-9090, www.tomharrisonmaps.com. *South Lake Tahoe Basin Recreation Topo Map*, published by Fine Edge Productions.

Finding the trail: From the **Y** in South Lake Tahoe (the intersection of US 50 and CA 89), travel south on US 50/CA 89 (they're one and the same along this stretch), going past the airport and the agricultural inspections station along the way. Proceed through the town of Meyers to CA 89. Turn left onto CA 89 (also known as New Luther Pass Road) and follow it uphill for 5.5 miles to the Big Meadows Trailhead and parking lot. Park and access the Tahoe Rim Trail from here. Note, the portion of the Rim Trail you'll be following is on the other side (south side) of CA 89.

Sources of additional information:

Olympic Bike Shop
620 N. Lake Blvd.
Tahoe City, CA 96145
(530) 581-2500
In addition to sales, service, and being a great source for local bicycling information, Olympic offers an amazing selection of rentals, from basic, quality models to exotic, full-suspension bicycles.

U.S. Forest Service
Lake Tahoe Basin Management Unit
870 Emerald Bay Rd.
South Lake Tahoe, CA 96150
(916) 573-2600; (916) 573-2674

Tahoe Rim Trail Association
P.O. Box 4647
Stateline, Nevada 89449
(775) 588-0686
TahoeRim@aol.com
www.tahoerimtrail.org

Notes on the trail: From the Big Meadows Trailhead parking lot on the north side of CA 89, begin pedaling south back toward the highway. Follow the Tahoe Rim Trail as it runs south and then diagonally crosses CA 89. Now on the south side of CA 89, the single-track Rim Trail starts off with a bang: a steep climb up a staircase-like stretch of granite boulders. This 0.25-mile section is extremely technical and only super-humans can probably ride it. The rest of us will more than likely hike-and-bike, grunting uphill for about 15 minutes. Hang in there—the rest of the ride and the spectacular scenery along the way makes it well worth your efforts now. Bypass a left trail that leads to Scott Lake.

Just when you think you're not having any fun, the trail levels and begins crossing Big Meadows, a pretty alpine meadow. During certain times of the year, depending on the previous winter's snowpack, the meadow is often carpeted by a glorious display of wildflowers, typically in late July or August. For the next couple of miles, the trail rolls up and down, and is more or less entirely rideable, devoid of any more terrifically steep climbs. The Rim Trail continues through a peaceful pine forest, still ascending with a couple of challenging uphills. The trail is mostly rideable thanks to its generally smooth condition. Persevere, for you soon reach the high point of the ride at a little over 2 miles from the Big Meadows Trailhead parking lot.

Enjoy a brief downhill cruise as you pedal through a red fir forest and pass granite and volcanic boulders. You may find the path somewhat difficult in some places and walking a few steps is an effective technique. Watch for an intersection and when you reach it, stay left on the Rim Trail towards Round Lake. (The right trail is Christmas Valley Trail and you'll be following it later.) In less than a half mile, you reach Round Lake, the first of two lakes on this adventure. Round Lake is a pretty, small alpine lake surrounded by willows, ideal for a snack break or picnic. If the day is hot, the lake makes a great swimming hole.

From Round Lake, it's about 2.9 miles to the end of the bike-legal portion of the Rim Trail, where it joins the Pacific Coast Trail. Continue following the trail around the left (east) side of the lake and begin climbing rigorously towards the ridge over patches of broken rock. It's technically challenging and you may have to walk a few steps or so. The narrow trail is generally rideable and it soon levels. The old aspen trees up here are big in diameter and during the autumn, they present a dazzling, fiery display of golds, reds, and yellows. You're now entering one of the biggest, prettiest alpine valleys and meadow systems in the Tahoe Basin. Like a huge dent in the rim and wall of tub-like Tahoe Basin, the glacial bowl here forms the source of the Upper Truckee River. If your timing is on, you'll be treated to a spectacular show of wildflowers carpeting the green meadows.

When you reach the Pacific Crest Trail, leave your bike at the intersection and hike southwest across the meadow for a short ways to one of the forks of the Upper Truckee River. There, you'll see an old but still active cow camp, marked by a beautiful, old, hand-built home sitting next to this terrific water source. Look east by southeast and you have a terrific view of the southern-most end of the Carson Range, anchored by Red Lake Peak at 10,061 feet. Immediately on the other side of the Range though out of view is Carson Pass and Kirkwood ski resort.

From the PCT, turn around and retrace your tracks past Round Lake and back to the Christmas Valley Trail intersection. This time, turn left onto Christmas Valley and descend alongside the tributary for about 0.2 mile to another trail junction, also on your left. The left trail runs for 1.2 miles up to Dardanelles Lake, and it's a worthy side trip. This gorgeous little lake sits in a beautiful basin and is a great place for a picnic or a swim.

From Dardanelles Lake, turn around and retrace you tracks back to Christmas Valley Trail. Go left onto Christmas Valley and descend steeply for about 2.8 miles, accompanied by a tiny branch of Upper Truckee River along the way. You soon cruise through a valley filled with aspen trees, especially spectacular when golden autumn leaves paint the landscape. Eventually, the trail intersects Old Luther Pass Road, also known as South Upper Truckee Road; turn right onto it. Climb for about 15 minutes and follow Old Luther Pass Road across CA 89 (New Luther Pass Road). This stretch of Old Luther Pass Road which is closed to vehicles leads to the Rim Trail and the Big Meadows parking lot. Total distance is 14.6 miles and includes the out-and-back stretch to the PCT and Dardanelles Lake.

Option: If adding more miles on non-technical terrain appeals to you, consider beginning your ride with a 5-mile, moderately ascending stretch on South Upper Truckee Road (this adds 10 miles total to the ride just described). The road is located between the KOA and Tahoe Pines campgrounds near the intersection of US 50 and CA 89. (CA 89 is also known as New Luther Pass Road). Begin by pedaling south for about 4.5 miles on South Upper Truckee, a lightly-used paved road. Portions of the road are closed to vehicles as it passes through a residential neighborhood and a lovely old ranch. The route runs through private property but through-access is allowed so long as you stay on the road. The quiet road eventually leads you across busy CA 89. Continue on the paved road (this segment closed to vehicles), and in about a mile, after an approximate 900-foot gain from US 50, you reach the Rim Trail at Big Meadows Trailhead and parking area. Proceed as described above.

RIDE 54 · Pine Nut Mountains Loops

AT A GLANCE

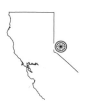

Length/configuration: 3 loops: 12-, 23-, and 32-mile; single-track and jeep fire roads

Aerobic difficulty: Moderately strenuous to strenuous; plenty of steep hills

Technical difficulty: Intermediate to advanced; rocky, steep ascents and descents; shortest loop is intermediate

Scenery: Tremendous views of the high desert and all its natural beauty and wildlife.

Special comments: This area is rapidly become a mecca for riders looking for something different or a quick escape from the snow-covered trails of the high Sierras. The two longer loops are not recommended for beginners.

Thanks goes to Keith Hart of Carson Valley Schwinn in Gardnerville, for submitting this ride. He and his store are one of the organizers of the annual Pine Nut Cracker, a NORBA-sanctioned mountain bike race which partakes of the route described below. Stop by his bike shop and pick up a map of the area before hitting the trail. His store is a great source for trail information, bike stuff, and repairs. A map is recommended since there's a mess of unsigned jeep roads and trails out there.

According to Keith, there's something on this route for riders of all abilities, from the sightseer looking to explore the areas around old silver mines, to a rider looking for some of the finest, fastest single-track anywhere. There are plenty of jeep roads that intersect this route and adventurous riders with plenty of water and time will enjoy exploring them. Following are three versions to this description: The 12- mile loop climbs some but is generally short and sweet and is well-suited for intermediate riders with excellent stamina. The 23-mile loop is more challenging with rocky and steeper climbs. You need to eat your Wheaties to enjoy it. Then, there's the 32-mile loop, which Keith calls the Pro/Expert Loop. You'll need more than your Wheaties on this version—it demands advanced bike handling skills over more rocky ascents and descents. Of course, walking is a proven technique that works nearly all the time.

And in case you're wondering, "Why would anyone want to ride here?" in the seemingly arid Pine Nut Mountains when the awesome trails of Lake Tahoe are right next door, here's the answer: It's the snow, baby. When the higher elevations are still covered with snow, the trails down here in the Pine Nuts and nearby areas are rideable. There are other reasons too, like getting away from the summer crowds so common on Tahoe trails. Highly skilled riders looking for something different and challenging find adventure here, too.

So what are the Pine Nuts? It's the figurative name locals use to identify their high desert mountains which consist of 362,000 acres in three counties: Douglas, Carson, and Lyon. Trails used on this ride are concentrated in Douglas County, southeast of Gardnerville, Nevada. Elevations here range from 4,300 to 9,400 feet. (Not to worry. This route doesn't climb that high.) Specifically, though, pine nuts are a product of pinyon pine trees. As a quirk of nature, the nut is significantly disproportionate to the size of the tree—big nut, small tree. Oddity or not, the nut played an important role in the lives of the Washoe and Piute Indians who roamed the semi-arid Nevada lands. Still harvesting the nuts for food like generations before them, the pine nut not only provides sustenance, it is a major part of their spiritual life, providing the focal point of many traditional ceremonies. Though you can buy pine nuts in the local super-markets, "nutting" is a popular recreational activity in September and October when the nuts are ripe. Incidentally, if you get hungry on the trail, don't plan on snacking on the nuts. They need to be cooked first to be digestible.

General location: About 30 miles east of South Lake Tahoe in Nevada, just a few miles south of Gardnerville.

Elevation change: For 12-mile, 23-mile, and 32-mile loops respectively: 800 feet; 1,700 feet; and 2,100 feet. Starting elevation and lowest point for all loops 4,700 feet. Highest point for short, medium and long loops, respectively: 5,550 feet; 6,700 feet; and 7,500 feet. Lots of steep and rocky ups and downs on the 23- and 32-mile loops.

Season: Early spring through mid-fall.

Services: None on the trail. Water, food and rest rooms at the 7-Eleven store about 3 miles from the trailhead. Other services in Gardnerville and South Lake Tahoe.

Hazards: Stay alert for rattlesnakes in the lower elevations. Because of extremely rocky conditions on the 23- and 32-mile loops, beginners should think twice about attempting either. Expect to share the trail with motorcyclists, off-road vehicle en-thusiasts, equestrians, and bikers.

RIDE 54 · Pine Nut Mountains Loops

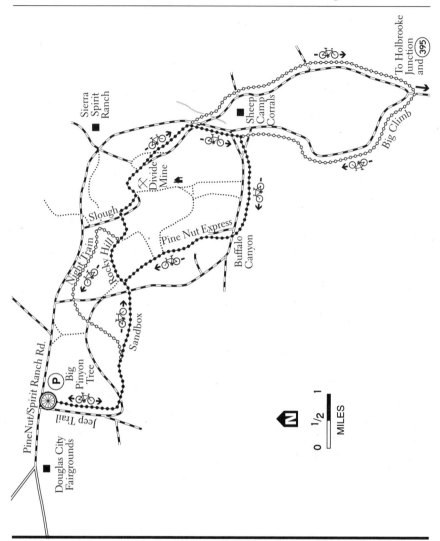

Rescue index: A fairly popular area, you may encounter other trail users who may be of emergency help. Though the nearest phone is at the Douglas County Fairgrounds, it may not be accessible as the grounds are not always open in between scheduled events. The reliable plan is to make your way back to the 7-Eleven where you can call 911. (You pass the store on the way to the trailhead at the fairgrounds.)

Land status: Bureau of Land Management.

Maps: Though BLM and USGS maps exist, the trails are not all depicted. The best map is the one created by Keith Hart, who has scouted the trails. Drop by his bike store, Carson Valley Schwinn, for a map and other trail information.

Finding the trail: Starting at the intersection of CA 89 and US 50 (also known as the Y) in South Lake Tahoe, head east on US 50 and into Nevada and drive for about 5.9 miles, to the intersection with Kingsbury Grade (NV 207). Go right onto Kingsbury and follow it about 18 miles to Gardnerville. From within the town, pick up US 395 and go south for about 2 miles to a signal light intersection with Pine Nut Road and Riverview Drive. There's a 7-Eleven store on the corner (a good place to pick up water and food). Turn left (east) onto Pine Nut and head for the Douglas County Fairgrounds. (If you don't want to drive your vehicle on dirt, park here at the fairgrounds.) Go about 1.5 miles and just before the fairground entrance, hang a left onto a dirt road marked Pine Nut Road 2 and Sierra Spirit Ranch. Proceed 1 mile on the dirt road and look for an outstandingly large pinyon pine tree next to a jeep road. (Some locals call this the "Pinyon Pine Tree Lot.") Park and begin pedaling from here.

Sources of additional information:

Bureau of Land Management
Carson City District
5665 Morgan Hill Rd.
Carson City, NV 89701-1448
(775) 885-6000

Carson Valley Schwinn
1504 Highway 395
Gardnerville, NV 89410
(702) 782-7077

Notes on the trail: Begin pedaling south on the jeep road for about 0.8 mile. There are several trails leading from the road. Stay on the main jeep road and at the top of a horseshoe curve bending left, look for a narrow trail peeling off on the right. You're now on what the locals call Sand Box, a single-track that begins as a steep downhill. Follow it; you'll feel like a kid in kindergarten again on this trail because it follows and crosses sometimes sandy creek beds. Keep in mind that what goes down must go up, so keep your granny gear handy. Sand Box continues for about 2.5 miles and leads to a rocky climbing section. Fondly referred to as Rocky Hill, this stretch is about a mile long. At the top, you earn a terrific view of the Carson Valley below. Riders of the 12-mile loop: make a left turn here at the top. Riders of the 23- and 32-mile loops: continue to the "mine climb."

Twelve-mile loop: Head north on Slough, a jeep road. In a short distance, it intersects Pine Nut Road (the main dirt road which leads past the fairgrounds). As you approach the intersection, keep your eyes peeled for Night Train, a single-track on your left. It's a fun, 2.5-mile stretch that parallels the main road heading west, ending at a jeep road. At this junction, you have several options to return to your car. The easiest way is via Pine Nut Road: Hang a right onto the jeep road here, then when you reach Pine Nut Road in a short distance, turn left and follow it back to the parking area. For the more challenging route, go across the road, bearing left at another intersection and eventually re-connect with Sand Box. Retrace your path on Sand Box and back to your car. Total distance is roughly 12 miles.

The 23-mile loop: From the top of the rocky hill, continue to head east on the single-track. Soon, it ends at a jeep road referred to as the "mine climb." Proceed to grind up the hill. When the road crests at a saddle, you will have reached one of the highest points of the lower Pine Nut Mountains. In the saddle is the closed, abandoned Divide Mine. (If you go exploring, there are other abandoned mines nearby. Though the mines are not boarded close, they're extremely unsafe, which means, for you and your buddy's sake, keep out!) Farther on this road, there is another picturesque spot over-looking the Carson Valley in the west and the smaller Pine Nut Valley in the east. Continue to head east on the jeep road which soon narrows to a single-track. When you reach an intersection with a jeep road, stay straight onto the jeep road and begin a short, steep hike-and-bike section. From there, carry on with the jeep road for about 3 miles. You soon reach a large four-way intersection with a creek flowing through its center. This intersection is known as Sheep Camp as evident by the corrals nearby. (Sheepherders use the corrals during the early spring and late fall.) At this intersection, the 23-milers and the 32-milers separate. (Mile-hungry, advanced riders, proceed across the creek instead. Directions continue below.) For you 23-milers, hang a right onto the improved dirt road and follow it for about 0.8 mile. Take the first jeep road on the right. In a short ways, bypass another jeep road coming in on your left. (32-milers: here is where your route rejoins the 23-mile route.) Now, gear down and begin a seemingly long 0.8-mile climb and then enjoy a long, fast downhill through Buffalo Canyon. Once you reach the bottom of the canyon, you immediately start climbing back up. Take a right onto another jeep trail, called Pine Nut Express which quickly narrows to a faster single-track. Carry on for about a mile until you come to a Y in the road. Bear left and continue down until you cross the familiar Sand Box trail. Hang a left onto Sand Box and retrace your path back to your car.

The 32-mile Pro/Expert Loop: From Sheep Camp, cross the creek and continue heading up the jeep road. Stay on the main road, bearing right at any questionable junctions. Keep climbing gradually for about 4.5 miles until you reach the crest. Located at the crest is a large, high meadow that looks down on a beautiful valley in the south toward Topaz Lake. Say good-bye to the main road and follow the faint jeep road which climbs on your right. (If you miss this turn and stay on the main road, you'll wind up in the valley and end up on US 395 near Holbrook Junction.) As you continue to climb the faint road, trail conditions become steeper and rocky but the real mountain goats on bikes won't mind. At the top, stay left and begin a fast descent back toward Sheep Camp. Just before Sheep Camp, make a hard left onto yet another jeep trail and continue back through Buffalo Canyon. Here, you rejoin the 23-mile route. Proceed as described above and return to your car after approximately 32 miles.

OTHER AREA RIDES

PEAVINE PEAK OUT-AND-BACK: Dominating the Reno horizon to the northwest is Peavine Mountain. There is a mess of jeep roads that crisscross the base of the mountain but the most popular—and arduous—ride is the one to the top. Located in Nevada, this is a serious hill climb measuring 7 miles one way (14 miles round-trip). You'll gain 3,000 feet in that 7 miles before you reach the turnaround point. Since most of the route is on gravel and jeep dirt roads, technical skills are not really tested in the outbound direction. The real challenge is staying in control on the downhill run, and for that reason, intermediate skills are required. The long climb between 5,200 and 8,300 feet elevation makes this a very strenuous ride. Along the way, the route leads around a canyon, past aspen groves and sites of abandoned gold mining camps that were active in the mid-1800s. Expect the terrain to be somewhat rugged—definitely not for the weak rider. Near the top of the ride, you have your choice of two peaks to bag, both of which sit close by. If you're feeling particularly bionic, bag 'em both. Whichever peak you choose, the view from it reportedly makes all that huffin' and puffin' worth it.

Finding the trailhead: From downtown Reno, find Virginia Street and head north, past McCarran and Parr Streets. Almost 5 miles from downtown, be sure to stay on North Virginia as it curves left (if you hit US 395, you've veered off Virginia). Stay on North Virginia for about 4 miles and keep an eye out for a wide gravel road on the left. This is the beginning of Peavine Peak Road. Park here, well off the road, and begin pedaling. (If you reach a big green water tank, you've gone about a half mile past the gravel road.)

Maps: Verdi 7.5 minute series.

For more information, contact: Any bike shop in Reno.

CARSON RIVER AND BRUNSWICK CANYON RIDES: If you live in the high country during the winter, it won't take long for you to yearn for bikeable, snow-free trails. When compared to Lake Tahoe, the Carson River Ride at 4,600 to 4,800 feet sees far less snow and is generally accessible year-round. Located a few miles east of Carson City, Nevada, in the desert highlands, Carson River Ride is configured like a lollipop (an out-and-back with a loop on the outer end) and measures about 10.5 miles round-trip. Other narrow dirt roads intersect the main road, so expect to do some exploring, which may add more miles to your adventure.

Finding the trail: The route follows narrow, rugged dirt roads, making intermediate level technical skills necessary. Though elevation gain is negligible (about 200 feet total), expect some steep but brief ups and downs. The Carson River Ride is completely on the north side of the river, sometimes within sight of it, other times a bit farther away and obscured. Essentially, the direction of travel is west to east toward a set of power lines just southeast of Empire Hill. When you reach the power lines, you can head back the way you came or explore other offshoot roads. Heartier riders with plenty of time can check out Brunswick Canyon on the south side of the river. Sharing the same starting point as the Carson River Ride, a primitive bridge (about a mile from the trailhead bridge) takes you to the other side of the river. The ride up and back Brunswick Canyon is not technically challenging, and bikers with intermediate skills can handle it. The climbing (more than 1,400 feet elevation gain) is the kicker. The general direction is north to south, past Sand Canyon Road and Bidwell Mine. A primitive camping area on Brunswick Canyon Road serves as the turnaround point, clocking in at 8 miles one way (16 miles round-trip). Many offshoot jeep roads offer hours and miles of additional exploration. On both rides, a word of caution: watch out for rattlesnakes.

Finding the trailhead: From Carson City, at the intersection of Carson Street (US 395) and William Street (US 50), go east on William about 4 miles to Deer Run Road. Head south on Deer Run for almost a mile to where it crosses Carson River on a bridge. Park here, before the bridge. Begin pedaling east on the wide gravel road on the north side of the river. In about a mile, a primitive bridge leads to the south side of the river, marking the beginning of the Brunswick Canyon ride as described above. If you want to tackle the harder of the two rides, continue over the primitive bridge. Otherwise, bypass this bridge and stay on the north side of the river.

Maps: New Empire and McTarnahan Hill 7.5 minute series.

For more information, contact: Any bike shop in Carson City or Reno.

HORSE CANYON/SILVER LAKE LOOP: For expert riders looking for a 20-mile-plus, technically challenging adventure in the high alpine country, this is it. Expect to grind up broken granite blocks, drop down 1- to 2-foot ledges at elevations ranging between 7,000 to 9,000 feet, all this amid a backdrop of wildflowers and magnificent vistas. At this altitude and on this terrain, everyone will push his/her bike up some portion of the ride. Located just east of Silver Lake, south of Kirkwood ski resort, between CA 88 and the Mokelumne Wilderness boundary, this area offers a number of rugged jeep and motorcycle roads and narrow trails from which to configure your own route. One of the more popular configurations is this loop, which begins at the Oyster Creek picnic area off CA 88 near the Silver Lake campgrounds. Begin by riding around the backside of the lake and then up some intensely technical single-tracks to the top of Squaw Ridge and the wilderness boundary. Once at the boundary, go left (northeast), skirting the edge of the wilderness area toward Scout Carson Lake and Horse Canyon Trail. Turn left onto Horse Canyon, and hang on for a fast and super-technical single-track downhill run to CA 88 and your car. Be sure to bring plenty of long-burning energy food and water—you'll need it.

Finding the trailhead: From South Lake Tahoe, go south on US 50 to CA 89. Go left onto CA 89 and head up and over Luther Pass to CA 88. Turn right onto CA 88 and travel for about 19 miles. Along the way, go through Carson Pass, past Caples Lake and Kirkwood ski resort, and then through Carson Spur. As you approach Silver Lake, look for the turnoff to the Oyster Creek picnic area and campground. Park here.

Maps: *South Lake Tahoe Basin Recreation Topo Map*, published by Fine Edge Productions; USGS Caples Lake 7.5 minute series.

For more information, contact:
Eldorado National Forest
100 Forni Rd.
Placerville, CA 95667
(916) 622-5061

SOME LOCAL BICYCLE SHOPS
& ORGANIZATIONS

Olympic Bike Shop
620 N. Lake Blvd.
Tahoe City, CA 96145
(916) 581-2500

CyclePaths Mountain Bike
 Adventures
1785 Westlake Blvd.
P.O. Box 887
Tahoe City, CA 96145|
(800) 780-BIKE or (530) 581-1171
www.cyclepaths.com

Paco's Truckee Bike & Ski
11200-6 Donner Pass Rd.
Truckee, CA 96161
(530) 587-5561

Lakeview Sports
3131 Harrison Ave.
South Lake Tahoe, CA 96150
(530) 544-0183

Tahoe Bike and Ski
2277 Lake Tahoe Blvd.
South Lake Tahoe, CA 96150
(530) 544-8060

Village Bicycles
800 Tahoe Blvd.
Incline Village, NV 89450
(702) 831-3537

Carson Valley Schwinn
1504 Highway 395
Gardnerville, NV 89410
(702) 782-7077

Tahoe Rim Trail Association
P.O. Box 4647
Stateline, NV 89449
(775) 588-0686
TahoeRim@aol.com
www.tahoerimtrail.org

Tahoe Area Regional Transit (TART)
(800) 736-6365; (916) 581-6365

THE HIGH COUNTRY OF THE EASTERN SIERRAS

Sitting higher than "Mile-High" Denver, Colorado, the mountain bike trails in this region range from 6,400 feet elevation at Mono Lake to over 11,000 feet at the top of Mammoth Mountain Bike Park. And believe me, if you're visiting from the flatlands, the air is noticeably thinner, no matter how strong you are at sea level. Since one of the most popular roads leading to the Eastern Sierras is through Yosemite National Park, a bike ride through Yosemite Valley shouldn't be missed by anyone, regardless of skill level and if you time it right during the day, you can avoid sharing the trail with hordes of tourists.

If checking out unusual geological features gives you a kick, you'll see some very cool evidence of Mother Nature at work along the Eastern Sierras. This is, after all, earthquake country, spiced with plenty of past volcanic episodes. This region includes two very different environments. There's fascinating though not very technical riding through the arid, sometimes sandy, desert-like terrain around surreal Mono Lake. One of the most saline inland lakes in all of North America, Mono beautifully reflects the clouds and subtle colors of the sky while mountains with volcanic craters stand guard nearby. Looking like something from outer space are tufa formations protruding from the lake and they're a must-see. Bike routes in the Mono vicinity are shadeless, which means summer riding can be very hot and dry. In contrast, about 20 minutes south in the Mammoth Lakes area, the terrain abruptly changes to thick, evergreen forests, marked by volcanic and earthquake features. Here, the bike trails are varied, from beginner to advanced, including outstanding trails in Mammoth Mountain Bike Park, arguably the best bike resort in California. From within the bike park, you reach another environment, the barren roof of Mammoth Mountain itself, perched above tree line at 11,053 feet, where you're eye-to-eye with distant snow-patched mountain peaks in the nearby Ansel Adams and John Muir Wilderness areas. To the west, as if to isolate this part of the state from the rest of California is the towering Ritter Range with its dramatically jagged Minarets piercing the sky. Spend a few days in laid-back, very unpretentious Mammoth Lakes and, if you're like me, you won't want to leave, or at least not until the next earthquake rattles through.

RIDE 55 · Yosemite National Park Bike Trail

AT A GLANCE

Length/configuration: 8-mile-plus out-and-back (4-plus miles each way); paved multi-use trail and closed paved vehicle road

Aerobic difficulty: Easy, all flat with one very short hill near Mirror Lake

Technical difficulty: Nontechnical, though riders should be comfortable sharing the trail with a lot of people

Scenery: Despite all the tourist traffic, Yosemite Valley is absolutely stunning. Sights along the bike trail include Lower Yosemite Falls, Mirror Lake, Half Dome, and the riparian environment along Merced River.

Special comments: Suitable for children, though they should be able to ride confidently on crowded trails. A longer option with more sites of interest can be pedaled, but since it involves riding with heavy traffic, youngsters are not recommended on this route.

A dmittedly, biking the paved trail through Yosemite Valley is not a real off-road adventure, nor is it technically challenging. But Yosemite National Park is not to be missed. If you've never been to Yosemite or if you're driving through it to reach Mono Lake, Mammoth, and other parts of the Eastern Sierras, this short, 8-mile out-and-back (4 miles each way) bike route is more than just a welcomed break from driving. The absolutely stunning sites you see along the way make it worth pulling the bike off (or out) of your car. The route weaves through the rich, riparian environment of the Merced River. Then there are Yosemite Falls and Lower Yosemite Fall — always impressive. A worthy side trip is to take the short hiking trail to the lower fall. After a whopping winter, the lower fall is particularly mighty and the spray from it can be drenching. At the far end of the bike route is Mirror Lake. The lake is in the natural process of filling with silt and drying up, eventually becoming a meadow. Its once-famed mirror reflections of the surrounding ridges are apt to not be as grand as in the past, but if you're lucky, the snow runoff may have elevated the water level just enough so that you can get a glimpse of that visual phenomena. And though you can see Half Dome, that uniquely shaped piece of granite from many places on the valley floor, the views from around Mirror Lake are especially awesome.

Unfortunately, the paved trail leads through the most congested area of the Yosemite Valley, namely Yosemite Village. Here, the Ahwahnee, an historic hotel and architectural gem, stands apart from the nearby campgrounds, the Village store, and food concession stands. (At least the tourist concessionaires are concentrated in one area and not spread out.) Expect to share the path with other trail users, including walkers (with or without baby strollers, and dog walkers), joggers, rollerbladers, and other bikers. Thus, your only real technical challenge is dodging tourists. Here's a tip: Invest in a handlebar bell. It's surprisingly effective and universal (lots of foreign tourists visit the park) yet friendly.

Though the 8-mile route described here follows a path separate from vehicles, you can ride all paved roads (unless posted closed to bikes). Just watch out for the

RIDE 55 · Yosemite National Park Bike Trail

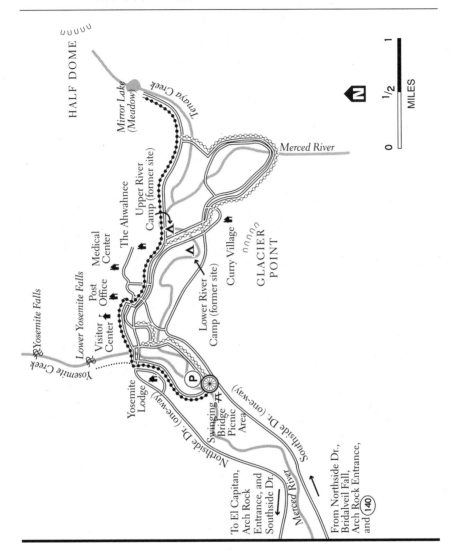

clueless motorists. Adult riders seeking more mileage and more scenic points of interest can ride the shoulder of Southside and Northside Drives, both of which are one-way vehicle roads leading in and out of Yosemite Valley, respectively. Pedaling Northside Drive takes you pass El Capitan, that sheer, vertical monolith of granite revered by technical rock climbers throughout the world. Bring binoculars, and you just might spot climbers defying gravity. About 1.5 miles past El Capitan, Southside Drive heads back to Yosemite Village. Along the way is Bridalveil Fall, a 62-story cascade of water which the Yosemite Indians referred to as "Pohono," or spirit of the puffing wind. A short, hiking-only trail is a worthwhile side trip.

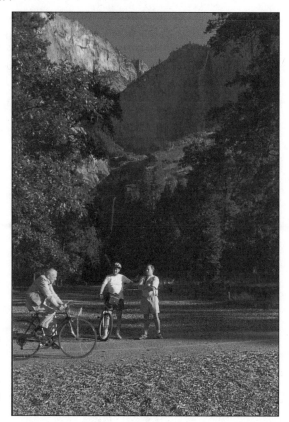

Enjoyed by walkers and bikers of all ages, this paved path runs past Yosemite Falls on its way to a hiking-only trail leading to the base of the falls. This senior cyclist obviously forgot his flashy yet functional helmet.

To avoid the seasonal summer crowds on the roads and the paved trails, ride early in the day. Or, visit late in the season, such as in September and October, after the hordes of tourists have left. Snowfall during the winter and spring deters fair-weather bikers in the off-season but imagine what a unique, solitary experience you'll have if you dress warmly before setting off on your bike. The Sunday brunch at the Ahwahnee is not to be missed, and that's a great motivator to ride early and ride hard before indulging in the famous late-morning feast.

General location: About 180 miles southeast of San Francisco, 88 miles east of Merced off CA 140.

Elevation change: Negligible change; Yosemite Valley and its paved trails sit at about 4,000 feet.

Season: Late spring through fall, though summer is crowded. The best time is during the off-season before Memorial Day and after Labor Day.

Services: Water, rest rooms, concession stands, formal and casual restaurants, medical clinic, showers, laundry facilities, a chapel, a museum, and a gas station can all be found in and around the Village. Both modest and pricey lodging is offered at Yosemite Lodge and the Ahwahnee. Canvas tents and rustic cabins are available in Curry Village for the budget-minded. Maintained campgrounds abound and reservations made well in advance are highly recommended. During the summer, rental bikes are available at Yosemite Lodge or Curry Village.

Hazards: As mentioned above, dodging other trail users will be the biggest hazard. Also, bears have long been a problem. If you have food in your car, be sure to store it in the trunk or completely covered and out of sight inside vehicles. The bears that frequent Yosemite Valley have been known to rip open vehicles if they suspect food is inside. Though a bear raiding parked cars is rare during the day, it's a good idea to play it safe by hiding food. Mountain lions live in the park, though sightings along this well-traveled path are rare. If you choose to pedal the longer-ride option, Northside and Southside Drives are heavily traveled and you'll need to ride defensively alongside motorists gawking at the scenery. Be alert for weather conditions which cause the water level of rivers and streams to rise rapidly.

Rescue index: You're bound to find other people visiting the park who may be of assistance. After all, Yosemite Valley is a popular destination. Alas, you're never away from civilization along this route. A medical clinic is located in Yosemite Village, near the post office.

Land status: Yosemite National Park.

Maps: *Yosemite Guide, Your Key to Visiting the Park*, a newspaper-type publication by the Yosemite Association, in cooperation with the National Park Service. *Yosemite National Park*, published by Tom Harrison Maps, 2 Falmouth Cove, San Rafael, CA 94901, (800) 265-9090, www.tomharrisonmaps.com. *Yosemite National Park*, published by Trails Illustrated, P.O. Box 4357, Evergreen, CO 80437, www.trailsillustrated.com. *Yosemite*, complimentary official park brochure, published by the U.S. Department of Interior, National Park Service.

Finding the trail: From Merced on US 99, head east on CA 140 for about 80 miles to the Arch Rock entrance of Yosemite National Park. CA 140 becomes El Portal Road as it continues into the park. About 5 miles from the entrance, you're forced to bear right onto Southside Drive, beginning a one-way road into the heart of Yosemite Valley. About 3 miles farther from where the one-way section began, drive past Bridalveil Fall and look for Swinging Bridge Picnic Area on your left. Park and access the signed bike trail from here.

Sources of additional information:

Yosemite National Park
Yosemite Public Information
U.S. Department of the Interior
P.O. Box 577
Yosemite, CA 95389
www.nps.gov/yose
(209) 372-0200

Recorded message for all types of information. If you want to speak to a live person, call Monday through Friday, 9 a.m. to 5 p.m.—and plan to be persistent.

Notes on the trail: Before hitting the trail, bring your bike lock and enough cash or a credit card in case you want to stop for a snack, a meal, or some memento from the visitor center. From the Swinging Bridge Picnic Area, pick up the paved bike path and begin pedaling away from Southside Drive, going over the Merced River and curving north. Follow the path through the meadow and soon go past Yosemite Lodge on your left. Cross Northside Drive, but, since this is the only way out of Yosemite Valley, be alert for approaching vehicles. On the other side of road, the paved path continues a few yards to Yosemite Falls. There's a bike rack here at the trail junction to Lower Yosemite Fall. The trail to the fall doesn't allow bikes, so you'll have to lock your bike here. The little half-mile walk is worthwhile.

When you return to your bike, head east on the paved path toward Yosemite Village. (If you want to ride the longer option, see the note at the end of this trail description.) Be prepared to share the trail with other folks who are also enjoying the surroundings. As you approach the Village, the trail becomes more congested. Expect the trail to be a bit convoluted here as it weaves past the museum, post office, Village store, and the Ahwahnee. Be patient and soon, after about 1.5 miles from Lower Yosemite Fall, the paved trail splits. The right split leads to Curry Village. You want the left split, which goes to Mirror Lake. Note that the Upper River campground used to be here; the 1997 flood destroyed it, and water level markers are posted.

After this intersection, upon taking the left split, the congestion subsides as you leave the madness behind. About a mile after the split, the paved trail ends and dumps you out onto a paved road. The road is closed to vehicular traffic except for shuttle buses. Still, if you're lucky, you won't encounter a bus as you climb a short but steep half-mile hill to Mirror Lake. As you power up the hill, keep an eye out for Half Dome looming in the distance on your right. There are some particularly spectacular views of it from this road, especially if you're riding late in the day and the sun is low, casting a warm light on its granite face. There's a hiking path leading to the north side of Mirror Lake. If you're looking for a nice picnic spot, check it out, after locking your trusty steed to the bike rack at the end of the road, of course. When you've had your fill, turn around and go back the way you came.

Longer option: From Lower Yosemite Fall, continue west on the bike path. In a short distance, the path ends. Hop onto Northside Drive and carry on due west. El Capitan will be looming on your right. Much farther beyond, Northside intersects Southside Drive. Make a hard left and follow Southside back toward Yosemite Village. Watch for Bridalveil Fall on your right. When you reach Swinging Bridge Picnic Area, you have a choice of direction. You can retrace the bike path to Lower Yosemite Fall, pick up the bike path on the other side of Northside Drive and head east to Mirror Lake. Or, you can continue sharing the road with motorists and follow Southside Drive into the Village.

RIDE 56 · Black Point at Mono Lake Ride

AT A GLANCE

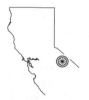

Length/configuration: 12.6-mile out-and-back with a loop; dirt roads

Aerobic difficulty: Easy; moderate if you're not acclimated to the high elevation

Technical difficulty: Not technical though there are scattered sandy spots

Scenery: Wide-open flatland of sagebrush. Geological sites of interest include Mono Lake viewed from various locations, the Black Point Fissures and the surrealistic tufa formations found at Mono City Park.

Special comments: Suitable for strong youngsters and kid trailers. There's no shade on the route and it does get hot here in the summer.

Although the route for Black Point at Mono Lake is basically an easy and non-technical ride, its surrounding landscape makes it one of the most interesting. Using mostly wide dirt roads, this 12.6-mile ride is configured as an out-and-back with a loop. The journey takes you to the lakeside base of Black Point, a barren mound of volcanic-cinders, topping off at 6,958 feet, about 5.4 miles from the starting point. But what can't be seen from the base are the fissures, a result of a volcanic eruption that occurred here some 13,000 years ago. As the cinder and ash cooled and hardened, an area near the top broke, forming cracks several hundred yards long, 20 to 50 feet deep, and a few feet wide. In this seemingly deserted landscape, small creatures such as rabbits, birds, coyote, lizards, and mice, to name a few, find welcome shade and shelter in the fissures. You can hike up to the fissures. It's a 45-minute hike over loose terrain, and if your lungs are not accustomed to the high elevation, it can be particularly arduous. Nevertheless, once at the top, the panoramic view looking over Mono Lake and Mono Craters in the south and the rugged snow-patched mountains in the west make it worth the effort.

You'll find the lake's edge at the base of Black Point to be a serene place. Several log poles lying on the ground make it a good spot to sit and observe the landscape. Though not dramatic like jagged granite mountain peaks, the landscape here is quietly beautiful, with the contrasting black and white islands of Negit and Paoha respectively, still sitting peacefully together after thousands of years. If the sky is cloudy, its reflections on Mono Lake can be absolutely stunning (and you'll wish you had your camera). Look at the proximity of the islands to the mainland and you'll begin to understand how the water level protects wildlife habitats. When the level drops, a land bridge emerges, providing unfettered access to predators of the islands' nesting birds and their eggs. Across the lake to its southern edge, you can see Mono Craters, and, if you're here in late spring, you may see snow-capped mountain ridges in the distance. There is life out there, living on the exposed lake bed: garter snakes, kangaroo rats, and lizards, to name a few. Mono Lake is also a major migration stop for birds, providing a feast of lake shrimp and massive swarms of non-biting brine flies. ("Mono" is an Indian word for "fly.") Don't be surprised if you see a flock of California seagulls here. About 85% of the entire state's seagull population use Mono Lake as a refueling station.

The lake itself is the remains of an ancient inland sea, approximately one million years old. Streams flowed into the lake for thousands of years, depositing minerals and sediment. At this altitude, copious evaporation resulted in increasingly higher concentration of dissolved salts. The flow of fresh water into the lake was—and still is—essential to sustaining the delicate ecosystem that evolved. Adding to the uniqueness of Mono Lake is its surreal waterscape dotted by its eerie stands of tufa (pronounced *too-fah*) along portions of the shoreline. These white towers of calcium carbonate (limestone) are a result of the highly alkaline and saline lake water commingling with fresh spring water bubbling up from under the lake bed. Some of the tufa date from 200 to 900 years old.

So what makes Mono Lake so controversial? Funny, what makes the lake so visually stunning is due in part to the strains placed upon it by the Los Angeles Department of Water and Power. In the early 1900s, as Los Angeles grew, demand for water escalated. Spearheaded by William Mulholland, whose goal was to convert the Los Angeles desert into an oasis, he managed to build aqueducts to transport water from Owens Valley (about 150 miles south of Mono Lake). Completely drained of its natural resource, Owens Lake turned into a toxic dust bowl, and Mulholland and his fellow Los Angelenos turned their sites farther north to Mono

RIDE 56 · Black Point at Mono Lake Ride

Lake. In 1941, aqueducts tapped into the four principle creeks draining into Mono Lake, diverting precious fresh water from the lake and decreasing the lake's water level. The delicate balance of fresh and salt water was disrupted, and super concentrations of salt in the lake brought the area's ecosystem to the brink of collapse. And so having witnessed the demise of Owens Valley, local and state citizens rallied to save Mono Lake by waging war over who has rights to control water in the region. In 1994, after numerous court battles which included a Supreme Court mandate to restore inbound creeks, the State Water Resources Control Board ruled in favor of a 17-foot rise in the water levels throughout the following 20 to 30 years. Though the controversy of water rights still exists as it always has since the days of Mulholland, at

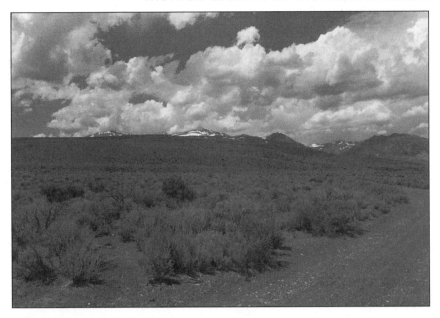

Wide-open, shadeless, gently rolling terrain of sagebrush and sand is the typical landscape around Mono Lake.

least Mono Lake is on the road to recovery. Ironically, had it not been for the decreased water levels, the surreal tufa which attracted significant state and national exposure would've remained submerged from our view.

General location: About 80 miles south of Lake Tahoe, on the northern edge of Mono Lake, just outside the eastern border of Yosemite National Park.

Elevation change: 200 feet; starting elevation and high point 6,600 feet; low point 6,400 feet. Mildly rolling terrain.

Season: Late May to October.

Services: Drinking water, rest rooms, and a lovely cultivated lawn area with picnic tables can be found at the Mono County Park. Interpretative displays and a walking trail through the tufa formations lead to the water's edge of Mono Lake. Limited services can be found at Lee Vining. Complete services available in Mammoth Lakes.

Hazards: There's no shade or suitable drinking water on this ride, and believe me, it can get real hot out there. Bring plenty of water and sun protection. Summer months often see afternoon thunder and lightning storms.

Rescue index: During the summer months, you're likely to encounter at least one touring motorist going to or coming from the Black Point Fissures located at the outer end of this ride. In case of an emergency, you should not wait for help to come by. Instead, you should find help either at the Mono County Park or on US 395 where you can flag down a passing motorist. The Mono Lake Visitor Center is about 3 miles south of US 395 and park rangers and staff are usually on duty.

Land status: Mono Basin National Forest Scenic Area and the Mono Lake Tufa State Reserve, U.S. Forest Service, and the California Department of Parks and Recreation. Some areas are owned by the city of Los Angeles. Many agencies are now actively working to save this unique region and include California Departments of Fish and Game, the U.S. Fish and Wildlife Service, and the Bureau of Land Management, to name few.

Maps: USGS Negit Island 7.5 minute series; *Eastern High Sierra Recreation Topo Map*, published by Fine Edge Productions, Bishop, California.

Finding the trail: From the town of Lee Vining, go slightly over 4 miles north on US 395. Turn right onto Cemetery Road. Descend a few yards and continue about a half mile to the Mono County Park. Park in the lot. Drinking water and rest rooms are available here.

Sources of additional information:

Mono Basin National Forest Scenic Area Visitor Center
P.O. Box 429
Lee Vining, CA 93541
(760) 647-3044

Center is located on the northern edge of Lee Vining, on the lake side of US 395. The Center offers outstanding interpretive exhibits, films, talks, and books. Definitely worth checking out if you're fascinated by Mono Lake and its surroundings.

Notes on the trail: Make sure you have plenty of water before starting the ride. You won't find any shade along the route and all creek water needs to be treated before consumption.

This a fairly easy ride in that it's hard to get lost on the few unmarked trails that crisscross this small area. If you ride without a map, keep the following landmarks in mind. The route is sandwiched between CA 167 on the north and Mono Lake on the south. Defining the west boundary is US 395 with the rugged mountains behind it dominating the western sky. In the east, if you find yourself riding very close to CA 167, (within a quarter mile or so), you're on your way around the entire lake via the Mono Lake Perimeter Loop on various dirt roads. It's an arduous 48-mile loop over lots of deep sand (don't attempt it without adequate preparation). Last but not least, the peak of Black Point sitting at 6,958 feet is an obvious landmark.

Having said that, begin by pedaling out the parking area and go right onto paved Cemetery Road. Upon passing the cemetery at about 1 mile, the smooth road gives way to a mostly hard-packed wide, dirt and gravel road, suitable for passenger vehicles. The road condition may be a bit washboardy and it's enough to keep you awake. Immediately bypass another dirt road signed "Do Not Enter," staying on the main road. Mono Lake is now somewhat hidden from view by the desert scrub-covered hills and the strong fragrance of sage fills your nostrils. Begin a steep climb (about 7% grade) and in less than a half mile, you reach the top of the ridge. You're now pedaling around the northwest side of Black Point.

At 2.8 miles, the road crosses Wilson Creek and reaches a major intersection with another dirt road. Hang a right onto the road, signed to Black Point. The road straight ahead is not signed and it's the road on which you'll be returning. A handful of minor trails and roads intersect the main road. If you're up for some exploring, do check them out but be forewarned that you may be in for some deep sandy spots. When you round the east side of Black Point heading south, another lesser road leads off on your left at about 4.7 miles. (This is the road we'll follow on the return loop.) In almost a mile, you reach the end of the road at an informational signboard, between Black Point and the lake.

After checking out the fissures and communing with nature, hop on your bike and retrace your bike tracks less than a mile to a minor road leading off toward the lake from the main road (yes, that one which was previously mentioned). Reaching this junction at about 6.2 miles, go right onto it. Don't expect to see any signs on this loop. The trail initially leads toward the lake, then curves left as you begin riding north. Many other lesser-traveled roads will intersect your more obvious road. Trail conditions are mostly semi-packed sand and gravel. Occasionally, you'll ride into a brief patch of deep, black, coarse sand, alternating with hard-packed, yellow-white dirt. This is a fun little ride spiced with a few ups and downs and double-tracks.

At about 7.2 miles, your road begins to parallel a barbed-wire fence. Continue past another dirt road signed "Dechambeau Pond Wetlands Restoration. A cooperative venture of the U.S. Forest Service, Ducks Unlimited, CalTran, and the Mono Lake Committee to restore seasonal wetland and moist meadowland." Look just to your left, due west and you'll probably see a concentration of birds swirling above a particular area in the nearby landscape, three ponds to be exact. A handful of other roads intersect here. The road you want is basically a well-traveled, mostly smooth, hard-packed dirt road paralleling the now familiar barb wire fence on your left.

Your main road and its companion barb wire fence curves west toward the mountain range. The road becomes a generously wide, hard-packed dirt road. You can pick up speed on this slightly descending stretch. At 9.8 miles, you close the loop at a familiar intersection. Wilson Creek runs through here and you see the "Black Point" sign again. From here, retrace your path back past the cemetery. You reach Mono County Park at about 9.8 miles.

Finally, lock up your bike and follow the walking path which leads through the tufa grove and out to the edge of the water. Bet you've never seen such a mess of flies as you do here.

RIDE 57 · South Tufa Out-and-Back

AT A GLANCE

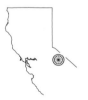

Length/configuration: 15.2-mile out-and-back (7.6 miles one way); dirt roads

Aerobic difficulty: Easy

Technical difficulty: Not technical

Scenery: This is the best place to see the tufa formations of Mono Lake.

Special comments: The route is a lightly traveled dirt road and it's well-suited for freewheeling youngsters and parents towing a kid-trailer.

This 15.2-mile out-and-back route (7.6 miles each way) is great for youngsters. The route consists of wide dirt roads that are basically level with very little car traffic, giving it a nontechnical and easy rating. But what makes this ride so cool for both kids and adults is the stuff you see! What better way to pique a kid's curiosity of geology than out in the field? The main attraction on this ride is the South Tufa Reserve and it's the best site to view these otherworldly rock formations. There, you'll find well-presented interpretive signs and a great walking-only trail through the tufa towers.

RIDE 57 · South Tufa Out-and-Back

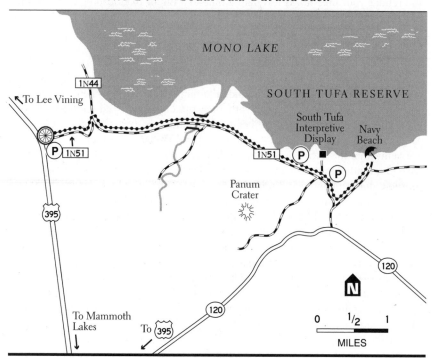

(For background information about the environmental and political significance of Mono Lake and it's unique tufa, see the introduction to Ride 56.) And for hearty riders, you have an option of checking out nearby Panum Crater, a sleeping volcano.

General location: About 80 miles south of Lake Tahoe, on the southern edge of Mono Lake, just outside the eastern border of Yosemite National Park.

Elevation change: Negligible change; mostly at 6,440 feet.

Season: Late May to October, or whenever the first snowstorm hits.

Services: Limited services can be found at Lee Vining. Complete services available in Mammoth Lakes. Swimming is allowed in the lake and the high concentration of salt makes you exceptionally buoyant (bring your own fresh water for rinsing). During the summer months, kayaks rentals are often available at both the South Tufa and Navy Beach locations. A self-guided nature trail, interpretive exhibits, toilets, and picnic tables are offered at South Tufa as well as occasional ranger-led hikes.

Hazards: There's no shade or suitable drinking water on this ride, and believe me, it can get real hot out there. Carry enough drinking water since none is available on the trail. All creek water needs to be treated before consumption. Summer months sometimes see afternoon thunder and lightning storms.

Rescue index: The South Tufa location attracts many sightseers and you should be able to find help there. A park ranger visits the site frequently. Otherwise, make your own way back to US 395 and back into Lee Vining for help.

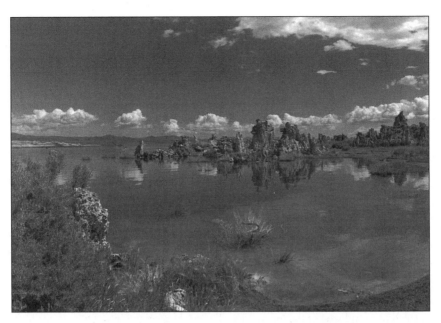

Otherworldly sculptures of tufa formations can be seen from the South Tufa Reserve.

Land status: Mono Basin National Forest Scenic Area and the Mono Lake Tufa State Reserve, U.S. Forest Service, and the California Department of Parks and Recreation. Some areas are owned by the city of Los Angeles. Many agencies are now actively working to save this unique region and include California Departments of Fish and Game, the U.S. Fish and Wildlife Service, and the Bureau of Land Management, to name few.

Maps: USGS Lee Vining 7.5 minute series; *Mammoth High Country Trail Map*, published by Tom Harrison Maps, 2 Falmouth Cove, San Rafael, CA 94901, (800) 265-9090, www.tomharrisonmaps.com; *Eastern High Sierra Recreation Topo Map*, published by Fine Edge Productions, Bishop, California.

Finding the trail: The route begins at the intersection of US 395 and road 1N151 (though some maps label it as 1N44), located about 1.7 miles south of Lee Vining. Essentially, it's the first dirt road on the left after passing CA 120 (Tioga Pass Road) on southbound US 395. Turn left here and park on the side of the road, well off the pavement. Alternatively, adults without children can start pedaling from the town of Lee Vining, riding the shoulder of busy US 395 to 1N151/1N44. Pack a bike lock so that you can enjoy the walking-only trail through the tufa towers.

Sources of additional information

Mono Basin National Forest Scenic
  Area Visitor Center
P.O. Box 429
Lee Vining, CA 93541
(760) 647-3044

Center is located on the northern edge of Lee Vining, on the lake side of US 395. The Center offers outstanding interpretative exhibits, films, talks, and books. Definitely worth checking out if you're fascinated by Mono Lake and its surroundings.

Notes on the trail: This is a fairly easy route to follow. On the outbound direction, Mono Lake is on your left. Start by cruising down a gentle hill over pavement. In a few yards, the pavement begins to disintegrate into a wide, dirt road. The route for the next 5 miles is mostly flat with a few easy ups and downs. Eerie tufa towers protruding out of the lake begin to come into view. Continue on the dirt road past a small overflow parking area on your left. At 5.5 miles, you reach the intersection of another wide dirt road with a bigger parking area straight ahead. Go left, toward the lake and bike as far as permitted toward the site known as South Tufa Reserve. Lock your bike and enjoy a short walk through the tufa "grove." Interpretive signs here enhance your visual discovery.

Back on your bike, retrace your tracks to the main parking area and continue past it. A little over 2 miles, another dirt road leads off on your left, signed Navy Beach. Turn left here and ride 1.4 miles to the beach, following signs along the way. Navy Beach is a favorite launching site of kayakers and kayak rentals are often available here. Swimming is allowed and the saltiness of the water makes you unusually buoyant. (Unfortunately, fresh water is not available here for rinsing off the salt.) From Navy Beach, hop back on your saddle and retrace your path back to your car.

On your return, consider taking a short side trip to Panum Crater, the northernmost volcano in a string called Mono Craters extending just south of here. Panum is located just southwest of the tufa reserve. Though there is a minor dirt road that leads from the reserve to Panum, the trail conditions are likely to be deep, tire swallowing sand. The best route includes a short 1.5 miles stretch on CA 120, a paved two-lane road. To get there from Navy Beach, return to the main dirt road which was signed "Navy Beach." Turn left onto the main dirt road leading away from the South Tufa Reserve and pedal almost a mile to CA 120 and turn right. Go about 1.5 miles due southwest to dirt road 1N200 and follow the sign to Panum Crater. Park your bike at the base and walk an easy trail up to the top. The crater contains an odd mess of volcanic material, created about 600 years ago by numerous lava swells that cooled and cracked. The view from the top reveals a sort of eerie moonscape and may even remind you of a Salvador Dali painting.

RIDE 58 · Hartley Springs Loop

AT A GLANCE

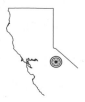

Length/configuration: 9.1-mile loop, counterclockwise; dirt and some sandy roads

Aerobic difficulty: Moderately strenuous with very steep climb at elevations above 8,200 feet

Technical difficulty: Easy to moderate, punctuated by several short stretches of soft dirt and sand

Scenery: Mostly forested shady riding. Part of the forest includes old-growth trees. A short excursion by bike or foot to the geological formation, Obsidian Dome, is nearby.

Special comments: The loop itself is somewhat signed though many unsigned minor trails and jeep roads intersect the route. Given the many other bike trails in the vicinity, this route is lightly used.

Located a little over seven miles south of the barren and arid Mono Lake Basin is richly forested Inyo National Forest. Here lies Hartley Springs Loop. If you've just ridden the routes at Mono Lake or plan to later, you'll witness a stark contrast in riding environments. If not for the tall red fir trees obscuring your view along this bike route, you would see, in the immediate distance, volcanic craters and buttes raising up from the seemingly lifeless lake basin. The forest around Hartley Springs campground, in fact, is populated by old-growth trees.

This 9.1-mile loop is a moderately strenuous ride on graded dirt roads through a peaceful and shady forest. Its technical rating is easy to moderate for the most part with the real technical challenge being a few short stretches that test your ability to maintain traction while riding up steep grades of soft pumice sand and dirt. Divided into thirds, the first 3 miles is a gradual descent punctuated with a short but steep hill, followed by another 3 miles of strenuous, steady climbing, gaining over 900 feet. Tremendous views of June Lake and Mono Lake in the distant north reward your huffing and puffing. The last 3 miles is essentially a sweet downhill run, traversing a gentle, forested slope before closing the loop at the primitive Hartley Springs campground. From within the shade of the forest, peek through the trees and you'll catch glimpses of the sun-baked arid lands to the east. Not quite as popular as other bike routes in Mammoth Lakes just south of here, the greatest draw to this forested ride is the lack of other trail users. It's likely you may be the only one on the loop when you ride. If you're like some cyclists, being out in the woods by yourself, accompanied by your trusty two-wheeled steed is one of the best benefits of mountain biking.

For those of you who like a little exploration and scrambling around geological formations, consider taking a short excursion to check out Obsidian Dome. The Dome is a mile-long chunk of black glass, towering 300 feet high. Located near the end of the loop, it's about 4-mile out-and-back (2 miles each way). Ride the short distance to the base of the Dome. Then, leave your bike at the parking area and hike up the rest of the way (a bike lock is recommended as this is a somewhat popular tourist stop). The craggy edges of the obsidian can be sharp and I'm sure they'd love to kiss your tires.

General location: About 90 south of Lake Tahoe, 10 miles south of Mono Lake and 10 miles north of Mammoth Lakes.

Elevation change: 960 feet; starting elevation 8,300 feet; high point 8,800 feet; low point 7,840 feet. Mostly gradual ascents and descents with some flat sections; several very steep but short climbs.

Season: June through October or when the first snowstorm hits.

Services: Campsites with fire grills, picnic tables, and pit toilets are available at Hartley Springs campground but drinking water is not, so bring plenty. Limited services available in Lee Vining 11 miles north on US 395. All other services can be found in Mammoth Lakes, about 10 miles south on US 395.

Hazards: The only real hazard is an occasional vehicle driving in or out of the campground.

Rescue index: Though not very remote, this route is not as popular as other trails in the area, so don't expect to see anyone else on the loop. In an emergency situation, you should make your way back to your car and head out to US 395 where you can flag down a motorist. The northern end of the loop closely parallels US 395 within 100 yards or so.

RIDE 58 · Hartley Springs Loop

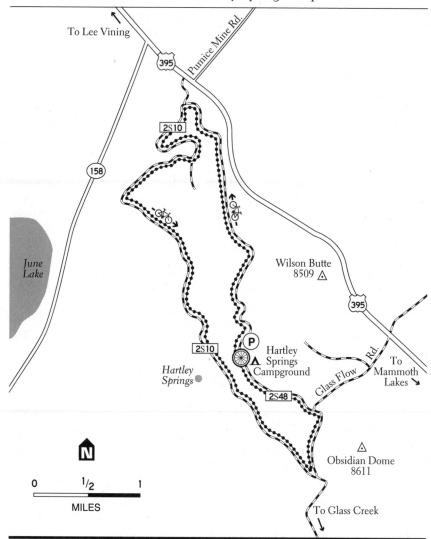

Land status: Inyo National Forest.

Maps: *Mammoth High Country Trail Map,* published by Tom Harrison Maps, 2 Falmouth Cove, San Rafael, CA 94901, (800) 265-9090, www.tomharrisonmaps.com. For handouts published by the national forest, stop by the Mono Lake Visitor Center in Lee Vining or contact the Inyo National Forest Mono Lake Ranger District (see "Sources of additional information" below). *Eastern High Sierra Recreation Topo Map,* published by Fine Edge Productions, Bishop, CA. USGS June Lake 7.5 minute series.

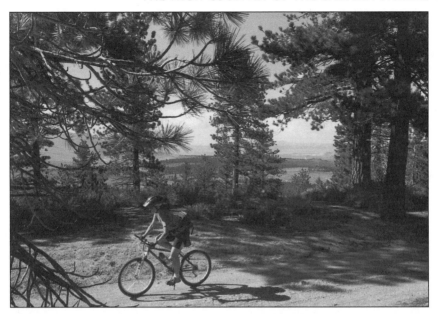

It's not likely you will see many trail users, if any, on this forested loop.

Finding the trail: The route is basically a north-south oblong loop and there are two places from which you can begin riding. The preferred spot is Hartley Springs campground near the southern end of the loop. The other spot is the north parking area located near the intersection of US 395 and Pumice Road on Forest Road 2s10. I recommend Hartley Springs campground as the starting point because you'll have about a 3.5-mile warm-up spin gradually descending terrain before tackling a steep 9%-plus grade hill. Starting at the north parking area, however, means you tackle that same steep hill immediately. That climb is an especially lung searing, thigh burning task when you factor in the elevation gains from 7,900 to 8,760 feet. If you're from much lower elevations, you'll really be affected by the thinner air.

To reach either trailhead, drive about 11 miles south of Lee Vining on US 395. Stay on US 395 and go 1 mile past June Lake Junction (basically an old gas station converted to a mini-mart) at CA 158. Watch for a sign indicating Pumice Mine Road on the left (east) side of US 395; directly across from it down on the right side of US 395 is the north parking area on dirt road 2s10. Park here and begin the grueling uphill grind. To reach the Hartley Springs campground trailhead, continue past Pumice Mine Road for about 2.5 miles farther. Look for a dirt road signed Glass Flow Road on right (west) side of US 395. Turn right here and follow it for almost a mile, at which point pavement resumes and you come to a signed intersection. At this intersection, you're now on the bike loop and Forest Roads 2s48 and 2s10 are marked. You also see a big brown sign here indicating directions to Hartley Springs campground, Obsidian Dome, and Upper Glass Creek. Turn right onto 2s48 and continue driving about a half mile to the campground. Park and begin your ride here.

Sources of additional information:

Inyo National Forest
Mono Lake Ranger District
Highway 120 (Tioga Pass Road)
P.O. Box 429
Lee Vining, CA 93541
(760) 647-3044
www.r5.pswfs.gov/inyo

Mono Basin Scenic Area
  Visitor Center
(half mile north of Lee Vining on
  US 395)
P.O. Box 429
Lee Vining, CA 93541
(760) 647-3044

Notes on the trail: This route is described in a counterclockwise direction. Though it could be ridden clockwise, I prefer to grunt, groan, and whine my way up the short, steep sandy section at the northernmost portion of the loop—a price I'm willing to pay in exchange for a longer, sweet, cruising descent toward the end of the ride.

Begin pedaling north on dirt road 2s48 (it's the continuation of the road on which you drove to reach the campground). The road is a narrow jeep road, mostly level with a few gradual ups and downs. It's technically smooth and easy as it weaves through the pine forest. Occasional tiny pieces of obsidian (black volcanic glass) in the road glint and catch your eye. Several other roads and trails intersect your path and being unsigned, it can get a bit confusing. Every so often, a tiny signpost labeled with a mountain bike symbol helps you stay on the loop. Such is the case for the first 3.2 miles, alternating between right and left turns as the signs direct you over gently descending terrain. Within these miles, somewhere along the way, 2s48 becomes 2s81 as it leads you up a short but steep sandy hill and brings you closer to US 395.

At 3.2 miles, you reach the intersection with another dirt road, 2s10. Immediately to your right is US 395, about 100 yards away. Go left onto 2s10, away from the highway and begin a very steep, (about 9% grade) sandy uphill push. Here's that arduous section I warned you about. It's easy to loose your traction, and I confess: I walked this section. Fortunately, this miserable stretch is less than a half mile. For the most part, the route traverses up the side of a wide canyon that surrounds the June Lake basin far below on your right. Once you reach the top, you're greeted by another bike sign directing you to the left. In a few yards, continue riding past signed dirt road 2s48 on your left. At about 5 miles, ignore a lesser trail peeling off on the right as you continue to head basically west. In a few yards, you reach an open vista point overlooking June Lake. Elevation here is 8,400 feet. Take a breather here and enjoy the view.

When you're good and ready, gear down and grunt up the last steep, somewhat sandy climb. Not to fret. It too is short, less than a mile with a welcome respite thrown in. At about 6.2 miles, you reach the high point of the loop at 8,700 feet. Now comes the reward: about a 2-mile sweet, gradual descent over smooth, mostly hard-packed dirt jeep road through the cool and shady forest. Fewer bike signs appear along this stretch and when in doubt, stay on the well-traveled jeep road, basically heading southwest.

At approximately 8.2 miles, the jeep road crosses a tiny creek. About 75 yards off the right side of the road is Hartley Springs with pure, crystal clear mountain water trickling out of a pipe shoved into the side of the slope. It's lush, cool, and mossy green here—and hungry mosquitoes are waiting for you to make an appearance. Back on your bike, continue a few yards farther past the creek and you reach a signed intersection with a hard hairpin turn to your left. (The road straight ahead leads to the Obsidian Dome. Follow it for a bit of a geological excursion if you wish.) Follow the hairpin curving left. At 9 miles, you reach the major signed intersection which you originally encountered when driving into the campground. Go left onto 2s48 and reach the campground in a few yards. You close the loop at 9.1 miles.

RIDE 59 · Inyo Craters Loop

AT A GLANCE

Length/configuration: 10.4-mile loop, clockwise; dirt jeep roads and some single-track

Aerobic difficulty: Moderate; strenuous if you're not accustomed to the higher elevation

Technical difficulty: Mildly technical

Scenery: A huge rock outcropping composed of black obsidian (volcanic glass), particularly glistening on sunny days. A short distance from the trail are several small craters of dormant volcanoes. Wide-open views of the western range, including the jagged Minarets.

Special comments: Suitable for strong youngsters if ridden as an out-and-back through Crater Flats in the first 4 miles. The ride can be lengthened by starting and ending at the Earthquake Fault (see Mountain View, Ride 63), or from the Daily Grind coffee joint.

Though not a technically challenging ride, Inyo Craters Loop is a favorite among the locals, from beginners to advanced riders. If you're a strong rider who's short on time but still want a work out, you can really crank up some speed since the mildly technical conditions encourage it. The route described here is a mere 10.4-mile loop, ridden in a clockwise direction, starting from the Inyo Crater Lakes parking area. Composed mostly of narrow jeep roads, some dirt single-track, and gravel roads, the route is lightly spiced with a confusing mess of dirt roads and single-tracks leading every which way. Fortunately, the bike route is adequately signed and orienting yourself to landmarks help you find your way. (If you want to do some exploring, I suggest you give yourself plenty of time and arm yourself with several maps. I have yet to find a map that accurately and clearly depicts all roads and trails.) For a real workout, lengthen the ride and make it a strenuous outing by starting from town or the Earthquake Fault (see Ride 63).

No matter how easy or tough you want to make it, Inyo Craters Loop offers pleasing terrain full of geological wonders. The basic ride as described here begins at the parking area of Inyo Crater Lakes, aptly named for the water-filled pits of several small volcanic peaks that blew their tops way before you or I were born. Originally estimated at about 1,500 years old, new evidence set the age of the blown peaks at about 600 years, making the craters one of the youngest geologic events in the Sierra Nevada range. Volcanic gases spewed tons of debris before creating the craters, one measuring 200 feet deep and the other 100 feet deep. Unlike other craters along this volcanic belt extending from Mono Lake in the north to Mammoth Mountain just south of here, these two are curiously not dry, managing to collect enough annual rainfall and snowmelt to form tiny lakes. Do check out the two craters, reached by foot (or bike), about 0.25 miles from the parking area via steep single-track trails. A

RIDE 59 · Inyo Craters Loop

To Mammoth Lakes

To Lee Vining

395

395

To Mammoth Lakes and 203

Mammoth Lakes Scenic Loop Rd

MILES

1/2

0

N

1

Obsidian Flat Campground

Deadman Campground

2529

3S22

3S22

3S29

3S89

Deer Mountain 8786

Inyo Craters

Crater Flats

P

To Mountain View Trail

3S22

third crater sits atop Deer Mountain, about 400 yards north of the two immediately accessible craters.

As you begin pedaling the loop, notice that the wide-open, seemingly barren meadows of pumice, set against the dramatic Ritter range and its jagged Minarets, is actually populated with delicate, tiny wild flowers and other vegetation. At the far end of the loop, as the route parallels small Deadman Creek in a gorge, look for a huge rock outcropping with a black face. That's black volcanic glass, called obsidian, and on a sunny day, it will be glistening.

General location: About 95 miles south of Lake Tahoe, about 4 miles northwest of Mammoth Lakes.

Elevation change: 460 feet; starting elevation 7,750 feet; high point 8,160 feet, low point 7,700 feet. Lots of rolling hills with stretches of flat terrain.

Season: June through October or when the first snowstorm hits.

Services: Pit toilets at the parking area. No water available. Water taken from creeks need to be treated. Three campgrounds—Obisidian Flats, Upper, and Lower Deadman Creek—are located on the loop; if you want to camp, check on availability first. All other services available in the town of Mammoth Lakes.

Hazards: Portions of the loop are well-traveled by passenger vehicles. Summers can be bloody hot, so carry plenty of water.

Rescue index: Mammoth Lakes is a popular summer vacation destination and the geological feature of the lakes attracts bikers and non-bikers alike. Though this is a somewhat popular bike route in the summer, it has the most use on weekends and late afternoons. For that reason, should an emergency arise on any point of the loop, don't expect help to come along any time soon. You should make your own way back to the parking area or the well-traveled Mammoth Lakes Scenic Loop (paved road 3S23) where your chances are greater of finding people who may be of help.

Land status: Inyo National Forest.

Maps: *Mammoth High Country Trail Map,* published by Tom Harrison Maps, 2 Falmouth Cove, San Rafael, CA 94901, (800) 265-9090, www.tomharrisonmaps.com; *Eastern High Sierra Recreation Topo Map,* published by Fine Edge Productions, Bishop, California. Some annual summer publications contain maps and are distributed by the Mammoth Lakes Visitor Center. Free map handouts are occasionally available, too. USGS Mammoth Mountain and Old Mammoth 7.5 minute series.

Finding the trail: The preferred parking area is at the Inyo Craters Lakes and it can be accessed in two ways: from the town of Mammoth Lakes or immediately off US 395 (traveling south from Mono Lake and Lee Vining).

To get to the town of Mammoth Lakes from US 395, go west on CA 203. Follow CA 203, also known as Main Street, through Mammoth Lakes. Travel 4 miles from US 395 and turn right (north) onto Minaret Road, which is still CA 203. Go about a mile to Mammoth Scenic Loop, a paved road; turn right here. Follow the Scenic Loop Road for about 2.7 miles to a dirt road turn-off signed to the Inyo Crater Lakes; go left (you may spot another small sign here identifying this dirt road as 3s29). Follow this dirt road for about a mile as it curves north, then west to a sort of 3-way intersection. Veer right on the main dirt road and take the middle road, following the sign to the lakes and the parking area. The parking area is reached in about 0.2 mile. Park here.

From Mono Lake and Lee Vining, travel south on US 395 to its intersection with Mammoth Scenic Loop Road, a paved two-lane road, and turn west (right) onto it. Drive about 3.3 miles to a signed dirt road turn-off to the Inyo Crater Lakes; go right (this is dirt road 3s29 and you may see this on a smaller sign). Follow the same directions to the parking area as above.

Sources of additional information:

Inyo National Forest Headquarters
873 N. Main St.
Bishop, CA 93514
(760) 873-2400

Inyo National Forest
Mammoth Ranger District
P.O. Box 148
Mammoth Lakes, CA 93546
(760) 924-5500
www.r5.pswfs.gov/inyo

Mono Basin National Forest Scenic
Area Visitor Center
P.O. Box 429
Lee Vining, CA 93541
(760) 647-3044
Center is located on the northern
edge of Lee Vining, on the lake side
of US 395. The Center offers outstanding interpretive exhibits,
films, talks, and books.

U.S. Forest Service
Mammoth Lakes Visitors Bureau
P.O. Box 48
Mammoth Lakes, CA 93546
(888) GO-MAMMOTH
Located at the entrance to Shady
Rest Park and Campground on CA
203, about 2.5 miles west of US 395.

Notes on the trail: Even though the Inyo Crater Lakes is a short 0.25-mile hike from the parking area, they're not visible from the parking area. You can either check out the craters now or after your ride.

From the parking area, hop on your bike and retrace your path back to the three-way intersection which you drove through before turning into this parking area. At the three-way intersection, look for mountain bike signs as well as road numbers. Don't follow road 3s29; instead, bear left and follow 3s22, heading in the opposite direction of a sign pointing to the lakes. This is the beginning of a clockwise loop. If you look at the loop as a clock face, you're beginning it at the number 6 position. If you ride with a bike odometer, set it to begin measuring distance here.

The route initially follows a semi-packed narrow dirt road, leading you past tall and fragrant pine trees. Be aware that other roads and trails will intersect the road you're on and for the next 4.2 miles, you want to stay on 3s22. Look for bike signs to help you stay on the loop. Almost a mile from the three-way intersection, the dirt road leads you into a small clearing with Mammoth Mountain looming majestically straight ahead in the southwest. Welcome to Crater Flats, a wide-open space of rolling terrain where the pine trees are stunted, thanks to the inhospitable soil. In fact, the ground is predominantly covered with fine white, gravel—pumice to be exact. The road is a delightful up and down cruise.

About a mile into the ride, a sign at a fork in the road directs you to go straight. The route is gradually curving west by northwest. The terrain opens up even more, bordered on your left by the Ritter range in the distant west. Immediately on your right, through the trees are huge steep mounds of rock outcroppings that look every bit like a tiny rugged mountain range. Still on 3s22, the road leads you into the forest again, becoming a bit more rugged with exposed rocks and tree roots.

The first creek crossing is reached at about 3.3 miles. Depending on the time of year, the creek may be shallow enough to ride through, otherwise, take advantage of a log bridge nearby. In a few yards, cross Deadman Creek via another log bridge, reached via a short single-track trail. On the other side of the creek, near a small picnic table, a dirt road runs in two directions. Look for a bike sign and follow its direction to go straight, due east, heading downstream with the creek paralleling the dirt road on your right. Though not identified as such, you're now on Deadman Creek Road, a somewhat wide dirt road. Maps don't clearly state if this is road 3s26 or 3s29. In any case, you should be pedaling due east. On both sides of Deadman Creek Road, several single-track trails peel off and rejoin in about 100 yards. Continue on and several more trails and dirt roads deviate from your loop route. It can be downright confusing here! Look for the trusty, though tiny, brown bike sign for guidance. At this point, about 4.1 miles into the loop, the route leads you through a small gorge. Keep your eyes peeled on the steep slope on your right, on the other side of the creek. You'll soon behold a huge patch of black volcanic glass. The material is obsidian and if the day is bright, it will reflect and refract the sunlight. Formed by rapid cooling of lava, obsidian readily fractures into shiny, curved surfaces. Native American Indians made use of its brittleness and shaped razor-sharp arrowheads for their spears.

At about 4.6 miles, you reach a big intersection. The road leading off to the left is 2s50. Stay straight on the main road as indicated by a mountain bike sign. Shallow patches of black gravel dot the road. Cruise past several campgrounds: Upper Deadman on the right and Obsidian Flat on the left. If you have shocks, zipping through the washboard road is a breeze. If not, you might want to slow your speed so as to not jar the eyeballs right out of your head. Your road widens a bit here while several other roads peel off.

You reach a well-signed intersection at 5.7 miles. The road you've been pedaling is 2s05. The intersecting road on the right is 2s29 (graced by a bike sign) and it leads to Mammoth Scenic Loop road. Turn right onto 2s29 and continue heading basically due east, now through a lovely pine forest. Many more dirt roads of varying sizes connect to your road. Fortunately, mountain bike signs are posted indicating where you need to make a turn or stay straight. When in doubt, stay on the main road. At about 7.3 miles, about 1.6 miles since turning onto 2s29, you reach another intersection signed with a bike symbol. Go right as indicated by the symbol. At this point of the loop, you're sort of at the number three position on the clock, having now ridden three-fourths of the loop.

At 9.8 miles, you come to an intersection with a lesser road. Though it's not signed here, look to the left, just a few yards ahead and you'll see a landmark: a fenced Unical Gas valve. Off in the distance on your left is Mammoth Mountain. In a few yards, a narrow, steep single-track signed with a bike symbol peels off on the right. If you didn't get enough huff and puffing, take this single-track. It's a shortcut to the parking area, trimming less than a half mile off the loop. Otherwise, stay on the main jeep road which is also signed by a bike symbol. At just over 10 miles, you close the loop by reaching the familiar three-way intersection near the parking area. Turn right and retrace 0.2 mile back to your car.

It's time to check out the craters if you didn't do so before the ride. Lock up your bike and walk the short distance to the craters. For those of you aching for more time in the saddle, you can pedal up to the crater's edge via a steep single-track accessed on the far northern end of the parking area. Either way, you'll find these tiny but odd water-filled craters and the accompanying interpretive sign interesting.

Optional add-on: Park at the Earthquake Fault and access the loop at the three-way intersection via dirt road 3s89. This out-and-back portion is slightly over 4 miles, adding a total of just over 8 miles to the above 10.4-mile loop, for a round-trip total of 18.4 miles. Steep climbs and sections of single-track on this portion make for a strenuous aerobic work-out requiring intermediate- to advance-level technical skills. (Refer to Ride 69, Mountain View Ride, for directions on how to access the trailhead at road 3s89. Read the "Notes on the trail," particularly at mile 3.7. Also check out my map.)

RIDE 60 · Easy Shady Rest Ride

AT A GLANCE

Length/configuration: 4.6-mile out-and-back with a loop, clockwise; paved bike path and dirt roads

Aerobic difficulty: Easy due to flatness

Technical difficulty: Mild except for occasional patches of soft dirt and sand

Scenery: Shady Rest Campgrounds, maintained ball fields, mixed conifer forests, wide open clearings and expansive views of the mountain ranges in the John Muir Wilderness and Mammoth Lakes Valley

Special comments: Great ride for young families and riders looking for a leisurely and short route. Suitable for kid-trailers and alley-cats.

Simply put, Easy Shady Rest Ride is a perfect bike outing for young families. It combines a lovely, car-free one-mile stretch of paved bike path with a 2.6-mile, all-dirt-road loop through a conifer forest and a wide-open sagebrush meadow. Total distance is 4.6 quiet miles away from vehicular traffic. Along the way, Shady Rest Park offers a kids' playground, softball fields, wooden tables, and rest room facilities—a great spot for a picnic after the ride. The terrain of the loop is mildly rolling, which is to say it's pretty much flat. The riding is mostly nontechnical over wide dirt roads with some scattered tiny patches of loose dirt and sand.

Following the bike path is obvious while the dirt loop at the end of the paved path, on the other hand, is not quite as easy. Though the loop is somewhat marked with colored identifying markers, a number of unmarked small trails and dirt roads crisscross the area. Which way to go? Don't let that keep you and your youngsters from enjoying this simple route. It's hard to get lost because the lay of the land makes keeping track of your direction a piece of cake. Just keep in mind that the loop is a slightly bent hot-dog shape, going east and west. On the outbound portion of the dirt loop, you'll cruise along the base of a hill. You won't be huffing and puffing up any steep sections, (if you do, you're off the loop and you're tackling the Knolls Loop, Ride 61). On the return portion of the loop heading basically west, the wide-open terrain enables you to keep your sense of direction because you can see CA 203 and the mountain range of the John Muir Wilderness on your left (south). I tell you all this because the few maps I have seen of this route don't show all the unsigned trails and roads. By reviewing the map shown here and heeding the few trail markers posted along the way, you'll have no trouble on this short outing. On all counts, this ride's a piece of cake!

General location: About 100 miles south of Lake Tahoe, in the town of Mammoth Lakes.

Elevation change: Negligible change; mostly at 7,700 feet.

Season: June through October or when the first snowstorm hits.

Services: Rest rooms and water available at the U.S. Forest Service/Mammoth Lakes Visitor Center as well as throughout Shady Rest Park and campgrounds. Soccer and softball fields, picnic tables, and playground facilities are located at

RIDE 60 · Easy Shady Rest Ride

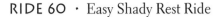

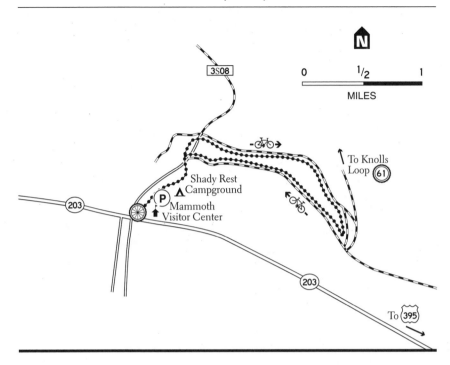

Shady Rest Park at the far end of the paved bike path. The campgrounds are maintained with piped water, barbeque pits, and rest rooms. There are 97 sites at New Shady Rest and 51 at Old Shady Rest. All other services available in town.

Hazards: The 1-mile stretch of paved bike path is popular with pedestrians and speeding kiddies on bikes, so heads up. Helmet required.

Rescue index: The paved bike path runs through the campground and is extremely popular in the summer, so you're likely to find people who may be of help. The dirt loop, however, sees fewer users, so in case of emergency, don't wait for help to come along—make your way back to Shady Rest Park, campground or the Visitor Center. Pay phone located at the Visitor Center.

Land status: Inyo National Forest.

Maps: Some annual summer publications contain maps and are distributed by the Mammoth Lakes Visitor Center. Free map handouts are occasionally available too. Also, along the paved bike path, look for signs that display a map of bike routes in the immediate vicinity.

Finding the trail: From the intersection of US 395 and CA 203 (Main Street), head west into Mammoth Lakes on Main Street. Go about 2.5 miles and turn right toward the U.S. Forest Service/Mammoth Lakes Visitor Center, Ranger Station, and the Shady Rest Campground. Park in the lot by the Visitor Center. Water, rest rooms, and tons of information can be found here.

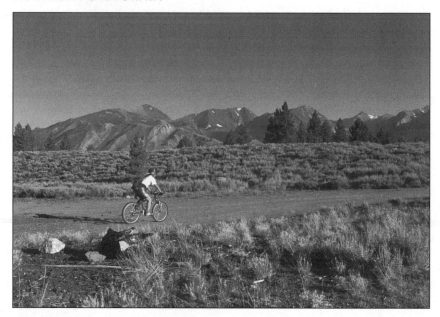

Enjoying an easy, wide-open spin with the peaks of the John Muir Wilderness in the distance.

Sources of additional information:

Inyo National Forest Headquarters
873 N. Main St.
Bishop, CA 93514
(760) 873-2400

Inyo National Forest
Mammoth Ranger District
P.O. Box 148
Mammoth Lakes, CA 93546
(760) 924-5500
www.r5.pswfs.gov/inyo

U.S. Forest Service
Mammoth Lakes Visitors Bureau
P.O. Box 48
Mammoth Lakes, CA 93546
(888) GO MAMMOTH
Visitor Center located at the bike path trailhead, at the entrance to Shady Rest Camp and Park off Main Street (CA 203)

Notes on the trail: Following the paved bike path is a no-brainer; the hot dog–shaped dirt loop is not as simple. From the Visitor Center parking lot, just hop onto the bike path and head north away from Main Street. The path is completely separate from the paved vehicle road. Cruise past the campgrounds and eventually, after about a mile, the path crosses a vehicle road and runs into Shady Rest Park. Here, you'll find a playground (with swings and monkey bars which sometimes exert a gravitational pull on kiddies), a soccer field, and several softball fields. There are also picnic tables and a rest room here.

Continue to follow the path as it crosses a paved road. The path cruises between the softball diamonds and soon ends at a parking lot. Look directly ahead, due east, for a handicapped parking sign. Immediately behind it is a wide dirt road. Take this dirt road and begin riding the hot dog–shaped loop in a clockwise direction. Right off the bat, lots of other dirt roads and single-track trails (signed and unsigned) intersect your route. Finding your way can be a bit confusing. When in doubt, stay on the wide dirt road. For the first 0.6 miles of the dirt road, as you descend ever so gradually through a pine forest, a single power line parallels your road overhead. Then, as you emerge from the trees into a clearing with almost 180-degree views of snow-capped mountain peaks in the south, the power line peels away from your road. On your left (north), the terrain immediately slopes uphill. Not to worry though, you won't be climbing any steep stretches. If you do, you're on the Knolls Loops (Ride 61) and not the Easy Shady Rest Loop.

A few hundred yards farther, at just over 2 miles from the Visitor Center, you reach a signed intersection as another power line joins you briefly. The left road is identified with a blue symbol signifying the Knolls Loop, while the green sign points right to the Shady Rest Loop. Go right and begin making a wide right turn through the open and gently rolling, sagebrush-covered meadow.

At about 2.4 miles, you come to another major intersection, though it's not signed here. The overhead power line deviates from your road. Stay right, effectively making a wide U-turn, heading sort of due south by southwest. In fact, look to your right across the meadow and you can see the road on which you pedaled out. A few yards farther and you reach another intersection. When we rode this route, the brown carsonite sign planted here had been snapped off—perhaps it's been replaced by the time you read this. In any case, bear right, basically staying straight and due west. The wide dirt road begins a gentle ascent as it passes several unsigned smaller trails. Stay on the main dirt road as it cruises into the forest, curving slightly southward. At 4.6 miles, you emerge from the forest and find yourself at the parking lot facing the softball fields. Cross the parking lot, pick up the paved bike trail and retrace your path back to the Visitor Center. Total combined mileage for the dirt loop with the bike path out-and-back is about 4.6 miles.

If you're looking for a big workout and you have time left in the day, consider riding the adjacent Knolls Loop, a 10-mile strenuous route. See the ride description that follows.

RIDE 61 · Knolls Loop

AT A GLANCE

Length/configuration: 10.7-mile loop, counterclockwise; dirt roads and a brief section on single-track

Aerobic difficulty: Strenuous due to long stretches of moderately steep climbing

Technical difficulty: Mild to intermediate; though the dirt roads are generally smooth and hard-packed, portions are soft-packed and sandy

Scenery: Panoramic views of the town of Mammoth Lakes, Lake Crowley, Mono Lake, Mammoth Mountain, and the surrounding ranges. Accessible rock outcroppings offer a great place for a snack break and fun exploration by foot.

Special comments: Bail-out optional trail shortens the ride. This loop can be ridden in either direction. Signboards posted near the visitor center and the campground describe this route in a clockwise direction.

There's not much to say about the Knolls Loop except that it's a favorite among locals. This 10.7-mile loop is a great after-work workout. Easily accessible from town, the hustle and bustle of city life is quickly replaced by the sounds of breezes blowing through the pine forests. The views from many rock outcroppings are soul-expanding and offer a bit of solitude for those seeking it. Composed mostly of dirt roads, the terrain is mildly intermediate. Occasional patches of soft dirt and pumice tease your bike handling skills and the uphills make the Knolls Loop a strenuous outing. Unlike other places nearby, this route doesn't lead you past any real geological wonders. Trail composition is mostly sandy pumice and somewhat hard-packed dirt. Occasionally, you'll spot obsidian chips (black volcanic glass) in the trail. There's even a big chunk of a rock outcropping that's composed of the black stuff.

The loop can be ridden in either direction. Riding it counterclockwise (as it's described here) means the downhills are longer and gentler while the climbing is steeper but shorter. Riding it clockwise makes faster, steeper but shorter descents and longer, gradual climbs. Located on the north side of town, the loop basically winds around several knolls. The counterclockwise direction begins with a one-mile cruise on the paved bike path through Shady Rest campground before climbing up behind impressive rock outcroppings. If you're not accustomed to the altitude here at Mammoth Lakes, your lungs and thighs will definitely scream on this ride.

Unsure if this loop is your cup of tea? You can always take the Sawmill Cutoff Road. It provides an option to shorten the loop or to reconfigure the route to your liking.

General location: About 100 miles south of Lake Tahoe, in the town of Mammoth Lakes.

Elevation change: 740 feet; starting elevation 7,700 feet; high point 8,280 feet; low point 7,540 feet. Lots of ups and downs with several long ascending and descending stretches.

Season: June through October or when the first snowstorm hits.

Services: Rest rooms and water available at the U.S. Forest Service/Mammoth Lakes Visitor Center as well as throughout Shady Rest Park and campgrounds. Soccer and softball fields, picnic tables, and playground facilities are located at Shady Rest Park at the far end of the paved bike path. The campgrounds are maintained with piped water, barbeque pits, and rest rooms. There are 97 sites at New Shady Rest and 51 sites at Old Shady Rest. All other services available in town.

Hazards: The 1-mile stretch of paved bike path is popular with pedestrians and speeding kiddies on bikes, so heads up.

Rescue index: Though the Knolls Loop is a well-known route, it's quite possible you won't see other trail users during your outing. In case of emergency, don't wait for help to come along. Depending on where you are on the loop, consider making your way back to the intersection of Sawmill Cutoff Road (3s08); it's a well-traveled dirt vehicle road and a motorist may pass by. Sawmill is also the shortcut back to Shady Rest Park, campground and the Visitor Center.

Land status: Inyo National Forest.

RIDE 61 · Knolls Loop

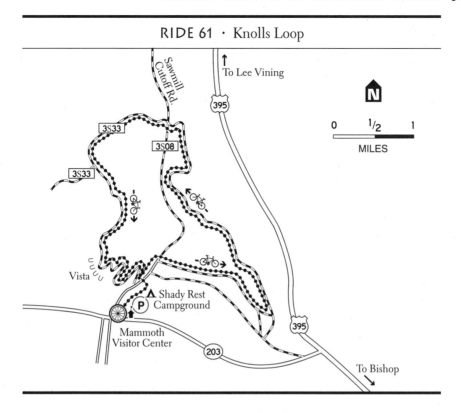

Maps: Some annual summer publications contain maps and are distributed by the U.S. Forest Service/Mammoth Lakes Visitor Center. Free map handouts are occasionally available too. Also, along the paved bike path, look for signboards which display a map of bike routes in the immediate vicinity. *Eastern High Sierra Recreation Topo Map*, published by Fine Edge Productions, Bishop, California.

Finding the trail: From the intersection of US 395 and CA 203 (Main Street), head west into Mammoth Lakes on Main Street. Go about 2.5 miles and turn right toward the U.S. Forest Service/Mammoth Lakes Visitor Center, Ranger Station, and the Shady Rest Campground. Park in the lot by the Visitor Center. Water, rest rooms, and tons of information can be found here.

Sources of additional information: See sources of additional information for Ride 60.

Notes on the trail: This 10.7-mile loop is described in a counterclockwise direction and starts on the paved bike path near the U.S. Forest Service/Mammoth Lakes Visitor Center. Begin by hopping onto the bike path and cruise 1 mile to Shady Rest Park. At the park, cross a vehicle road and follow the path to its terminus between two softball diamonds and into a parking lot. Facing east from the ball fields, look for a blue handicapped parking sign. Directly behind this sign is a narrow dirt road leading into the forest, running due east. (Incidentally, look left to the far end of the parking lot and there you see a wide dirt road signed 3s08. Though not named as such, this is the Sawmill Cutoff Road and it intersects the Knolls Loop at the north end of the loop, about 2.5 miles up. Remember this road—it's a good bail-out road to shorten the ride or to seek emergency assistance.)

A word of caution: Navigating your way through Knolls Loop is confusing since quite a few unsigned single-track trails and dirt roads crisscross the route. Maps I have seen only add to the confusion because not all trails are accurately indicated, if at all. Fortunately, many intersections on the route are signed by a brown carsonite post decorated with a blue "Knolls" label and a white biker symbol. Generally speaking, these signs are useful in helping you stay on the loop. (When we pedaled this route, we encountered several carsonite signs that were blank and another one ambiguously laying on the ground at an intersection.) The fact of the matter is, there are different ways to access the Knolls Loop and starting on this dirt road behind the handicapped parking sign is one of them.

That said, as you leave the parking lot, ignore the signed single-track trail that immediately crosses your road. Stay on the dirt road as it leads you through the forest over mostly flat and semi-packed terrain. A single power line parallels your road. In just over a half mile, you emerge from the forest and skirt a sizeable clearing with CA 203 and the snow-capped mountain ranges of the John Muir Wilderness off in the distance on your right. On your left, the terrain immediately slopes up steeply toward a bank of towering rock outcroppings. At about 2 miles from the Visitor Center, (about a mile from the softball fields), you reach a signed intersection. Say good-bye to the power line as you follow the Knolls sign to the left. Drop your gearing and get ready to huff and puff up the steepest section of the ride, about an 8–12% grade. Bear down. It's only for a short distance, about a half mile. Maintaining traction is a challenge because the trail condition is likely to be soft dirt and sand with tiny pieces of obsidian (black volcanic glass) dotting the trail. Persevere. The jeep road curves to the north, leading you up and behind rock outcroppings, and you feel like you're doubling back in the direction from which you came. If you're not accustomed to the altitude, your lungs and thighs may beg for mercy. As you continue the uphill march on this knoll—on bike or by foot—views of the Mono Lake basins appear on your right and the town of Mammoth Lakes and the Mammoth Mountain Bike Park on your left. Finally, at about mile 3, you reach the top of the steepest section. Take a breather and explore the rock outcroppings if you'd like. The view northeast toward Mono Lake, and south to the John Muir Wilderness and Mammoth Lakes is expansive. Many trails and jeep roads intersect your route, not all of which are signed. Stay on the main route and watch for biker and the Knolls carsonite markers.

Enjoy a gradual downhill run, bypassing a lesser jeep road on your right. At about mile 3.5, at the bottom of the short descent, you reach a major intersection. Stay right, heeding the Knolls sign. At this point, you're looking directly into the town of Mammoth Lakes far below. Continuing on, the terrain cruises up and down. You come to another signed intersection at about 4.6 miles. Go right and in a few yards, reach another signed intersection. This time, go left, following the Knolls sign. By now, you're at the top of another knoll amid pine trees and the view to the south is tremendous. Another short downhill run and at the bottom, at almost 5 miles, you come to another signed intersection. Stay straight and in a few yards, another intersection appears. The Knolls sign directs you to stay straight, bearing slightly left.

At about mile 5.4, you reach a major intersection. There are at least 3 other roads converging and signs are everywhere. The road running left and right is 3s08, which is the Sawmill Cutoff Road. (As mentioned earlier, this is the bail-out shortcut that leads to the softball fields parking lot in 2.5 miles.) The road straight ahead is 3s33, a passenger car dirt road which leads to the Mammoth Scenic Loop Road, and signed by the now familiar Knolls bike marker (this is the road you want). Gradually ascend the dirt road and watch out for occasional cars. At about mile 6.5, you reach the high point of the loop. Approximately 0.3 miles farther, you find another major intersection. Here, the Knolls marker directs you to go left, turning off road 3s33. From here, now heading mostly south, the rest of the ride is basically a downhill cruise, weaving through forested terrain and small clearings that are sometimes dotted with wildflowers. Continue following the Knolls markers through several more intersections.

At 8.3 miles, keep an eye out for a sign pointing to the Vista Point. You can pedal or hike the short steep distance, about 100 yards. In any case, as you peer through the pine trees, you're rewarded with an expansive view of the town, Mammoth Mountain, the surrounding snow-capped peaks, and a bit of Lake Crowley. Return to the main trail and resume your downhill run. In just over 9 miles, an unsigned road intersects your road. Veer right and begin looking for and following blue diamond markers tacked to trees.

At 9.6 miles, another unsigned road comes in on your left and telephone poles begin paralleling your road, now a narrow jeep road. Once again, stay straight, bearing right and follow the poles as it curves to the left, still gently descending through the pine forest. In a few yards, you reach another unsigned intersection. Stay on your road, going straight and under the phone line. Say good-bye to the phone line as it follows the other road.

Finally, at 9.8 miles, you see another Knolls marker at yet another intersection. This time, the sign points to a single-track trail. At this intersection, off on your left in the bushes is an abandoned, rusting cab of a truck. Hop onto the single-track, follow it through the forest and, in a short while, your trail parallels a paved road on the left. Soon, it leads you past a huge sign that describes the various biking trails in the vicinity. The asphalt road here is the paved portion of the Sawmill Cutoff Road and leads to the softball fields as well as to the park entrance in town. Continue farther, keeping Sawmill on your left. Go past the turn-off to the Old Shady Rest campground. At 10.7 miles, the single-track ends as it crosses Sawmill. Hop onto the paved bike path and make your way back to the visitor center and your parked car. Total distance of the Knolls Loop is approximately 10.7 miles.

RIDE 62 · Horseshoe Lake Loop

AT A GLANCE

Length/configuration: 1.9-mile loop, counterclockwise; single-track trail

Aerobic difficulty: Easy

Technical difficulty: Mildly technical, though some sections at the beginning are punctuated with abrupt dips and beginners might want to walk through them.

Scenery: Filtered views of lovely little Horseshoe Lake as seen from within a pine forest. A sandy beach near the end of the loop offers a wide-open view of the snow-capped mountain peaks of the John Muir Wilderness.

Special comments: An easy trail well-suited for freewheeling kiddies and true beginners who have basic bike-handling skills. This trail is also re-ferred to as the Waterwheel Trail.

Unless you're a youngster or a true beginner with little single-track riding experi-ence, you may find this sweet loop so tame it's downright boring. The loop is only 1.9 miles long and skirts the forested perimeter of lovely Horseshoe Lake, a pris-tine little lake sitting at 8,900 feet. Except for a short, steep, roller-coaster section near the beginning, the trail is level and composed of almost all single-track trail. Technically, it's mild and manageable by anyone with minimal bike handling skills. And so what if it's all over too soon? Ride the loop again.

Like many mountain bike trails at Mammoth Lakes, the surrounding environ-ment makes Horseshoe Lake Loop a worthwhile ride. Horseshoe Lake is basically un-developed, except for a small campground. Because there are no boat ramps, boat rentals, and no resort, the lake is fairly quiet. Picnic tables and sunny sandy beaches, especially near the end of the loop, offer relaxing spots to enjoy views of the snow-capped mountain peaks of the John Muir Wilderness. In early summer, creek cross-ings are likely to reveal a stunning display of wildflowers commingling with the lush green understory which line the trickling streams. (There are about eight tiny creek crossings, some of which have a convenient wooden bridge in place.) And like other sites in the area, Horseshoe Lake has its own geological wonder. From the parking lot at the beginning of the loop, you may notice an area of dead Jeffrey pine trees dotting the barren terrain. No, it wasn't fire or disease that caused the demise of the trees, but rather carbon dioxide gas dissipating up from the soil, no doubt a by-product of natural underground activity induced by the area's volcanic rumblings. Strangely enough, this hostile terrain is only right at the beginning of the loop while the rest of the route weaves through healthy, fragrant pine forest.

General location: About 100 miles south of Lake Tahoe, a couple of miles south-west of the heart of Mammoth Lakes.

Elevation change: Negligible change; mostly at 8,900 feet.

Season: June through October or when the first snowstorm hits.

Services: Picnic tables, barbeque pits, rest rooms, and piped water available at the campground. This would be a great camping adventure for kids. All other services available in the town of Mammoth Lakes.

Hazards: The first half mile of the narrow single-track trail runs through several short and steep ravines. Cyclists who are unsure of their bike handling skills may want to dismount and walk the few yards through these sections. Also, watch for oncoming traffic from other bikers and hikers. There's a short section of the loop where you have the option of riding the shoulder of paved Lake Mary Road. If you do, watch out for vehicular traffic, which can be frequent during the summer.

Rescue index: This is a popular trail in the summer and chances are good you'll meet other trail users who may be of emergency help. Otherwise, you're likely to find help back at the parking lot or on Lake Mary Road.

RIDE 62 · Horseshoe Lake Loop

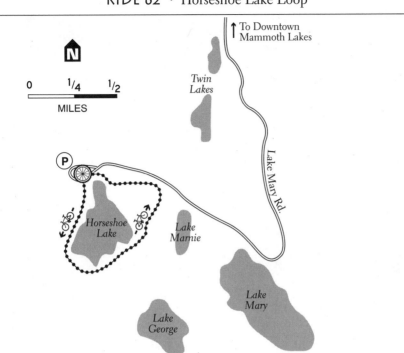

Land status: Inyo National Forest.

Maps: *Eastern High Sierra Recreation Topo Map*, published by Fine Edge Productions, Bishop, California. Some annual summer publications contain maps and are distributed by the U.S. Forest Service/Mammoth Lakes Visitor Center. Free map handouts are occasionally available too.

Finding the trail: From the town of Mammoth Lakes, head west on Main Street (CA 203). At its intersection with Minaret Road, continue straight through and Main Street becomes Lake Mary Road. Follow Lake Mary Road as it curves past Twin Lakes and Lake Mary. After 5 miles, the road ends at Horseshoe Lake in the parking lot.

Sources of additional information: See sources of additional information for Ride 60.

Notes on the trail: Begin pedaling through the parking lot, going south directly away from Lake Mary Road. Look for a single-track trail, just past the rest rooms and the small campground. In a few yards, you'll spot a mountain bike sign. While there is at least one sign that identifies this trail as Waterwheel Trail, you won't see it signed Horseshoe Lake Loop. Why is that? Who knows. Horseshoe Lake Loop is a far more descriptive title and that's probably why it sticks in people's minds.

In the first 0.5 miles, within a Jeffrey pine forest, the single-track skirts the edge of the lake on your left, ranging from 30 to 100 feet away. The trail leads you up and down short, steep ravines and you may want to dismount and walk through any difficult spots.

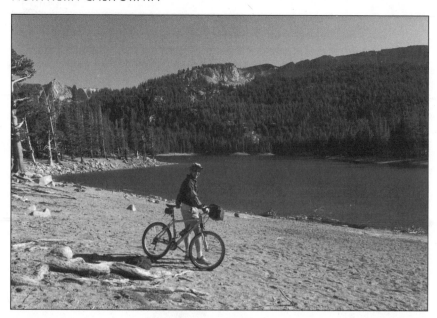

Tiny Horseshoe Lake features a short single-track, perfect for kids and timid beginners hoping to improve their technical skills.

If you're riding early in the summer, you will likely cross a number of tiny creeks, some of which have a small wooden bridge in place. Other single-tracks peel off from your trail toward the water and you can ignore them. Stay on the main trail. So long as the lake is on your left, you won't get lost.

At almost a mile, the single-track leads you past the stone foundation of a house destroyed by fire. The fireplace is the obvious evidence. From this point, the trail turns away from the lake. For the next 0.4 miles to the intersection with Lake Mary Road, you catch only glimpses of the lake through the forest. When you reach the paved Lake Mary Road, you have the option of riding on the far shoulder of the road which will take you back to the parking area in less than a mile. (If you do, be alert for vehicular traffic.) If you don't relish the idea of riding pavement, then look left for a dirt single-track trail lying just before the road. Follow the trail through the forest and at about 1.7 miles, you reach a sandy beach that offers a wide-open view to the south of the lake and the John Muir Wilderness. It's a great spot to relax and snooze in the warm sun or have a picnic. Continuing on, you reach the parking lot at 1.9 miles. If you feel the ride ended way too soon, ride the loop again.

RIDE 63 · Mountain View

AT A GLANCE

Length/configuration: 5.7-mile point-to-point; single-track and dirt jeep road (Option: 9.3-mile loop, clockwise; includes pavement)

Aerobic difficulty: Moderate; strenuous if you're not acclimated to the higher altitude

Technical difficulty: Mild to intermediate, due to stretches of sandy pumice trail conditions

Scenery: Stunted whitebark pines and trail composed of white volcanic pumice make it easy to imagine you're riding in snow. The Earthquake Fault, a geological site, is definitely worth checking out.

Special comments: Mountain View trail is fairly well-signed. This route can be easily combined with several other nearby trails, extending the mileage considerably for a great intermediate- to advanced-level outing (see "Notes on the Trail" for add-on suggestions).

It was the end of the day and the sun was just about to disappear behind the Ritter Range. For the sake of time, my husband, Bruce, volunteered to ride the Mountain View Trail while I took on the mundane task of measuring mileages by car, scouting alternate routes, and picking him up a the end of his fun ride. ("So many trails, so little time," was a frequent grumbling of mine.) And so, based on his report, here's what riding the Mountain View trail was like.

Starting from the Minaret Summit Vista overlook at 9,175 feet, Mountain View is a 5.7-mile trail that basically descends through a drainage, punctuated by several short stretches of moderately strenuous climbing, ending at the Earthquake Fault. (Though geologically misnamed, the "fault" is really a volcanic cooling fissure.) The trail threads through an odd-looking pygmy forest of whitebark pine trees, caused by the nutrient-poor, gray-white pumice soil on which the trees so stoically survive. Suitable for strong beginners with some single-track handling skills, Mountain View combines mostly narrow single-tracks and short stretches of abandoned jeep roads. The route is about 65% downhill and 35% uphill and being so well-signed, "it's hard to get lost," according to Bruce. This route can be enjoyed as a point-to-point, a loop, an out-and-back, or as an add-on to other rides. Described below is the point-to-point version.

General location: About 100 miles south of Lake Tahoe on the east side of the Sierras in, in Mammoth Lakes.

Elevation change: 500 feet; starting elevation and high point 9,200 feet; low point 8,700 feet. Mostly downhill with a brief section of moderate climbing.

Season: June through October or when the first snowstorm hits.

Services: None found on the trail. Pit toilets at Minaret Summit Vista and Earthquake Fault. All services are available in the nearby Mammoth Mountain Bike Park or in the town of Mammoth Lakes. The closest services (snack bar, delis and restaurants, bike rental, clothing and accessories shop, as well as drinking water, rest rooms, phones, and first aid) is at the Bike Park.

RIDE 63 · Mountain View

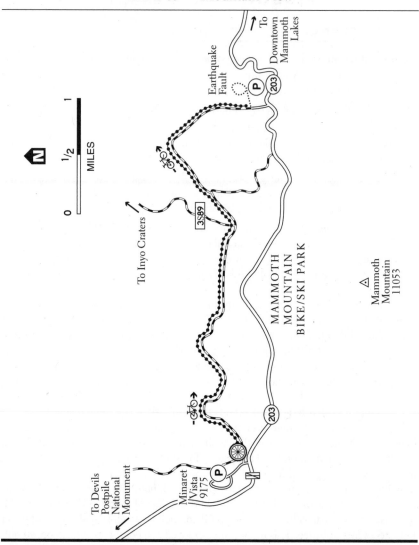

Hazards: A short stretch of single-track skirts a steep drop-off. Loop riders, watch out for cars on CA 203.

Rescue index: Not a heavily used trail, don't rely on other trail users for help or you may be waiting a long time. During the summer, the ranger booth on CA 203 that controls vehicle traffic to the Devils Postpile is manned during the day. So, in case of emergency and if you're not too far from the trailhead, you're sure to find help at the ranger booth. Farther down, about 5 miles from the overlook trailhead, a 1-mile bail-out dirt road leads south to CA 203. Once on the heavily traveled highway, you can flag down a passing motorist. The Earthquake Fault is a popular tourist spot and you're likely to find visitors who may be of help.

Land status: Inyo National Forest.

Maps: Some annual summer publications contain maps and are distributed by the Mammoth Lakes Visitor Center. Free map handouts are occasionally available too. USGS Mammoth Mountain and Old Mammoth 7.5 minute series.

Finding the trail: From the intersection of US 395 and CA 203, go west on CA 203 toward the town of Mammoth Lakes. Continue through town and go right onto Minaret Road, still following CA 203. Immediately go past the Daily Grind, a popular local coffee joint housed at the Travelodge motel and in just over a mile, you reach the turn-off to the Earthquake Fault. If you plan to do this ride as a loop, park here in the small paved lot, next to this geological wonder, and begin pedaling uphill on CA 203 (there's a wide shoulder) to the trailhead at Minaret Summit Vista overlook, reached in 3.6 miles. Otherwise, for a point-to-point ride, park your end shuttle car here at the Earthquake Fault and drive your second car up CA 203 to the overlook, passing Mammoth Mountain Bike Park's main entrance along the way. Go right into a road leading to the overlook parking lot, just before the forest ranger–controlled entry booth. Upon turning, immediately notice a big brown sign stating "San Joaquin Jeep Rd, Bike Trail." This is the trailhead. Dirt parking is limited here and I suggest parking in the paved lot a few yards up the road, at the overlook where a sweeping view of the Ritter Range and the Minarets is awesome. Begin your ride by pedaling back down to this point.

Sources of additional information:

Mammoth Mountain Bike Park
P.O. Box 24
Mammoth Lakes, CA 93546
(888) 4-MAMMOTH
(760) 934-2581
www.mammoth-mtn.com/bike.htm

U.S. Forest Service
Mammoth Lakes Visitors Bureau
P.O. Box 48
Mammoth Lakes, CA 93546
(888) GO-MAMMOTH
Visitor Center located at the bike path trailhead, at the entrance to

Shady Rest Camp and Park off Main Street (CA 203)

Inyo National Forest Headquarters
873 N. Main St.
Bishop, CA 93514
(760) 873-2400

Inyo National Forest
Mammoth Ranger District
P.O. Box 148
Mammoth Lakes, CA 93546
(760) 924-5500
www.r5.pswfs.gov/inyo/

Notes on the trail: For loop or point-to-point riders, the dirt portion of your ride begins at the trailhead found behind the San Joaquin Jeep Rd, Bike Trail sign. It's immediately on your right as you turn off CA 203 to the overlook. Once on the trail, the route is well-signed.

Mountain View trail starts off as a dirt jeep road and leads down into a drainage. Immediately keep an eye out for a sign identifying the trail you're on as Mountain View. Before long, the road becomes a narrow single-track, colored by gray-white pumice and cruises alternately through forest and small clearings.

At almost a mile, cross over a little stream on a wooden bridge. The area is populated by a forest of stunted whitebark pine trees. The single-track weaves through the forest and the trail conditions in the turns are likely to be soft with fine pumice. Ride through several large clearings, about 100 yards in diameter, totally covered with pebbly white pumice.

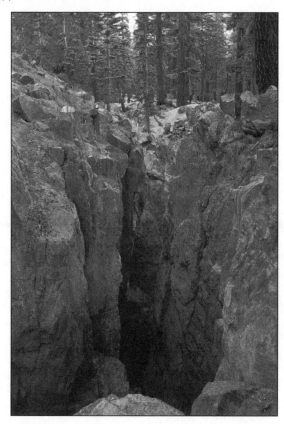

Located at the end of
Mountain View, the
Earthquake Fault is
worth a look (it's really a
volcanic fissure).

For those of you who are unaccustomed to the altitude, the slight rise in terrain encountered at almost 2 miles will feel like a major climb (though it really isn't). Persevere, the burning in your lungs and thighs is short-lived. Continue pedaling through the sometimes sandy trail, going through the oddly stunted forest and small clearings. At about 3 miles, the trail widens into a dirt jeep road. Follow the dirt road for a few yards and soon make a sharp left (signed). The trail here becomes a narrow single-track again.

At about 3.3 miles, cross another small stream over a well-made wooden bridge and continue following the single-track. The trees here are taller and more normal-sized. In about 0.2 mile, cross a third stream, which is slightly larger than the first two. Climb out of the stream bank and at 3.7 miles, you reach a signed intersection. The left trail (3s89) leads to Inyo Craters. If you're an aerobically strong and intermediate-skilled rider, here's your chance to add on a great ride. (See the trail description for Inyo Craters Loop, Ride 59.) Follow the right trail, signed to Mammoth Mountain and Mountain View. The route quickly becomes a jeep road again. Stay with the jeep road as it climbs somewhat steeply, about 6% grade for about a half mile.

At about 4.2 miles, follow a left turn sign indicating the continuation of the Mountain View trail, now a single-track again. The trail continues to climb gently as it traverses a steep hillside. When you're able, take your eyes off the trail (or stop for a moment!) and savor the view of the distant mountain ranges to the north and northwest: Deadman Pass, the San Joaquin, and Ritter Ranges. On a late afternoon ride, when the sun is low in the west, the silhouette of the jagged Minarets are particularly striking against the sky.

At about 5 miles, the trail splits and a sign points you to the left. (A right turn here is the shortcut to CA 203, reached in about a mile.) Gradually descend through the forest and at 5.7 miles, the dirt trail ends at the asphalt turn-off road which leads to the Earthquake Fault. Go left and find your end-shuttle car at the parking area.

Lock up your bike and take a short walk to inspect the Earthquake Fault. Geologists now believe this long trench was actually a cooling fissure related to a nearby volcano and not a result of an earthquake. The fissure is about 30 yards deep and likely to still contain some snow hiding in the shadows on the floor, even in the middle of summer.

RIDE 64 · Off The Top—Mammoth Mountain Bike Park

AT A GLANCE

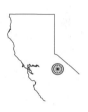

Length/configuration: 8.7-mile point-to-point, accessed by gondola; single-track and some dirt roads

Aerobic difficulty: Easy, virtually all downhill

Technical difficulty: Mild to almost intermediate. Sections of the narrow single-track weave around trees, up and down twisty dips, and thread through tight hairpins.

Scenery: From 11,053 feet, your jaw will drop from the wide-open panoramic views of the snow-patched mountain ranges in the John Muir and Ansel Adams Wildernesses.

Special comments: Located in the Mammoth Mountain Bike Park, a ticket must be purchased to use the lift, gondola, and shuttle van. The insanely steep and technically challenging Kamikaze Downhill can be accessed off this route. (See options discussed at the end of this profile.)

There are some dyed-in-the-wool cyclists who blow off mountain biking at a ski resort, calling anybody who takes a chair lift up to the top a wussy. Part of the sport, they proclaim, is being out in the wilds of nature, facing the raw terrain and exerting yourself 'til you're breathless. Well, the fact of the matter is, not everyone feels that way and plenty of people have an unforgettable time riding at ski resorts–turned–bike parks. But fun is fun and the price of a lift ticket is worth it, especially if the trails are spectacular. Mammoth Mountain Bike Park is arguably the best lift-operated resort in California. Unlike other bike parks, Mammoth has plenty of terrain for all abilities, boasting over 70 miles of single-track and a well-run shuttle-van and lift system. Cyclists of all abilities will definitely enjoy Off The Top, a mostly single-track trail that is, for the most part, a complete downhill run back to the main lodge. Never a boring ride, it's got exhilarating, expansive views of snow-patched mountain ranges and deep canyons. When you begin, literally, off the top of the Mammoth Mountain Summit at 11,053 feet, the trail has you traversing 45-degree slope that's vast and barren—you're way above timberline after all. It's here that you feel that thrilling tinge of vertigo. As you gradually descend the south face of the summit, your bike handling skills are put to the test by tight switchbacks filled with soft pumice dirt. See if you can skillfully maneuver through the turns without dabbing your foot. After about three miles of soul-expanding wide views, the trail descends into the quiet conifer forest, leading to the far western edge of the Bike Park. Here, Off The Top ends and you have a choice of several trails. For this outing, we opted for Beach Cruiser, another easy- to intermediate-level single-track that weaves through trees, punctuated with small dips and occasional exposed tree roots before reaching our starting point at the Bike Center.

General location: About 100 miles south of Lake Tahoe on the east side of the Sierras.

Elevation change: 2,153 feet loss; starting elevation 11,053 feet; low point 8,900 feet. Long, sweet descent with some level stretches.

Season: Late June to September and possibly into October.

Services: Mammoth Mountain Bike Park runs lifts, gondolas, and a reliable van-shuttle service for riders and their bikes. The shuttle runs every half-hour, sometimes more frequently if lots of people are clamoring to hop on board. Park use-fee, which entitles you to use all transportation services, cost from about $26 for adults, and $15 for children. Most services are available at the main lodge or nearby and include snack bar, delis and restaurants, bike rental, clothing and accessories shop, as well as drinking water, rest rooms, phones, and first aid. Accommodations of every comfort level available nearby and many local establishments offer lodging and bike packages. All services independent of the bike park are also available in the decidedly hip town of Mammoth Lakes.

Hazards: Other than the extreme terrain, the only real hazard is sharing the road with mountain bikers who are speedier than you. Conversely, if you're determined to beat the clock, watch out for slowpokes who like squeezing their brake all the way down the run. Off The Top is a narrow single-track with just enough room for one rider. Needless to say, passing requires someone to pull off the side of the trail.

Rescue index: This is a popular route and you're sure to find other trail users who might be of help. Bike patrollers employed by the Bike Park and equipped with walkie-talkies cruise all routes. Emergency phones throughout the park makes finding help fairly easy.

Land status: Inyo National Forest.

Maps: Mammoth Mountain Bike Park map.

Finding the trail: From the intersection of US 395 and CA 203, go west on CA 203 toward the town of Mammoth Lakes. Continue through town and go right onto Minaret Road, still following CA 203. Go past the Daily Grind, a popular local coffee joint housed at the Travelodge motel, and in about 4 miles, you reach the Bike Park's main entrance. The Mammoth Mountain Inn is located on the right, across from the park. Park in the huge lot. If you're staying in town, consider catching the Bike Park's shuttle van to the main lodge. Ride to the shuttle pick-up point at the Daily Grind/Travelodge (6209 Minaret Rd. near Canyon Blvd. and Footloose Sports). Bike Park tickets can be purchased at the Daily Grind.

RIDE 64 · Off The Top—Mammoth Mountain Bike Park

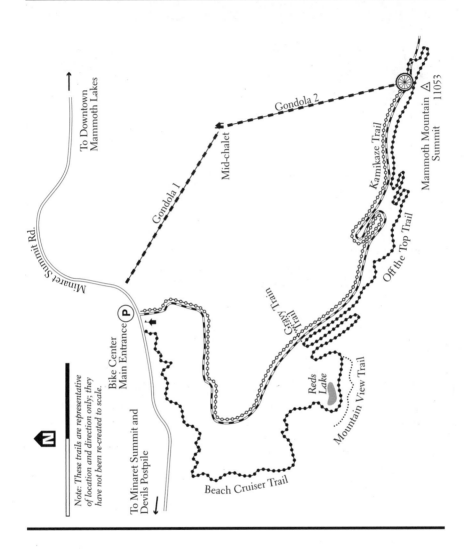

Sources of additional information:

Inyo National Forest Headquarters
873 N. Main St.
Bishop, CA 93514
(760) 873-2400

Inyo National Forest
Mammoth Ranger District
P.O. Box 148
Mammoth Lakes, CA 93546
(760) 924-5500
www.r5.pswfs.gov/inyo/

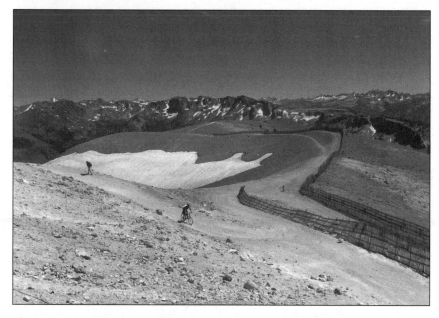

This ride begins at Mammoth Mountain's summit, sitting at 11,053 feet, way above timberline where the view is breathtaking.

U.S. Forest Service
Mammoth Mountain Bike Park
P.O. Box 24
Mammoth Lakes, CA 93546
(888) 4-MAMMOTH
(760) 934-2581
www.mammoth-mtn.com/bike.htm

U.S. Forest Service
Mammoth Lakes Visitors Bureau
P.O. Box 48
Mammoth Lakes, CA 93546
(888) GO-MAMMOTH
Visitor Center located at the bike
path trailhead, at the entrance to
Shady Rest Camp and Park off Main
Street (CA 203)

Notes on the trail: Before embarking on this adventure, consider your tire pressure. The dominant composition of the trails at the Bike Park is rocks, pumice, and sand. A bike patroller suggests riding with a tire pressure between 28 and 34 psi; "anything close to 40 psi is too high."

From the main lodge and bike center, follow the signs to the gondola house. As you hop into the gondola, attendants hook your bike to the outside of the car. Enjoy the views as the gondola takes you up to Mid-Chalet. Stay in the car and continue up to the Mammoth Mountain summit. As you exit the gondola house, now way above timberline at 11,053 feet, you're struck with an awesome panoramic view to the south of the John Muir and Ansel Adams Wildernesses. Follow the directional signs here pointing left to Off The Top trail. (An immediate right puts you on Kamikaze.)

Having found Off The Top, the trail leads you down the back (south) side of the summit, becoming a narrow, loosely packed, single-track trail as it hugs the wide-open slope. If you're riding in the early summer, there's likely to be tiny wildflowers dotting the otherwise barren, grayish-white pumice slope. Keep your eyes on the trail as you maneuver through roughly 10 tight, often sandy switchbacks. Pulling off the side of the trail to let speedsters pass gives you a chance to take in the spectacular views along this awesome trail.

At 3 miles from the summit, you descend below timberline. The single-track trail continues to be somewhat challenging with a series of short, shallow dips, kind of like a widely spaced washboard. Feel free to whoop and holler as you guide your trusty two-wheeled steed and "ride the pegs" (standing on your pedals and butt off the saddle as you ride through rough terrain). Let your elbows and knees absorb the bumps. The trail narrows in some spots and some tree roots are exposed, just the thing to keep you alert.

After 5.5 miles, Off The Top basically ends at a messy junction of several trails: Beach Cruiser, Mountain View, and Gravy Train, all rated easy to intermediate. Take your choice of trails—each ultimately leads you back to the main lodge. Choosing Beach Cruiser, the trail gently drops into a remote and tiny valley toward Reds Lake. At 5.6 miles, you reach the Mountain View trail junction. Stay on Beach Cruiser by hanging a left. In about 3 miles, you're back at the main lodge, next to the Gearhead Deli, a perfect place to grab a snack or take a break. Then make your way back to the gondola and check out more great trails.

Mountain View option: If you want a great 180-degree view of the western ridge-line, follow Mountain View out of the Bike Park, toward Minaret Summit Vista, a well-placed overlook on the other side (north side) of CA 203. There, you'll have a great view of the Minarets, a set of jagged fingers of granite that interrupt an otherwise calm mountain ridgeline. Several challenging mountain bike trails are accessed from the summit, including Mountain View to the Earthquake Fault, as described in Ride 63. To return to the Bike Park from the summit, follow CA 203 downhill a couple of miles to the bike park entrance. Though there's a decent shoulder, watch out for car traffic.

Kamikaze Downhill option: Truth be told, the Kamikaze Downhill wasn't my cup of tea. The scenery wasn't remarkable—in fact, there are far better runs in the bike park with jaw-dropping views than this one. But, hey, not everyone rides for the scenery. If your idea of a truly awesome biking experience is hinged purely on sheer speed and the more vertical the better, you'll love this run. The famed Kamikaze Downhill is one of the more popular NORBA races on the west coast. Devoid of obstacles, Kamikaze is nothing but a plain old wide fire road, mostly smooth, hard-packed dirt. Usually covered with a thin layer of loose dirt and gravel, the route is steep. Did I say steep? Yes, that's steep as in starting at 11,053 feet and plunging 2,153 feet in 3.5 miles. But oh what a trail. The real fun—and attraction—of Kamikaze is to see how fast you can get down the hill, all in one piece, and that means laying off the brakes and picking the best, fastest line down the slope. The winning times (in minutes and seconds) of the 1998 NORBA Championship for women and men, respectively, were 4.51 and 4.22. That's hurling down the hill on a two-wheeled contraption at 70+ mph. If you can come within 10 seconds or beat these times, then you certainly belong in NORBA's big girls and boys league.

RIDE 65 · Paper Route & Big Ring— Mammoth Mountain Bike Park

AT A GLANCE

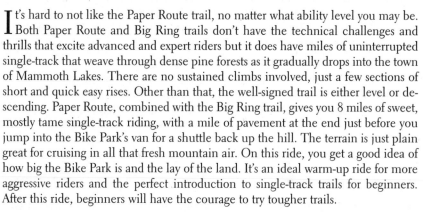

Length/configuration: 9.1-mile point-to-point; single-track and about a mile of paved road

Aerobic difficulty: Easy

Technical difficulty: Mild

Scenery: Single-track travels through a mix of dense forest and open ski runs.

Special comments: Located in the Mammoth Mountain Bike Park, a ticket must be purchased to use the lift, gondola, and shuttle van. Great for young families, including alley-cat riders. Not suitable for kid-trailers.

It's hard to not like the Paper Route trail, no matter what ability level you may be. Both Paper Route and Big Ring trails don't have the technical challenges and thrills that excite advanced and expert riders but it does have miles of uninterrupted single-track that weave through dense pine forests as it gradually drops into the town of Mammoth Lakes. There are no sustained climbs involved, just a few sections of short and quick easy rises. Other than that, the well-signed trail is either level or descending. Paper Route, combined with the Big Ring trail, gives you 8 miles of sweet, mostly tame single-track riding, with a mile of pavement at the end just before you jump into the Bike Park's van for a shuttle back up the hill. The terrain is just plain great for cruising in all that fresh mountain air. On this ride, you get a good idea of how big the Bike Park is and the lay of the land. It's an ideal warm-up ride for more aggressive riders and the perfect introduction to single-track trails for beginners. After this ride, beginners will have the courage to try tougher trails.

General location: About 100 miles south of Lake Tahoe on the east side of the Sierras.

Elevation change: 890 feet loss; starting elevation and high point 8,900 feet; low point 8,300 feet. Mellow downhill.

Season: Late June to September and possibly into October.

Services: Mammoth Mountain Bike Park runs lifts, gondolas, and a well-coordinated van-shuttle service for riders and their bikes. The shuttle runs every half-hour, sometimes more frequently if lots of people are clamoring to hop on board. Park use-fee, which entitles you to use all transportation services, cost from about $26 for adults, and $15 for children. Most services are available at the main lodge or nearby and include snack bar, delis and restaurants, bike rental, clothing and accessories shop, as well as drinking water, rest rooms, phones, and first aid. Accommodations of every comfort level are available nearby and many local establishments offer lodging and bike packages. All services independent of the Bike Park are also available in the decidedly hip town of Mammoth Lakes.

Hazards: You may encounter some vehicular traffic as you cruise through a residential neighborhood on the last mile to the shuttle pick-up at the Daily Grind.

RIDE 65 · Paper Route & Big Ring—Mammoth Mountain Bike Park

To The Daily Grind and Shuttle Stop

Canyon Blvd.

Paper Route

Big Ring

To Downtown Mammoth Lakes

Big Ring

Chair Lifts

Paper Route

Downtown

Chair Lifts

Chair Lifts

Gondola 1

To Devils Postpile

P

Bike Center

N

Note: These trails are representative of location and direction only; they have not been re-created to scale.

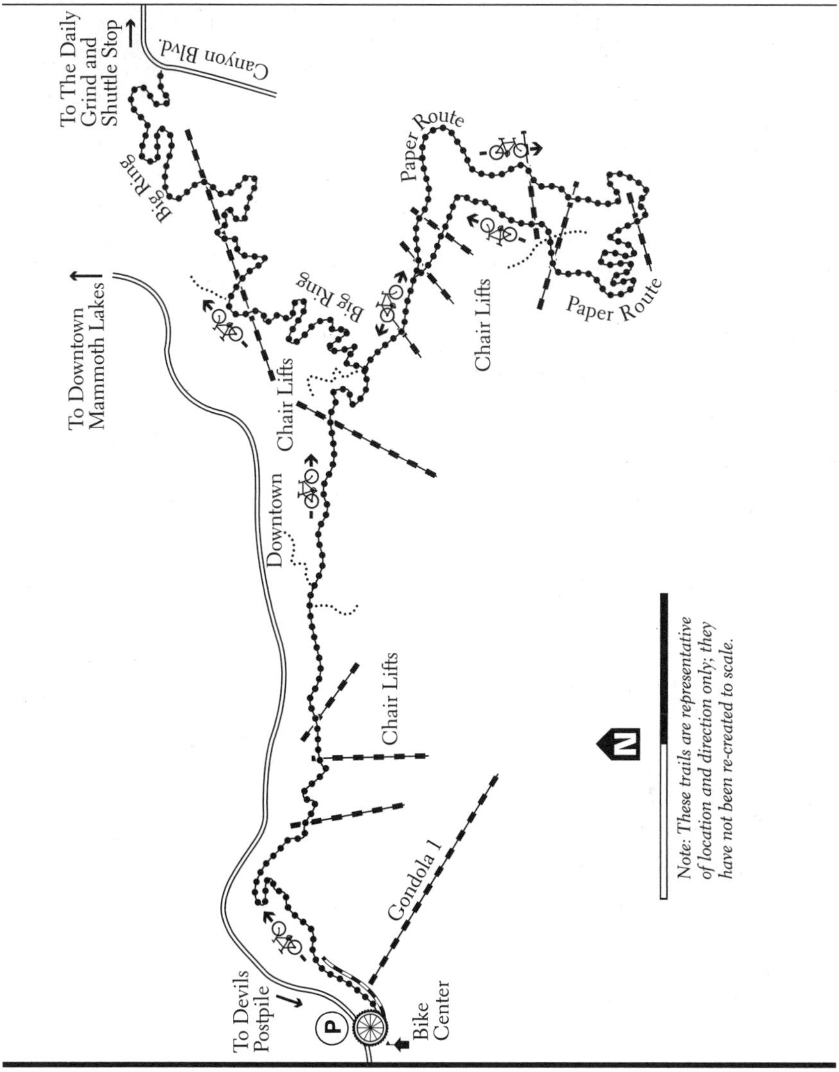

Rescue index: This is a popular route and you're sure to find other trail users who might be of help. Bike patrollers employed by the Bike Park and equipped with walkie-talkies cruise all routes. Emergency phones throughout the park make finding help fairly easy.

Land status: Inyo National Forest.

Maps: Mammoth Mountain Bike Park map.

Finding the trail: From the intersection of US 395 and CA 203, go west on CA 203 toward the town of Mammoth Lakes. Continue through town and go right onto Minaret Road, still following CA 203. Go past the Daily Grind, a popular local coffee

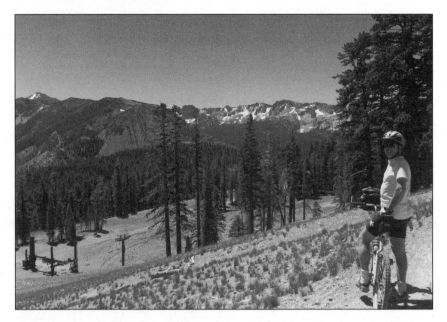

Paper Route travels through the southeast portion of the bike park, ultimately offering a view of the water that put the "Lakes" in Mammoth Lakes.

joint housed at the Travelodge motel, and in about 4 miles, you reach the Bike Park's main entrance. The Mammoth Mountain Inn is located on the right, across from the park. Park in the huge lot. If you're staying in town, consider catching the Bike Park's shuttle van to the main lodge. Ride to the shuttle pick-up point at the Daily Grind/Travelodge (6209 Minaret Rd. near Canyon Blvd. and Footloose Sports). Bike Park tickets can be purchased at the Daily Grind.

Sources of additional information: See sources of additional information for Ride 64.

Notes on the trail: From the main lodge and Bike Center, head east (left as you face Mammoth Mountain), toward the gondola house. Go under the gondola cable and follow the signs for Paper Route. Before you know it, you're on a narrow trail weaving through the trees. Some of the initial turns are tight, forcing you to control your speed and pay attention to your maneuvering skills. Bypass other trails that intersect Paper Route, at least for now—come back to them on another run. Be aware that some portions of Paper Route are designated one-way.

At about 3 miles, you reach the intersection with Big Ring at a tiny covered deck with a picnic table and a water cooler. Paper cups are provided for your convenience. We pass this way again later and pick up Big Ring at that time. But for now, continue following Paper Route as it leads you on a wide, twisty loop along the eastern midsection of Mammoth Mountain. Views of the snow-patched range within the John Muir Wilderness emerge and the cruising is easy. Heed one-way signs. You reach the far end of the loop at about 4 miles, where you have a great view of Twin View Lakes and several other watery gems. For the next half mile, you get to huff and puff a bit as you regain some elevation. The switchbacks tame an otherwise strenuous ascent and in no time, you're cruising level terrain again.

The Follow Me trail intersects Paper Route at about 5.2 miles, and if you're aching for something slightly more challenging, try it. Otherwise, stay on Paper Route and at 6.3 miles, you've returned to the tiny covered picnic table and water cooler. Here, the slightly more challenging Big Ring single-track trail begins. Watch out for oncoming bikers because it's a two-way trail. Big Ring is a bit steeper, has tighter curves, and slightly rougher trail conditions. And for a real cheap thrill, a couple of shallow (very shallow, no more than 8 feet deep) drop-offs are included. Still, beginners can usually conquer Big Ring—and love every inch of it. The trail cuts across a wide-open ski run that's strewn with dark red lava rock. Patches of loose, finely ground lava rocks in the path try to grab your tire and slow your speed. Soon after that, the trail ends at the pavement next to the Canyon Lodge (closed during the summer), in a residential neighborhood. Follow wide Canyon Boulevard to the left, leaving the dirt trail literally behind you. In less than a mile, Canyon intersects Minaret Road. Hang a left and go a few yards to the Daily Grind, a coffee joint housed at the Travelodge. Order up a *latté* to-go and wait for the next shuttle van to take you back up the hill to the main lodge for another round of downhill fun.

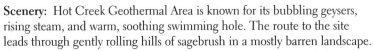

RIDE 66 · Hot Creek Hatchery Road to the Hot Springs

AT A GLANCE

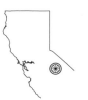

Length/configuration: 4.6-mile out-and-back (2.3 miles each way); dirt road with some stretches of pavement

Aerobic difficulty: Easy due to very negligible elevation gain

Technical difficulty: Not technical due to smooth road conditions

Scenery: Hot Creek Geothermal Area is known for its bubbling geysers, rising steam, and warm, soothing swimming hole. The route to the site leads through gently rolling hills of sagebrush in a mostly barren landscape.

Special comments: Suitable for youngsters and kid-trailers. Heartier riders looking for their own private hot springs will be glad to know this area is crisscrossed by other dirt roads, some of which may lead to secluded springs.

One of the most active volcanic regions in California is the Mammoth Lakes region along the eastern side of the Sierras. Though the underground is constantly moaning and groaning, locals aren't worried. In fact, they cherish a great by-product of the earth's rumpling: numerous hot springs that dot the landscape. What could be better than soaking in a heated swimming hole with an expansive view in the west of snow-capped mountain ranges reaching into to the blue sky? Free of charge too! Well, the answer is a hot spring all to yourself, devoid of other skinny-dippers. That said, many of the hot spots favored by locals are not publicized, much less revealed. You'll have to explore and find them on your own.

This 4.6-mile out-and-back ride (2.3 miles each way) leads to one of the most well-known hot springs in the region. Paralleling Hot Creek, Hot Creek Hatchery Road is a hard-packed dirt road, as smooth as a pancake. Elevation gain is practically nothing as it leads you through wide-open, gently rolling hills of sagebrush and scrub. Though the road is well-traveled, it's generously wide and well-suited for young families.

Kids of all ages are likely to enjoy checking out Hot Creek State Fish Hatchery, home to millions of young trout (located at the ride's starting point, open daily to the public). Hot Creek is an officially designated Wild Trout Stream since a huge population of native trout thrive here. Hot Creek Ranch (along this route) caters to the angling crowd, offering cabins, a fly shop, and easy access to fishing spots (catch-and-release only).

How about a good soak in the warm waters of Hot Creek? Bring your swimsuit and a bike lock. You'll find changing rooms and rest rooms at the geo-thermal site. A short walking trail and boardwalk provide easy access to the hot springs.

General location: About 3 miles southeast of the town of Mammoth Lakes.

Elevation change: Negligible change; mostly at 7,100 feet.

Season: June through October.

Services: Changing room and rest rooms near the thermal site. There is no drinking water, so bring plenty. All other services in Mammoth Lakes.

Hazards: Stay alert for frequent vehicular traffic throughout the ride. Fortunately, the washboard surface of the dirt road will slow motorists. Wear eye protection as the road is often dusty during the summer. Dipping in the thermal pools is at your own risk (12 people have died and numerous more injured). If you decide to partake of the soothing water, *use extreme caution!* Stay alert for sporadic pollution in the creek and sudden changes in water temperature. Children must be supervised at all times as some areas of the pool can be lukewarm initially but quickly become hot to the point of scalding. Get out of the hot springs *immediately* if there's an earthquake or tremor as water temperature can change abruptly. Stay away from the site during seismic alerts as the grounds may become more unstable. Watch out for broken glass; wear foot protection at all times, in and out of the water. Access to the springs is closed from sunset to sunrise. Heed all signs—*no kidding!*

Rescue index: Being a popular swimming hole, you're likely to find help from passing motorists or visitors at the spring. For emergency phone calls, Hot Creek Ranch and the Hatchery may be able to offer assistance.

Land status: Inyo National Forest.

Maps: *Mammoth High Country Trail Map,* published by Tom Harrison Maps, 2 Falmouth Cove, San Rafael, CA 94901, (800) 265-9090, www.tomharrisonmaps.com; *Eastern High Sierra Recreation Topo Map,* published by Fine Edge Productions, Bishop, California; USGS Whitmore Hot Springs 7.5 minute series. Some annual summer publications contain maps and are distributed by the U.S. Forest Service/ Mammoth Lakes Visitor Center. Free map handouts are occasionally available too.

Finding the trail: From the intersection of US 395 and CA 120 (the main road leading out of Mammoth Lakes), travel south on US 395 for about 3 miles to Hot Creek Hatchery Road, also signed to the airport. Go left onto the Hatchery Road, a paved road, and in just under a mile, you reach the hatchery. Park in the lot and begin pedaling from here.

RIDE 66 · Hot Creek Hatchery Road to the Hot Springs

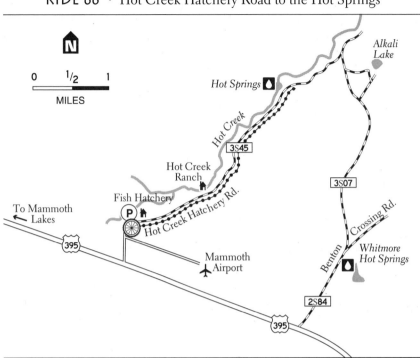

Sources of additional information:

Inyo National Forest Headquarters
873 N. Main St.
Bishop, CA 93514
(760) 873-2400

Inyo National Forest
Mammoth Ranger District
P.O. Box 148
Mammoth Lakes, CA 93546
(760) 924-5500
www.r5.pswfs.gov/inyo/

Hot Creek Ranch
Rural Route 1, Box 206
Mammoth Lakes, CA 93546
(760) 924-5637

U.S. Forest Service
Mammoth Lakes Visitors Bureau
P.O. Box 48
Mammoth Lakes, CA 93546
(888) GO-MAMMOTH
Visitor Center located at the bike
path trailhead, at the entrance to
Shady Rest Camp and Park off Main
Street (CA 203)

Notes on the trail: Following this route is so easy, you really don't need a map. On the other hand, if you plan to explore other dirt roads beyond the Hot Creek Geothermal Area, be sure to bring a map. If you plan on taking a dip, bring a bike lock in addition to your swimsuit and foot protection (to wear while in the hot springs).

From the hatchery parking lot, continue following the paved road which you came in on, going east. In less than a mile, the pavement becomes a dirt road and may be somewhat washboardy, depending on when it was last graded. Just shy of a mile, the road leads through the Hot Creek Geologic Site gate. Pavement resumes as you cruise past "Fisherman's Trail" parking lot, then becomes dirt again. At 2 miles from the hatchery, bypass a dirt road leading off on the left, staying on the main road. In a few yards, you reach the main parking area above the hot springs. Lock your bike here before walking down to the hot springs.

After checking out this bubbling and steaming site, return to your car by reversing direction. If you're up for more riding, exploring, and even finding a hidden hot springs to have all to yourself, consult your map and continue east on the dirt road on which you pedaled in. Reportedly, there are several more hot springs, one at Little Alkali Lake and another about a mile before the intersection of 2 roads: unsigned dirt road 3s07 and paved Benton Crossing Road (FS 2s84). Whitmore Hot Springs, a well-known pool maintained by the county, is located at this intersection. Once you've reached Whitmore, you can either reverse direction and retrace your path back past Hot Creek Geothermal Area and eventually back to your car at the hatchery. Or, you can return to your car by finishing this ride as a loop. To ride the loop, continue heading southwest on paved Benton Crossing Road. When you reach US 395 in about a mile, go right and ride 2.5 miles to Hot Creek Hatchery Road. Hang a right here and you're back at your car in less than a mile. This loop is approximately 11 miles.

OTHER AREA RIDES

BODIE HISTORIC STATE PARK: OK, this is not really a mountain-bike ride, but, hey, it's the best way to check out this exceptional ghost town. Occupying about 160 acres (roughly half a square mile), Bodie is a former gold-mining town that is well maintained in a state of "arrested decay." With your trusty two-wheel steed, you'll see more than most visitors to this internationally popular site. (We met a couple who had come all the way from France just to see this place after hearing so much about it.) If you have children with you, getting them to ride (in a kid-trailer or on their own bike) beats hearing them whine about "all that walking." There are many fascinating buildings and artifacts to behold. You could spend a couple of hours here. If you're an aspiring photographer, you're likely to find plenty of interesting subjects. Sitting at 6,400 feet elevation in the hills east of US 395 near the Nevada state line and north of Mono Lake, Bodie is mostly flat. Except for the buildings, the area is completely without shade. Very informative self-guided tour brochures available at the state park entrance. The surrounding dirt roads have been known to attract mountain bikers, and if you want to ride them, check with a ranger at the state park before doing so. A 17-mile dirt route (one way) can be ridden due northwest from Bodie to Bridgeport (follow Masonic Road—also known as Geiger Grade—to Aurora Canyon Road, then go west). Expect to gain about 2,600 feet on your way to Bridgeport. If you can, leave a shuttle car in Bridgeport. Otherwise, you'll have to either backtrack or pedal the shoulder of busy US 395 south to County Road 270 and then east to Bodie. Either way, it's about 33.4 miles or 36.7 miles round-trip, respectively. Not exactly a great bike ride but if you gotta ride, have at it.

Finding the trail: From Lee Vining, travel north on US 395 about 20 miles to CA 270 (Bodie Road, a wide, sometimes washboardy dirt road). Head east on CA 270 about 13 miles to Bodie State Historic Park. Park in the designated parking lot. Small entry fee is charged.

Maps: USGS Bodie SE, Bodie SW, and Bodie NW 7.5 minute series.

For more information, contact:

Bodie State Historic Park
P.O. Box 515
Bridgeport, CA 93517
(760) 647-6445

DEADMANS PASS: This short, 5-mile out-and-back (2.5 miles each way) starts from Minaret Vista (the same trailhead as the Mountain View ride described earlier in this chapter). The dirt road that the route follows is basically nontechnical. It's the elevation that's a kicker: if you're unaccustomed to the altitude, you'll feel it. Starting at roughly 9,200 feet, the trail climbs 1,000-plus feet to more than 10,000 feet in 2.5

miles. Perhaps the spectacular vista you'll have of the Minarets, the Ritter Range, peaks in Yosemite, Ansel Adams Wilderness, and Mono Basin will distract you from the burning pain in your lungs and thighs.

Finding the trail: The trailhead is the same as Mountain View (Ride 63). Refer to that ride for directions. Just like Mountain View, Deadmans Pass begins a few yards on your right immediately after turning off of CR 203 into the parking lot. You will have driven past the trailhead when you park in the lot next to the rest rooms.

Maps: USGS Mammoth Mountain and Old Mammoth 7.5 minute series.

For more information, contact:

> Inyo National Forest
> Mammoth Ranger District
> P.O. Box 148
> Mammoth Lakes, CA 93546
> (760) 924-5500
> www.r5.pswfs.gov/inyo/

ROCK CREEK LAKE RIDE: There are two great rides located about 15 miles south of Mammoth Lakes, immediately next to US 395, near the tiny town of Tom's Place. This ride is a 22-mile loop that climbs paved Rock Creek Road. It then returns on technically challenging four-wheel-drive dirt road and trail running over Tamarack Bench and through Sand Canyon. It takes place between 5,000 and 10,000 feet. If you're short on time or lacking high-altitude endurance, you can enjoy this adventure as a 14-mile point-to-point ride (requiring two shuttle cars), which will effectively eliminate most of the climbing. Advanced technical skills are a necessity as the narrow dirt road and trail can be deeply rutted from runoff and just downright gnarly.

Finding the trail: From Mammoth Lakes, head south on US 395 for almost 15 miles to Tom's Place. Hang a right (west by southwest) onto Rock Creek Road (this is the road that leads to the lake and campground) and immediately park in a paved area alongside US 395, near Crowley Lake Drive. For one-way riders, place your end-shuttle car here, then drive the second car, your bikes and buddies up toward Rock Creek Lake. Park in the day-use parking lot, and begin pedaling toward Tom's Place.

Maps: USGS Mt. Morgan and Tom's Place 7.5 minute series.

For more information, contact:

> Inyo National Forest
> White Mountain Ranger District
> 798 North Main Street
> Bishop, CA 93514
> (760) 873-2500

LOWER ROCK CREEK TRAIL: This is the other ride that also begins near Tom's Place, less than a mile farther than the above ride. Lower Rock Creek can be ridden as a point-to-point or loop configuration. The attraction of this ride is its 8-mile stretch of single-track alongside the wooden creek. Starting from a trailhead almost a mile southeast of Tom's Place, the direction of travel is along the creek, basically downhill toward Paradise Lodge, on an often very narrow trail which is frequently used by hikers and fishing enthusiasts. The first 3.3 miles of the single-track stretch reportedly requires intermediate skills with several bailouts onto Lower Rock Creek Road (the single-track actually crosses the road twice). The next 4.7 miles is much more technical with some very challenging spots, with no bailouts, and ends at Paradise Lodge—advanced skills needed. To make a loop, just hop onto the road and follow it uphill back to Tom's Place trailhead. Total loop distance from a bail-out point is 6 to 7 miles round-trip, and 16 miles from Paradise Lodge.

Finding the trail: From Mammoth Lakes, head south on US 395 for about 15 miles to Tom's Place. Go about 0.25 miles farther and take the Swall Meadow, Lower Rock Creek turnoff to the west (right side) of US 395. Less than 100 yards south of US 395, on the west side of Lower Rock Creek Road, look for a small dirt pulloff marked by a Inyo National Forest sign indicating parking for day-use. Park here. Access the trail on the east side of Lower Rock Creek Road. To enjoy this trail as a one-way ride, leave an end-shuttle near a bailout (about 3 miles down the Lower Rock Creek Road, on the shoulder) or roughly 8 miles down the same road near—but not at—Paradise Lodge (please don't block any driveways).

Maps: USGS Rovana and Tom's Place 7.5 minute series.

For more information, contact:
Inyo National Forest
White Mountain Ranger District
798 North Main St.
Bishop, CA 93514
(760) 873-2500

SOME LOCAL BICYCLE SHOPS & RELATED BUSINESSES

Mammoth Mountain Sporting
  Goods
Sierra Center Mall
Old Mammoth Rd.
Mammoth Lakes, CA 93546
(760) 934-3239

Footloose Sports Center
Corner of Canyon and Minaret
Mammoth Lakes, CA 93546
(760) 934-2400

Mammoth Mountain Bike Clinics
  with Cindy Whitehead
Mammoth Mountain Bike
  Promotions
P.O. Box 9165
Mammoth Lakes, CA 93546
(760) 924-2955
Certified by USA Cycling as an Elite Coach in 1997, Cindy Whitehead conducts instructional camps, clinics, and women's weekend events.

THE EAST BAY AREA

Hard to believe that just minutes from one of the country's most populous and congested area are outstanding mountain bike trails—and lots of them for riders of every ability. Bravo to the forward-thinking citizens who in 1934 created the East Bay Regional Park District for the purposes of preserving open spaces, watersheds, foothills, and marshlands—all in the name of maintaining the area's natural beauty. And it's a good thing because in 1999, the population of the East Bay grew to a whopping 2.3 million. One shudders to think that this side of the San Francisco Bay could easily be solid cityscape. Under the jurisdiction of Contra Costa and Alameda Counties, the gems of the East Bay Area include 50 parks and 20 regional trails, scattered from the shores of the Bay, east over rolling ridges to the Livermore Valley and the flatlands of the delta region. Though bikes are not allowed on all trails and in all parks, there's still plenty from which to choose, including Mt. Diablo State Park and a handful of locally maintained parks.

While Interstates 680 and 580 contribute greatly to the growth of the East Bay, they also provide easy and quick access to the parks, unless of course you're stuck in rush-hour traffic. Both interstates run parallel, mostly north and south, essentially separated by a series of semi-forested rolling ridges. I-580 is the less scenic highway on the far western edge of this region, running through a solid blanket of city after city, from Fremont in the south to Oakland, Berkeley, and Richmond in the north. A few minutes immediately east of I-580, sandwiched between the two interstates are a series of adjoining parks, forming a nearly solid chain in which ambitious riders can pedal its 31-mile-plus length (one-way). Numerous other trails can be accessed along the way and riders of all abilities and endurance can find trails to their liking. I-680 is the more scenic route, snaking through Fremont and then north through Pleasanton, Walnut Creek, and Concord. Noticably more suburban than the congested I-580 corridor, I-680 passes by many other parks as well as towering Mt. Diablo State Park, home of the highest point in the East Bay. If you're a bionic rider, you'll undoubtedly sense Mt. Diablo quietly issuing a challenge to you and your bike to conquer it. The rest of us mortals who don't feel the challenge will find plenty of other trails well suited to our abilities, from paved bike paths, to dirt roads and a few single-tracks.

RIDE 67 · Mount Diablo–Mitchell Canyon Loop

AT A GLANCE

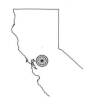

Length/configuration: 15-mile loop, counterclockwise; fire roads, a single-track trail and paved road

Aerobic difficulty: Very strenuous due to elevation gain

Technical difficulty: Mostly intermediate with significant stretches of advanced terrain due to steep descents over loose trail conditions

Scenery: On a clear day, a sweeping 360-degree view encompasses an astounding 40,000 square-miles which, according to geographers, is second to the view from Africa's Mount Kilimanjaro.

Special comments: Not recommended for beginners. In the summer, get an early start and bring lots of water as it gets bloody hot out here.

The Mount Diablo–Mitchell Canyon Loop is a heck of workout. Not for the weak or beginning biker, this 15.2-mile counterclockwise loop gains about 3,215 feet in the first 7.7 miles on wide, smooth fire road. This initial stretch doesn't require much technical ability but it definitely demands exceptional stamina and climbing legs of steel. Once you reach the summit—and though you may gag at hearing the following refrain a thousands times before—the view is really worth it, especially on a clear day typically after a strong, cleansing rain. Even if the atmosphere is not ideal, just think how good and smug you'll feel when car-bound tourists at the summit ask you where you began your ride. They will admire your fitness when you tell them you made it up to the top on your own steam—guaranteed. After sufficiently gawking at the view from the summit overlook, the way back down will put your technical abilities to the test. The challenge is maintaining control of your speed and traction while descending a significantly steep, curvy single-track trail over loose dirt and gravel. Throw in a few spots of heart-stopping drop-offs and it's enough to make intermediate riders think twice about walking. Though the single-track stretch is short, the subsequent fire roads are just as steep and loose—the kind of terrain that separates the intermediate from the advanced riders.

Besides this loop route, there are a number of other bike trails within Mount Diablo State Park and the neighboring regional parks. Many configurations are possible, ranging from easy to very strenuous in endurance, and from mild to advanced in skill requirements. If you venture out beyond this loop, know that mountain bikes are limited to fire roads with a few exceptions of single-track trails. Most single-tracks are hiking-only—please obey all signs. To find out which single-tracks permit bikes, check with the ranger station.

Aside from the trail conditions, Mount Diablo is an oasis of nature towering over the sprawling East Bay Area. Wildflowers are abundant in the spring, from February to April. You may see wildlife such as black-tail deer, raccoons, gray foxes, rabbits, coyotes, badgers, bobcats, and tarantulas on this loop. Mountain lions, though rarely seen, reside here as well. Of special geological note is the composition of the mountain. One to two million years ago, Mount Diablo was part of the ocean floor. Rock underneath the ocean floor estimated to be over 160 million years old was violently

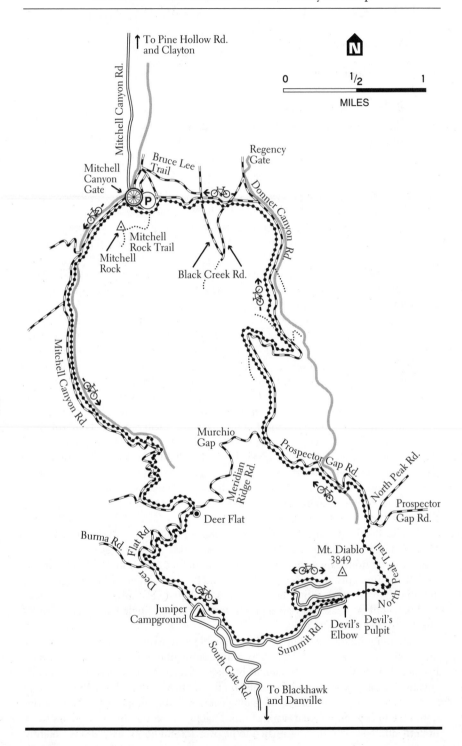

To Pine Hollow Rd. and Clayton

N

0   1/2   1
MILES

Mitchell Canyon Rd.

Bruce Lee Trail

Regency Gate

Mitchell Canyon Gate

Donner Canyon Rd.

P

Mitchell Rock Trail

Mitchell Rock

Black Creek Rd.

Mitchell Canyon Rd.

Murchio Gap

Meridian Ridge Rd.

Prospector Gap Rd

North Peak Rd.

Prospector Gap Rd.

Deer Flat

Burma Rd.

Deer Flat Rd.

Mt. Diablo
3849

North Peak Trail

Juniper Campground

Summit Rd.

Devil's Elbow

Devil's Pulpit

North Peak Trail

South Gate Rd.

To Blackhawk and Danville

pushed up through six to eight miles of overlying rock and soil. In the process, sections of the rock were jumbled, some turning completely upside down, trapping sea creatures as well as saber-tooth cats and three-toed horses. When you reach the summit, check out the stone blocks that make up the observation tower. The blocks were quarried here and you can see bits of embedded fossilized shells.

General location: East of San Francisco, across the bay, about 10 miles east of Walnut Creek.

Elevation change: 3,280 feet; starting elevation 580 feet; high point 3,840 feet; low point 560 feet. Most of the climbing is long and within the first 7.5 miles to the summit. After that, it's mostly downhill.

Season: Year-round. Best time to ride is April to May when the wildflowers are blooming profusely and the grasslands are still green. Summers tend to be hot and dry so start early in the day and bring lots of water. The state park has been known to close during days of high fire danger.

Services: Drinking water and rest rooms available at the Mitchell Canyon parking area, the summit building atop Mount Diablo, and the Juniper Campground near the summit. A pay phone is also located at the summit building. Passenger cars can be driven all the way up to the summit on a paved road. Other than these places, there are no other services anywhere along the route. All services can be found in Walnut Creek and Clayton.

Hazards: Occasional poison oak and rattlesnakes. Be sure to bring lots of water, especially on warm days. The exposed grasslands and trails of upper Mitchell Canyon become sun parched and dusty, and shade is a rare occurrence. Sunscreen is strongly recommended. Watch out for other hikers, equestrians, and other bikers. When riding the paved road section to the summit, stay alert for cars.

Rescue index: The steepness of Mitchell Canyon and your area of travel means you'll see few trail users. So, in case of an emergency, don't expect help to come along anytime soon. You should be self-reliant and prepared to make your own way to either the trailhead at the Mitchell Canyon north parking area ranger station or to the Mount Diablo summit. At both places, you are likely to find someone who may be of help. A pay phone is located at both Mitchell Canyon parking area and the summit. The northeastern edge of the loop skirts the edge of residential homes in the Regency development and several trails lead into these neighborhoods. Also, there is a fire station located about 1.75 miles north of the Mitchell Canyon parking area at the intersection of Mitchell Canyon and Clayton Roads.

Land status: Mount Diablo State Park.

Maps: *Trail Map of Mount Diablo State Park and Adjacent Parklands*, published by Mount Diablo Interpretive Association, about $6.00. *Mount Diablo State Park*, as published by the State of California Department of Parks & Recreation, about $1.00.

Finding the trail: From Walnut Creek, take the Ygnacio Valley Road/Main Street exit off I-680. Follow Ygnacio Valley Road east, crossing North Broadway to Pine Hollow Road. Ygnacio Valley intersects Pine Hollow at about 6.7 miles from the North Main–Ygnacio Valley intersection. Turn right onto Pine Hollow and drive for another 1.7 miles to Mitchell Canyon Road. Hang a right onto Mitchell Canyon and in about a mile, it leads you into Mount Diablo State Park. A half mile farther, you reach the entrance booth where you'll need to self-register for day use of the parking area. Cost is about $2.00. There is potable water, picnic tables, a pay phone, and rest room facilities here as well as the park ranger station. Park and begin pedaling from here.

Sources of additional information:

Mount Diablo Interpretive
   Association
P.O. Box 346
Walnut Creek, CA 94597-0346
(510) 927-7222

Mount Diablo State Park
96 Mitchell Canyon Rd.
Clayton, CA 94517
(510) 837-2525

Notes on the trail: Though this loop can be ridden in either direction, general consensus among locals is to ride it counterclockwise, starting on Mitchell Canyon Road, a wide, smooth fire road. In that way, you'll pedal the steep single-track portion as a descent, which is decidedly more fun for advanced technical riders. Bring a quarter or two for the telescopes at the summit overlook—definitely a must if it's a clear day.

Pick up the signed fire road at the southern end of the parking area and head toward White Canyon, Juniper Campgrounds, Deer Flat Trail, and the summit. This is Mitchell Canyon Road and it's a smooth, non-technical dirt road that immediately begins climbing moderately. The next 7.7 miles south is an arduous climb to the summit, gaining a little over 3,200 feet with road grades ranging from 2% to 9%. Fortunately, there are a few short, flat stretches along the way that give your burning lungs and stressed leg muscles a break. Mitchell Canyon Road follows little Mitchell Creek up through the canyon. Though the hillside is a mixture of grasslands dotted with oak, pine, and laurel trees, the road is mostly exposed. If you're riding on a warm, dry day, this is the stretch where you'll really feel the heat. Bypass several dirt roads leading off on your right and continue on the main fire road toward Deer Flat.

At 2.2 miles, the road steepens and indeed, this is the beginning of the steepest portion of Mitchell Canyon Road. Persevere as you grind up the smooth dirt road through a series of switchbacks. It'll be over soon. Take a break if you need to and tell your riding buddies you're stopping just to take in the view of the Clayton Valley and Mitchell Canyon below behind you to the north. When you reach the junction of another fire road signed Deer Flat Road at about 3.5 miles, the worst is over and you will have climbed 1,300 feet to an elevation of 1,990 feet. From here, according to a sign, the road on your right is Deer Flat Road and leads to Juniper Campground in 1.5 miles. This is the road you want. *Make sure you don't miss this turn* as the straight-ahead, seemingly obvious fire road is unsigned Meridian Ridge Road, running to Murchio Gap.

Deer Flat Road continues the uphill march though generally not as steep as the last couple of miles. As you continue along a ridge, you have a glimpse of downtown Walnut Creek over your left shoulder. Begin traversing around the south side of the ridge and continue past signed Burma Road, a dirt road leading off on your right. Stay on Deer Flat Road and about a half mile from the Burma Road junction, you enter Juniper Campground. Go through the gate onto the pavement. There are rest rooms and drinking water here. Follow the paved road as it climbs gently through the campground. Right before the road intersects paved Summit Road, there is a great overlook on your right, through the trees and still within the campground, that offers a 180-degree view toward the west. If it's a clear day, you should be able to see the San Francisco Bay shimmering in the distance.

Hang a left onto Summit Road and stay alert for cars. From here to the summit, the road is paved and there's not much of a shoulder. Follow the road past Muir

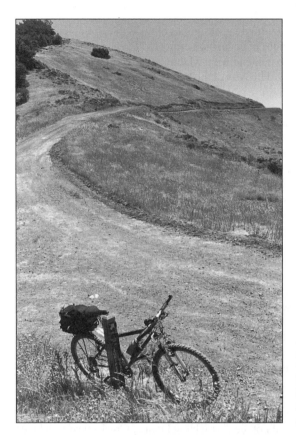

The viewpoint from Moss Rock Ridge is a good place to catch your breath after conquering the steepest ascent of this loop.

picnic area on your left, and, in a few more yards, you reach a left hairpin turn called Devil's Elbow. Here, at the bend in the road, two single-tracks take off on your right. The far right track is signed Summit Trail and is hiking only. The near right trail is the North Peak Trail and that's the single-track which you'll be following after you come back down from the summit. The summit is about a mile from here, so stay on the paved road, following it through the hairpin and bypassing a dirt road leading to the Diablo Communication Center on your left. Ride past the day-use parking lot on the right and continue the moderate climb for a few more yards to the Summit Building. At 7.5 miles, you've made it to the top! The summit sits at 3,849 feet and is the high point of this loop ride. Consider yourself lucky if it's a clear day because you'll have a sweeping 360-degree view. Telescopes are available for your viewing pleasure (25¢) and you might even see Half Dome in Yosemite. The building and overlook tower houses a museum and visitor center. Check out the stones that make up the observation tower. These stones were quarried from this mountain and contain embedded fossils—a testament to the tremendous geological events that created this mountain millions of years ago.

After you've thoroughly recovered from the climb and/or had enough time enjoying your surroundings, retrace your path down the pavement to Devil's Elbow and the North Peak trailhead. At 8.8 miles, you begin descending North Peak, the only single-track portion of this loop—and it's technically challenging. The trail is a narrow single-track that rolls sharply up and down as it hugs the mountainside. Expect the trail conditions to be intermittently steep, about 8% grade and mostly covered with loose dirt, rocks, and semi-buried larger chunks of rocks the size of tennis balls and basketballs, and brief sections of deep, bare drop-offs. There are also water bars and a few exposed tree roots to contend with. Maintaining traction and controlling your skid is the order of the day. The view of the San Joaquin Valley sprawling below on your right is expansive—if you can bear to take your eyes off the trail, that is. Walking works and will enable you to see the view as well as the Devil's Pulpit, a monolithic rock towering above the North Peak Trail. Watch out for poison oak along this stretch—they're even lurking in the shade of a fragrant stand of laurel trees at 9.5 miles. When you come out from the laurel trees, look behind and above toward the summit overlook—that gives you a sense of how much you've descended in the last 1.6 miles. The single-track continues to drop steeply and at 9.8 miles, you reach the signed intersection with Prospector Gap Road, a fire road, running left and right. North Peak Trail continues through the intersection, climbing severely uphill. Not to worry—that's not part of this loop.

Hang a welcome left onto Prospector. The fire road descends steeply, about 9% grade in some brief stretches, and the terrain is likely to be loose dirt and gravel. Rain ruts cross as well as run downhill with the road, forming tiny canyons that, for some reason, seem to have a gravitational pull for your front wheel. Fight the pull as you deftly descend the exposed road and at about 10.7 miles, bypass Middle Trail, a hiking-only trail. Less than a half mile farther, hang a hard right onto signed Meridian Ridge Road toward Donner Canyon Road. The trail condition of Meridian is similar to Prospector Gap Road—loose, very steep and challenging. The pitch varies from moderate to extremely steep for a short distance.

The technical challenge softens significantly at about 12.5 miles, near the junction of Cardinet Oak Road and Donner Canyon Trail, a fire road. Turn left here onto Donner Canyon Trail and head toward the Regency Gate. Bypass other hiking trails on your left and right. Heard but not seen is trickling Donner Creek on your right. At about 13.2 miles, continue past the hiking trail leading to the Donner Cabin Site on your right. The riding is smooth and easy now and more fire roads intersect Donner Canyon Trail. Following the correct road becomes a bit of a challenge here as the roads are not always signed. You reach a major fork at about 13.8 miles where an unsigned fire road takes off on your left and the straight-ahead leads to the Regency Gate in the Regency residential development. Make the hard left and follow the fire road due west, riding up and down rolling, grassy hills. By now, straight ahead in the distance is an unsightly rock quarry, a yellowish-white scar in the flank of a nearby mountainside. At about 14 miles, Back Creek Trail crosses your path and a sign here indicates you've been riding Bruce Lee Trail (named in memory of a dedicated trail builder) and that the Mitchell Canyon staging area is 0.84 mile. You're on the right track. Continue on Bruce Lee, crossing a dry creekbed, then begin climbing a short, steep stretch. At the top of the climb, a signed fire road runs left and right. The left path is signed, indicating Mitchell Rock Trail while the right is the continuation of Bruce Lee to Mitchell staging area. Say good-bye to Bruce Lee and go left toward Mitchell Rock. (You can certainly take the right trail which is a more direct route to the parking area, cutting less than a half mile off the loop.) The trail rolls up and down over sometimes soft-packed dirt. At the next signed intersection, hang a left, still following the trail to Mitchell Rock. A few yards beyond that, at another signed junction, go right following Mitchell Rock Trail to Mitchell Canyon Road. (The straight-ahead trail is Mitchell Rock Trail to Eagle Peak Trail and is hiking only.) Follow the fire road as it leads through a patch of oak trees. Signed Bruce Lee Trail leads off on the right; bypass it. Shortly thereafter, you close the loop by rejoining Mitchell Canyon Road, the fire road you originally rode up on, next to the parking area. Go right here and finish in the parking lot. Total mileage, including the out-and-back stretch on the pavement to the summit is approximately 15 miles.

RIDE 68 · Shell Ridge–Stage Road Dirt Ride

AT A GLANCE

Length/configuration: 11.7-mile out-and-back with a loop, counterclockwise; fire roads

Aerobic difficulty: Moderate with occasional short, steep ups and downs

Technical difficulty: Mild with a short section of barely intermediate terrain over slabs of rock

Scenery: Wide-open grassy, rolling hills that offer a glimpse of nearby Walnut Creek. Deep canyon and creekside vegetation covered by a peaceful oak forest.

Special comments: Youngsters and adults towing kid-trailers may enjoy the beginning portion, turning around when they've had enough. Strong, advanced riders can combine this ride with the Mount Diablo–Mitchell Canyon Loop (Ride 67). Note: A loosely enforced park regulation requires bells on bikes.

Near the base of domineering Mount Diablo is this little gem of open space, the Shell Ridge Recreation Area. What a great backyard the residences of Walnut Creek have. Owned and managed by the city of Walnut Creek, the trails here are easily accessible. But the best part of Shell Ridge is riding possibilities are expanded because its trails run into adjacent Mount Diablo State Park and Diablo Foothills Regional Park. You can configure your own route, making them as long or short as you like. Your ride can be leisurely or a tough all-day workout.

The ride presented here takes advantage of the adjoining parks and gives beginners and intermediate riders a thoroughly satisfying adventure without having to tackle the steepness of riding up Mount Diablo. Riders need only have basic bike handling skills and good endurance to enjoy this 11.7-mile out-and-back-loop ride. The fire roads that make up this route are generally hard-packed, becoming dusty during the summer and incredibly muddy during wet days. Leading you through wide-open rolling, grassy hills and deep forested creek canyons, it's hard to get bored on this ride, even if you're an expert rider. If you're a hard-core rider looking for a workout that will challenge you technically and aerobically, consider linking this ride with the Mount Diablo–Mitchell Canyon Loop (see previous ride description). But, before you pedal off and make up your own configuration, you absolutely, positively must have your own map. *Trail Map of Mount Diablo and Adjacent Parklands*, published by the Mount Diablo Interpretive Association is outstanding (see Sources of Additional Information below).

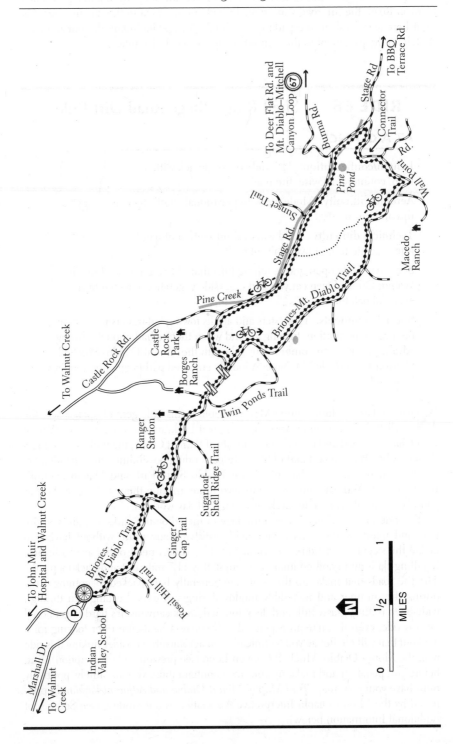

General location: East edge of Walnut Creek, about 30 miles east of San Francisco.

Elevation change: 580 feet; starting elevation and low point 300 feet; high point 880 feet. Lots of flat riding in between long ups and downs.

Season: Year-round though several long portions of the route become ankle-deep, thick mudpits during wet weather. Wait at least a week or two after a heavy rain.

Services: None on the trail. All services can be found in Walnut Creek.

Hazards: Poison oak is prevalent along Stage Road set within a cool shady forest along Pine Creek. Rattlesnakes live here as do rarely seen mountain lions. Watch out for other trail users as the area around the trailhead is extremely popular with runners and walkers, with or without their dogs. Equestrians enjoy these trails too.

Rescue index: The trailhead next to the Indian Valley School is set within a residential neighborhood, making it a popular after-work destination. Chances are you'll meet other trail users, especially on the weekends, who may be of help. Borges Ranch and Macedo Ranch, about 3 miles and 5 miles respectively from the trailhead, is accessible by car and a phone for emergencies is likely to be available at both places. Castle Rock Park, about a half mile off the loop is also accessible by car and is a popular park during the weekends. John Muir Hospital is within 15 minutes from the trailhead.

Land status: Shell Ridge Recreation area, maintained by the city of Walnut Creek; Diablo Regional Park, maintained by the East Bay Regional Park District; and Mount Diablo State Park.

Maps: *Trail Map of Mount Diablo State Park and Adjacent Parklands*, published by Mount Diablo Interpretive Association, about $6.00.

Finding the trail: From I-680 in Walnut Creek, take the Ygnacio Valley Road/Main Street exit and head east by northeast. Drive for about 1.2 miles to Homestead Avenue. Turn right onto Homestead and then make the first left onto Marshall Drive. Follow Marshall through a residential neighborhood about 1.5 miles to its end at Indian Valley School. Park near the trailhead. Avoid parking in front of anyone's house as the nearby residents don't welcome trail users who leave their car at their front door. Cars have reportedly been vandalized by irate residents.

Sources of additional information:

Walnut Creek Open Space
1035 Castle Rock Rd.
Walnut Creek, CA 94598
(510) 943-5854
The ranger station is located near Borges Ranch and is accessible a short distance off the bike route.

Mount Diablo State Park
96 Mitchell Canyon Rd.
Clayton, CA 94517
(510) 837-2525

Diablo Foothills Regional Park
East Bay Regional Park District
2950 Peralta Oaks Ct.

P.O. Box 5381
Oakland, CA 94605-0381
(510) 562-PARK or (510) 635-0135

Mount Diablo Interpretive
  Association
P.O. Box 346
Walnut Creek, CA 94597-0346
(510) 927-7222

Bicycle Trails Council of the
  East Bay
P.O. Box 9583
Berkeley, CA 94709
(510) 420-1617

Notes on the trail: Following this route is fairly easy as many of the trails and their intersections are signed. Harsh weather sometimes obliterates the information displayed on the wooden posts. Generally, the route is an east-west out-and-back with a loop. The loop is ridden counterclockwise though it can be ridden in reverse just as easily. Note too that when you pass through a cattle gate—and there are several— leave it as you found it, either open or closed.

Begin by going through the gate in front of the Indian Valley School. The terrain is fairly open here and there are several trails radiating from this gate. The trail you want parallels the cyclone fence on your right, descending gently. After a few yards, the trail forks. Take the left fork which leads you away from the fence, now directly behind you. About a half mile from the trailhead, bypass the signed Fossil Hill Trail on your right. The signpost here tells you you're on the Briones-to–Mount Diablo Trail. Continue east on the Briones–Mount Diablo Trail, cruising up and down brief rolling hills. In another half mile, veer right onto Ginger Gap Trail, a brief double-track trail that rejoins the Briones–Mount Diablo Trail near a pond in about 0.3 mile. Back on the Briones–Mount Diablo Trail, continue pass Joaquin Trail and go through a gate. Joaquin Pond is just on your right over a berm.

Climb up a short but steep stretch and at just over 2 miles, bypass the signed Sugarloaf–Shell Ridge Trail on your right. Bear left, staying on Briones–Mount Diablo Trail, still rolling over open, grassy hills. You're gradually climbing up the side of a ridge and if you look behind, you can see the valley in which Walnut Creek lies. Almost a half mile from the last trail junction, go past signed Twin Ponds Trail on your right. A few yards farther brings you to a gated fence. The fence roughly marks the boundary line between Shell Ridge Recreation Area and Mount Diablo State Park. Just before the gate is the trail that leads down to Borges Ranch. Ignore that trail and go through the gate, now entering the state park.

Still on the Briones–Mount Diablo Trail, you're now heading toward Macedo Ranch. You're in cattle territory and the fire road may be deeply rutted by cow hooves, making for a bumpy, irritating ride. In almost a half mile from the last gate, about 3 miles from the Indian Valley School trailhead, go through another gate. On the other side of the gate is a signed intersection. Now begins the counterclockwise loop. The left fire road is signed Shell Ridge Loop Trail to Buckeye Ravine Trail. You'll be returning to this point via Shell Ridge Loop Trail. For now, bear right and continue on Briones–Mount Diablo Trail, still heading east. Still in open, rolling terrain, the dirt road may be rugged due to millions of deep hoof prints (obviously a favorite cattle trail). Cruise past another pond and at 3.3 miles, bypass a trail leading off on your right. You've basically reached the high point of the ride along this stretch, about 880 feet. When you reach a fork with a narrow single-track trail peeling off on your right, follow either trail as they rejoin in a few yards around a hill. Don't forget to check out the view behind you. Here, looking down between the hills is Walnut Creek and Concord.

At approximately 4.8 miles, still on the Briones–Mount Diablo Trail, a signpost tells you that the left hiking-only trail leads to Stage Road while the straight-ahead fire road leads to Wall Point Road. Continue toward Wall Point and in 0.3 mile, you indeed reach the beginning of that trail, another fire road. Bypass the trail on the right leading down to Macedo Ranch and bear left onto Wall Point Road. Down on your right you see Macedo Ranch and nearby residential neighborhoods. About a half mile farther, in the shade of a few oak trees, go through a gate and left onto a wide connector trail. Here, the trail is white-ish, blonde, hard-packed dirt and gravel. You've left the wide-open range and begin descending into a forested creek canyon, clearly a different environment now. Pine Pond sits a little below in the ravine on your left.

At just over 6 miles, the wide trail ends as a single-track at a gate. Go through the gate and come to a multi-signed intersection. The right trail is signed Pine Creek Trail and leads to BBQ Terrace Road; this same trail is also signed Stage Road to Diablo Ranch. Pine Creek Trail and Stage Road are one and the same, running both left and right at this intersection. Pine Creek Trail is a much more applicable name than Stage Road since this narrow dirt road parallels Pine Creek. For whatever reason, Stage Road is the name that sticks in people's mind. No matter. Turn left onto Stage Road/Pine Creek Trail.

This is arguably the prettiest part of the ride in that you travel through a lush, forested creek environment. In about 0.4 mile from the left turn, go past Pine Pond on your left and Burma Road leading off on your right. (For those of you aching for more of a challenge and more mileage, Burma Road is the linking trail to the Mount Diablo–Mitchell Canyon Loop, Ride 67.) For the next mile, Stage Road/Pine Creek Trail crosses the creek in several places. If you're riding early in the year or after a great deal of rain, expect to see the creek invade the road along this stretch. In fact, if you're riding when the ground has not completely dried, boy oh boy, are you in for a treat. Lovely Stage Road/Pine Creek Trail turns into an ankle-deep mudpit, stretching almost a half mile. It loves to swallow bike tires and yours is no exception. What makes this tremendously annoying is that you must drag your bike through the mud, because riding is impossible. Why trudge through the mud? Poison oak lines both sides of the road and forces you to endure the quagmire. So it's face the mud or pay for it later.

Hopefully, you won't have to deal with such conditions. When you reach the regional park boundary line, go through the gate and cross the main flow of the creek. Incidentally, the creek is a good place to try and wash off any poison oak oil you may have gotten on your skin and bike. After the crossing, pedal through a level small clearing on the hard-packed dirt road. Still riding within a canyon, Stage Road slowly leads you uphill. There's a short stretch of intermediate terrain, made so by semi-buried slabs of smooth boulders in the trail. On your right, down near the creek is a small open meadow alongside an old, abandoned spillway.

When you reach the next intersection, the signs here indicate Castle Rock Trail on your right and Stage Road to Shell Ridge Loop on your left. Bear left, staying on Stage Road. (When I rode here last, parts of the signs were missing. Hopefully, the signs have been replaced with accurate ones.) Begin a gradual climb up the hard-packed dirt road, still within the shade of the forest and canyon walls. About 0.2 mile beyond the intersection, look for a picnic table sitting underneath several shady oak trees on your left. It marks a signed trail junction of Shell Ridge Loop running both straight and left. Turn left and begin climbing a somewhat steep hill. Bypass Buckeye Ravine Trail, a former ranch road that has degraded into an incredibly steep, extremely narrow single-track which is now open to bikes. If you're game, try tackling Buckeye. It takes you up to the same spot as the tamer Shell Ridge Loop Trail.

Whichever route you take, the climb leads you out of the ravine and into open terrain. In less than a mile from the picnic table intersection, you close the loop by reaching the Briones–Mount Diablo Trail. Hang a right here and retrace your path through several gates. Bypass the side trail to Borges Ranch and eventually return to the trailhead at Indian Valley School. Your total ending mileage is about 11.7 miles.

RIDE 69 · Black Diamond Mines Loop

AT A GLANCE

Length/configuration: 9-mile out-and-back with a loop; fire roads and some pavement

Aerobic difficulty: Moderately strenuous due to steep climbing sections

Technical difficulty: Mildly technical

Scenery: Rolling, grassy hills in and above an undeveloped valley. During the spring, the hills are refreshingly green with abundant wildflowers.

Special comments: Greathouse Portal Visitor Center, located inside an abandoned mine, is a worthwhile stop. Riders made of steel can connect to the Mount Diablo–Mitchell Canyon Loop (Ride 67) and other trails in the Mount Diablo State Park and surrounding regional parks.

Many of the fire roads in Black Diamond Mines Regional Preserve allow bikes but most of them are short out-and-back stretches. The ride described here is a loop with a short out-and-back and the combined mileage is 9 miles round-trip. Rated mildly technical, the fire roads are generally smooth and hard-packed, devoid of obstacles. Though the park is open year-round, riding in the spring is the prettiest, when the open rolling hills and valley floor are covered with fresh green grass and wildflowers. Just be sure to let the park dry out after a heavy rain. From the trailhead, a nearly one-mile stretch leads up to the beginning of the seven-mile counterclockwise loop. The first half of the loop route drops down into a peaceful valley, leading past several historic mine sites. The route through the valley is basically a sweet, flat trail and you can really pick up speed here. The second half of the ride involves lots of climbing back up to the ridge on smooth fire roads. Riders of all technical abilities—from basic to advanced—and with great endurance and strong climbing muscles will enjoy this ride.

The history of this area goes way back. Three groups of Indian who spoke the Bay Miwok language lived here: the Chupcan, Volvon, and Ompin tribes. Spanish, Mexican, and American settlers arriving after 1772 managed to destroy most of the culture and lifestyle of the Indians. In the 1860s, the hills became known for their rich deposits of coal—"black diamonds." Immigrants hoping to capitalize on the precious resource flooded the region and five coal mining towns thrived: Nortonville, Somersville, Stewartville, West Hartley, and Judsonville. Nearly four million tons of coal was mined here, making it California's largest coal mining operation at that time. Eventually, rising production costs and competing new energy sources closed coal mining operations and the once bustling towns died. In the 1920s, underground sand mining began near the old Nortonville and Somersville town sites. Controlled by the Hazel–Atlas Glass Company in Oakland, the Nortonville mine supplied foundry sand to the Columbia Steel Works in nearby Pittsburg for glassmaking. After mining more than 1.8 million tons of sand, operations slowed and eventually succumbed to foreign competition. Some miners found new life in ranching, mostly raising cattle. In the early 1970s, the East Bay Regional Park District began acquiring land here.

RIDE 69 · Black Diamond Mines Loop

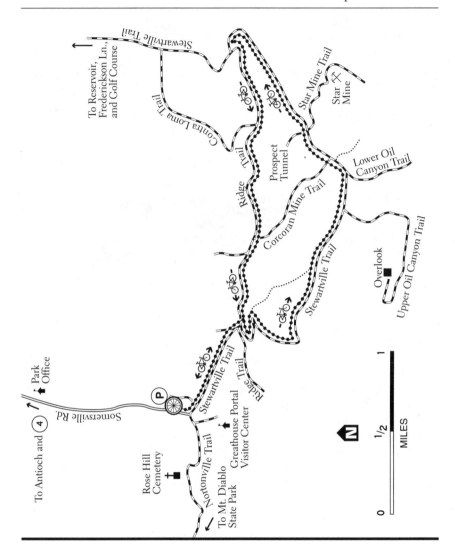

Today, descendants of the original mining families still graze cattle in the preserve. A healthy wildlife population lives here including deer, opossums, foxes, bobcats, and lots of lizards. Rarely seen mountain lions also reside here. Over 100 species of birds have been sited, including the rare golden eagle. The preserve offers summertime activities, including hikes, concerts, naturalists' presentations, and historical programs.

General location: About 55 miles northeast of San Francisco.

Elevation change: 860 feet; starting elevation 450 feet; high point 985 feet; low point 125 feet. After surmounting the first hill, the route descends, then flattens for the about 5 miles, followed by a series of steep hills along a ridge.

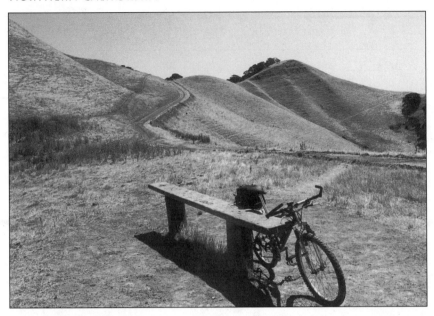

This loop begins and ends at this junction of Stewartville and Ridge Trails. The Ridge Trail leading downhill (on the left of this photo) closes the loop on this ride.

Season: Year-round.

Services: Drinking water and pit toilets available at two parking areas: next to the park office adjacent to the entry booth and at the trailhead. Drinking water can also be found near the old Somersville town site picnic area and Greathouse Portal, about 0.1 mile from the trailhead. Campgrounds with rest rooms are available at Stewartville Backpack Camp and Star Mine Group Camp. The Greathouse Portal is a former sand mine that is now used as the Visitor Center, housing excellent interpretive displays and historical artifacts. A well-made video revealing the history of the area can be viewed there. The park rangers even let you park your bike inside the cool mine—a pleasant respite after a hot day of riding. During the summer, the preserve offers concerts and plays in the park.

Hazards: The preserve is home to a variety of wildlife, including rarely seen mountain lions. Stay alert. Rattlesnakes enjoy sunning themselves on the trails when the weather's warm, typically in the spring. So, look before you place your hand, sit, or step, even around picnic grounds. Rattlers are not usually out during very hot weather. The park closes at dusk.

Rescue index: During the popular spring months, you're likely to see hikers and other trail users, especially on the weekends. Otherwise, for emergencies, you'll need to make your own way back to the Somersville trailhead, parking area, or park office near the main entrance booth. You might find help at the Greathouse Portal Visitor Center, although it is only open seasonally. If you're near the eastern end of the route, seek help by following Stewartville Trail northward, down to Frederickson Lane, then turn right toward the municipal golf course, about a mile from the park boundary.

Land status: Black Diamond Mines Regional Preserve, maintained by the East Bay Regional Park District.

Maps: *Black Diamond Mines Regional Preserve*, the official park map.

Finding the trail: From I-680 near Concord, head east on CA 4 toward Pittsburg and Antioch. Take the Somersville exit, after Pittsburg but before Antioch. Drive south on Somersville Road for about 1.6 miles toward the hills and at a sharp left turn, continue straight, entering Black Diamond Mines Regional Preserve. Continue on Somersville for almost 3 miles to the main entrance, marked by the pay booth. Seasonal parking fees may be enforced, about $3. The park office is located here and water and rest rooms are available. Continue driving south on Somersville for another 2 miles to the parking area. Park and begin pedaling from here.

Sources of additional information:

Black Diamond Mines Regional
  Preserve
5175 Somersville Rd.
Antioch, CA 94509
(925) 757-2620

East Bay Regional Park District
2950 Peralta Oaks Ct.
P.O. Box 5381
Oakland, CA 94605-0381
(510) 562-PARK or (510) 635-0135

Notes on the trail: Before hitting the trail, consider bringing a flashlight. It comes in handy if you want to explore Prospect Tunnel, a 400-foot former coal mine, 200 feet of which is open to the public.

Finding the route is easy because the trails are fairly well-signed and accurately depicted in the official park map. Basically, the route is a counterclockwise loop which you access via a 1-mile stretch. When you close the loop, you then retrace your path on the 1-mile stretch back to your car. Since your surroundings are wide-open, grassy, rolling hills and flat valley floor, nearly devoid of trees throughout, you can easily see most of the route. The ride initially rises over a ridge, descends into a peaceful, wide-open valley, cruises along the valley floor, then climbs steeply up along the same ridge to close the loop. All the trails that make up this route are really fire roads. In fact, narrow single-track trails are hiking-only trails and are generally marked. Bikes are allowed only on dirt roads unless otherwise posted. There are several gates on this route and when you go through them, remember to leave them as they were—open or closed.

So, starting from the parking lot, pedal to the south end of the lot and pick up the signed Stewartville Trail on your left. Stewartville is a fire road, wide, smooth, semi-hard-packed and easy to ride. The trail heads southeast and begins a moderate climb up to the nearby ridge top, almost a mile away. Short sections of level or gently sloping terrain offer brief respite from the climbing. At the ridge top, next to a gated fence, Ridge Trail leads off on your right, paralleling the fence. (A trail peels off behind your left shoulder, signed to park boundary. Ignore it.) Go through the gate, still on Stewartville Trail, and notice Ridge Trail also running steeply uphill on your left. You'll be coming down that stretch on your return to this spot when you close the loop. There's a wooden bench here overlooking the valley below. From here, you can see Stewartville Trail cutting through the valley floor. You'll be riding that stretch in no time.

Now begins your moderately steep, curvy descent into the valley. On this stretch, the composition of the trail may be loose with small broken chunks of dried mud. That combined with the steepness may challenge your ability to maintain control and you may want to walk a few yards to more stable terrain.

At about 1.8 miles from the starting point, you reach the valley floor. A signed trail on your right leads to the park boundary. Bypass it, staying left on Stewartville Trail as it continues to gently descend. Here begins a sweet, easy, and gently rolling stretch through the valley. At 2.6 miles, Stewartville crosses over a tiny creek. Immediately pass Miners Trail, a hiking-only path on your left. Go over another creek which may be dry. Ride through a gate at about 3.2 miles. A few yards beyond it, Upper Oil Canyon Trail, another fire road, leads off on your right. (Upper Oil Canyon Trail leads to an overlook in about 1.2 miles and bikes are allowed on it. Some steep climbing is involved, but hey, at least you get to come back down it. Check it out if you'd like. Also here at this intersection is a backpack campground in which rest rooms are available.)

Continue following Stewartville Trail heading east on basically flat terrain. About 0.3 mile beyond Upper Oil Canyon is Lower Oil Canyon Trail on your right. (It too permits bikes and is a 1.3-mile out-and-back, each way. Worth checking out if you have the time or inclination.) Stay on Stewartville, still heading east, cruising past a corral on your left. A few yards farther, go through a gate after cruising past Star Mine Trail, a hiking-only path. At 3.9 miles, Corcoran Mine Trail leads steeply up-hill on your left. (Bikes are allowed on Corcoran and it's a shortcut to Ridge Trail. Taking it will cut almost 4 miles off this ride. But it's a mean, steep, and narrow trail up to the ridge.) A few yards farther, still following Stewartville Trail, Star Mine Trail rejoins your road, only this time, it's a wide gravel road. At this point, you're at the lowest point of this ride, elevation 125 feet. Star Mine Group Camp is located here. Take a slight side trip here by turning right onto Star Mine. Go past the camp-ground, riding down and up and around for about 0.6 mile to Star Mine, located on the right. Though there's not much to see of this coal mine except for a small, fenced cave entrance, you can still imagine the grueling, underground working conditions that once thrived here from the 1860s to the turn of the century. Turn around and retrace your path back to Stewartville Trail. (The bikeable portion of Star Mine Trail continues south for another half mile to the park boundary.)

Back on Stewartville, go right and continue heading east. (Incidentally, here's an opportunity for some exploring if you'd like. Prospect Tunnel Trail is almost directly across from Star Mine Trail on the left side of Stewartville Trail. Prospect allows bikes and leads up to a former coal mine, stretching 400 feet long. You can actually explore 200 feet of the tunnel but you'll need a flashlight.) The route now begins its gradual climb out of the valley, gently curving to the northeast. Underneath your tires, the trail contains some broken pieces of asphalt mixed with the dirt and gravel. As you rise above the valley floor on your right, you get a glimpse of the flatlands around the San Joaquin River Delta.

When the trail curves to nearly due west at about 6 miles, it's payback time. Here, Ridge Trail intersects Stewartville on your left and runs steeply uphill about 9% grade. Take a deep breath, downshift and turn left. (If you wanted to extend your ride by almost 2 miles, you could continue on Stewartville, bearing right. After about a half mile, hang a left onto Contra Loma Trail and pedal about 1.2 miles to its inter-section with Ridge Trail. Don't think this extension lets you bypass any of the steep terrain on Ridge. It doesn't. If anything, the climbing on Contra Loma is steeper and slightly longer.) As you grind away, look up toward the ridge line and you feel like you're riding right into the sky. For the next 2 miles, you'll gain 670 feet before clos-ing the loop at Stewartville Trail near the beginning trailhead. In the meantime, get-ting there is an aerobic challenge. Like many trails that run along a ridge, Ridge Trail rolls up and down a bunch of steep hills, (about 9 hills, but who's counting?), ranging from 7% to 11%-plus grade. Fortunately, the trail is somewhat forgiving. Level and gentle stretches offer your legs and lungs some respite, albeit way too brief. The wide-open sweeping views of the valley below on your left and the flatlands on your right help keep your mind off the arduous task. At 6.8 miles, about 0.8 mile since leaving Stewartville Trail, Contra Loma Trail intersects Ridge on your right. (This is part of the extension previously mentioned.) Continue on Ridge and after a long hill, as the trail traverses the exposed slope just below the ridge line, go past Corcoran Mine Trail on your left (about a mile after Contra Loma Trail). A few yards farther, ignore a trail on your right which leads to the park boundary. After one more short hill, the intersection at Stewartville Trail down below comes into view. Let your two-wheeled steed fly down the hill and pop you right up the last incline to the intersection. Turn right onto Stewartville, closing the loop at 8.3 miles. From here, retrace the last 0.7 mile back toward the trailhead and ultimately your car.

If the Greathouse Portal Visitor Center is open, do check it out. The staff allows bikes to be rolled into the cool tunnel which houses the interpretive displays and artifacts. An excellent video is also shown about the region and its coal and glass mining industry during the late 1800s. (Their hours are very limited, generally 9 a.m.–3:30 p.m. on the first and third Saturdays of each month.) As you finish the ride, you can reach the Greathouse Portal Visitor Center by hanging a left onto Nortonville Trail immediately before the picnic and parking area. Direction signs are posted along the way. It's located almost a mile from the parking lot. If you continue pedaling west on Nortonville, you would reach the historic Rose Hill Cemetery in about a half mile, and eventually Mount Diablo State Park in about 6 miles, where many other bike trails are available.

RIDE 70 · Briones Crest Loop

AT A GLANCE

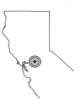

Length/configuration: 8-mile loop, clockwise; wide single-track, double-track, and fire road

Aerobic difficulty: Moderately strenuous due to lots of short, steep climbs

Technical difficulty: Mildly technical

Scenery: Rolling grassy hills and views of Concord, marshlands, and the retired naval ships in Suisun Bay at the mouth of the Sacramento River

Special comments: Lots of short ups and downs make this a great training ride to build climbing legs. Come on! Power through the climbs without shifting gears!

You would think that for a park that's so close to cities such as Walnut Creek, Lafayette, Martinez, and Concord, the views from the peaks and ridges from within Briones Regional Parks would be filled with developed cityscapes. So it's a pleasant surprise to discover that the views are mostly of rolling hills and watershed lands. Though there is a stretch in which the mothball fleet of naval ships in the Suisun Bay is visible, this 8-mile loop ride is a favorite of locals wanting a quick getaway from the hustle and bustle of the city. Fire roads make up the loop and in some sections, the trail looks more like a wide single- or double-track. Technically, the terrain is mild, though a few rain ruts add a bit of spice to an otherwise smooth route—perfect for beginners. The hills, on the other hand, are steep but very brief, and fairly strong stamina is necessary in order to enjoy the ride.

Like many other nearby parks and open spaces, Briones Regional Park is part of the East Bay Municipal Utility District (EBMUD), the agency that governs valuable watershed land in its task to keep the East Bay from becoming thirsty. The name is attributed to Felipe Briones who, in 1829, built a home near what is now the Bear Creek gate entrance. He cultivated the land and raised cattle. After his untimely death in 1840, the boundaries of the Briones' land were frequently contested by subsequent owners and the state of California. In 1906, the People's Water Company acquired much of the area for watershed attributes. The East Bay Municipal Utility District acquired People's Water Company in 1916 and constructed the nearby San Pablo Dam in 1923. Finally, in 1957, EBMUD, in conjunction with Contra Costa County, deemed the watershed of Bear Creek an open space park and named it Briones. Today, Briones Regional Park provides many recreational uses, attracting more than just mountain bikers. Equestrians and hikers are frequent visitors to the park. Black-tailed deer, coyotes, red-tailed hawks, and rarely seen mountain lions are but a few of the park residents.

General location: About 40 miles east of San Francisco, just north of Lafayette and Orinda.

Elevation change: 785 feet; starting elevation and low point 700 feet; high point 1,460 feet. Lots of short but steep hills.

Season: Year-round. In mid- to late summer, along the first-half of the loop, star thistle bushes are apt to be over 4 feet tall, encroaching the narrow fire road—and they're decorated with blood-thirsty tiny thorns. Riding through this gauntlet can be painfully annoying.

Services: None on the route. Parking fee required seasonally. Drinking water, rest rooms, and picnic tables at the trailhead at Bear Creek Staging Area. Campsites and archery range available. All other services in Lafayette and surrounding towns.

Hazards: On rare occasions, mountain lions may be spotted. Stay alert for rattlesnakes sunning themselves on the trails, especially when the weather's warm, typically in the spring. Look before you place your hand, sit, or step, even around picnic grounds. Rattlers are not usually out during very hot weather. Also see comment about star thistles above in "Season."

Rescue index: The park is a popular horseback riding site and you may meet a rider or two on the trail, even during the weekdays. Early weekday evenings and weekends bring out more bikers and hikers so your chances are good of finding someone who may be of help. There are many trails on the loop route that lead back down to the Bear Creek Staging Area and provide shortcuts for emergencies. On the farthest east side of the loop, several trails lead down to well-traveled roads where you can flag down a passing motorist for help.

Land status: Briones Regional Park, maintained by the East Bay Regional Park District.

Maps: *Briones Regional Park*, the official park map.

RIDE 70 · Briones Crest Loop

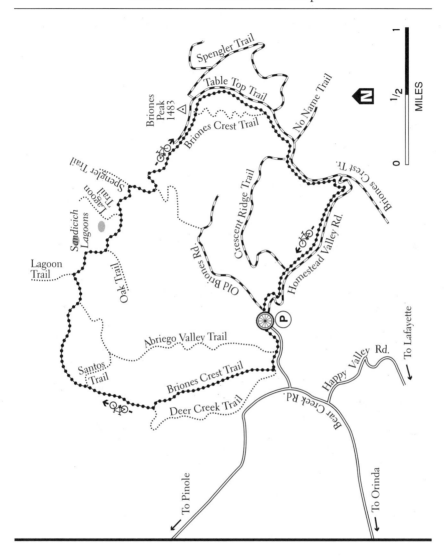

Finding the trail: From I-80 or I-680, head east or west respectively on CA 24 toward Orinda and Lafayette. If you're driving east on CA 24, take Camino Pablo Road north toward San Pablo Reservoir. Just before the reservoir, go right onto Bear Creek Road and follow it past Happy Valley Road to the park entrance. Just inside the main entrance is the Bear Creek Staging Area, a parking lot large enough to accommodate a dozen or so horse trailers. As you pull into the lot, keep an eye out for a trailhead with about 5 descending steps—this is your trailhead. Park in the lot.

Sources of additional information:

East Bay Regional Park District
2950 Peralta Oaks Ct.
P.O. Box 5381
Oakland, CA 94605-0381
(510) 562-PARK or (510) 635-0135

Notes on the trail: From the Bear Creek Staging Area, say "hello" to and be respect-ful of the equestrians who may be saddling up here. Pedal out toward the north end of the parking lot and look for the trailhead with the descending steps. You won't see the steps until you're practically right on top of them. Though the trail is not identified, it immediately climbs and leads to Deer Creek Trail and Briones Crest Trail after paral-leling the paved road for a few yards. A sign identifies Briones Crest Trail at a hard right turn. Take the right here and begin climbing a very steep but short rise. The trail is normally a narrow fire road and may look more like a wide single- or double-track dur-ing various times of the year. If you're riding during the dry season, it's likely to be hard-packed, possibly with some rain ruts. And so begins a long series of steep ups and downs on Briones Crest Trail, roughly following a ridge through mostly wide-open ter-rain. The steepness of the ascents and descents range from flat up to 10%-plus grade. Fortunately, those sections are mostly less than a mile long.

Within a mile, at the top of one of the climbs, go through a cattle gate, leaving it the way you found it—open or closed. Here, you have about a 360-degree view of the nearby rolling hills and Abreigo Valley immediately on your right. A few yards farther, go through another gate, still on Briones Crest Trail. As you continue to gain elevation, you can see Abreigo Valley Trail down in the valley along with its several campgrounds. Bear right, bypassing Deer Creek Trail and through another gate. Soon, as you pass Costa Peak (sitting at 1,235 feet) on your left, look northeast and you have a view of Briones Crest Trail rolling up and down the hilltops.

At about 1.5 miles, continue past unsigned Santos Trail on your right. There are several lesser trails leading off in this vicinity and when in doubt, stay on Briones Crest Trail, the main fire road, which sometimes resembles a wide single-track. A barb wire fence begins paralleling your trail and you soon go through an opening and into the John Muir Wildlife Area. (The area is unsigned but it's indicated on the park map.) Still within wide-open space, looking northeast, you can see the sur-rounding marshlands and the mothball fleet of naval ships in the bay. Abriego Valley Trail intersects your Briones Crest Trail by coming through a fence on your right. Stay left on Briones Crest and continue the now familiar ups and downs, briefly ac-companied by fencing on your right. At 2.5 miles, continue past the western trail-head of Lagoon Trail and cruise through a small stand of oak and laurel trees—one of several rare patches of shade on this loop. Sandicich Lagoons, marked by two ponds, sit just below on the left as you pass the intersection of Mott Peak Trail on your right. By now, as the loop route leads southeast, you have a view of Concord, Walnut Creek, and Mount Diablo sitting below in the distance. A little over 3 miles, enjoy a quick descent, zipping past the other end of Lagoon Trail on your left. Almost a half mile farther, you reach a **T** intersection with Spengler Trail on your left. Stay right on Briones Crest Trail and begin climbing toward Briones Peak, the highest point of the ride.

Continuing on Briones Crest Trail, go past Old Briones Road on your right. (Incidentally, Old Briones is another popular biking trail.) Portions of Briones Crest

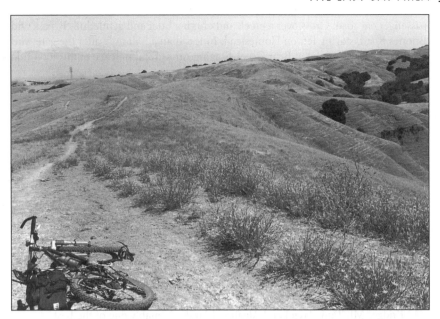

This view of Crest Trail, rolling up and down the hilltops, gives you a hint of what to expect.

here make up the Ivan Dickson Memorial Loop. At about 4 miles, a barb wire fence appears and parallels your trail on the left. The route skirts the Briones Peak sitting at 1,483 feet, and a short side-trip up to the top yields a 360-degree view. You may see several unsigned single-track trails leading off of Briones Crest and you may be tempted to bike it but remember: bikes are only permitted on fire roads in this park.

Very soon after passing the peak, enter a shady patch cast by oak and fragrant laurel trees, followed by a welcoming short downhill stretch. At the bottom of the hill, just before a gate, Briones Crest Trail curves to the right. Say good-bye to Briones Crest and stay straight, going through the gate. Bear left onto Table Top Trail and then, in a few yards, bear right, still on Table Top, bypassing an unsigned left-hand trail. At this point, almost 4.4 miles from the beginning of your ride, now back in wide-open terrain, you can see Mount Diablo dominating the ridges immediately to the southeast. Ride past a bunch of communication dishes (actually, they look more like huge, flat drums than dishes) and proceed downhill. Let your wheels roll, picking up momentum to pop you up the next short but steep hill—maybe you won't need to crank the pedals to reach the top. Continue through several more similar roller-coaster hills, generally descending. At just over 5 miles, stay on Table Top Trail as you bypass Spengler Trail on your left. A few yards farther, Table Top merges into Briones Crest Trail coming in on your right. Follow Briones Crest and after several more brief hills, go through a gate. Soon after the gate, ignore both No Name Trail on your left and Crescent Ridge Trail on your right. Then, following a brief downhill cruise, hang a right onto Homestead Valley Trail, at just over 6 miles.

Homestead Valley is a fire road masquerading as a double-track trail and descends gradually and easily over mostly hard-pack terrain. Stay alert for rain ruts, especially in the shade of the surrounding oak trees. Eventually, the road leads you past Bear Creek Trail on your left (hikers and equestrians only) and then the western end of Crescent Ridge Trail. Stay left on Homestead. Go through a gate onto a dirt, passenger car road. Cross over a creek and climb a brief and gentle hill. Bypass Old Briones Road, staying left on Homestead. In less than a half mile after the gate, you return to the parking lot at Bear Creek Staging Area. Total mileage of this loop ride is about 8 miles.

RIDE 71 · Tilden–Wildcat Canyon Loop

AT A GLANCE

Length/configuration: 13.5-mile loop, clockwise; fire road and paved path

Aerobic difficulty: Moderate with some moderately strenuous sections due to steep, short climbs

Technical difficulty: Mildly technical

Scenery: Spectacular views to the west of San Francisco, the Bay, both Oakland–San Francisco Bay Bridge and Golden Gate Bridge, Mt. Tam, Angel and Alcatraz Islands. Arguably one of the best places to catch a sunset in northern California is a spot on this loop.

Special comments: Easily accessible Nimitz Way is ideal for youngsters and kid-trailers. Note: A loosely enforced park regulation requires bells on bikes.

This 13.5-mile loop, ridden clockwise, offers something for every level of rider, including youngsters on their own bike or in a kid trailer. The ride begins in Tilden Regional Park, then crosses into adjacent Wildcat Canyon Regional Park and tours the park perimeter before re-entering Tilden. Most of the loop requires barely moderate endurance although there is a three-mile stretch in the middle of the loop which contains numerous nasty little hills that are quite steep. Comprised mostly of smooth, mildly technical fire roads and a small stretch of paved multi-use trail, the loop has many access points. Strong, adult beginners and all other level of adult cyclists can ride the entire loop starting from Big Leaf picnic ground or Inspiration Point.

If you have the kiddies in tow, you can ride one of two out-and-back stretches. From Big Leaf picnic area, the first 4.8 miles, punctuated with one steep 20-yard climb, is suitable for kid-trailers and youngsters, making it a fun out-and-back ride of 9.6 miles round-trip. From Inspiration Point, the path is paved and runs 3.8 miles one-way (7.6 miles round-trip) and is suitable for youngsters and kid-trailers. Though much of the loop can accommodate kid-trailers, you need super-bionic strength in order to surmount a bunch of nasty, little hills.

And speaking of those hills, tackling the climbs is rewarded by an incredibly expansive view of San Francisco and the Bay, with all its notable landmarks such as the Golden Gate Bridge and Mt. Tam. Sunsets from a particular spot on the loop are undeniably gorgeous. As for the rest of the route, the loop offers a variety of terrain. The first part of the ride leads you through a lush, rich riparian environment alongside Wildcat Creek. If you're quiet, you may see a number of resident rabbits hopping down the trail. The next portion of the loop climbs up to the sunset viewpoint, leading you up wide-open rolling, grassy hills, sparsely covered by live oak. Pedaling up and down short hills along the ridge, the loop eventually mellows and becomes a paved multi-use trail, rolling through fragrant eucalyptus and laurel groves. The final stretch leads you through another thick riparian environment before closing the loop.

Tilden Regional Park is one of the oldest areas of the East Bay Regional Park District (EBRPD), having opened to public recreational use in 1936. It was named in honor of Major Charles Lee Tilden, a park founder and the first president of the EBRPD Board of Directors. Tilden Regional Park offers a lot of fun opportunities, especially for children. The park offers pony rides, miniature steam train rides, a fully-operational old-fashioned carousel, swimming at Lake Anza, botanical gardens, and an Environmental Education Center which offers interpretive programs and nature walks. The Brazil Building, constructed by Works Progress Administration crews during The Great Depression, today houses the interior of the Brazilian exhibit from the 1939 World's Fair.

Unlike Tilden, Wildcat Canyon Regional Park is largely undeveloped and covers 2,428 acres. Historically, the Alvarado staging area on the northwestern end of Wildcat Creek Trail dates back to before 1772 when Native Americans lived here. Archeological findings show several Native American villages were located here. In the mid-1800s, Spanish explorers claimed the land on behalf of their king. The early 1900s saw the National Park Service construct facilities in its "rustic park architecture" and included a dance platform, open-air pavilion and extensive artistic stone masonry work. Though most of the facilities fell into disrepair and disappeared, the remaining stone masonry is now included in the National Registry of Historic Places. Eventually, pressure from growing cities increased the demand for water. The value of the Wildcat Canyon environment with all its streams and springs became the center of attention in the battle over water rights. On its way to becoming a park, Standard Oil, in 1966, drilled exploratory oil wells. The results were not promising and in 1967, the East Bay Regional Park District acquired much of the land which now makes up Wildcat Canyon Regional Park. Today, efforts are underway to restore the region with native grasses throughout the hills and re-establish native rainbow trout in the creek. Geologically speaking, Wildcat Canyon has been shaped by landslides and slumps. To this day, numerous small earthquake faults continue to shape this park and, if you have keen eye, you can see evidence of it along the northwest end of Wildcat Creek Trail.

General location: About 30 miles east of San Francisco, in the hills above Berkeley.

Elevation change: 550 feet; starting elevation 375 feet; high point 925 feet; low point 325 feet. Loop starts off with gently sloping terrain, then climbs a series of nasty little hills along the ridge before descending onto a mellow, paved path.

Season: Year-round although large portions of the dirt fire roads are likely to be muddy during wet months. The paved multi-use trail is rideable year-round.

Services: Drinking water available at Big Leaf picnic and parking area. Picnic tables and rest rooms can be found at Big Leaf and Lone Oak sites. Inspiration Point at the south end of the paved multi-use path, adjacent to Wildcat Canyon Road has rest rooms and an information signboard where map flyers can usually be found. Another source for the park's map flyers is at the Visitor Center/Environmental Education Center/Little Farm location, about 0.25 mile from the Big Leaf parking area. Though not on the route itself, a pay phone and snack bar are located about 0.6 mile from the Big Leaf parking area, at the merry-go-round carousel site. Kiddie attractions within Tilden Regional Park include Pony Rides, Little Train (miniature steam train which

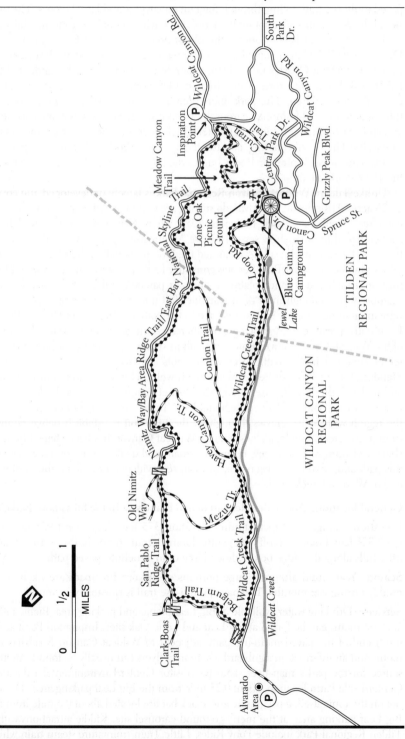

offers rides along one of the park's scenic ridge), and swimming at Lake Anza (with seasonal lifeguard and snack bar). Adult attractions include an 18-hole golf course, Environmental Education Center (excellent exhibit and interpretative programs of the Wildcat Creek watershed), botanical garden, Brazil Building (a historic facility available for social events). All other services can be found in the greater Oakland-Berkeley metropolitan area.

Hazards: To access the dirt loop from the parking area at Big Leaf picnic ground, you'll be pedaling a few yards on Central Park Drive, so watch out for vehicles. Expect to share the trail with other trail users, especially on Nimitz Way, the paved multi-use path. Yield to hikers and equestrians. Poison oak grows here, so stay on the trail. Though rarely seen, stay alert for rattlesnakes and mountain lions.

Rescue index: Your chances of finding other trail users who may be of help are excellent everyday during the popular summer months. In the off-season, you're likely to encounter other trail users particularly near the loop's starting point and on the paved Nimitz Way, usually in the late afternoon as many locals like to enjoy a stroll or quick ride after work. The loop is accessible by four trailheads located on well-traveled vehicle roads. Making your own way down to the nearest road in order to flag down a passing motorist is always possible.

Land status: Tilden Regional Park and Wildcat Canyon Regional Park, both maintained by the East Bay Regional Park District.

Maps: *Tilden Regional Park* and *Wildcat Canyon Regional Park*, the official park maps.

Finding the trail: From the Berkeley, take I-580 north from the San Francisco–Oakland Bay Bridge (I-80). Almost 3 miles from the bridge, take the University Avenue exit and follow it toward the university. Go left onto Shattuck Avenue and drive for almost 2 miles to Marin Avenue. Hang a right on Marin, following it northeast for about a half mile to Spruce Street. Go left onto Spruce and follow it as it winds up to the intersection of Grizzly Peak Boulevard, Wildcat Canyon Road, and Canon Drive. Bear left onto Canon Drive and enter Tilden Regional Park. Veer right as Canon becomes Central Park Drive near the Pony Rides. Directly across Central from the Pony Rides is Big Leaf picnic area. Park on Central, in front of the rest rooms and drinking fountain and begin pedaling from here.

For direct access to the paved Nimitz Way, don't turn left onto Canon Drive. Instead, go right onto Wildcat Canyon Road and follow it as it winds through the western edge of Tilden Regional Park for about 2 miles to its junction with South Park Drive. Stay left, still on Wildcat Canyon Road, now curving north and cutting through the center of the park. Your reach Inspiration Point in about a mile. Park here. (Note: Nimitz Way is also known as the Bay Area Ridge Trail and the East Bay National Skyline Trail.)

From Walnut Creek, Lafayette and Orinda, take CA 24 west. Take the San Pablo Dam Road exit and head north (the south direction at this exit is Moraga Way). Follow San Pablo for about 4.7 miles then go left onto Wildcat Canyon Road. Stay on Wildcat for about 2.5 miles to Inspiration Point parking area. If you want to ride only the paved Nimitz Way, park here and access the trail near the mouth of the parking lot. You can also park here and begin riding the clockwise loop. Otherwise, continue on Wildcat Canyon as it cuts through Tilden Regional Park. After about a mile, go past South Park Drive, staying right on Wildcat Canyon. Follow Wildcat Canyon as it winds through the edge of the park. At almost a mile from South Park

Drive, go right onto Central Park Drive. Drive past the merry-go-round carousel and in about a half mile, you reach Big Leaf picnic area, located across the road from the Pony Rides. Park in front of the rest rooms and drinking fountain and begin pedaling from here.

Sources of additional information:

> East Bay Regional Park District
> 2950 Peralta Oaks Ct.
> P.O. Box 5381
> Oakland, CA 94605-0381
> (510) 562-PARK or (510) 635-0135

Notes on the trail: From the Big Leaf picnic grounds, facing the Pony Rides, begin pedaling south (left) on paved Central Park Drive for a few yards. Watch out for cars and bear left onto a paved road which leads to Lone Oak picnic grounds and Blue Gum Group Camp. A sign indicating "Bike access" displayed near Lone Oak indicates you're heading in the right direction. Beyond the picnic grounds, still on a paved road, look for a dirt fire road just past the rest room facilities. Though you won't see a sign identifying this wide and smooth fire road as Loop Trail, this is the trail you want. Hop on it and begin a gentle climb.

Continue on Loop Trail and enter the Tilden Nature Study area through a gate. Stay on the fire road, cruising past a drinking fountain on your left and then a trail leading to New Woodland Camp on your right. Your surroundings are made up of fragrant laurel and eucalyptus trees and the road is likely to be somewhat shady. Bypass several lesser trails, including a signed one to Nimitz Way. When in doubt, stay on the main, well-traveled fire road. Many of the lesser trails, incidentally, are often signed off-limits to bikes. At a little over 1.1 miles, enjoy a brief gentle descent to the T intersection with Wildcat Creek Trail, lying next to Jewel Lake. Though Wildcat Creek Trail is not signed, Loop Trail which you've been riding, is identified. It's peaceful and serene here—hard to believe that you're in the heart of one of the busiest metropolitan areas in the entire country. Turn right onto Wildcat Creek Trail, a wide, hard-packed, smooth fire road. (Drinking fountain, rest rooms, and a park bench available at this intersection.)

For the next mile, the fire road gently descends as it follows Wildcat Creek which is hidden in the thick bushes on your left. You can really pick up speed on this stretch. Eventually the forest gives way to wide-open terrain of gently rolling hills on your right. At just over 2 miles from your car, you enter Wildcat Canyon Regional Park. There's a sign posted here, possibly with some complimentary map flyers (good to know if you're without a map). From this point, the trail begins rolling up and down short rises, including one that's about 10% steepness. Not to worry—it's about a 20-yard grind. Bypass unsigned Havey Canyon Trail and, at about 3.5 miles, bypass Mezue Trail, both on your right. (Incidentally, Harvey Canyon allows bikes though it's subject to seasonal closure. It climbs a steep 1.5 miles to Nimitz Way. A shortcut, Havey trims 5 miles off the loop.) Continue on Wildcat Creek Trail as it parallels a rich riparian forest of alder, willow and bay laurel trees, and water-loving flora. As you zip down this stretch, try not to run over or scare the daylights out of the many resident gray-brown rabbits scooting off the trail. At a little over 4 miles, you reach the lowest point of the loop at 325 feet just before the fire road turns to pavement. You won't have to watch out for traffic as the road is abandoned, but you need to stay

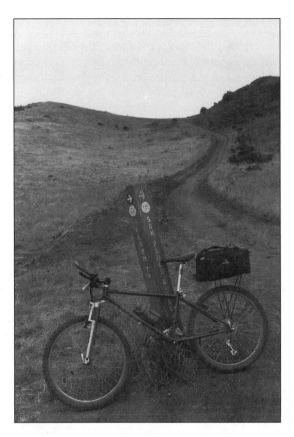

Yep, the route grinds up
this hill on San Pablo
Ridge Trail.

alert for speed bumps. This road was deserted a while ago due to small earthquake
faults lying below. Wildcat Creek Trail alternates between pavement and dirt. At 4.9
miles, after reaching the top of a short climb on pavement, you'll be tempted to fly
downhill. Have at it but keep your eyes peeled for Belgum Trail near the bottom,
leading off on your right.

Hang a right onto Belgum and begin a rolling climb to the San Pablo Ridge.
Belgum is another paved road that runs abruptly uphill for about 30 yards, goes
through a cattle gate, then becomes dirt road. (Remember to close the gate.) There
are a couple of oddly placed palm trees near here. Now begins the arduous task of
climbing up a bunch of humbling, steep, short hills. The pedaling is hard work but
worth all that huffing and puffing because at about 5.7 miles, nearly at the ridge line,
the unobstructed view looking west is incredible. Arguably one of the best places in
all of Northern California to catch a sunset, the panorama includes San Francisco,
the Golden Gate and Oakland–San Francisco Bay Bridges, Angel and Alcatraz
Islands, and Mt. Tam. There's even a park bench here, evidence that others feel the
same way about the view.

A few yards beyond the park bench, you reach the top of the ridge. Typical of ridge
trails, this dirt road rolls up and down, ascending and descending sometimes severely
steep slopes. In less than a half mile from the park bench, bypass a single-track trail
on your right. Two paths lead off on your left. The far left is signed Clark Boa Trail;
ignore it. Follow the near-left, obvious fire road, signed toward San Pablo Ridge Trail,

also referred to as the East Bay Skyline Trail. From this junction, let your wheels fly downhill to a fork at the bottom. Take the right fork, signed San Pablo Ridge Trail. Yep, it's the one that shoots straight up about 18% grade! Fortunately, the steepness lasts for about 0.2 mile. When you reach the top, take a breather and mentally vow to milk all the subsequent downhills for all they're worth because they're all followed by steep but short uphills. At 7 miles, you pass a surveyor's marker and you can see down both sides of the ridge. To the west is the San Francisco Bay, and to the east is San Pablo Reservoir and rolling hills. About a half mile farther, you finally reach the high point of the loop, sitting at about 925 feet, near where San Pablo Ridge Trail merges into signed Mezue Trail.

Continue on Mezue Trail, passing an old cattle corral on your right. Go through a gate and in a few yards, Mezue turns into Nimitz Way, a paved multi-use trail. Most of the strenuous climbing is behind you now. Nimitz continues to roll up and down but in a much more gentle nature. Stay on Nimitz Way all the way to its end at Inspiration Point and Wildcat Canyon Road. Along the way, stay alert for several cattle guards which lie across the paved path. Incidentally, the grassy land through which Nimitz Way passes is part of a "Grazing Demonstration Project" conducted by local agencies, a resident cattle rancher, and the University of California. The project uses controlled livestock grazing as a management tool to enhance native grasses which include purple needle and California oat grasses as well as a variety of wetland flora.

At around 9.6 miles, Nimitz Way runs into Tilden Regional Park. Continue on Nimitz Way as it cruises through a grove of fragrant eucalyptus and redwoods. You reach the end of the paved path next to Inspiration Point and Wildcat Canyon Road at 11.6 miles. Just before the gate which bars vehicles from Nimitz Way, Curran Trail, a narrow dirt road, leads down on your right. Drop down the side of Nimitz Way onto Curran and follow it 0.2 mile to Meadow Canyon Trail. Highly prone to storm damage, expect Curran to be a bit rougher than any other part of the loop thus far. Turn right onto Meadow Canyon and enjoy an easy descent on a wide fire road as you cruise around a creek drainage, shaded by tall grasses, live oak, bay laurel and eucalyptus trees and through a lush riparian environment. It's a sweet trail and at 13.3 miles, it ends at Lone Oak picnic grounds where you close the loop. Go left onto the pavement and follow it a short distance back out to Central Park Drive. Hang a right here and return to your car. Total miles for this great loop ride is about 13.5 miles.

RIDE 72 · East–West Ridge Loop

AT A GLANCE

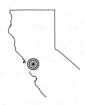

Length/configuration: 9.7-mile loop, clockwise; fire roads and small stretch on pavement

Aerobic difficulty: Moderately strenuous due to a portion of steep but short climbs

Technical difficulty: Mildy technical with a long stretch of somewhat advanced rocky section

Scenery: 100-foot high, 2nd and 3rd growth redwoods, the offspring of ancient redwoods that used to smother these hills. Site of Rainbow trout which are descendants of a pure strain of native trout found in nearby San Leandro Creek drainage.

Special comments: Depending on your ability, the loop can be ridden in either direction. The clockwise direction is suitable for strong beginners while the reverse is enjoyed by intermediate-advance level riders. Strong riders who wish to tow a kid-trailer will find an out-and-back portion to be a great workout. Note: A loosely enforced park regulation requires bells on bikes.

It's refreshing to know that from the bustling cities of the East Bay, just minutes from Oakland, you can get out into the "woods," away from the city madness. Redwood Regional Park is a gem. Here, you can enjoy a great workout, riding this 9.7-mile loop, comprised of mildly to moderately challenging fire roads. And for added spice, there's a 2.8-mile stretch that technically advanced bikers will love. But that's not to say strong beginners should avoid this route. This loop can be ridden in whatever direction suits your ability. If you're a strong beginner with only basic bike handling skills, go for the clockwise direction. If you're an adventurous intermediate or advanced rider, you'll find the counterclockwise direction to be more fun and challenging. The clockwise direction lets you savor a fast, mildly technical 3.3-mile descent, followed by a 2.8 somewhat advanced technical uphill section. The technical section is made challenging by irregularly shaped and sized large slabs of rocks, effectively creating a sort of stair-stepping terrain, spiced with short drops and some loose dirt and rock. You need to be able to control your speed when descending this technical stuff, and for that reason, the counterclockwise direction will appeal to stronger, more skilled riders. Of course, beginners can walk down this section, but then, that means a long climb up to East Ridge Trail. Though the following ride description is written going clockwise, counterclockwise is easy to follow, so long as you have an official park map.

Unlike adjacent parks immediately to the north, you won't be impressed by any outstanding views. Instead, be impressed by your imagination for here, ancient redwoods once covered these ridges and the Redwood Creek canyon below. Indeed, millions of years ago, redwood trees covered most of North America. Climatic changes gradually reduced the expanse of those trees. As people moved into California in the 1800s, fueled by the promise of gold, logging operations grew to meet the demand for building materials. In the mid-1800s, a redwood grove occupying five square miles was stripped, leaving a "sea of stumps" by 1865. It is reported that at one time, several champion redwood trees were used as navigational landmarks by ships sailing under the Golden Gate Bridge. Today, though the forest is far less dense than it used to be, it is populated by direct descendants of these ancient trees representing second and third generations.

On a slightly different note, Redwood Creek which runs through the heart of Redwood Regional Park, is actually registered as Historical Landmark No. 970 in honor of the Rainbow trout which was first named here as a uniquely separate species. Redwood Creek is a spawning ground for the rainbows and efforts are still underway to ensure the longevity of that breed and its environment. Fishing, of course, is not allowed here.

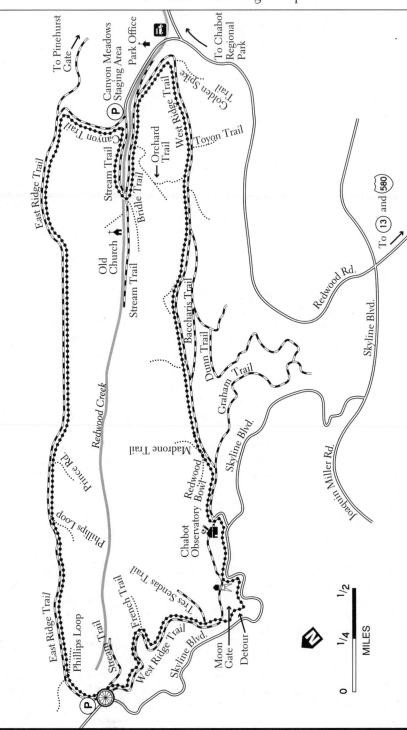

Canyon Meadows Staging Area
Park Office
To Pinehurst Gate
To Chabot Regional Park

Canyon Trail
Stream Trail
West Ridge Trail
Golden Spike Trail
Orchard Trail
Toyon Trail

East Ridge Trail

Old Church
Bridle Trail
Stream Trail

Redwood Creek

Baccharis Trail
Dunn Trail
Graham Trail

Skyline Blvd.
Redwood Rd.
Skyline Blvd.

To 13 and 580

Prince Rd.
Phillips Loop

Madrone Trail
Redwood Bowl

Chabot Observatory

Joaquin Miller Rd.

East Ridge Trail
Phillips Loop
Stream Trail
French Trail
Tres Sendas Trail
West Ridge Trail
Skyline Blvd.

Moon Gate
Detour

N

0   1/4   1/2
MILES

General location: About 20 miles east of San Francisco, in the hills above Oakland.

Elevation change: 805 feet; starting elevation 1,280 feet; high point 1,365 feet; low point 560 feet. The first half of the clockwise loop is mostly descending. The second half makes up for elevation loss by climbing often steep, technical portions of West Ridge Trail.

Season: Year-round, though wet months produce somewhat sticky, muddy trail conditions.

Services: Drinking water, rest rooms, and pay phone available at both Skyline and Canyon Meadow Staging Areas. Picnic tables and rest rooms can be found at Canyon Meadow and near the archery range. The Chabot Observatory, near the archery range, is scheduled for opening in mid-2000 and will have water and rest room facilities available. All other services can be found in the neighboring greater Oakland metropolitan area.

Hazards: Stay alert for other trail-users, especially when riding through curvy sections where your view of on-coming traffic is obscured by thick, tall bushes. Watch out for poison oak and rarely encountered rattlesnakes.

Rescue index: Your chances of finding other trail users who may be of help are excellent everyday during the popular summer months. In the off-season, you're likely to encounter other trail users usually in the late afternoon (many locals enjoy a stroll or quick ride after work). The loop is accessible by four major, frequently used staging areas: Skyline Gate, Pinehurst Gate, Canyon Meadow (main park entrance), and Chabot Observatory. In an emergency, you can make your own way to these locations and if need be, flag down a passing motorist. Canyon Meadow Staging Area is accessed via the main park entrance, where the park office and fire station are in the immediate vicinity. Phones are located at Canyon Meadow as well as Skyline Gate and Chabot Observatory.

Land status: Redwood Regional Park, maintained by the East Bay Regional Park District.

Maps: *Redwood Regional Park*, the official park map.

Finding the trail: From the intersection of I-580 and CA 13 in Oakland, take CA 13 north. Go about a mile, turn right onto Redwood Road, and head north into the hills. In about a mile, hang a left onto Skyline Boulevard, also known as Joaquin Miller Road. Stay on this road for about 0.75 mile and keep your eyes peeled for Skyline going right and separating from Joaquin Miller. Follow Skyline for almost 2.5 miles as it winds up and pass Chabot Observatory and residential homes. The Skyline Gate Staging Area is on the right side of the road (east side). Park here.

Sources of additional information:

East Bay Regional Park District
2950 Peralta Oaks Ct.
P.O. Box 5381
Oakland, CA 94605-0381
(510) 562-PARK or (510) 635-0135

Notes on the trail: This is a fairly easy route to follow as the trails in this park are generally well-signed. Many trails, which lead down into the creek drainage from East Ridge Trail are off-limits to bikes and are so marked. Likewise, many routes that lead off the northeast side of West Ridge Trail are closed to bikes while several trails on the southwest side permit bikes. All along the way, signs are posted at nearly all trail intersections.

From the Skyline Gate Staging Area, pick up East Ridge Trail on the far north edge of the parking lot. East Ridge is an obvious, wide, smooth dirt fire road. This mildly technical road is occasionally accented by rain ruts, potholes, and brief patches of loose dirt and gravel. Bypass all other lesser trails which lead off on both sides of the road. Generally speaking, the terrain rolls gently up and down, mostly descending. A couple of steep but short rises may require a lower gear or you can just power up them. Spruce, pine, redwood, live oak, bay laurel, madrone, and eucalyptus trees, and thick chaparral bushes grow in profusion on both sides of the road. In the distance far below on your right lies Redwood Creek canyon, though the thick vegetation obscures any significant view.

About 3 miles into the ride, at the bottom of a downhill, go right onto Canyon Trail. (Staying straight on East Ridge runs to the Pinehurst Gate Staging Area.) Continue descending on Canyon. Keep your speed in check and be alert for other trail users as the trail narrows slightly, is a bit curvy, and your view is obscured by thick, tall vegetation. Stay away from the bushes especially if you don't get along with poison oak.

In less than a half mile, you reach the Canyon Meadow Staging Area, an obvious landmark with its numerous picnic tables and parking lot. Here, Canyon intersects a simply signed bike trail. According to the park map, this bike trail is Stream Trail going left and right. Hang a right onto Stream and cruise past the playground area and Orchard picnic grounds. There are interpretive signboards here displaying information about stream restoration. The park is still in the process of reintroducing native Rainbow trout into the creek. (Don't even think of it—fishing is not allowed.) Bypass Lupine Trail and cross the creek on a bridge. At 3.6 miles, Stream intersects Bridle Trail on your left. But before making the hard left onto Bridle, take a short side-trip to the old church site by staying straight on Stream Trail which is now paved. This paved road is used by authorized park vehicles only and chances are you won't encounter any cars or trucks. The paved road leads you into the cool, shady redwood forest and in less than a half mile, you reach the old church site. Only the foundation of the church remains but you can imagine what a great spiritual spot this must have been with ancient redwoods towering overhead. Retrace your path back to Bridle Trail.

At the junction of Stream and Bridle Trails, a sign indicates West Ridge Trail is reached via Bridle. So, bear right and follow Bridle, a level, narrow dirt road which parallels a fence and the creek on the left. Bypass Orchard Trail, which is signed off-limits to bikes. West Ridge Trail is the next trail leading off on your right and it's payback time. West Ridge immediately climbs steeply, about 10% grade and the terrain becomes technically more rugged with some scattered loose rocks and dirt. Maintaining traction is a challenge. In the summer and during dry spells, expect this stretch to be dusty. Along the way, fortunately, there are brief sections of level or gentle slopes that offer your climbing muscles brief respite. Ignore Golden Spike Trail on your left and continue the uphill grind. Watch out for poison oak here among the eucalyptus and live oak. Soon, the trail is enlivened with large slabs of semi-buried chunks of boulders. Bypass several smaller trails peeling off both sides of West Ridge Trail, many of which are off-limits to bikes. Baccharis Trail, at 6 miles, leads off on your left and allows bikes. (Baccharis parallels West Ridge for about 0.7 mile before rejoining West Ridge. It also leads to Dun and Graham Trails, which allow bikes. If you want, you can

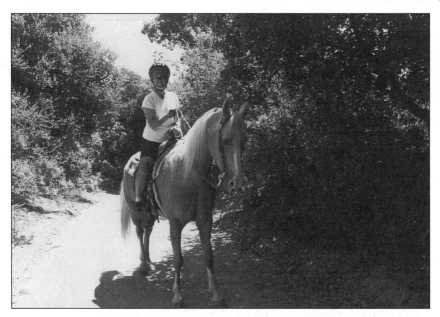

While ascending West Ridge Trail, I was persuaded by a friendly equestrian to try his mode of transportation.

add a couple more miles by riding these trails before they rejoin West Ridge Trail.) When you pass Chown Trail (no bikes), West Ridge gets a bit more rugged with more semi-buried large rocks and slabs of boulders stair-stepping up the hill. Riding up is a challenge and walking most certainly gets you up the trail. Continue past Fern, Baccharis, and Madrone Trails.

When you reach the Redwood Bowl—a small clearing with picnic tables—the difficult terrain is over. At 7.5 miles, you reach the archery range and Chabot Observatory. As of this writing, the Observatory is still under construction and completion is slated for June, 2000, at which time this portion of West Ridge Trail will be slightly re-aligned and re-opened. In the meantime, follow the temporary detour signs. Finding the detour trail and staying on it gets a bit convoluted here. Basically, hang a left onto a small paved road near the construction offices and ride down to Skyline Boulevard. Go right onto Skyline with the Observatory construction now on your right. Follow Skyline for about 0.6 mile, passing a water tank up on a hillside on your right. Keep your eyes open for a small single-track trail leading off Skyline on your right. Expect to see a temporary West Ridge Trail detour sign displayed here. Hop onto this dirt trail and follow it as it parallels Skyline. At a point when you think the trail dumps you back onto Skyline, look for a right curve leading to a gated fire road. Go past the gate onto the narrow fire road. You're now back on the original West Ridge Trail.

West Ridge now rolls along gently, generally heading uphill. Stay on the main fire road, passing Tres Sendas, French and Stream Trails along the way. After cruising through shady stands of redwoods, bay laurel and spruce trees, you reach Skyline Gate Staging Area. Total mileage is about 9.7 miles.

RIDE 73 · Lafayette–Moraga Trail

AT A GLANCE

Length/configuration: 15-mile out-and-back (7.5 mile each way); paved trail

Aerobic difficulty: Easy due to smooth trail condition and little elevation gain

Technical difficulty: Not technical, though riders need to be comfortable sharing the path with other trail users

Scenery: Pleasant residential neighborhoods alongside busy, well-separated St. Mary's Road. The last mile near the south end of the trail in Moraga runs through more wide-open spaces amid grassy rolling hills.

Special comments: A great after-work, quick aerobic ride for adults, and a well-suited route for freewheeling kids and kid-trailers. Note: A loosely enforced park regulation requires bells on bikes.

This 7.5-mile (one-way) paved trail is the shared gem of the communities of Lafayette and Moraga. Deemed one of, if not the most successful trail conversion in the Rails-To-Trails Conservancy program in the country, the Lafayette–Moraga Regional Trail is a much-appreciated path that attracts nearly 500,000 users per year. Not surprising, the value of homes lucky enough to border it have risen, more than homes several blocks away. Easily accessible from many locations along the route, you can ride the trail in its entirety for a 15-mile round-trip mild workout. Or, you can ride whatever portion you like, turning around whenever you please— great to know if you have youngsters who get tired or bored easily.

Originally a portion of the San Francisco–Sacramento Railroad, this paved trail was born out of the two communities' cooperation with the Central Contra Costa Sanitary District, East Bay Municipal Utility District, and Pacific Gas & Electric Company. Opened in 1976, the trail makes use of established utility easements alongside Las Trampas Creek and is a fine example of dual land-use.

General location: About 30 miles east of San Francisco, between the communities of Lafayette and Moraga.

Elevation change: 260 feet; starting elevation and low point 140 feet at the north end; high point 400 feet at the south end.

Season: Year-round.

Services: Ample parking at 5 staging areas (listed in order from north to south): Olympic Boulevard/Reliez Station Road (the northern-most end of the trail), Lafayette Community Center, St. Mary's Road Staging Area, Moraga Commons, and Valle Vista (the southern-most end of the trail). Rest rooms can be found at all staging locations except St. Mary's Road, and Olympic/Reliez. Rest rooms at the Lafayette Community Center are available only from 9 a.m. to 5 p.m. Water available at Moraga Commons and Lafayette Community Center. Though not really a staging area, an additional site at the intersection with Foye Drive, about a mile from the north end of the trail, offers water and rest rooms. Drinking water can be found behind the fire station on the west side of the trail, about 2.9 miles from Olympic/Reliez trailhead. Picnic

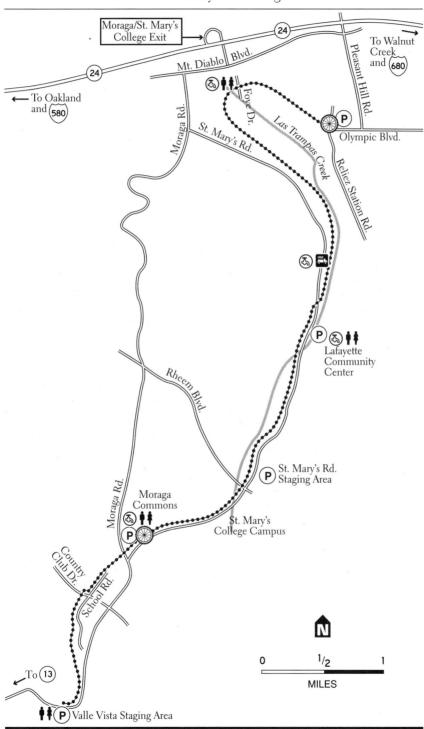

table located at St. Mary's Road Staging Area. Moraga Commons has picnic tables and maintained playground. Other services nearby on St. Mary's Road which parallels the path. On hot summer days, you may encounter enterprising youngsters selling cold lemonade along the trail.

Hazards: This is an immensely popular multi-use trail used by walkers (including dog-walkers and baby strollers), roller bladers, bikers, and joggers. Equestrians are permitted though they don't seem to frequent the path. Youngsters should be comfortable with sharing the trail with others. Watch out for vehicle traffic as the paved trail crosses driveways and residential streets. Be aware that many don't have stop signs or signal lights. There are fewer street crossings along the 2.4-mile stretch from Moraga Commons toward Lafayette Community Center, and so, young families may want to park and start riding from Moraga Commons in order to take advantage of this less interrupted section. Helmets required.

Rescue index: A popular trail, even early in the day, you will meet other trail users who can offer assistance. Many homes border the trail and the residents are generally friendly, helpful, and likely to place an emergency phone call for you. A fire station is located on the west side of the trail, about 2.9 miles from Olympic/Reliez trailhead.

Land status: Lafayette-Moraga Regional Trail, maintained by the East Bay Regional Park District.

Maps: *Lafayette-Moraga Regional Trail*, the official park map.

Finding the trail: CA 24 is the east-west connector between I-580 and I-680. Whether you're traveling from San Francisco or Walnut Creek, head east or west respectively, on CA 24 to the Moraga Road/St. Mary's College exit. Make your way to the south side of CA 24 and onto Mount Diablo Boulevard. Mount Diablo parallels CA 24. You need to decide from which staging area you want to begin riding because when you intersect with Mount Diablo upon exiting CA 24, you will either go left or right.

Moraga Commons is the preferred staging area if you have very young, freewheeling children with you. To reach this area, go right onto Mount Diablo Boulevard and immediately move over to the left lane. At the next signal intersection, turn left onto Moraga Road. Follow Moraga Road south as it winds up the hill toward Moraga. At 4.6 miles from Mount Diablo Boulevard, look for Moraga Commons at the intersection of Moraga Road and St. Mary's Road, on the northeast corner. The obvious clue is a very inviting, well-maintained grassy playground area. Park in the lot and begin pedaling north toward Lafayette. This is the best stretch for youngsters and if they get tired of riding, just turn around and return to Moraga Commons where they are likely to become re-energized by the playground facilities.

The Olympic Boulevard/Reliez Station Road Staging Area at the northern-most end of the paved trail is the best place to park if you're looking for a long, aerobic workout. To reach this area, go left onto Mount Diablo Blvd. and travel about a mile to Pleasant Hill Road. Hang a right onto Pleasant Hill and drive about 0.8 mile to Olympic Boulevard. The staging area—a maintained parking lot—is on your left. Park here.

Sources of additional information:

East Bay Regional Park District
2950 Peralta Oaks Ct.
P.O. Box 5381
Oakland, CA 94605-0381
(510) 562-PARK or (510) 635-0135

Rails-To-Trails Conservancy
California Chapter
26 O'Farrell St., Suite 400
San Francisco, CA 94108
www.railtrails.org
(415) 397-2220

Notes on the trail: Since this out-and-back trail is accessible from a number of lo-cations, including from within residential neighborhoods, you can make this ride as long or short as you like. The length of the trail, for the most part, runs through quiet, pleasant neighborhoods, between the backyards of houses on public utility easements, frequently crossing quiet residential streets. Speed limit is 15 mph. Helmets required. That said, here are a few notes of what you'll find along the trail.

Of the 1.7-mile section south of Moraga Commons, a 0.3-mile stretch uses resi-dential streets and sidewalks. Though traffic is light, you'll still be sharing the road with vehicles. After that, the final 1.4 miles to the southern end of the path is no-ticeably more rural, surrounded by open, grassy, gently rolling hills, and far fewer homes bordering the path. This part of the trail is decidedly less used and is also the prettiest in that you're leaving the traffic and man-made developments behind.

The 2.4-mile section between Moraga Commons north toward Lafayette Com-munity Center is crossed by a handful of quiet vehicle roads. The trail itself parallels St. Mary's Road, a busy two-lane road and is consistently well-separated by natural landscaping. If you have young, freewheeling children with you, this is the best stretch to ride since encounters with vehicles are less that other sections of the trail.

The 3.2-mile section between Lafayette Community Center to the northern trail-head at Olympic Boulevard crosses numerous quiet, residential streets in Lafayette and that means you won't be able to cruise along at a fast, uninterrupted clip. Besides, the speed limit is 15 mph. It's still a pleasant ride as this is where the paved trail is shady and runs between the backside of many homes alongside Las Trampas Creek.

OTHER AREA RIDES

ANTHONY CHABOT REGIONAL PARK: You'll find this park just minutes off I-580, about 20 minutes from downtown Oakland, in the hills above San Leandro. Part of the East Bay Regional Park District (EBRPD), this park is anchored in the south by 315-acre Lake Chabot and is popular with boaters, fishing enthusiasts, and campers. The park itself is over 4,900 acres, and the majority of trails allow bikes (please obey all signs). A 4.5-mile paved trail alongside the lake is popular with young families. Rest rooms, picnic tables, and a snack bar are nearby. If you have intermediate technical skills and moderate endurance, and you're looking for a workout, check out the park's 14.5-mile loop designated as a bike route. It leads to some of the more remote areas of the park and through quite a variety of terrain consisting of dry native chaparral, hillsides dotted with live oak, fragrant groves of eucalyptus, and peaceful valleys—what an oasis for the heavily populated East Bay. About 10% of the loop is paved multi-use path; the rest is dirt, usually dry and dusty. Many other trails off the loop allow bikes, and you can add more miles by exploring them. Note: A loosely enforced park regulation requires bells on bikes.

Finding the trail: From northbound I-580, take Fairmont Drive exit in San Leandro and make an immediate left, then an immediate right onto Fairmont Drive. Fairmont soon merges with Lake Chabot Road. Follow the signs to the marina located on your left. Parking in the marina lot requires a small fee; free parking outside the lot is allowed, though it may be time-restricted—look for signs. Suggested direction of travel for the loop is counterclockwise. Hop on the loop at the marina and follow the East/West Shore Trail (paved multi-use trail) to the right, toward Live Oak and Honker Bay Trails.

Map: Provided free by the EBRPD and available at most entrances, gates, and main trailheads. A map is a necessity as there are many trails that connect to the loop.

For more information, contact:
East Bay Regional Park District (EBRPD)
2950 Peralta Oaks Ct.
P.O. Box 5381
Oakland, CA 94605
(510) 562-PARK or (510) 635-0135

MISSION PEAK REGIONAL PRESERVE: Located in the steep hills behind Fremont, this preserve is home to one of the toughest hill climbs in the Bay Area. From the popular Stanford Avenue staging area in Fremont, you'll climb over 2,100 feet in a mere 3 miles (6 miles round-trip). But, oh, what an effort. The general consensus is that climbing Mission Peak is downright painful. No one rides it just for pure fun, and bikers who are brave enough to tackle it do so for the workout. The view from the top is spectacular and on clear days, you can see Mt. Tamalpais in the north, Mt. Diablo and the Sierra Nevadas in the northeast, Mt. Hamilton in the south, and the Santa Cruz Mountains in the west, not to mention the Bay. The bike route to the top is a combination of fire roads and single-tracks. Intermediate technical skills are needed (controlling your speed and not skidding on the fast downhill run is important, especially when hikers and other trail users are present). Summer can be brutally hot and dry. If you must ride, do so early in the day or late in the afternoon. Heavy rains leave the trails and roads extremely muddy, so give them ample time to dry out.

Finding the trail: From northbound I-680 or I-880, take the Mission Boulevard exit in Fremont and head east. Follow Mission to Stanford Avenue (Weibel Winery at this intersection). Make a right onto Stanford and follow it to its dead end at the trailhead. Be sure to have a map, as there are several ways to reach Mission Peak from Stanford Avenue. If you want a slightly easier, less challenging but longer approach to the Peak, start from the Ohlone College staging area. To reach that trailhead, use the same directions as above but continue past Stanford Avenue for a short distance. Turn right into the campus and make your way to the east boundary of the campus. The trailhead you want is Spring Valley Trail or Peak Trail.

Map: Provided free by the EBRPD and available at most gates and main trailheads. If this is your first time here, a map is a must.

For more information, contact:
East Bay Regional Park District (EBRPD)
2950 Peralta Oaks Ct.
P.O. Box 5381
Oakland, CA 94605
(510) 562-PARK or (510) 635-0135

PLEASANTON RIDGE REGIONAL PARK: Known for great climbs and some killer-downhills, this 3,163-acre park occupies Pleasanton Ridge on the west side of I-680 and Pleasanton. A 20-mile-plus ride can be easily configured in these lovely hills. Mostly comprised of well-maintained dirt roads, you'll need intermediate technical skills. Very strong beginners with the right attitude will enjoy many of these trails too, although the Sinbad Canyon area does include some technically challenging single-tracks. Views of the Livermore Valley are magnificent from these oak-covered hills. If you ride in the spring, your workout will be amid splendidly carpeted hills of lush green grass. Summer can be unbearably hot, dry, and dusty. A suggested route is this: Oak Tree Trail up toward the ridge, then right on Ridgeline Trail. Follow it northwest past Castlewood Country Club. Go left onto Thermalito Trail and close the loop back at the top of Oak Tree Trail and return. If you have more time on your hands and are aching for more miles and technical challenge, head toward Sinbad Canyon by following Ridgeline instead of turning left onto Thermalito. This public-access trail skirts a stretch of private property, so be sure to stay on the trail. After your spin around Sinbad Creek Trail, retrace your tracks on Oak Tree Trail.

Finding the trail: From San Jose, travel north on I-680. As the highway runs past Fremont, it veers northeast for about 5 miles, then heads north again, at which point keep an eye out for the Sunol Boulevard/Castlewood exit. Take this exit and make your way to the west side of I-680 toward the ridge. Bear right and continue on Castlewood Drive and then a left on Foothill Road. Follow Foothill to the Oak Tree Trail staging area. Park here. Be sure to pick up a map at the staging area. Begin by following Oak Tree Trail up toward the ridge.

Map: Provided free by the EBRPD and available at most gates and main trailheads.

For more information, contact:
East Bay Regional Park District (EBRPD)
2950 Peralta Oaks Ct.
P.O. Box 5381
Oakland, CA 94605
(510) 562-PARK or (510) 635-0135

JOAQUIN MILLER PARK: Unlike the majority of parks in the East Bay, this park is not part of the East Bay Regional Park District. Rather, it's part of the city of Oakland Office of Parks, Recreation, and Cultural Affairs division. The trail network at Joaquin Miller measures over 15 miles, and get this: most of the bikeable trails are narrow enough to be considered single-tracks through forests of young redwoods! And right next to Oakland! What an Oasis. Serious bikers concede that these trails require advanced technical skills. There are logs, roots, and rocks to hop over, steep climbing turns, drop-offs, jumps, and sections that you're likely to walk. Imagine that—extreme single-track in the East Bay and everybody sharing the trail. This is not to say that hikers, dog-walkers, equestrians, and bikers enjoy a perfect marriage. Some trail users would like to see bicycling banned from the entire park, if not some of the trails. That said, be sure to exercise exceptional trail etiquette, saying a friendly "hello" to other trail users when you meet them on the narrow paths. Stay on designated trails. Being courteous means we'll all be able to enjoy these challenging single-tracks for many years to come. Thank the Bicycle Trails Council of the East Bay (BTCEB) for being instrumental in keeping the park open to bikers. (The BTCEB is active in forging positive biker-park relations and trail maintenance. It urges all bikers to volunteer. See below for contact information.) The recommended route in this park is the loop on Sunset Trail to Big Trees Trail, pedaling through stands of redwood trees along the way. Then hop on Sequoia Bay View Trail to Cinderella Trail, which is reportedly so steep that you're bound to walk up part of it. Cinderella eventually cuts back to Sunset Trail, and your reward is a spectacular view of the Bay Area.

Finding the trail: In Oakland, from the I-580 and CA 13 junction, go briefly north on CA 13 to the first exit, which is 35th Avenue/Redwood Road. Go east on Redwood, past Safeway, and up into the hills to Skyline Boulevard. Turn left on Skyline and continue about a half mile past the ranger station on your right. Bear left onto Joaquin Miller Road and then right on Sanborn Drive. Park at the Community Center. Joaquin Miller Park is on the Oakland side of Skyline Boulevard. Across Skyline from Joaquin Miller is the Roberts Recreation Area of Redwood Regional Park.

Map: Free map available at Joaquin Miller Community Center, down at the bottom of the park off Joaquin Miller Boulevard.

For more information, contact:

City of Oakland
Office of Parks, Recreation, and
   Cultural Affairs
1520 Lakeside Dr.
Oakland, CA 94612
(510) 238-3187
Ask them to send you a map, or pick
one up at the Community Center.

East Bay Regional Park District
   (EBRPD)
2950 Peralta Oaks Ct.
P.O. Box 5381
Oakland, CA 94605
(510) 562-PARK or (510) 635-0135

SOME LOCAL BICYCLE SHOPS
& ORGANIZATIONS

Martinez Cyclery
4990 Pacheco Blvd.
Martinez, CA 94553
(925) 228-9050
www.martinezcyclery.com

Missing Link Bicycle Shop
1988 Shattuck Ave.
Berkeley, CA 94704
(510) 843-7471

Solano Avenue Cyclery
1554 Solano Ave.
Berkeley, CA 94707
(510) 524-1094

Pioneer Bike Shop
11 Rio Vista Ave.
Oakland, CA 94611
(510) 658-8981

Castro Valley Cyclery
20515 Stanton Ave.
Castro Valley, CA 94546
(510) 538-1878

Psycho Cycles
1578 Washington Blvd.
Fremont, CA 94537
(510) 770-1878

Cal Bicycles
2106 First St.
Livermore, CA 94550
(925) 447-6666

Clayton Valley Bicycle Center
5411 Clayton Rd.
Clayton, CA 94517
(510) 672-2522

East Bay Regional Park District
   (EBRPD)
2950 Peralta Oaks Ct.
P.O. Box 5381
Oakland, CA 94605
(510) 562-PARK or (510) 635-0135

Bicycle Trails Council of
   the East Bay
P.O. Box 9583
Berkeley, CA 94709
(510) 466-5123 or (510) 420-1617

East Bay Bicycle Coalition
P.O. Box 1736
Oakland, CA 94604
(510) 433-7433

Grizzly Peak Cyclists
Berkeley, CA
(510) 528-8099

San Francisco Bay Trail
P.O. Box 2050
Oakland, CA 94604
(510) 464-7900
www.abag.ca.gov

This trail system is planned to be a continuous 400-mile recreational trail that encircles the entire Bay Area. Unlike the Bay Area Ridge Trail system, the Bay Trail will link the shorelines of all nine counties surround the San Francisco Bay via paved multi-use paths, dirt trails, bike lanes, sidewalks, or signed bike routes. As of the end of 1999, 210 miles of the Bay Trail have been completed. Almost every section of the trail system thus far is open to bikes as allowed by local jurisdiction. For more information, including maps, check out their Web site or contact them at the address listed above.

THE NORTH BAY AREA—
MARIN COUNTY

This small region defining the northern end of the San Francisco Bay is worthy of a chapter all to itself. History was made here. Marin County, after all, is considered by many to be the birthplace of mountain biking. Lucky for us that so many fat tire pioneers played together in this region, their camaraderie the by-product of their desire to just have fun ridin' and racin'. It was also inevitable that the growing number of Marin County bike enthusiasts would encounter what no other region in the state—and perhaps in the country—had yet: trail access issues. Hikers claimed cyclists were destroying the beauty and solitude of the environment, citing illegal trails were being carved into the public lands. Bikers wanted more than just technically tame fire roads to pedal. Concerned groups of citizens from all points of view organized in an effort to forge peaceful co-existence policies. Today, cyclists enjoy a fragile peace with non-biking groups, thanks to the efforts of local advocacy groups, such as the Bicycle Trails Council of Marin (BTC). In the interest of keeping that peace intact, Joe Breeze, one of the sport's celebrated pioneers and a local resident, makes an appeal worth repeating: ". . . Marin, especially Mt. Tamalpais, is a beachhead for national mountain bike access issues. While riders everywhere should ride responsibly, irresponsible riding in Marin has a pronounced effect on access issues locally and nationally." That said, all riders—visitors and locals alike—are urged to obey the speed limit in effect over all of Marin County's trails and dirt roads: 15 mph tops and 5 mph on curves and when passing. On paved vehicle roads, heed posted speed limits and ride single-file. If you drive your car to reach a ride, avoid parking in front of private residences and do not block roadways or driveways. Better yet, use public parking lots and ride to the trail. If you aren't familiar with what it takes to be a responsible rider, take a moment and read the section titled "Trail Etiquette" in the front of the book.

Let's switch gears and talk about the historical significance of Marin County. It sort of "started" with a race down a dirt road called Repack. And who better to tell the story than someone who was there: Joe Breeze, one of the founding fathers of our sport as we know it today. Joe is credited with building the first modern mountain bike frames using all new parts. In October, 1977, he rode his first ever "Breezer" bike to victory at Repack. He's been designing and building his Breezer mountain bikes ever since, and they're ridden by cognoscenti worldwide. Sincere thanks to Joe who graciously gave his permission to reprint the following speech he made to a gathering of bike enthusiasts at the top of Repack on the occasion of the 20-year anniversary of that first race.

FROM REPACK TO THE WORLD: TWENTY YEARS
(Read at the top on October 21, 1996)

Here we are gathered at what could be called the cradle of mountain biking. It was 20 years ago to the day at this very spot that Repack, the race, came into being. And it was from Repack, that what was later to be called mountain biking, went national.

Now, people have been riding off-road since the advent of the bicycle, but the key to the mountain bike's success was the balloon tire, which was popularized by Schwinn in the 1930s. 26 x 2.125—that was the key. The big wheel with the big cross-section. The balloon tire fired the imagination for how far one could go off-road.

But that would have to wait. The then new double-tube balloon-tire bike fueled the bike boom of the 1930s and 1940s—on the road. And yes, there have been people riding off-road since the advent of the balloon tire. All around the country, in isolated pockets, off-road activity would come and go. Neighborhood kids in the Alleghenies, a canyon clan up in the Ozarks—many places. They'd catch the bug for a summer or maybe play at it sporadically over the course of a few years, but inevitably they'd go on to something different. Same is true of Marin County where there were many isolated occurrences.

It took another bike boom, in the 1970s, to make the difference. The obvious hit that mountain biking is today would have you believing that once someone figured out the correct formula there was no stopping it. Well, the correct formula wasn't one bike. It was a mountain called Tamalpais, people who loved the outdoors, and an inexhaustible supply of bikers that kept momentum going.

My first encounter with 26 x 2.125 balloon tires was in the late 1960s. Friends at Tam High had such bikes, but I must say I scoffed at them. What clunkers! Then I heard about the Canyonites in Larkspur. They were even more into it, and even had races. I believe the Canyonites are responsible for planting the major seed.

By 1973, mainstream cycling in the form of Velo Club Tamalpais and friends had caught the ballooner bug and this was the beginning of the inexhaustible supply of riders. For a bunch of roadies with a major jones for cycling and an in-depth knowledge of all the roads between the Golden Gate and the Russian River, it was like a whole new country was discovered right at our doorstep.

Being proficient at riding off-road tends to be largely due to handling skills, and with this competitive lot it was only a matter of time before someone said they were fastest downhill. Repack was discovered by Fred Wolf and other Ross Valley friends in the early 1970s. By 1976 after many a coaster brake had been repacked, the race was born. Fred and Charlie Kelly rounded up a Navy chronometer and an alarm clock and Alan Bonds egged on the others. In fact, it was Alan who won that first Repack race twenty years ago.

Word quickly traveled through the towns around the mountain and Repack became an instant magnet for those wishing to display their handling prowess. So eager were we to compare handling skills, the first nine Repack races were held on the average of one a week.

Repack was the crucial event in the development of mountain biking. Here for the first time, Mount Tam bikers were all drawn together on a regular basis to share their stories and share their ideas about the new bike. This cross-pollination of ideas spurred the bike's evolution and solidified the sport.

In all there were twenty-four Repack races. Twenty-two of them were held in 1976 to 1979, mostly in the fall as the road-race season wound down.

Racing generated new excitement and an event to focus on. Racer and reporter Owen Mulholland spread the word out of Marin with his story, "California bikies are 'mountainside surfin' " in *VeloNews*, February 10, 1978. Then in January 1979, San Francisco's KPIX-TV shot that segment for "Evening Magazine." It eventually aired around the country on CBS affiliates. In 1979 Charlie published a story in *Outside* magazine. The word was out of Marin and before the nation.

So Repack not only catalyzed interest in fat-tire, off-road riding around Mt. Tam, it created nationwide attention for the fledgling sport, and that no doubt instantly renewed the interest of all those people around the country who had earlier ridden balloon-tire bikes off-road. We were now all in the right place, at the right time.

The part I like best about this whole mountain bike thing is that while "we were just having fun," we were birthing an activity that has greatly popularized a vehicle that can be so beneficial to our individual health in the recreational sense and one that is so beneficial to our world health in the utilitarian sense.

Thank you Repack. — *Joe Breeze* © 1998 by Joe Breeze. All rights reserved.

RIDE 74 · Angel Island Double Loop

AT A GLANCE

Length/configuration: 10.4 miles total, loop within a loop (Perimeter Road loop 7 miles on paved and gravel road; Upper Fire Road Loop 3.4 miles on dirt fire road), both can be ridden in either direction

Aerobic difficulty: Both loops are easy with a few short, gentle hills

Technical difficulty: Perimeter Road Loop is nontechnical; Upper Fire Road Loop is moderately technical due to potholes and rain ruts

Scenery: Expansive views of Bay Area cityscape in all directions. Historic military sites dating back to The Civil War, World War II, and the Cold War. The North Garrison, site of an infamous Chinese immigration station is now a museum. Arrive at the island via a ferry boat ride.

Special comments: One of the best, all-day outings for young families and adult riders of all abilities.

If you have a fondness for San Francisco, you'll love the views from Angel Island. Though this ride is not very challenging, riders of all ages, abilities, and strengths will love this outing. This ride consists of a loop within a loop. The larger, easiest loop follows Perimeter Road which encircles the entire island. Also referred to as the Lower Loop, the road is mostly paved with a long section of gravel. Entirely free of vehicles, the seven-mile Perimeter Road Loop is easy and mostly level with a few short, gentle hills. Young families with freewheeling kids and kid-trailers find this a perfect outing. If you're a dirt-lover wanting more of a challenge, you have to treat yourself to the Upper Fire Road Loop, a narrow fire road, situated about 150 yards higher than the Perimeter Road Loop. It's only slightly more challenging but the

RIDE 74 · Angel Island Double Loop

views and leaving the crowd below on the lower loop makes it a worthwhile ride. A bit more rugged with some ruts and potholes, adventurous beginners with little technical skills will enjoy it. Whether you ride one or both loops, you can easily spend a full day here when the weather is warm and sunny. Half the fun of this outing is taking the ferry from any one of four Bay Area ports.

Sitting in the San Francisco Bay, just inside the Golden Gate Bridge, Angel Island is larger than Alcatraz Island. Though not as well-known as Alcatraz, Angel Island is a profound repository of our nation's military and immigration history. The island's known historic past began centuries ago with the Miwok Native Americans fishing and hunting here. In 1775, a few years after the discovery of this well-protected bay in 1769,

Lt. Juan Manuel de Ayala dropped anchor at the island's cove (which now bears his name) and claimed the land Spanish territory. Like other Catholic explorers, he named the land "Isla de Los Angeles" (Island of the Angels). In the early 1800s, sea otters in the waters off the island attracted Russian hunters while cattle grazing was introduced by the Mexican government. In 1859, the U.S. federal government acquired the island and from that time on, through the Civil War, World War II, and the Cold War, the island served as a strategic military and defense post. Eventually, Angel Island became known as "the Ellis Island of the West" with the founding of the Immigration Station at the North Garrison. From 1910 to 1940, the U.S. Immigration processed almost 200,000 immigrants here, mostly Chinese. Many were detained here for months, sometimes over a year, enduring prison-like conditions and treatment, before being allowed entry into the U.S. or deported. Today, the historic buildings that remain have been preserved as museums and it's definitely worth a visit. There, you'll find historic displays among the barracks and other processing buildings. Keep a sharp eye out and you'll find poems of Chinese characters scrawled on the walls, no doubt lamenting about the love ones left behind in the old country and how dismal life was while waiting in this "no-man's land." On the west side of the island is Camp Reynolds, also known as the West Garrison, a battery dating from 1863 which served as military housing and offices. One of the largest collections of Civil War–era buildings, the camp housed a large contingent of union soldiers stationed here to protect munitions sites in Benicia across the bay as well as the gold and silver deposits in the Sierra Nevadas. Today, the park service schedules Civil War reenactments and cannon firings on weekends during the summer months to commemorate this island's service to the nation during the 1800s. On the east side of the island is Fort McDowell, also known as the East Garrison. Buildings here date from the Spanish-American War and for many years after, served as the military's West Coast processing center for thousands of incoming and outgoing soldiers during both world wars. On the south side, closed to the public is the Nike Missile Site, the island's connection to the Cold War. Throughout the island, many of the historic buildings are in a state of arrested deterioration, waiting for more funding for restoration.

So, head for the nearest ferry, with or without your bike. Bike rentals for everyone, including tandems and kid-trailers are available on the island. It's a perfect way to enjoy the outdoors and learn a bit of history, too.

General location: Right smack in the middle of San Francisco Bay, between San Francisco and Oakland.

Elevation change: Negligible change; lower loop from 0 to 300 feet; upper loop from 300 to 450 feet.

Season: Year-round, though ferry service is limited to weekends during the winter months.

Services: Ferry service, which allows bikes, is the only way to get to the island and is available from several Bay Area locations (see "Finding the trail"). During the summer months, convenient services include a well-stocked snack bar (including beer!), bike rentals (including Zap® electric bikes and tandems, kid-trailers for bikes, and helmets), picnic grounds, barbeque pits, running water (potable), rest rooms throughout the island, and a visitor center with sundries (such as sunscreen, film, etc.). There are also volleyball courts and a baseball diamond (by reservation). In the off months, service is limited and it's a good idea to call to confirm what's open for business. Historic military and cultural sites are generally open though some sites such as the immigration museum at the North Garrison are open during specific hours and days. The historic chapel at Fort McDowell East Garrison is available for weddings. Environmental campsites are available and reservations are required. Park rangers are on duty year-round. All other services located in any of the Bay Area cities.

Hazards: Several spots on the Upper Fire Road Loop skirt steep drop-offs. Using a bike lock is recommended while you explore historical sites on foot. Though there are many hiking trails on the island, bikes are allowed only on the Perimeter Road and the Upper Fire Road. Watch out for poison oak if you explore any of the hiking trails. Summer weekends attract hordes of people. Fortunately, they generally stay close to Ayala Cove where the ferry dock, snack bar, and picnic grounds are located. Nevertheless, you have no choice but to ride through this congested area in order to access Perimeter Road.

Rescue index: During the popular spring and summer months, especially on weekends, you're likely to meet other trail users who may be of help on the Perimeter Road and at the historic sites. Phones as well as service personnel can be found at Ayala Cove. Park rangers are on duty generally year-round.

Land status: Angel Island State Park.

Maps: *Angel Island State Park*, official park map, specifically the environmental camping handout. Also *Marin Bicycle Map*, published by Marin County Bicycle Coalition; (415) 488-1245.

Finding the trail: Unless you have your own private boat, the only way to access Angel Island is by public ferry. Year-round ferries depart San Francisco, Vallejo, and Tiburon. They also run from Oakland/Alameda during the summer only. During the off-season, schedules vary and service is typically on weekends and holidays. Travel time varies depending on where you board the ferry and is generally less than an hour. The shortest ride is about 15 minutes from Tiburon. Ferry services are offered generally during the daylight hours, with the last returning ferry in the late afternoon. Call for current information, schedules, fares, location, and where to park your car. San Francisco Bay Cruise: (800) 229-2784, (415) 773-1188, out of state (415) 546-2896; San Francisco Blue & Gold Fleet: (415) 705-5555; Angel Island–Tiburon Ferry: (415) 435-2131; Vallejo Ferry: (707) 643-3779; Oakland/Alameda Ferry: (510) 522-3300.

Sources of additional information:

Angel Island State Park
P.O. Box 318
Tiburon, CA 94920
(415) 435-1915; (415) 435-5390

For picnic ground reservations and camping, call Destinet at (800) 444-7275.

For info about bike rental, kayaking, and tram tours, call Angel Island Company at (415) 897-0715. For info about the historic buildings, tours, and upcoming events (including cannon firings!), call (415) 435-3522 or (415) 435-1915.

Notes on the trail: Let's face it, you can't really get lost on Angel Island. The main road that surrounds the entire island is Perimeter Road. Once you disembark at the ferry dock in Ayala Cove, hop on your bike and make your way through the crowd of people, following the walkway toward the snack bar, picnic grounds and around the cove. On the inland side of the picnic grounds, follow signs indicating the bike route. Make a hairpin left turn onto a wide dirt trail and begin a short, steep climb through

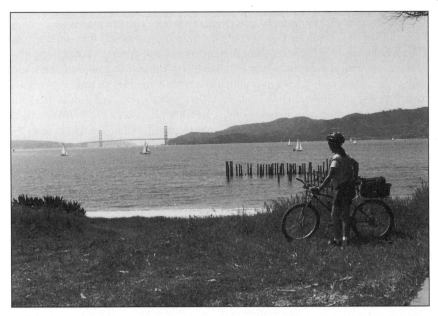

Linda checks out the view of the Golden Gate near Point Stuart at Camp Reynolds off the Perimeter Road.

the shady forest of oak and eucalyptus trees. In less than a half mile, you reach paved Perimeter Road. From here, you begin the Perimeter Road Loop by going either left or right, clockwise or counterclockwise, respectively. Either way, you'll eventually return to this point. For this description, go right (counterclockwise).

The cruising is easy on wide, paved Perimeter Road. At 1.2 miles from the edge of the Ayala Cove picnic grounds, a dirt trail leads down toward Camp Reynolds, also known as the West Garrison. A huge contingent of soldiers was once stationed here in the 1890s and old, mostly abandoned buildings and barracks are all that remains. You can ride down to the water's edge. A couple of picnic tables are available here as well as rest rooms and drinking water.

Return to the Perimeter Road and continue your counterclockwise direction. In a short while, the pavement turns to gravel. Go past an unpaved road leading up on your left and in a few yards, past the Rock Quarry. At about 3 miles, a minor fire road peels off on the left toward Battery Drew. This side trail rejoins the Perimeter Road in less than a half mile, and though it climbs steeply for a few yards, the effort is worthwhile just to get away from other trail users and to enjoy a fast, albeit short, dirt downhill run. An old, abandoned military battery stands overlooking the south bay.

Back on the Perimeter Road, continue on and at about 4 miles, you reach a four-way intersection. The dirt road running steeply up on your left is one of two bikeable trails that lead up to the Upper Fire Road Loop. The right paved road leads around the Nike Missile Site and is likely closed to the public. At this intersection, say goodbye to other trail users by turning left onto the steep, dirt road. You may have to dismount and push your bike, especially if the terrain is deeply rutted by past rainstorms. In about a 100 yards, you reach the Upper Fire Road and the terrain levels considerably. (You can go either left or right—you'll still complete this upper loop by returning to this point.)

This description continues by going left, clockwise. The fire road is much more rugged than the Perimeter Road but adventurous beginners will have no problem. Though the fire road has some short stretches of ups and downs, and brief drop-offs, there are no real significant climbs or hazards to sweat over. Beginners just remember: dismounting and walking over difficult sections is an effective technique. At just over 5 miles, a hiking-only trail leads uphill on your right toward Sunset Trail and Mount Livermore. Bypass it and continue heading basically north then east on the fire road. Bypass another hiking-only trail intersection. You'll notice that here on the north side of the island, the vegetation is lush and shady.

Continue meandering due east and at about 6 miles, you can see down into Ayala Cove and Tiburon across the north bay. Go past the "Domestic Water Supply" storage area and descend a few yards to an intersection with another fire road leading off on your left, at roughly 7 miles. This fire road is another bikeable trail connecting the Perimeter Road to the Upper Fire Road loop. Bypass it, staying right on the dirt fire road you've been following. In less than a half mile, a hiking-only trail leads up to Mount Livermore and shortly after that, you complete the upper loop. Go left back down the steep dirt road toward Perimeter Road. Hang a left onto the gravel road and continue your counterclockwise direction on a gravel road. (The real Perimeter Road continues straight toward the Nike Missile area. In 1998, storm damage forced the closure of this portion of the loop and diverted all trail users to this alternate gravel road.)

As you approach Fort McDowell, also known as the East Garrison, your route descends through a shady, fragrant forest of eucalyptus trees. There are historic buildings as well as a picnic area here. Eventually, you make a hard left and find yourself back on paved Perimeter Road as you cruise past more historic structures as well as the chapel. The cruising is easy and at almost 9 miles, a side road leads down toward the immigration station, also known as the North Garrison and China Cove. If the museum is open, it's a worthwhile historical visit. After the U.S. Immigration Service moved off the island to San Francisco, German and Japanese prisoners of war were housed here from 1942 to 1946.

After your history lesson, continue on Perimeter Road and in almost 10 miles, you close the loop. If you want more of a workout, ride all or part of the loops again, this time without stopping. Otherwise, retrace your path back toward the picnic grounds and Ayala Cove, just in time to catch your ferry. Make sure you get on the right ferry or you may find yourself clear across the bay from where your car is parked.

RIDE 75 · Tennessee Valley Double Loop

AT A GLANCE

Length/configuration: 12.6-mile double loop (North Loop 5.6 miles; South Loop 7 miles), both clockwise; dirt roads and short stretches on single-track and pavement

Aerobic difficulty: Mostly moderate with several stretches of strenuous hills

Technical difficulty: Mild with some intermediate spots due to obstacles and ruts

Scenery: Mostly open terrain, which means you can see a great distance. Sights include secluded Gerbode Valley and spectacular expansive views of the Pacific Ocean and parts of the East Bay and San Francisco.

Special comments: Out-and-back rides on either loop, as well as a side-trip down to Tennessee Cove are suitable for beginners and young families. The entire route is like a figure-eight and because both loops originate in the same parking lot, you can ride one loop, then decide if you want to tackle the other one.

Located in the Marin Headlands section of Golden Gate National Recreation Area, secluded Tennessee Valley is easily accessed from US 101 and Highway 1 (CA 1). It's hard to believe that this naturally pristine area is less than a half hour away from one of the nation's most bustling, crowded metropolitan areas. The beach access, fire roads, and trails make Tennessee Valley a popular area for equestrians, hikers, bikers, and young families.

The two loops presented here is really a figure-eight route. Since the main parking area is located right smack in the middle of the "8," beginners can try one instead of both. With decent endurance, novices and beginning mountain bikers with some technical skill can ride both loops, walking over a few spots of brief rugged, more difficult terrain. Both loops are adequately signed though a good map is suggested. The North Loop (Coyote Ridge Trail) is 5.6 miles, clockwise, with breathtaking, expansive views of the Pacific and the rugged shoreline. Riding mostly dirt fire road over roller-coaster hills and a mile stretch of intermediate technical single-track, elevation gain on the North Loop is over 1,000 feet—not exactly a great ride for beginners who lack endurance. The South Loop (Marincello-Bobcat Trails) is seven miles, clockwise, over mostly easy dirt fire road. The climbing, though not as much as the North Loop, is still a challenge because the road rising out of Gerbode Valley is unrelenting for over a mile. The valley itself is wonderfully peaceful, filled with singing birds—it really is hard to believe that San Francisco is just on the other side of the southern ridge. Beginners with little single-track riding experience may find Old Springs Trail, near the end of the South Loop, to be a somewhat challenging but definitely enjoyable section. Just remember, walking over loose, rocky spots is a technique that always works.

Of special note is the Golden Gate Raptor Observatory (GGRO), a cooperative program of the Golden Gate National Park Association and National Park Service. Marin Headlands attracts over 15,000 birds each year, showcasing the largest concentration of raptors on the northern Pacific Coast. The best place to view these soaring creatures is at Hawk Hill, accessed via a hiking and biking trail about a half mile off the South Loop. Best viewing times are between 10 a.m. and 3 p.m., September and October. The GGRO sponsors hawk-watching groups at Hawk Hill from September through November. Fall migration talks and other related activities are also offered.

General location: About 4 miles north of San Francisco.

Elevation change: North Loop: 1,011 feet; starting elevation 200 feet; high point 1,031 feet; low point about 20 feet. Route descends initially, then climbs a series of steep, short hills, interspersed with brief level sections before descending a long section back to the parking lot. South Loop: 915 feet; starting elevation 200 feet; high

RIDE 75 · Tennessee Valley Double Loop

point 925 feet; low point about 10 feet. Route starts with a moderate ascent, followed by a long descent into the valley floor, then regains lost elevation via a long unrelenting moderate climb back up to the parking lot.

Season: Year-round.

Services: Public phone, pit toilets, and picnic tables available at the Tennessee Valley Road main parking lot. Campsites available at Haypress, Hawk, and nearby Bicentennial campgrounds.

Hazards: Watch out for other trail users especially on the single-track portions of both loops. Equestrians favor these trails and bikers should always give horses a wide

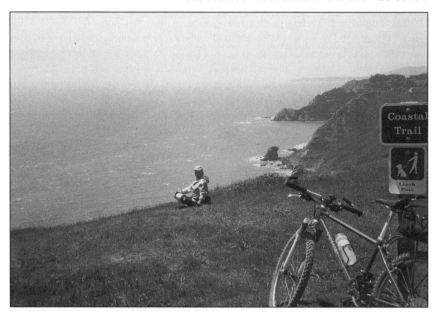

Just two miles into the North Loop ride, Bruce takes a break to appreciate a stunning view of the Pacific and the rugged shoreline far below.

berth. Approach horses slowly or stop; ask for permission to pass before doing so. Bobcats reside here, hence the name of one of the trails. If you venture down to tiny, black-sand Tennessee Valley Beach—or any other nearby beach for that matter—beware that the surf and rip currents can be treacherous (not that the water is warm enough for swimming in). Check tide tables before venturing to isolated beaches as rising tide can trap you against towering cliffs with no escape route. The land along the coastal cliffs are likely to be unstable and may crumble and slide at any time. Stay safely away from the edge, especially when soaking in the views at an overlook.

Rescue index: Both loops are popular with hikers, equestrians, joggers, and strolling young families. During the weekends, chances are good you will find help from other trail users. Weekdays, however, you may have to wait a long time before someone comes a long. In that case, you should make your way back to the Miwok Stables parking area at the end of Tennessee Valley Road where you'll find a public phone and perhaps other people. If you're near the southern end of the South Loop, you may find help on Bunker Road, which is the road that leads to the Marine Mammal Center, the Headlands Institute, and Rodeo Beach, as well as a public bus stop.

Land status: Golden Gate National Recreation Area.

Maps: A *Rambler's Guide to the Trails of Mt. Tamapalis and the Marin Headlands*, published by The Olmsted & Bros. Map Co., (510) 658-6534. *Marin Bicycle Map*, published by Marin County Bicycle Coalition; (415) 488-1245. *Golden Gate National Recreation Area*, official park map and brochure, published by the National Park Service.

Finding the trail: From San Francisco, head north over the Golden Gate Bridge. Go through the Waldo Tunnel and proceed about 2.2 miles farther to the exit for Stinson Beach/Mill Valley/Highway 1 (CA 1, also known as Shoreline Highway).

Follow Highway 1 for less than a mile and then turn left onto Tennessee Valley Road. Go about 2 miles to where the road ends at a gate adjacent to a large parking area. Park and begin pedaling from here. Though you can access this figure-eight loop at a number of other places, this parking area is popular and there are conveniences here (rest room, picnic table, and phone). If arriving by bike from San Francisco, pedal across the Golden Gate, then make your way through Sausalito via a bayside bike path. Pedal north, then west to the Marin Headlands via a connector trail near the Rodeo Avenue exit (off US 101), or via Donahue Street near where Highway 1 and US 101 separate. You reach the South Loop on Bobcat Trail near Hawk Camp.

Sources of additional information:

Sausalito Cyclery
No. 1 Gate 6 Rd.
Sausalito, CA 94965
(415) 332-3200
At Bridgeway and Gate 6 Road, on the Mill Valley–Sausalito bikeway on the north end of town near US 101.

Golden Gate National
   Recreation Area
Marin Headlands Visitor Center
Fort Barry, Building 948
Sausalito, CA 94965
(415) 331-1540 or (415) 561-5656
http://www.nps.gov/goga

The Golden Gate Raptor
   Observatory
Fort Mason, Building 201
San Francisco, CA 94123
(415) 331-0730

The Marin Headlands Visitor Center
(415) 331-1540

Bicycle Trails Council of Marin
P.O. Box 13842
San Rafael, CA 94913
(415) 479-5482

Notes on the trail: Both loops begin and end at the parking area next to Miwok Stables.

The North Loop: Begin by following paved Tennessee Valley Road, heading west past the gate. This is a gentle descent and you can really pick up speed on this short, almost 1-mile cruise on pavement, so watch out for other trail users. After passing several hiking-only trails, the pavement ends at a fork. The left fork is signed "No Bikes" and continues as pavement for a few yards, then becomes dirt. It's an alternate route to Tennessee Beach via a meadow. The right fork is signed Coastal Trail to Muir Beach and it's the continuation of Tennessee Valley Road, a smooth, mildly technical, dirt fire road. Take this right fork, bypass several other lesser trails on your left, and begin a series of steep but short climbs. Fortunately, the steepness mellows in some spots, giving your leg muscles welcome relief. As you rise above the Tennessee Valley and its tiny lake, the view is open amid low shrubs of fragrant sagebushes and you catch a glimpse of the Pacific Ocean.

At about 2 miles from the parking lot, you reach a windy, grass overlook poised above a cliff. Get off your bike and walk a few yards toward the edge. (Use extreme caution and be aware of unstable, loose ground.) The view is absolutely spectacular with the Pacific spanning 180-degrees and white surf crashing into the rugged coastline far below. Elevation here is 590 feet. When you hop back on your bike, bypass a lesser hiking trail leading off of the main dirt road, signed Coastal Trail and off-limits to bikes.

Continue your uphill march, descending in a few stretches but mostly climbing. You top the mother of all hills when you reach an intersection of several trails. The first trail to your right, signed Fox Trail, is off-limits to bikes. A few yards farther on your left is a tiny unsigned hiking trail and a fire road. (It leads down to Muir Beach and bikes are allowed.) From this wide-open vantage point, look behind you and, if it's not foggy, you'll see the tip of San Francisco's skyline signature, the Transamerica pyramid, peeking over the ridge. Bear right onto signed Coyote Ridge Trail (actually a narrow dirt fire road). Along the way, you bypass Middle Green Gulch Trail peeling off on your left.

Staying on Coyote Ridge, climb up another steep stretch and at 1,031 feet, you reach the high point of the North Loop. (Actually, the highest point is just a few yards up the hill off the loop, on the left side of the fire road.) From here, you have a 360-degree view of the entire north Bay Area. You can see the towers of the Golden Gate Bridge just rising over the southern ridge. Looking east, you can see Angel Island, both the Oakland–San Francisco Bay and Richmond Bridges as well as the Berkeley Hills and Oakland. Distance from the parking lot to here is about 3.3 miles.

From this point, the rest of the loop is basically downhill interrupted by a few short stretches of level and moderate climbing. Leave the high point by following Coyote Ridge Trail as it descends over mildly technical terrain, spiced by a few rain ruts. The narrow fire road hugs the northern slope of a hill as it descends. Bypass other trails as they are hiking-only trails. In a few minutes, the fire road leads you through a fragrant, shady eucalyptus forest and past a water tank on your left. Continue about 0.2 mile farther to a signed intersection. Take the right fire road, signed Miwok Trail and climb a short, steep hill. At the top of this hill in a clearing, a hiking-only trail tapers into your trail. Bear left and follow Miwok Trail as it climbs another short but steep hill.

At about 4.5 miles, you top the final hill. From here, the next mile is a fun, rolling downhill back to the parking lot. Your intermediate technical skills will be tested as the terrain is somewhat rugged. There are rubber water bars and a few patches of loose rock to ride over. The trail begins as a fire road and quickly narrows into a wide single-track, bounded on both sides by tall bushes as it weaves down the slope. Tiny dips in the trail, when taken at high speeds, will get you some "air." Enjoy, but watch out for other trail users. There are several hairpin turns with steps set in to control erosion along this stretch. The fun descent ends as you ride through a eucalyptus forest and over a tiny wooden bridge. You arrive back at the parking lot at 5.6 miles.

The South Loop: Begin by pedaling toward Miwok Stables at the southeast corner of the parking lot. Adjacent to the stables' entrance, go left through a gate onto Marincello Road, a wide dirt fire road. The first mile is a moderate, mildly technical climb over mostly open terrain. As you gain elevation, glimpses of the East Bay, Tiburon, San Rafael, and the Richmond Bridge appear. The steepness mellows significantly near the top of the ridge. If you're riding in late spring, you may see a fragrant mass of yellow scotchbroom covering the hillside on your right. At just over 1.5 miles, Bobcat Trail (off-limits to bikes) tapers into your fire road from behind your right shoulder. This is the high point of the South Loop. Carry on with the gradual climb and you can begin to see some of the tips of tall skyscrapers in San Francisco and the towers of the Golden Gate Bridge beyond the southern ridge. Bypass all other trails that lead off from the fire road. At almost 2 miles, Hawk Camp trail which leads up to Hawk Hill takes off on your right. (Hawk Hill is a prime raptor-watching spot and the trail allows bikes.)

At 2.2 miles, after some short rolling ups and downs, a sign finally appears indicating the fire road you're pedaling is now the Bobcat Trail. Still a smooth, easy fire road, Bobcat Trail begins the long, sweet descent down into Gerbode Valley. As you pedal along the valley floor, you will undoubtedly see a road traversing up a steep hillside straight ahead on the other side of the valley. Yep, you'll be taking that path back up and out of the valley. From the valley floor, it looks steeper than it really is. Go through a small eucalyptus grove, bypassing several trails leading off on your left (both of which lead to Rodeo Valley, Rodeo Lagoon, Cronkhite Beach, and Bunker Road). Stay on Bobcat, bearing right through a curve to a signed T intersection. Here, Bobcat intersects Miwok Trail running both left and right. Hang a right here and begin the 1.2-mile climb out of the valley.

When you reach the junction with Wolf Ridge Trail (no bikes), you're almost finished with the climbing. About 0.2 mile farther over one more steep but short hill, Old Springs Trail takes off on your left. Lucky for you, the fire road straight ahead runs up a steep hill measuring about 10% grade and is signed "No Bikes." Turn left onto Old Springs, going over a wooden bridge. The next 1.3 miles is a twisty, wide single-track, bounded on both sides by low bushes. Old Springs, for the most part, is a sweet, curvy descent with some spots of very rugged, loose rock and dirt. Beginners may want to walk over a couple of rocky drops. The trail ends with a short, steep stretch into Miwok Stables. Go through the stable, bearing left and toward the parking lot. Finishing mileage for the South Loop is 7 miles.

RIDE 76 · Mt. Tam Loop via Old Railroad–Eldridge Grades

AT A GLANCE

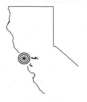

Length/configuration: 13.2-mile loop, counterclockwise; fire road and paved road

Aerobic difficulty: Moderate due to gradual, sustained climbing

Technical difficulty: Mildly technical with a 2.6-mile section of intermediate-rated rocky trail conditions

Scenery: From Mt. Tam's East Peak, the view includes the Pacific Ocean, San Francisco and the Bay, Angel Island, and the East Bay; on clear days, you can see the Farallon Islands and Mt. Diablo.

Special comments: The first 8.25 miles can be ridden as an out-and-back (16.5 miles round-trip) and is perfect for strong beginners. One of the most popular rides in the Bay Area, solo riders are never far from emergency assistance. The West Point Inn, especially on pancake breakfast Sundays, is a popular mountain biker joint. Mt. Tam is where mountain biking was born!

Mount Tamalpais, fondly referred to by locals as Mt. Tam, is well-known as *the* mountain biking playground of the entire Bay Area. It offers majestic views, is rideable year-round—even in wet weather—and riders of all abilities can enjoy many of its trails. This 12-mile clockwise loop is a classic, making use of the ever popular, well-traveled Old Railroad Grade, a mostly smooth, mildly technical wide road that was a railway bed in the late 1800s and early 1900s. The gradients were between 5–7%, and for us bikers, that means it's an easy climb for even the strongest beginners. In fact, beginners can just pedal the Old Railroad Grade up to the top of Mt. Tam, specifically East Peak, take in the views of the San Francisco Bay and Pacific Ocean, then turn around and head back down the same way. Intermediately skilled riders, on the other hand, can test their abilities by riding down rocky and steep Eldridge Grade. Eldridge starts off as a gnarly 2.6-mile section before mellowing out into mildly technical terrain. There are numerous places from which to access Mt. Tam. This one starts and finishes in the town of Mill Valley.

In 1896, the Mill Valley & Mt. Tamalpais Scenic Railway was constructed over an 8.25-mile route that crept up to the summit. Visitors from all over the world rode the small but mighty locomotives to the top. They enjoyed the magnificent views and indulged in wine and food at the Tamalpais Tavern, constructed by the railway. Though the service was a popular attraction, financial success was never fully realized. In 1924, spurred by the popularity of automobiles and buses, Ridgecrest Boulevard was completed and it provided visitors easy access to Mt. Tam without riding the train. The onset of the Great Depression only served to deter more riders, and in 1929, the final blow came when a fire destroyed a locomotive and the hotel. Today, West Point Inn, built in 1904 as a station for the Mt. Tamalpais Railway and the Bolinas Stage (coaches), still attracts lovers of the mountain. Run by the West Point Inn Association, a non-profit volunteer organization, breakfasts are served (mostly on weekends) and are extremely popular with local hikers and bikers. During the summer, a fund-raising pancake breakfast is offered on the second Sunday of each month between May and October. Pedal up here on a Sunday and you'll discover the West Point Inn is a popular meeting place for bikers.

But there's more to Mt. Tam than meets the eye. Yes, there's a lengthy network of rideable trails (actually dirt roads) weaving through Mount Tamalpais State Park and its adjacent lands, providing numerous ride configurations for short or all-day outings. That's certainly is a major draw. But the lure of Mt. Tam—what makes it a must-ride—is the fact that mountain biking was born here. This area was—and still is—the backyard for Joe Breeze, Gary Fisher, and many other bicycle-building pioneers. (Joe reports that his first balloon-tire ride was on the Old Railroad Grade back in 1973.) Anybody who loves the sport and lives in California or the nearby states is bound to pedal these trails, sooner or later.

General location: About 10 miles north of San Francisco.

Elevation change: 2,140 feet; starting elevation and low point 200 feet; high point 2,340 feet. Basically, one big hill climb.

Season: Year-round.

Services: West Point Inn is a restaurant and lodge favored by locals and is run by the West Point Inn Association. Located about one-third of the way (1,780 feet) up the Old Railroad Grade, it serves a popular pancake breakfast on each second Sunday from May through October, from 9 a.m. to 1 p.m., first-come, first-serve, about $6 per person. Refreshments, water, and rest rooms are available on most weekends. At the top of Mt. Tam, at the East Peak to be exact, you'll find more than just water

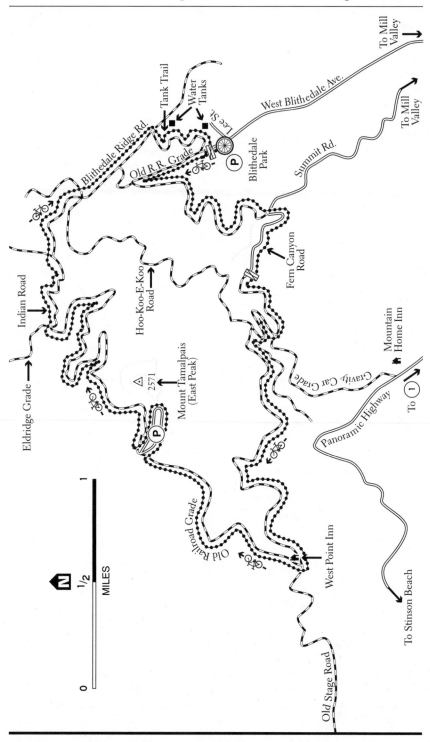

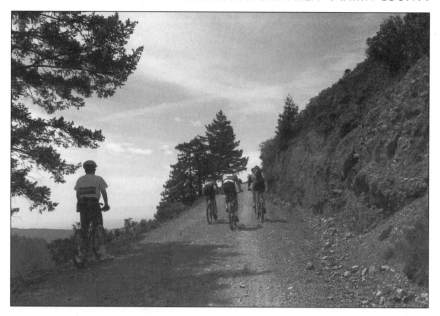

Popular Mt. Tam can be a hard workout or a leisurely ride for bikers of all skills and levels, and it's the place to pedal if you're a solo biker wanting to meet like-minded people.

fountains and rest rooms. There's a visitor's center, a gift shop, and a snack bar that serves chili dogs, ice cream novelties, energy bars, bagels, candy bars and sodas. (Yup, it's a popular tourist spot, totally accessible via a paved road.) There are picnic tables with a great view here—and it's a favorite place to hang out and check out all the other bikers that make it up to the top. Other than these two places, there are no services on the route. All services are available in the surrounding communities: San Rafael, Mill Valley, and San Francisco.

Hazards: The speed limit here on Mt. Tam is 15 mph, 5 mph when passing other trail users, and it's enforced by rangers equipped with radar. All trails here are immensely popular with hikers and bikers, so expect to encounter lots of traffic. Several short stretches of the route use somewhat well-traveled, paved vehicle roads. You're likely to see more vehicular traffic at the top at East Peak.

Rescue index: Most every day of the week, you're likely to meet other trail users who may be of assistance. There is a phone at West Point Inn as well as at the top at East Peak, which is accessible by cars and emergency vehicles.

Land status: Marin Municipal Water District, Marin County Open Space District, and Mount Tamalpais State Park.

Maps: *A Rambler's Guide to the Trails of Mt. Tamapalis and the Marin Headlands,* published by The Olmsted & Bros. Map Co., (510) 658-6534. *Marin Bicycle Map,* published by Marin County Bicycle Coalition; (415) 488-1245. *Mount Tamalpais State Park,* official park map and brochure.

Finding the trail: Locals begin their ride from within the town of Mill Valley. Parking your car in the downtown area, however, is a risky affair since parking is metered or timed. The ride description presented here starts off near Blithedale Park, at the northern end of West Blithedale Avenue. From San Francisco, travel north on US 101 about 6 miles from the Golden Gate Bridge. Go past the Highway One/Stinson Beach exit. Take the East Blithedale/Tiburon Boulevard exit. Follow East Blithedale to the west side of US 101 and head toward Mill Valley. Continue on East Blithedale toward town and it eventually becomes West Blithedale Avenue at Throckmorton Avenue. Follow West Blithedale, which soon becomes Ralston as the road curves and runs into Blithedale Park, a tiny park hidden within a quiet residential neighborhood. Leave your car anywhere near the park, taking care to not block anyone's driveway or mailboxes. Begin riding from here.

Sources of additional information:

Marin Municipal Water District
220 Nellen Ave.
Corte Madera, CA 94925
(415) 924-4600

Mount Tamalpais State Park
801 Panoramic Highway
Mill Valley, CA 94941
(415) 388-2070

Bicycle Trails Council of Marin
P.O. Box 13842
San Rafael, CA 94913
(415) 479-5482

Marin County Open Space District
Parks and Recreation Department
Marin Civic Center
San Rafael, CA 94903
(415) 499-6387

West Point Inn
1000 Panoramic Highway
Mill Valley, CA 94941
(415) 388-9955
Located on Old Railroad Grade

Notes on the trail: Before hitting the trail, consider bringing a bike lock and cash for a snack bar break. You just might want to linger at the West Point Inn for a while or check out the view from a walking-only path at East Peak.

Pedal north on West Blithedale. In a few yards, the pavement ends at a gated dirt road. This is the beginning of Old Railroad Grade. Go through the gate and as you begin the gentle climb, stay left on the main dirt road, bypassing other trails that lead off on your right. In about two miles, Old Railroad Grade becomes paved Summit Road and then immediately becomes Fern Canyon Road (but you wouldn't know it if you missed seeing the street sign.) Nevertheless, follow the paved road, bearing right, passing Temelpa Trail, a hiking-only trail on your right. A few yards later, the pavement ends at a metal gate and becomes dirt Old Railroad Grade once again. A sign here indicates you're now entering the Mount Tamalpais Watershed.

Old Railroad Grade continues its gradual uphill climb and in just over 4 miles, you reach a signed **T** intersection. Take the dirt road to the right, which leads to West Point Inn and East Peak. In a few yards, you'll see the old Mesa Station platform at the foot of the famous "Double Bowknot" gravity car grade. Soon, you reach the intersection with Hoo-Koo-E-Koo Trail. Go left, following Old Railroad Grade. The road traverses the south side of Mt. Tam and as you gradually gain elevation, a view of San Francisco and surrounding communities emerges on your left. Bypass all lesser trails—they're designated hiking-only.

You reach West Point Inn about 2 miles after the Hoo-Koo-E-Koo intersection. Water, beverages, and rest rooms are available here during most weekends. (See "Services" above for information about a fabulous pancake breakfast served on

Sundays.) Continue past West Point Inn and in almost 2 miles, Old Railroad Grade ends at paved East Ridgecrest Boulevard. Go right onto the pavement, keeping right at the split, and climb less than a half mile to the parking area and the East Peak gathering point. If it's a sunny day, picnic tables here provide a great spot on which to take a break and even people-watch. Sedentary tourists motor up here to take in the view and bikers love to hang out on the picnic tables and see who else biked up the hill, not that it's an overly arduous climb. Here, you'll find water and rest rooms, as well as a snack bar. But the best prize of all is the expansive vista seen via a walking path. It's worth checking out here but you'll want to throw a lock on your bike first.

When you've had your fill of tourists and the like, head back through the parking lot to where Old Railroad Grade popped you out onto the pavement. Across the road from there, a few yards away on your right is the beginning of Eldridge Grade. It's a narrow dirt road leading down from the pavement. This portion of the trailhead is fairly rocky, steep and downright gnarly—definitely not for beginners. (If you're not up to the challenge, just retrace your path down Old Railroad Grade. It's about 8.25 miles back down to Blithedale Park, 16.5 miles round-trip.)

Otherwise, hop on Eldridge Grade and begin a technical downhill run over rocky, and somewhat rutted terrain. Expect the trail to be an obstacle course, strewn with patches of loose rock and dirt as well as other bikers and hikers grunting up toward you. Walking is an option and will most certainly get you down the more difficult sections. The first 2.6 miles of Eldridge Grade is the most demanding. Go through three hairpin turns in less than 0.5 mile. After passing Wheeler Trail on your right, Eldridge Grade intersects Indian Fire Road. Hang a right onto Indian Fire Road, a wide, mildly rugged dirt road, and follow it about half a mile to another intersection. Here, a sign refers to the dirt road straight ahead leading to Phoenix Lake, (the site of more outstanding bike routes). Ignore that road (but vow to explore it at another time). Instead, make a hard right turn and follow the fire road 0.1 mile farther to yet another intersection. Signs here indicate Blithedale Ridge Road is straight ahead, bearing left. The right dirt road is a hairpin turn onto Hoo-Koo-E-Koo Trail. (How can you forget a name like that? This is the east end of Hoo-Koo-E-Koo and you passed its western end much earlier in the ride. Bikes are allowed.)

For now, go straight, veering left and follow Blithedale Ridge Road, going up a steep but very brief hill. Before you know it, you've topped the rise. Fly downhill and ignore several other trails on your right leading away from the main road. In about a mile from Hoo-Koo-E-Koo, a wide dirt road runs off on your right. It's unsigned but if you look down that road a short way, you'll see a couple of short telephone poles and maybe a glimpse of a water tank. This is what the locals refer to as Tank Turns Trail. Go right onto this unnamed fire road and continue a gentle downhill cruise. After passing two water tanks, the dirt road becomes pavement for a few yards as it runs through a tight turn, then changes to dirt again. A few yards farther, your trail runs into Old Railroad Grade at a left turning hairpin. Follow the hard left turn and in about 0.3 mile, go through a wooden gate at the bottom. When you hit real pavement, you're on West Blithedale Avenue. From here, continue on West Blithedale toward Blithedale Park and to wherever you left your car. Total mileage is about 13.2 miles.

RIDE 77 · Bolinas Ridge Fire Road

AT A GLANCE

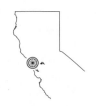

Length/configuration: 22.2-mile out-and-back (11.1 mile each way); dirt road sometimes masquerading as double-track

Aerobic difficulty: Moderately strenuous due to numerous hills

Technical difficulty: Mild

Scenery: Wide-open rolling grazing land; cool, shady redwood forest with some old-growth trees, views of misty Inverness Ridge on the Point Reyes peninsula, Tomales Bay, Bolinas Lagoon, and the town of Bolinas.

Special comments: Suitable for strong beginners who want to improve gear-shifting skills. Young families may enjoy riding it as a much-shortened out-and-back. Steep uphill stretches may force some kids (and beginners) to dismount and walk.

The Bolinas Ridge Fire Road is such an easy trail to follow, you probably won't need a map. It's well signed and the route is an obvious dirt road. Basically a hard-packed dirt and gravel road, masquerading as a double-track in some spots, its general smoothness makes it mildly technical terrain. Though there are numerous steep hills, none are unforgivingly long, generally about a quarter-mile in length. Riding the route as an out-and-back from north to south is mostly uphill with steepness up to a 9% grade, forcing some beginners and youngsters to dismount and walk. Not to worry. There are plenty of welcomed flat and coasting sections throughout. Keep in mind that as you grind up all those rolling hills of open pasture and carry on into a redwood forest, the return from south to north is mostly downhill. Unobstructed views of nearby ridges make the return simply exhilarating. A popular route, riders of all abilities enjoy the Bolinas Ridge Fire Road, riding it in any number of configurations. Though the following trail description is written as a 22.2-mile out-and-back (11.1 mile each way), other configurations are possible, such as a shorter out-and-back, turning around at any point; a point-to-point requiring a shuttle car; as a loop which incorporates paved Sir Francis Drake Boulevard, CA 1, and Bolinas-Fairfax Road; or as an add-on to any of the other nearby biking routes. Though Point Reyes National Seashore is the gem of western Marin County, only limited mountain biking is allowed here in the park. Of all the legal bike trails available, many are rated easy to moderate aerobically, and mostly mild technically. Most of these trails are suited for youngsters. (Visit the Bear Valley Visitor Center and ask for an official park map and their handout on suggested rides.)

Unlike other regions in northern California, the Point Reyes peninsula is a land of shakes, rattles and rolls. This is earthquake country! Plate tectonics is the name of the dance here as two land masses—the Pacific and North American plates—subtly bump and grind against each other. The stretch at which the two plates collide and rub make up the San Andreas Fault Line, running north and south. Highway 1 (CA 1), closely parallels the fault line, crisscrossing it along the rift zone. To the west of the fault line, the eastern edge of the Pacific plate pushes and slides northward

RIDE 77 · Bolinas Ridge Fire Road

against the other plate. As a result, land is forced above sea level, forming the Point Reyes peninsula (most of which is designated the Point Reyes National Seashore). The peninsula along with the Pacific Plate continues its slow migration north toward Alaska at a rate of about two inches a year. The North American plate east of the fault line travels much more slowly, moving west against the peninsula. The subtle dance builds pressure along the fault line and relief eventually comes in the form of hundreds of small tremors. Occasionally, the land surface breaks from the stress and the two plates actually shimmies a significant distance, resulting in a major earthquake. At the Bear Valley Visitor Center, fine interpretative displays give you more insight into the area's geological history. If you have time—and can bear to part with your

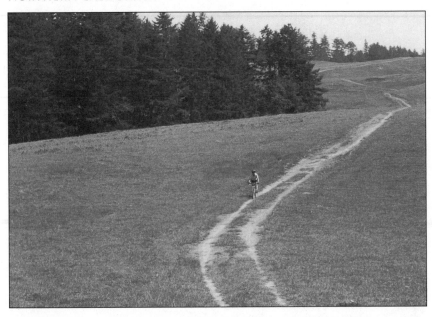

The return to the north trailhead is mostly descending on gently rolling hills.

bike—take the Earthquake Walk, a hiking-only trail that follows the Rift Zone Trail (located near the Visitor Center). There, you'll see markers that literally show how much both plates have shifted over time.

General location: About 25 miles north of San Francisco, along CA 1.

Elevation change: 1,310 feet; starting and low elevation about 360 feet; high point about 1,670 feet. Lots of hills, so you gain and lose elevation repeatedly.

Season: Year-round.

Services: None on the trail. Some services in Olema and Point Reyes Station, about 1 to 2.5 miles toward the west. Nearby Samuel P. Taylor State Park, about 2 miles to the east, offers fine campgrounds, rest rooms, water, and picnic tables. Complete services can be found in San Rafael and surrounding cities of eastern Marin County.

Hazards: Occasional poison oak along the road.

Rescue index: This is a popular route year-round. During the summer and weekends, your chances of finding a trail user who may be of help are better than other times of the year. Nevertheless, you should be self-reliant. If no one comes along, make your own way to either trailheads both of which are located next to frequently traveled roads, and flag down a passing motorist. The fire road is easily accessible by emergency vehicles.

Land status: Golden Gate National Recreation Area, managed by Point Reyes National Seashore.

Maps: *Point Reyes National Seashore,* official park map and brochure published by the National Park Service. Other handouts at Bear Valley Visitor Center. *Marin Bicycle Map,* published by Marin County Bicycle Coalition; (415) 488-1245. *Trail Map of*

Point Reyes National Seashore, published by Tom Harrison Maps, 2 Falmouth Cove, San Rafael, CA 94901, (800) 265-9090, www.tomharrisonmaps.com.

Finding the trail: To get to the north trailhead from San Francisco, drive north on US 101 across the Golden Gate Bridge. Take the Sir Francis Drake Boulevard exit south of San Rafael and follow it as it winds its way through San Anselmo, Fairfax, and then through Samuel P. Taylor State Park. Stay on Sir Francis Drake for a little over 4 miles past the state park main entrance to almost the top of the hill before Olema. On the east side of the hill, keep an eye out for a tiny, narrow dirt pulloff on the south side of the road, next to a wooden pedestrian gate and a trailhead sign. (Actually, the pulloff is a wide dirt shoulder.) Park off the pavement and begin pedaling here. You'll need to hoist your bike over the gate or barbed-wire fence.

To ride as a point-to-point, set-up your return shuttle-car at the north trailhead and begin pedaling from the south trailhead. (If you'd rather do more climbing than descending, start at the north end and arrange your shuttle cars accordingly.) To get to the south trailhead, there are two approaches. You can take Sir Francis Drake Boulevard into Fairfax and pick up Bolinas-Fairfax Road (it's a paved street simply signed Bolinas Road in Fairfax—not the same road as in nearby San Anselmo). Follow Bolinas Road as it winds up and over the shoulder of Pine Mountain and across Alpine Dam, arriving at the forested south trailhead in about 10 miles. Or you can follow US 101 north from San Francisco to Highway 1 (CA 1). Continue on Highway 1 north toward Bolinas. At the northern end of the Bolinas Lagoon, go right onto unsigned, paved Bolinas-Fairfax Road. Follow it for about 4.3 curvy miles uphill to the south trailhead, located on your left amid the shade of a redwood forest.

Sources of additional information:

Point Reyes National Seashore
National Park Service
Point Reyes, CA 94956

Bear Valley Visitor Center
Bear Valley Rd., just north of Olema
(415) 663-1092

Bicycle Trails Council of Marin
P.O. Box 13842
San Rafael, CA 94913
(415) 479-5482

Notes on the trail: At the route's northern trailhead (Sir Francis Drake Boulevard), begin by hoisting your bike over the pedestrian gate or barbed-wire fence. Surrounded by wide-open, gently rolling hills, pedal the single-track a few yards down and then up to the Bolinas Ridge Fire Road. Go left onto the fire road. The entire 11.1-mile road contains numerous short hills to grind up and cruise down, some of which vary in pitch from flat to 9%, though most of them are about 8%. The road surface you encounter at the beginning is fairly indicative of the terrain throughout. You're rewarded with sweeping curves and views of the nearby mountain ranges from atop Bolinas Ridge. Go through several cattle gates, leaving them the way you found them—opened or closed. If it's a warm, sunny day, don't expect to see any shade until about 4.6 miles. Don't get too excited about it though—the shade is cast by a row of about four closely spaced eucalyptus trees.

Bypass all other trails that intersect the fire road, going past Jewell Trail after 1.3 miles from the start, and Shafter Bridge Trail after 5 miles. At about 5.6 miles, you experience a major environmental change as you enter a redwood forest. It's cool, lush and shady here and the surrounding vegetation changes to ferns and thick understory. Most of the redwoods here are young-growth but once in a while, you spot a sizable one, almost the width of a Volkswagen Beetle. There are a few sawed stumps here too, the only evidence that tall and mighty trees once stood here. A few semi-exposed tree roots awaken your bike-handling skills.

At just over 6 miles, Randall Trail, a dirt fire road, drops down on your right. Bypass it, staying on the main fire road. (Incidentally, Randall Trail allows bikes and it's a favorite route of strong bikers who climb it. From Highway 1, it ascends 920 feet in 1.7 miles to the Bolinas Ridge Fire Road.) Continue past McCurdy Trail, a wide single-track that descends on your right down toward Highway 1. (Bikes are allowed on McCurdy and it, too, is another favorite of hearty bikers, ascending 1,270 feet from Highway 1.) When you cruise past a water tank on your left, you're about 2.5 miles from reaching the south trailhead at Bolinas-Fairfax Road. A little over a mile farther, you begin climbing out of the forest. As you begin the last descent, you might catch a great glimpse of Bolinas far below on your right and Pine Mountain Ridge on your left. Bolinas Ridge Fire Road terminates at the south trailhead after climbing a half-mile stretch back into the forest.

To return, turn around and go back the way you came. Though there are a few uphills in this direction, you've earned your reward—a mostly downhill run back to the north trailhead.

RIDE 78 · Barnabe Peak Loop and Devil's Gulch

AT A GLANCE

Length/configuration: 9.8-mile loop with an out-and-back, counterclockwise; mostly dirt fire road with short stretch on vehicle road and bike path

Aerobic difficulty: Loop is moderately strenuous due to exceptionally steep hills; out-and-back is easy

Technical difficulty: Mildly technical though the extreme steepness of some hills makes it a challenge to stay on the bike

Scenery: Lush, shady forest along creeks, rising to ridge of open grassland dotted with oak trees. On clear days, you can see the Pacific Ocean, Point Reyes National Seashore, and Mount Tamalpais. Papermill Creek is home to spawning silver salmon during the winter.

Special comments: The out-and-back along Devil's Gulch and the paved bike path are perfect for young children and kid-trailers.

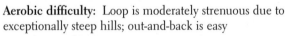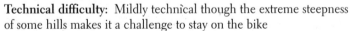

The loop ride up to Barnabe Peak from the main area of Samuel P. Taylor State Park demands great stamina but little technical skill. Though the peak tops out at 1,466 feet, the highpoint of this counterclockwise loop sits just below it at about 1,400 feet. Starting from Papermill Creek within the park's cool and shady main picnic area, the trail climbs 1,320 feet in about three unrelenting miles. Be sure to eat your Wheaties because some portions of the journey to the peak measures more than 13% steepness. For strong beginners, staying on your bike and not popping wheelies becomes the technical challenge of the day. The reward for all your grunting and

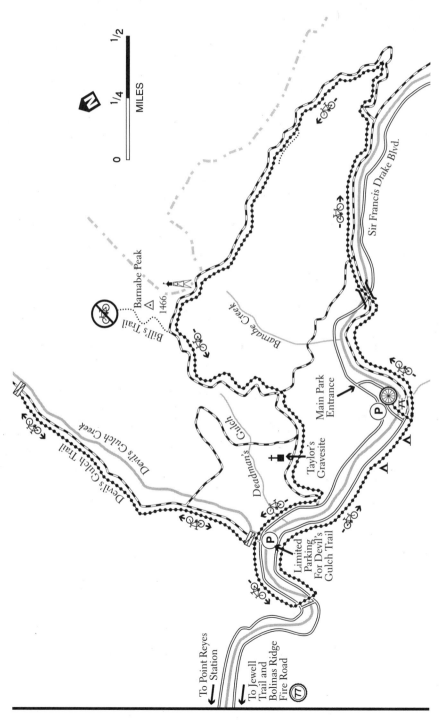

0   1/4   1/2

MILES

Barnabe Peak

Bill's Trail

1466

Barnabe Creek

Deadman's Gulch

Devil's Gulch Creek

Devil's Gulch Trail

Taylor's Gravesite

Main Park Entrance

Sir Francis Drake Blvd.

P

P

Limited Parking For Devil's Gulch Trail

To Point Reyes Station

To Jewell Trail and Bolinas Ridge Fire Road

77

groaning is a 2.5-mile downhill on a smooth wide fire road back to Sir Francis Drake Boulevard—you might not ever have to crank the pedal! After that and before you close the loop, ride a short and very easy 1-mile out-and-back stretch on Devil's Gulch Creek Trail (a 2-mile round-trip stretch). Finish the entire ride by cruising the paved bike path along shady Papermill Creek. Both Devil's Gulch Creek Trail and the paved path are well-suited for novices and young children.

Many parks in the state park system have historic backgrounds and Samuel P. Taylor Park is no exception. Like many ambitious entrepreneurs who recovered from gold-rush fever, Samuel Penfield Taylor bankrolled several business enterprises with about $5,700 worth of gold dust in August, 1852. He built a papermill here and produced newsprint for many San Francisco dailies as well as fine paper and square-bottom paper bags (a popular novelty at the time). Elsewhere in this canyon, Taylor operated a black-powder mill but that venture ended his dream of entrepreneurial fame when it literally blew up in 1874. He never reopened the powder mill. In that same year, a narrow-gauge railroad was built, easily connecting this canyon with the Point Reyes–Tomales Bay area. Perhaps his greatest endeavor that lives on, sort of, is Camp Taylor, a resort hotel that offered outdoor camping as an attraction. In the late 1870s and early 1880s, Taylorville, as it was called then, became a popular weekend retreat. Today, the idea of Camp Taylor lives on as Samuel P. Taylor State Park, which today encompasses over 2,600 acres and still attracts weekend crowds throughout most of the year.

General location: About 60 miles north of San Francisco.

Elevation change: 1,300 feet; starting elevation 120 feet; high point 1,400 feet; low point 100 feet. The loop is essentially one big, nasty hill climb, interspersed with brief, mellow stretches, followed by an unrelenting downhill. The out-and-back is a very gentle uphill ride with plenty of level stretches.

Season: Year-round.

Services: Drinking water, rest rooms, hot showers, picnic areas, public phone, and 60 maintained campsites within the main entrance of the state park. Various other services such as eateries and grocery stores available in nearby towns. All other services available in San Rafael, about 20 miles east.

Hazards: Watch out for occasional poison oak, especially along Devil's Gulch Creek Trail. During the summer months, the paved bike path through the campground can become congested with youngsters on bikes and walkers (including baby-strollers). Part of the route follows Sir Francis Drake Boulevard on a tiny shoulder for 0.5 mile, and it is a well-traveled vehicle road, often with speeding motorists. Ride this portion with extreme caution! Getting to the Devil's Gulch Creek Trailhead is a safety challenge; see "Finding the trail" for a cautionary note.

Rescue Index: Most of this ride is on the dry and steep north side of the creek canyon. That means you won't encounter many other trail users, if any at all, who may be of help. Should you need emergency help, you might find assistance at the fire lookout, located at the route's high point. Otherwise, you'll have to make your own way back to the campground or flag down a passing motorist on Sir Francis Drake Boulevard.

Land status: Samuel P. Taylor State Park.

Maps: *Samuel P. Taylor State Park*, official park map published by the California Department of Parks & Recreation, available at ranger station for a small fee. *Marin Bicycle Map*, published by Marin County Bicycle Coalition; (415) 488-1245.

Finding the trail: From the city of San Rafael, drive 15 miles west on 3rd Street to 2nd Street to Red Hill Boulevard, which merges into Sir Francis Drake Boulevard as you go through San Anselmo. Continue through the towns of Fairfax, Woodacre, Forest Knolls, and Lagunitas. As you cross into the state park boundary, the road begins weaving through an increasingly dense redwood forest. The ranger kiosk and main entrance is on your left, on the south side of Sir Francis Drake, 2.5 miles beyond Lagunitas. Summer weekends tend to be busy and, if you're not camping, rangers may ask that you park outside the main entrance, alongside Sir Francis Drake (which means you avoid paying the day-use fee). Wherever you park, begin pedaling by accessing the paved bike path at the Redwood Grove Picnic Area, located inside the main park entrance on the south side of Papermill Creek (also known as Lagunitas Peak). Note: Redwood Grove Picnic Area is not the same as the Main Picnic Area.

If you want to ride Devil's Gulch Creek Trail with youngsters, the one and only safest way to reach the trailhead is to drive there. Yep, even if you're camping in the park. The only other way to reach it is by foot (or bike) via shoulderless Sir Francis Drake Boulevard—and that, to me, is a dangerous alternative. So, to reach the trailhead, drive out of the main park entrance and go left onto Sir Francis Drake. Travel 1 mile and look for a small dirt parking area on the left side (creekside) of the road, directly across Devil's Gulch Creek Trail. Cautiously turn left and park here. (Note, this trail is actually a paved road that may be closed by a wide gate.) To begin the ride, hold back the kiddies and cross with your bikes when it's safe.

Sources of additional information:

Samuel P. Taylor State Park
P.O. Box 251
Lagunitas, California 94938
(415) 488-9897

Bicycle Trails Council of Marin
P.O. Box 13842
San Rafael, CA 94913
(415) 479-5482

Notes on the trail: If it's a sunny, summer day, don't be fooled by the coolness found in the shade of the redwood forest alongside Papermill Creek. Most of the loop is located on drier, south-facing slopes and it gets boiling hot out there, so bring plenty of water. Following and staying on the proper route to the Ridge Trail trailhead is your biggest challenge. This ride description begins and finishes on the south side of Sir Francis Drake Boulevard, near the ranger station. So, from within the Redwood Grove Picnic area, look for a paved bike path and follow it east. In a few yards, you reach a metal gate. Go through the gate and almost immediately, the paved path ends and a wide dirt trail begins. Young-growth redwood trees here shade the path as it parallels Papermill Creek, winding through the lush creek canyon. At 0.5 mile, go up a bridge and over Sir Francis Drake Boulevard. After the bridge, continue following the easy and wide dirt trail due east. The creek, which has crossed underneath Sir Francis Drake as well, is now on your right, sandwiched between your dirt trail and the road. Your unsigned trail is a hard-packed, smooth dirt, fairly wide multi-use trail.

You're on the right trail when you come to a signed intersection at about 0.7 mile from the Redwood Grove Picnic Area. Here, the sign indicates Madrone Group camping area in 0.9 mile, Barnabe Trail 1.7 miles, Devil's Gulch in 2.2 miles—all in the direction behind you. The Ridge Trail, on the other hand, is reached in 0.6 mile straight ahead. Continue on this flat dirt trail and sure enough, at about 1.3

miles, an unsigned trail leads steeply uphill on your left, about 13% grade. The only sign here states that if you stay on the flat trail, you'd reach Mt. Tam in 12.6 miles. This left trail is Ridge Trail according to the park map.

Take a deep breath and gear down as you take this left trail—the unnamed Ridge Trail. Here is where staying on the route is a no-brainer but the going gets tougher. For the next 2 miles, you begin climbing out of the creek canyon and its cool redwood forest. The first mile is a steep pull, softened by a few brief mellow inclines. Your only real technical challenge on this mildly rough, hard-packed road is staying on your bike despite the extreme steepness. If you're not accustomed to riding these kinds of cruel inclines, not "popping wheelies" will be your technical challenge. The terrain is more open, dry and less shady as you begin to rise above tiny valleys on your right. Just when you think you've had enough, you reach the ridge and though the trail continues to ascend, the grade is merciful. Typical terrain on ridges is a roller-coaster ride and the Ridge Trail is no exception. In just over 3 miles, you get your first glimpse of the fire lookout, a somewhat modern structure.

As you torture yourself up the last nasty hill toward the lookout, you'll probably become so focused that you won't notice a tiny sign indicating you're leaving the state park boundary. Not to worry. Just stay on the fire road and at about 3.3 miles (from the beginning at Redwood Grove picnic area), you finally reach the lookout. (Actually, you're at the base of the hill upon which the lookout sits, about 50–100 feet up. The lookout is a working station and visitors are not invited, so don't bother to tackle the extra distance to it.) Elevation here at the base is about 1,400 feet, the high point of this ride. If you're lucky to have a clear day, you can see Drake's Bay, the Pacific Ocean, Point Reyes National Seashore, and Mount Tamalpais.

From here, it's darn-near all downhill, baby. And you've earned it. At the base of the lookout, bear left onto a fire road and re-enter the state park. Too bad the descent is so short, only 1.3 fast miles all the way down to Sir Francis Drake Boulevard on mostly wide fire road. Though this dirt road is not signed in the field, the map labels it Barnabe Trail. As you fly down the hill, watch out for loose patches of gravel, especially as you zip through curves over steep inclines. On your way down, bypass Bill's Trail, a hiking-only trail at about 3.8 miles. A dirt road appears on your right at about 4.3 miles; ignore it. Continue down Barnabe Trail and intersect Sir Francis Drake Boulevard at about 4.6 miles.

Hang a right onto this somewhat busy vehicle road and pedal the narrow shoulder for 0.3 mile. Immediately after going over Devil's Gulch Creek, turn right onto a paved side road toward the horse corral. Cruise around a wide metal gate and in a few yards, the pavement ends and becomes a wide dirt road. You're now on Devil's Gulch Trail, a wide, smooth, technically easy route that closely parallels Devil's Gulch off on your right. The environment on this trail is completely different from what you just rode. Here, the vegetation is lush with ferns and water-loving plants and aromatic bay laurel trees. It's totally shaded here amid the sound of trickling Devil's Gulch. In contrast to that, the terrain on your left is grassy rolling hills, totally exposed to the parching sun if not for a few stands of oak trees. There's a tiny trail next to the creek and you'll be tempted to pedal it but don't. It's a hiking-only trail. Besides, an agonizing week of oozing, itching poison oak blisters is a lot to pay for a short 1.1 mile single-track thrill. At about 6.8 miles (still measuring from Redwood Grove Picnic Area), bypass a horse corral. Continue following Devil's Gulch Creek upstream, still on your right, and at 6.8 miles, you reach the end of the trail at a locked gate and fence within the shady forest—a great spot for a break.

When you're ready, turn around and go back the way you came, enjoying a fast descent to Sir Francis Drake Boulevard. You reach Sir Francis Drake at just over 8 miles. Cautiously make a right onto shoulderless Sir Francis Drake. Immediately look for a bridge, which spans Papermill Creek, on the other side of the road, about 0.2 mile farther and just before a blind curve. Watch for cars as you carefully and quickly cross both lanes of traffic, possibly stopping and waiting for a safe moment. Walking is recommended.

Head across the bridge, going through a gate, and pick up the paved bike path. The paved path runs both left and right and for those of you wanting miles, read about the add-ons below. For those of you with nothing to prove, bear left on the sedate bike path and follow it through the shady redwood forest. At approximately 9 miles, you cruise past the site of the old paper mill and a few yards farther, the Fish Ladder in the creek. (Spawning runs of the silver salmon occur annually, beginning in November while the steelhead trout run is usually between February and March. And it's quite a sight to behold!) At 9.7 miles, you reach the Redwood Grove Picnic Area and close the loop. From here, make your way back to your car.

For optional miles, here are two possibilities, both of which involve turning right onto the bike path at the bridge.

1. If you want easy, flat miles, go right toward the town of Tocaloma for about 2.5 miles and then turn around.

2. If you're still aching for a real challenge today, consider tackling Bolinas Ridge Fire Road, as described in Ride 77. To access that ride, hang a right on the bike path and pedal about 0.7 mile to Jewell Trail that peels off on the left. Follow Jewell as it climbs for about a mile to Bolinas Ridge Fire Road. Enjoy!

RIDE 79 · Pine Mountain–Repack Loop

AT A GLANCE

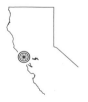

Length/configuration: 19-mile loop; clockwise; fire roads, dirt roads, and pavement; (several options exist: 5-mile Repack Road loop and 13-mile all-dirt loop)

Aerobic difficulty: Strenuous due to steep climbs over rugged terrain

Technical difficulty: Intermediate with some advanced sections over rocky and loose terrain. Repack Road is not recommended for beginners as it is an extremely steep, uneven, and somewhat loose dirt trail.

Scenery: Views of rolling open hills, a pygmy cypress forest, and remote mountain ranges in the heart of Marin County

Special comments: Repack Road was, arguably, the site of the first mountain bike race in the entire country. Truly the Mother of all historic mountain bike races in the country, this is a must-ride for serious bikers.

With an average steepness of 12% and pitches of up to 30%, this 2.1-mile screaming downhill stretch of the overall loop is definitely not for beginners. Repack is a rocky, loose and often dusty narrow dirt road marked by rain ruts. The rest of the loop around Pine Mountain is not as technical though there are some advanced technical sections of brief duration. So what? Walking up or down them is always an acceptable technique, which means even strong adventurous beginners can ride most of this loop. Throughout the entire loop, the terrain climbs steeply up and down, gaining and losing about 1,600 feet. Lying in the Marin Municipal Water District (MMWD) and Marin County Open Space, the route leads you up and down several ridges, through many different ecosystems, and offers a splendid view of the northern San Francisco Bay and beyond. Plenty of downhill stretches over remote terrain, especially the area around the secluded backside of Pine Mountain, make the huffing and puffing up the steep sections worth it.

But hey, this isn't just any bike ride. If ever there was a "classic" ride in northern California, the Pine Mountain–Repack Loop is it. This ride has been the site of the Thanksgiving "Appetite Seminar" since 1974, but that's not its claim to fame. Repack Road was the site of the reportedly first-ever mountain bike race on the West Coast, having been staged in 1976 using old clunker bikes equipped with one-speed, balloon-tires and coaster brakes. The winning time was posted by early mountain bike pioneer, Gary Fisher, with a winning time of 4 minutes, 22 seconds. (The time, reportedly, still stands as the fastest time down Repack.) Referred to as Cascade Canyon Road on some maps, the road was dubbed Repack due to the fact that many racers had to repack their old coaster brake hubs after burning them out during the race. In 1977, Joe Breeze, another local bicycling pioneer and entrepreneur, built the first real successful batch of modern mountain bike frames. Did they think then that their modified two-wheeled contraptions would become a multi-million-dollar outdoor activity with an international following?

General location: About 55 miles north of San Francisco.

Elevation change: 1,600 feet; starting and low elevation about 120 feet; high point 1,720 feet. Lots of long hill climbs interspersed with mellow sections, followed by descents toward Kent Lake. Then comes a series of climbs up to San Geronimo Ridge before an extreme drop back down into town.

Season: Year-round though some roads are subject to closure by the fire marshall during times of high fire danger. Summer is extremely hot so riding in the morning or early evening is preferred.

Services: None on the trail. Most services available in the town of Fairfax; all services in San Rafael.

Hazards: During the summer, the trail can get unbearably hot, especially along exposed, shadeless sections of the route and wearing sunscreen is a must. Be sure to carry plenty of water. Several tiny creeks offer water but it must be treated before drinking. Though rarely seen, stay alert for mountain lions.

Rescue index: This ride runs through somewhat remote watershed land. Though this is a well-known route, don't expect to meet other trail users who may be of help during an emergency—you may be waiting a long time. You should make your own way back to the Pine Mountain–Azalea Hill trailhead or to the Elliot Nature Preserve at the end of Repack Road at Cascade Drive. The Preserve is popular with hikers and dog-walkers since it borders a residential neighborhood in the town of Fairfax.

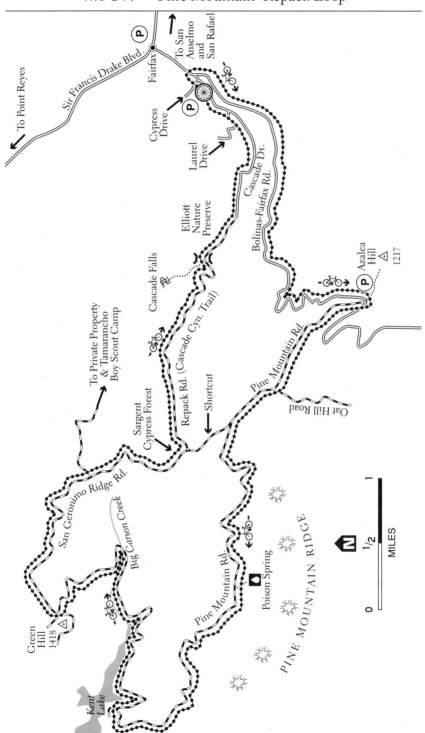

Land status: Marin Municipal Water District, Mount Tamapalis Watershed and Marin County Open Space.

Maps: A *Rambler's Guide to the Trails of Mt. Tamapalis and the Marin Headlands,* published by The Olmsted & Bros. Map Co., (510) 658-6534. (The route is not completely shown on the map. A stretch less than a mile on the northern-most edge of the route runs off the map.) *Marin Bicycle Map,* published by Marin County Bicycle Coalition; (415) 488-1245.

Finding the trail: The trailhead is within the town of Fairfax, located 4 miles west of San Rafael. From San Francisco, drive north on US 101 and take the San Anselmo/Sir Francis Drake Boulevard exit. Follow Sir Francis Drake due west through San Anselmo to Fairfax. Once in Fairfax, finding the Bolinas-Fairfax Road is a bit difficult. Look for the town's movie theater and public parking lot, both of which are located on Broadway which parallels the south side of Sir Francis Drake. Make your way left off Sir Francis Drake to Broadway and look for Bolinas Road (same as Bolinas-Fairfax Road) one block west of the theater. The public parking lot is on Broadway at the beginning of Bolinas Road. Consider packing a lunch on this ride. Several sandwich shops are located in town. You can park in the public lot or continue a short ways up to a tiny maintained town park in the residential neighborhood. To get to the town park, turn south onto Bolinas Road and in less than a half mile, turn right onto Cascade Drive. Follow Cascade for about 500 yards to the Cypress Drive junction and the tiny town park. You'll find street parking here, not a parking lot. Park and begin pedaling from here.

Sources of additional information:

Marin Municipal Water District
220 Nellen Ave.
Corte Madera, CA 94925
(415) 924-4600 or (415) 459-5267

Sunshine Bicycle Center
737 Center Blvd.
Fairfax, CA 94930
(415) 459-3334

Located one block east of the theater, Center Blvd. is the east extension of Broadway.

Bicycle Trails Council of Marin
P.O. Box 13842
San Rafael, CA 94913
(415) 479-5482

Notes on the trail: Before heading out for this ride, be sure to bring plenty of water, snacks, and a good map, either the *Marin Bicycle Map* or the Olmsted Brothers map (see "Maps" above). Although this is a famous ride, don't expect to see the route well-marked.

From the tiny town park at the junction of Cascade and Cypress Drives, begin by descending back down Cascade to Bolinas Road. Watch for residential traffic and turn right onto Bolinas, a two-lane narrow paved road with moderate traffic. The road immediately begins to climb, varying from 2% to 7% grade with a few welcome level sections. Continue on Bolinas past a hiking trail leading to Concrete Pipe and Phoenix Lake. A few yards farther, ride past Sky Oaks Road which leads to Lake Lagunitas, Bon Tempe Lake and the water treatment plant. At just over 2 miles from your starting point, go past Meadow Club and its golf courses. From this point, Bolinas Road leads you into the Mount Tamalpais Watershed of the MMWD. In almost 1.5 miles from the Meadow Club (3.4 miles from your starting point), after topping the ridge near Azalea Hill, you finally reach the junction of signed Pine

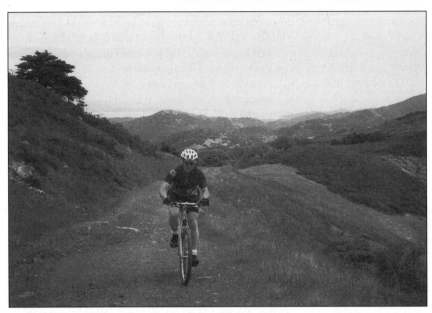

Unlike Repack Road, Pine Mountain Road, pedaled here by Bruce, can be enjoyed by most riders with decent stamina and intermediate skills, even strong beginners with the right attitude.

Mountain Road leading off on your right toward the northwest amid a wide-open panorama of rolling hills. A double metal gate closes off this wide fire road and across from it, up a few yards on the left of the paved road, is a small dirt parking area at the trailhead to Azalea Hill. (If you want to do this ride without going down Repack Road, you could park your car here, making the Pine Mountain Loop a 13-mile, all-dirt ride.)

Say good-bye to paved Bolinas Road and hello to dirt. Hop onto Pine Mountain and wake up your technical ability. The fire road is rugged with semi-buried and loose rock, interspersed with long stretches of hard-packed dirt. For the next 2.8 miles, the road is devoid of shade, mostly surrounded by low bushes. Climb up and down steep but short stretches as you follow the ridge line up to Pine Mountain. In some stretches where the road is so strewn with rocks ranging from golf ball to cantaloupe size, frequent use by bikers and hikers has blazed a sort of single-track through the obstacle field. Don't forget to look back for a wide view of the northern San Francisco Bay.

At about 4.5 miles, go past unsigned Oat Hill Road leading off on your left. This junction is signed "Pine Mountain" straight ahead. Continue straight and about a half mile farther you reach another junction, also signed "Pine Mountain," this time to the left. (For riders who park at the Pine Mountain–Azalea Hill parking area and plan to ride the 13-mile all-dirt loop option, skipping Repack, the right unsigned "shortcut" road is the trail you'll be returning on. For riders who only seek the thrill of screaming downhill on Repack on the 5-mile loop option, hang a right, taking this shortcut to the top of Repack. You reach Repack in about 0.3 mile.) The rest of you die-hards, bear left onto Pine Mountain Road. About 1.5 miles farther, you reach Pine Mountain, the high point of the entire ride at elevation 1,720 feet. Climb the extra 40 feet to the top for the view. Notice the 150-year-old stone walls erected to separate the Mexican Land Grants. Don't be fooled into thinking that all the hard work is behind you. Even though the fire road begins descending down the back side of Pine Mountain, toward Kent Lake, there are plenty of short and steep climbs to come.

The ecosystem begins to change from a dry, semi-arid landscape to a lush, shady forest of fragrant laurel, oak, and mixed conifer trees. Watch out for occasional poison oak along the road. Cruise past Poison Springs hiking trail on your left and continue grinding up and smiling down a bunch of steep little hills. Still basically descending toward Kent Lake, you begin to see young-growth redwoods growing among the other trees and standing above lush understory. At just over 9 miles from your starting point in town, the shady road descends into a sharp unsigned hairpin fork, that is, a hard turn to the right as well as to the left. Make the right hairpin turn and in a few yards, you should see a green carsonite signpost marked "PM2." Don't expect to see a large body of water making up Kent Lake as the forest is dense here, effectively obscuring your view. Follow the road as it traverses a thickly forested slope, passing many other green signposts, marked "PM3," "PM4," and so on. The road eventually begins climbing out of the drainage. If you're riding early in the year, you're likely to ride through several trickling streams along this stretch. At about 10.5 miles, just after green signpost PM8, the sound of a brisk running stream can be heard down on your left. Almost a mile farther, the road leads you through a wet crossing through Big Carson Creek and then up a south-facing slope. Erosion has washed part of the road down into the ravine, narrowing the road in several places. As you grind up the road, look left and you can see a portion of the road on which you just rode.

At 12.4 miles from your starting point in town (about 9 miles from the Pine Mountain Road trailhead at Azalea Hill), you reach a major, unsigned four-way intersection of obvious dirt roads, near the Green Hill summit. The road straight ahead descends and the left climbs gently toward the southwest. Take the right turn, climbing up a steep stretch, due north. Though the road is unsigned, you're on San Geronimo Ridge Road and the trail condition is fairly technical due to rocky conditions, loose gravel, and steepness. As you continue up to the ridge, the forest thins and you can see distant ridges across a valley off on your left. In that valley runs Sir Francis Drake Boulevard and you can faintly hear its roar of traffic. Carry on following the well-traveled dirt road as it leads uphill toward the ridge. About a mile from the four-way intersection, the road runs underneath a power line and goes through an opening in a dilapidated barbed-wire fence. Your view here is expansive now that you're on the top of the ridge amid rolling, open hills.

Stay on the well-defined dirt road, still rocky and rugged. At about 14 miles, bypass an unsigned dirt road descending on your left. Almost a mile farther, ride through the pygmy Sargent Cypress Forest, a short 600-yard stretch of short trees with a somewhat thick canopy. Just as you leave the cypress forest, the dirt road junctions with the top of unsigned Repack Road, also known as Cascade Canyon Trail. (For bikers riding the 13-mile loop, continue straight, bearing right on San Geronimo Ridge Road, and in about 0.2 mile, you intersect with Pine Mountain Loop. Go left and retrace your path back to the trailhead and your car.)

Turn left onto Repack. At this junction is the beginning of the famous downhill race! A small hill beyond this tame road obscures your view of the dangers which lurk just over the top. It's definitely not for beginners. The trail condition is loose and rocky, spiced with rain ruts and some fairly steep sections verging on 30%. Bounded on both sides by tall bushes, this narrow dirt road drops about 1,300 feet down toward

Cascade Creek in about 2.1 miles. Nowadays, the speed limit is a radar-controlled 15 mph. When you reach the creek and the "Finish Line" rock, at almost 17 miles, go right over the bridge and continue the dirt road as it leads through the Elliot Nature Preserve. The Preserve dirt road crosses the creek four times, though the creek may be dry depending on the time of year. If the creek is raging, walk your bike on the unrideable (posted "No Bikes") single-track to the left of the first stream crossing. When you exit the Preserve through a wooden gate, bear right onto the paved residential street. Though it's not signed here, the road is Cascade Drive. Continue the gradual descent on Cascade for about 1.4 miles. You finally reach your car next to the tiny neighborhood park at about 19 miles.

RIDE 80 · China Camp Shoreline—Ridge Loop

AT A GLANCE

Length/configuration: 10.5-mile loop, counterclockwise; with optional trails to shorten or lengthen the distance

Aerobic difficulty: Mostly moderate with a long, easy stretch on wide, flat single-track

Technical difficulty: Mildly technical with some intermediate sections of deeply rutted and steep, loose terrain

Scenery: Views of San Pablo Bay, the East Bay hills, Mount Diablo, Angel Island, and San Francisco.

Special comments: Portions suitable for beginners and gutsy young, freewheeling children. Kid trailers not recommended.

For mountain bikers, China Camp State Park can be considered an exception in the state park system because nearly all trails here allow bikes. It's a small park, only 1,512 acres, but if you love cruising, moderate single-track, you just might find true love here. The route described is based on a 10.5-mile loop, most of which is on hard-pack single-track trails. Most of the route is mildly technical, manageable by beginners wanting to develop their single-track riding skills. Beginners can ride the first 4.5 miles as an out-and-back, for a total distance of 9 miles with a maximum elevation gain of less than 150 feet. Hardier riders can tackle the full loop, ascending and descending about 800 feet on sometimes steep but short hills, or even venturing off on other trails at various junctions on the loop.

Along the way, the single-track trail hugs slopes of hills forested by live oak, madrone, and incredibly aromatic California laurel and eucalyptus trees, and meanders through rolling grassy meadows. And yes, you get views of the marshlands, San Pablo Bay, the north bay and the regions across the bay, and glimpses of San Francisco. During the summer, the trails in this park are hard-packed and even dusty in some places. Conversely, wet days are likely to result in muddy, slippery conditions. Meadows display wildflowers in late spring.

Located three miles east of downtown San Rafael and about 30 miles north of San Francisco, China Camp is an immensely popular destination for bikers, hikers,

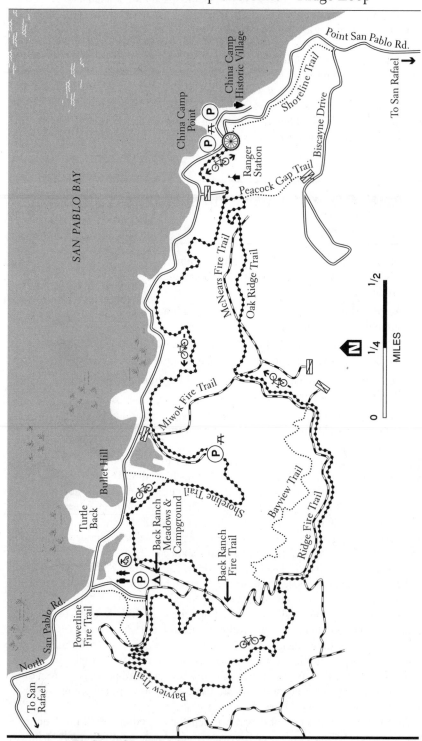

Point San Pablo Rd.

China Camp Historic Village

China Camp Point

To San Rafael

Shoreline Trail

Biscayne Drive

Ranger Station

Peacock Gap Trail

SAN PABLO BAY

McNears Fire Trail

Oak Ridge Trail

Miwok Fire Trail

½

¼

N

0

MILES

Bayview Trail

Ridge Fire Trail

Bullet Hill

Shoreline Trail

Turtle Back

Back Ranch Meadows & Campground

Back Ranch Fire Trail

North San Pablo Rd.

Powerline Fire Trail

Bayview Trail

To San Rafael

equestrians, campers, and picnickers year-round, especially on summer weekends. During a summer outing, the trail users I met were mostly bikers—singles, twosomes and groups, each one grinning and having a fun, rollicking time. There were folks on clunkers and others equipped from head to saddle with accessories equal to a college semester's tuition.

And speaking of tuition, get yourself a free, quick history lesson by visiting the informative museum at the China Camp Village after the ride. Here, preserved historic buildings take you back to the time when shrimp harvesting was the key in the establishment of a booming Chinese community. The tiny museum is well worth the visit. Before or after your history lesson, enjoy a refreshment from the snack bar there. Picnic tables are right smack on the pebbly beach, with an expansive view of the East Bay. If you didn't get enough riding, other trails await your exploration.

General location: 3 miles east of downtown San Rafael; about 30 miles north of San Francisco.

Elevation change: 670 feet; starting elevation and low point 80 feet; high point 750 feet. The first half hovers between 80 and 200 feet. The second half climbs roughly 500 feet in a little over 2 miles. Thereafter, the loop descends through a series of short ups and downs.

Season: Year-round.

Services: Drinking water, rest rooms, pay phones, and ample fee parking at Back Ranch Meadows Campground and China Camp Village. Interpretative museum and snack bar at China Camp Village during the summer. Free parking allowed in designated dirt parking pulloffs alongside North San Pedro Road and Point San Pedro Road. Camping in designated campgrounds permitted. All other services available in San Rafael.

Hazards: Hunting is not allowed inside the park boundaries but in the fall shotguns can be heard and duck hunters maybe seen in the outlying marsh area. When riding the single-track, stay alert for oncoming trail users (bikers, hikers, and equestrians).

Rescue index: This park is highly popular with other trail users especially on the weekends. Trails inside the park are generally within 1 mile from the one and only major road. Rangers on duty during the spring, summer, and fall.

Land status: China Camp State Park.

Maps: *China Camp State Park*, official park brochure. *Marin Bicycle Map*, published by Marin County Bicycle Coalition, (415) 488-1245.

Finding the trail: From either north- or southbound US 101, take the North San Pedro Road exit, which is adjacent to the Frank Lloyd Wright–designed Marin County Civic Center. Follow North San Pedro east as it approaches the northern edge of the San Pedro peninsula. North San Pedro winds its way east and enters China Camp State Park after 3 miles. Continue on North San Pedro past Back Ranch Meadows Campground to China Camp Village. Park in the dirt parking lot, adjacent to a commemorative stone plaque outside the entry driveway into China Camp Village. (North San Pedro Road becomes Point San Pedro Road after China Camp Village. If you reach Bicayne Drive, you've just exited the park and missed the suggested parking area.)

Sources of additional information:

China Camp State Park
Route 1, Box 244
San Rafael, CA 94901
(415) 456-0766

Start to Finish
1820 Fourth St.
San Rafael, CA
(415) 459-3990
Rents bikes.

Performance Bicycle
Montecito Shopping Center
369 Third St.

San Rafael, CA 94901
(415) 454-9063

Mike's Bicycle Center
1601 4th St.
San Rafael, CA 94901
(415) 454-3747

Bicycle Trails Council of Marin
P.O. Box 13842
San Rafael, CA 94913
(415) 479-5482

Notes on the trail: Begin by pedaling to the right (west) on the shoulder of North San Pedro Road for about 50 yards to a single-track trail on the left (south) side of the road. It's signed the Village Trail and is an easy, wide, hard-packed, dirt single-track. Follow it through a couple of switchbacks as it gradually climbs to a junction with Shoreline Trail in almost 200 yards. Upon reaching the intersection, the trail levels off. Continue straight onto Shoreline; do not make a hard hairpin turn to your left.

From here, stay on Shoreline Trail for just under 5 miles, following signs to Back Ranch Fire Trail and Back Ranch Meadows campground. Little technical skill is required for this section of the loop and beginners will grow accustomed to single-track riding in no time at all. The trail leads past China Camp Park Ranger Office at about 0.5 mile and then past Peacock Gap Trail at about 0.8 mile.

At about 2.5 miles from the trailhead, still on the single-track, you reach the intersection with the Miwok Fire Trail, as well as a dirt vehicle road. Cross the Miwok Fire Trail and turn left onto the dirt road, following it as it gently climbs to the Miwok Meadows Group Day Use area. Pick up the single-track Shoreline Trail again on the other side of the parking lot, where you see a sign marked "Shoreline Trail to Back Ranch 1 mile."

As you gently climb Shoreline Trail toward the Back Ranch Fire Trail, the path becomes a bit more technical with semi-buried small chunks of rough rock and a few exposed tree roots. The trail is still hard-packed, easy riding, and varying from a 4- to 8-feet wide. Continue past Bullet Hill Trail and Turtleback Nature Trail.

As you approach the Back Ranch Meadow Campground parking lot, you come to a fork that's signed. The right fork leads to the campground while the left is the continuation of Shoreline Trail. Stay left on Shoreline as it skirts around the southern edge of the campground. Cross Back Ranch Fire Trail (actually a dirt road) and follow Shoreline around the west side of the campground. Eventually, the trail skirts the western edge of the main parking lot behind the rest rooms. (How convenient!) Facilities available here include drinking water and pay phones.

At this point, you have ridden about 4.5 miles from the trailhead. The rest of the loop is slightly more challenging as the climbs are a bit steeper and sustained, and the trail condition is somewhat more technical in a few spots. Beginners can turn around here and retrace their path on Shoreline Trail back to China Camp Village.

Elevation here at the campground parking lot, next to the rest rooms, is about 130 feet. Continuing on, look behind the rest rooms for an unsigned fire road leading

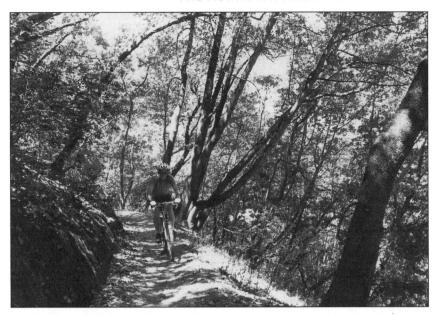

Single-track trails through shady slopes, combined with open meadows and fire roads, make China Camp a favorite with local cyclists.

west and follow it for about 200 yards, pedaling on pavement for a minute or less. Clues to the trail you want get a bit convoluted for the next 0.2 mile, but persevere. Keep an eye out for power lines overhead and signs to Bay View Trail. Immediately to the left of the paved road, look for a brown metal gate across a dirt fire road and make your way around it. There may or may not be picnic tables here, but at least there is an intersection of trails. The trail sign states that you're on Powerline Fire Trail and that it leads you to the junction of Bay View Trail. And guess what? There are power lines overhead! The trail on your left, running left and right (south and north) is Shoreline Trail. You're on the right track.

Follow Powerline Fire Trail (about 40 yards wide) as it begins a somewhat moderate, mildly technical climb through the forest. In less than a half mile, you reach the signed intersection of Powerline Fire Trail and the single-track Bay View Trail. At this point, you've pedaled about 5 miles from the trailhead at China Camp Village and elevation here is about 255 feet.

Hang a left onto hard-packed Bay View Trail and begin a moderate climb as the single-track traverses up the forested slope, aided by switchbacks. The trail becomes increasingly more technical thanks to the narrowness, the tightness of the switchbacks, the slightly more rugged path, and the thrilling drop-offs in a few places. After about a half mile, the climb is less steep and the trail becomes nontechnical.

Continue the gentle climb and at about 6.4 miles, another single-track trail makes a hard hairpin turn up and to your right. Though it's unsigned here, this trail leads north out of the park and into San Pedro Mountain Open Space Preserve. It eventually connects with Bay Hills Drive (definitely worth exploring). At this junction, take Bay View Trail as it continues to the left, crossing a tiny stream on a well-made footbridge.

At about 7 miles, approximate elevation 670 feet, Back Ranch Fire Trail crosses Bay View Trail, running downhill on your left and steeply uphill on your right. Hang a right here onto Back Ranch and grind your own narrow path up and past the deep ruts. In 0.3 mile, 220 feet higher, you reach Ridge Fire Trail, elevation 750 feet approximate. This is pretty much the high point of the loop. Turn left onto Ridge and keep an eye out for glimpses of San Francisco off on your right. You might even see the tips of the towers of the Golden Gate Bridge if it's not shrouded in fog. Ridge is mildly technical although there are several very steep roller coaster sections covered with a layer of loose, soft dirt.

When you reach the intersection of Bay View Trail (its eastern end) at about 8 miles, you will have dropped about 420 feet. Bypass Bay View and stay on Ridge Fire Trail for almost a half mile to a major signed intersection. Turn left here onto Miwok Fire Trail for a few yards and then hop onto Oak Ridge Trail, a sweet, mildly technical single-track leading off on your right.

Follow Oak Ridge Trail as it cruises gently downhill, crossing McNears Fire Trail twice before it intersects Peacock Gap Trail at about 9.7 miles. Go left onto Peacock Gap for about 200 yards to Shoreline Trail. At this point, you've just completed the loop. Make a hard right onto Shoreline and retrace your path back to your car. If you have time, check out historic China Camp Village.

OTHER AREA RIDES

MT. TAM NORTH SIDE LOOP: This is a strenuous ride that requires intermediate technical skills. Composed of dirt fire roads and pavement, this 25-mile-plus loop is on Marin Municipal Water District land.

Finding the trail: (same as Pine Mountain–Repack Loop) Begin pedaling from the public parking lot in Fairfax. The route essentially goes up Bolinas-Fairfax Road to Porteous Avenue to Deer Park. Follow the dirt road to Boy Scout junction, then to Five Corners and up to Lagunitas Lake via Shaver Grade and Sky Oaks Road. Go almost completely around the lake, counterclockwise, to Eldridge Grade. Follow Eldridge past the east peak of Mt. Tam and continue down East Ridgecrest Boulevard (a paved road) toward Rock Springs and eventually to Laurel Dell fire road. Follow Laurel Dell through Potrero Meadows down to Rocky Ridge fire road, and then across the Bon Tempe Dam and spillway. Below the spillway, turn right up the gravel road and continue less than a half mile to Sky Oaks Road. Turn right, and in about 100 feet, a left turn down Shaver Grade will make your loop complete. It's almost all downhill to Fairfax. If you're short on time or if it's a busy trail day, you may want to opt on taking a left down Bullfrog Road below the spillway at Bon Tempe Dam. Stay on Bullfrog around to the Sky Oaks Ranger Station and then onto pavement to Bolinas-Fairfax Road. Go right onto Bolinas-Fairfax and follow it back into town and your parked car.

Maps: A *Rambler's Guide to the Trails of Mt. Tamapalis and the Marin Headlands*, published by The Olmsted & Bros. Map Co., (510) 658-6534. Or *Marin Bicycle Map*, published by Marin County Bicycle Coalition, (415) 488-1245.

For more information, contact:

Marin Municipal Water District
220 Nellen Ave.
Corte Madera, CA 94925
(415) 924-4600

Mount Tamalpais State Park
801 Panoramic Highway
Mill Valley, CA 94941
(415) 388-2070

POINT REYES NATIONAL SEASHORE: The long, meandering ride through this great park is made up of a bunch of easy, short trails in out-and-back configurations on paved roads. Trails that allow bikes are Marshall Beach, Abbott's Lagoon, Bull Point, Sunset Beach, Estero, Drakes Head, Muddy Hollow, Bear Valley, and a portion of the Coast Trail.

Finding the trail: Park at the Bear Valley Park Headquarters on Bear Valley Road near the junction of CA 1 and Sir Francis Drake Boulevard in Olema.

Maps: Pick up a free map at the park headquarters. *Trail Map of Point Reyes National Seashore*, published by Tom Harrison Maps, 2 Falmouth Cove, San Rafael, CA 94901, (800) 265-9090, www.tomharrisonmaps.com.

For more information, contact:

Point Reyes National Seashore
National Park Service
Point Reyes, CA 94956

Bear Valley Visitor Center
Bear Valley Rd., just north of Olema
(415) 663-1092

SOME LOCAL BICYCLE SHOPS & ORGANIZATIONS

Bicycle Trails Council of Marin (BTC)
P.O. Box 494
Fairfax, CA 94978
Phone & Fax: (415) 488-1443
www.btcmarin.org
Probably the most active local mountain-bike advocacy group in Northern
California, this nonprofit, all-volunteer organization was formed in 1987 with
the purpose of dealing with long-brewing trail user conflicts and land-use issues.
Dedicated to promoting safe and responsible riding, BTC is at the forefront of
educating bikers and all other trail users of local regulations and proper trail
etiquette; the organization also works to increase the acceptance of bicycling
as a legitimate and environmentally sound use of land. To that end, BTC is
politically active and works hard to maintain an effective relationship with
various land agencies. They're always in need of volunteers.

Marin County Bicycle Coalition (MCBC)
P.O. Box 35
San Anselmo, CA 94979
(415) 488-1245
www.bikadelic.com/mcbc
A local organization dedicated to both road and mountain biking, with the
purpose of "promoting bicycling for everyday transportation and recreation."
In 1999, the MCBC published *Marin Bicycle Map for Road, Mountain, and
Transit Biking*, the first comprehensive bicycle map for Marin County. This map
was prepared by Cartographics of San Francisco and mountain bike pioneer Joe
Breeze. Available at many Marin County bike and bookstores as well as bike
stores in San Francisco.

Sausalito Mountain Bike Rental
803 Bridgeway
Sausalito, CA
(415) 331-4448

Sausalito Cyclery
No. 1 Gate 6 Rd.
Sausalito, CA 94965
(415) 332-3200

Bicycle Odyssey
1417 Bridgeway
Sausalito, CA 94965
(415) 332-3050

Angel Island Tram Tours
On Angel Island
(415) 897-0719
They also cater events.

Mill Valley Cycleworks
369 Miller Ave.
Mill Valley, CA 94941
(415) 388-6774

Start to Finish
116 Throckmorton Ave.
Mill Valley, CA 94941-1910
(415) 388-3500
Rents bikes.

Village Peddler
1161 Magnolia Ave.
Larkspur, CA 94939
(415) 461-3091
Rents bikes.

Caesar's Cyclery
29 San Anselmo Ave.
San Anselmo, CA 94960
(415) 721-0807

Pacific Bicycles
275 Greenfield Ave. (at Sequoia)
San Anselmo, CA 94960
(415) 457-9775

Sunshine Bicycle Center
737 Center Blvd.
Fairfax, CA 94930
(415) 459-3334
Rents bikes.

Cycle Analysis
At Fourth and Main Sts.
(Highway 1)
Point Reyes, CA
(415) 663-9164
Mostly seasonal rentals.

Start to Finish
1820 Fourth St.
San Rafael, CA
(415) 459-3990
Rents bikes.

Performance Bicycle
Montecito Shopping Center
369 Third St.
San Rafael, CA 94901
(415) 454-9063

Mike's Bicycle Center
1601 4th St.
San Rafael, CA 94901
(415) 454-3747

Bike Hut
459 Entrada Ave.
Novato, CA 94949
(415) 883-2440

Pacific Bicycle
132 Vintage Way
Novato, CA 94945
(415) 892-9319

Classcycle
1531-B South Novato Blvd.
Novato, CA 94945
(415) 897-3288
Rents bikes.

Bicycle Factory
1111 Grant Ave.
Novato, CA 94945
(415) 892-5538

THE WEST BAY AREA

The San Francisco Peninsula is like a slender finger protruding north along the San Andreas fault line, anchored at the northern-most tip by everyone's favorite city by the bay, San Francisco (fondly referred to as "The City" by locals). The Santa Cruz Mountains begin just south of the City running south and splitting this narrow strip of expensive real estate, creating two distinctively different west and east halves. The western portion is shaped by steep, forested terrain, bounded by the Pacific Ocean. Life on the Pacific side is laid back, sort of like the unhurried attitude of Highway 1 snaking along the coast through the quiet communities of Pacifica, Half Moon Bay, Pescadero, and all the way down to Año Nuevo State Reserve, home of equally laid back northern elephant seals. Summers are often foggy, so much that Pacifica is the self-proclaimed Fog Capital of California—and proud of it. The east side of the peninsula is quite a different story. A solid, smothering blanket of urban sprawl forms the northern end of "Silicon Valley," clinging tightly to terra firma amid the gridlock and stressed infrastructure caused by abundant jobs and over-population. This is where you'll find South San Francisco, San Bruno, Burlingame, San Mateo, and Palo Alto. Traffic congestion and air pollution ignore county lines and continue down into the South Bay Area of Santa Clara County.

Like blood veins that feed the peninsula, the east half is served by two paralleling major highways—beautiful Interstate 280 and industrial US 101. To the west of I-280 is Skyline Boulevard, a two-lane road that rolls along the spine of the highest ridge that divides the peninsula. Together, I-280 and Skyline make it possible to reach places of solitude, quickly and easily, unless you get caught in rush-hour traffic. Not unlike the East Bay, pockets of open space make living on the Peninsula bearable for us average income folks. Thanks to the Midpeninsula Regional Open Space District (MROSD), there are 23 open space preserves, many of which allow mountain biking. With over 41,000 acres of foothill and flatlands along the bay shore, the MROSD encompasses over 330 square miles. The rides described in this chapter are along Skyline and offer something for riders of every ability. And let's not forget San Francisco. Swap your knobbies for slicks and you're ready for a great sightseeing road ride through the City, pedaling soft hills and flat stretches. Despite the rat race, the Peninsula is still a nice place to be.

RIDE 81 · Tour of San Francisco and the Golden Gate

AT A GLANCE

Length/configuration: 18 miles, a loop with out-and-back; mostly paved streets and paved bike paths

Aerobic difficulty: Moderate due to some brief hills and mileage

Technical difficulty: Not technical, though you should be comfortable riding with automobile traffic

Scenery: Dramatic views from the Golden Gate Bridge, including the Marin Headlands. Beaches along the Pacific Ocean, Golden Gate Park and the Presidio, affluent San Francisco homes, and the Palace of Legion of Honor.

Special comments: Golden Gate Park is perfect for taking the kiddies; all other portions of the route not recommended. The Bridge may be suitable for young children who ride confidently and have great bike handling skills but constant parental attention is required. Kid-trailers on the Bridge are not recommended.

How many times have you driven over the Golden Gate Bridge, saw cyclists zipping along on the sides and said to yourself, "I want to ride my bike across the Golden Gate some day," but just didn't know exactly were to start or where else you'd go? Well, pop a couple of slick tires onto your mountain bike and check out this unforgettable 18-mile ride. So, what if it's nontechnical and all on pavement. Hard-core riders will enjoy this easy spin as much as beginners due to the fact that San Francisco is arguably the most gorgeous city in all of North America. Sure, the City—as she's fondly called by locals—is built on a bunch of hills. But not to worry: the route described here offers plenty of level, easy riding with a few steep but oh so brief hills. This is a ride you do for the urban scenery, not the technical challenge.

I won't begin to describe the dramatic views from and of the Golden Gate Bridge with the San Francisco Bay, Pacific Ocean and Marin Headlands in the background. You just have to come see for yourself. Culturally speaking, the route offers a lot. Cruise through one of the City's prime pieces of real estate, the Presidio. Former home to the Sixth U.S. Army, it was founded in 1776 by the Spanish and is now managed by the National Park Service. Tours of the Presidio's natural and historical features are offered at the Visitor Center on Montgomery Street. Then there's Fort Point, one of the few Civil War–era forts west of the Mississippi, constructed in the 1850s. The fort's location was put to good use during World War II as a part of an underwater mine operation to protect the Golden Gate Bridge and the Bay. Self-paced audio tours and videos are shown often and give insight into the fort's past. Located practically underneath the Bridge, a video describing its construction is featured here. The Palace of Legion of Honor is an impressive museum with over 4,000 years' worth of ancient and European art. If you're into paintings by Van Gogh, Rembrandt, El Greco, and Monet, or sculptures by Rodin, you'll want to lock up your bike and venture inside for an hour or two. In Golden Gate Park, there's the M.H. de Young and Asian Art Museums,

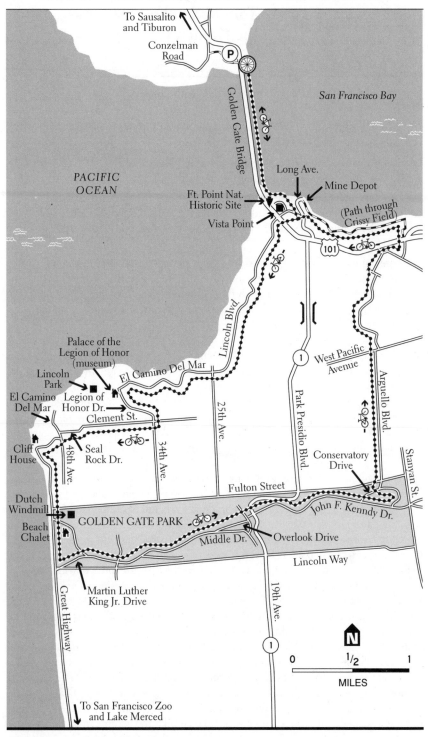

To Sausalito and Tiburon

Conzelman Road

San Francisco Bay

PACIFIC OCEAN

Golden Gate Bridge

Long Ave.

Mine Depot

Ft. Point Nat. Historic Site

(Path through Crissy Field)

Vista Point

101

Lincoln Blvd.

Palace of the Legion of Honor (museum)

Lincoln Park

El Camino Del Mar

El Camino Del Mar

Legion of Honor Dr.

Clement St.

25th Ave.

West Pacific Avenue

Arguello Blvd.

1

Park Presidio Blvd.

Cliff House

48th Ave.

Seal Rock Dr.

34th Ave.

Conservatory Drive

Stanyan St.

Dutch Windmill

Fulton Street

Beach Chalet

GOLDEN GATE PARK

Middle Dr.

John F. Kenndy Dr.

Overlook Drive

Lincoln Way

Great Highway

Martin Luther King Jr. Drive

19th Ave.

1

N

0   1/2   1

MILES

To San Francisco Zoo and Lake Merced

Steinhart Aquarium, Conservatory of Flower, Academy of Sciences, Morrison Planetarium, Shakespeare Garden (with its occasional free live performances presented outdoors in the summer), Japanese Tea Garden, Bison Paddock, soccer games, polo events, and on and on. On Sundays, a portion of John F. Kennedy Drive, one of the park's main roads, is closed to vehicular traffic. It's the place to be, especially on a sunny afternoon, when people-watching is at it's finest. And if the wildlife in Golden Gate Park is too much for you, there's the San Francisco Zoo, described here as a two-mile out-and-back add-on (four miles round-trip). Whew! No dirt on this ride but, hey, there's more to life than riding dirt.

General location: San Francisco.

Elevation change: 400 feet; starting elevation 255 feet; high point 400; low point at sea level.

Season: Year-round.

Services: Pit toilet at starting point. All services available on the route or not far off the route.

Hazards: Expect all portions of the route to be busy. When on automobile routes, expect lots of traffic and watch out for cars parking and pulling out of parking spaces as well as opening car doors. Expect this kind of traffic hazard particularly around the Cliff House and in Golden Gate Park. The bike/walkway which runs across the Golden Gate Bridge is fairly well-traveled. Some sections on the bridge are narrow, just enough space for two passing bikers. The path going around the bridge's two towers are tight, narrow and blind so be sure to slow down and stay on your side of the path. Watch out for walkers on the bridge (although on weekends, bicyclists and pedestrians are separated to the west and east side, respectively). Even so, many serious cyclists zip across the Golden Gate on their way to the famed dirt mountain bike trails in the Marin Headlands so be sure to stay to the right. Expect lots of tourist congestion near the vista point at the San Francisco end of the bridge, especially on sunny weekends. In Golden Gate Park, weekend crowds are apt to be large when the sun is out. That means expect to dodge lots of kiddies on bikes and kid-trailers on the bike trail.

Rescue index: You'll most likely have no trouble enlisting the help of a passer-by. Since the route is entirely in town, finding a phone isn't difficult.

Land status: Golden Gate National Recreation Area, the city of San Francisco, and San Francisco Recreation and Parks.

Maps: Any good San Francisco map that shows the streets in detail.

Finding the trail: This route can be accessed from any number of points on the route. The trick is to find parking that isn't timed and is free.

For this ride description, we parked at the northern end of the Golden Gate Bridge. So, if you're coming from north of San Francisco, travel south on US 101. About a mile before the Bridge, continue past the Bridgeway Boulevard exit and, shortly thereafter, through Waldo Tunnel. Take the first exit after the tunnel, which is the Sausalito exit. (If you reach the Toll Plaza, you've gone too far.) Look for a brown sign directing you to the Golden Gate National Recreation Area. Go a few yards and turn right onto Conzelman Road and then immediately hang a left into the paved parking lot, following a sign marked "Trailhead." This parking area is within 100 yards of the northern end of the Golden Gate Bridge.

If you're already in San Francisco, you would be better off parking at Fort Point Historic Site parking lot off Lincoln Boulevard near Long Avenue, close to the south end of the Golden Gate Bridge. By parking here, you avoid paying the bridge toll and sitting in traffic crawling over the bridge. The described route passes this parking lot twice—at the beginning of the ride and near the end. That means you can ride over the Golden Gate as an out-and-back at the beginning or at the end of the bike tour.

Sources of additional information:

San Francisco Recreation and Parks
McLaren Lodge
Golden Gate Park
Fell and Stanyan Streets
San Francisco, CA 94117
(415) 666-7200
McLaren Lodge is open weekdays, or send a $2 check to receive materials (call to confirm cost).

Golden Gate National Park
    Association
(415) 556-2236

The Presidio
National Park Service
(415) 556-0865

Fort Point National Historic Site
Marine Dr., under the south end of
    the Golden Gate Bridge
(415) 556-1693

San Francisco Zoo
Sloat Blvd. and 45th Ave.
(415) 753-7061

California Palace of the Legion of
    Honor
Lincoln Park
Clement St. and 34th Ave.
(415) 863-3330

Lots of information can be found on the Internet. Try key words "San Francisco parks" or: http://civiccenter.ci.sf.ca.us/recpark/location.nsf/

Notes on the trail: Before you hop on the saddle for your urban adventure, find that sturdy bike lock. You won't regret bringing it because there will be plenty of attractive places at which to stop. How about a refreshment, snack, or a meal? A neighborhood coffee joint for a quick latté? A cultural visit to a museum, aquarium, conservatory, or the zoo? What about bringing a camera? There are lots of photo opportunities on this ride. And bring money just in case you see something you can't do without (but save $3 for the Golden Gate Bridge toll if you're planning to drive into the City after your ride).

Starting from the north end of the Golden Gate Bridge, begin pedaling by hopping onto the trail leading over the Golden Gate Bridge. Heed the posted signs regarding which walkway allow bikes. (On Saturday and Sunday, bicyclists are restricted to riding the west side of the bridge and pedestrians on the east side. The rest of the week and during the night you're free to ride whichever side you like. The walkway on the other side of the bridge is accessed by a narrow path which runs underneath the bridge.) The bridge spans the mouth of the bay and is 1.7 mile long. The walkway is narrow with just enough room for two oncoming cyclists to pass. Stay right and slow down as you curve around the tight turns at the foot of the towers.

Riding on the west side, the walkway curves sharply right and down once you reach the end of the Golden Gate. Stay on the paved path and bypass the Coastal Trail peeling off on your left (it's off-limits to bikes). Follow the path around and under the bridge. After emerging from under the bridge, bear left at a fork and watch out for lots of pedestrian traffic. (The right fork leads up to a popular vista point and it's worth a look if you can stand the bus loads of sightseers.)

Though it's not signed as such, you've just entered the former military reservation known as the Presidio, one of the City's prize pieces of real estate. Begin a gradual descent and coming up on your left is a dirt pulloff—it's a classic location to snap a picture of the Golden Gate. Go past a narrow turn-off leading to the Golden Gate Gift Shop. Follow the brown sign indicating Fort Point to the left while staying on the paved path. At about 2.2 miles, after a gradual descent, you reach the gravel parking lot for Fort Point National Historic Site on your left. (Incidentally, you can park and start your ride here if you don't want to drive over the Golden Gate.) The bike path ends here, running right smack into Lincoln Boulevard. Hang a right onto Lincoln and begin riding up the wide shoulder. Take care because Lincoln is a busy street and the shoulder width varies from three feet to a thin paint strip. Immediately bypass a major driveway that leads to the vista point and gift shop. At 2.3 miles, say good-bye to the maddening crowd as you follow Lincoln underneath US 101.

For the next 1.5 miles, Lincoln Boulevard cruises up and down. Begin climbing a gradual hill and go through the intersection with Merchant Road, staying on Lincoln. At 2.7 miles, the climbing mellows and on your right, you have a terrific view of the mouth of the bay with the Marin Headlands off in the distance and the Golden Gate now behind you. Lincoln basically skirts the edge of the water which is now about 100 yards below you, alongside Baker Beach. After a few more stretches of ascents and descents, Lincoln leaves the Presidio and at the intersection with 25th Avenue, it becomes El Camino Del Mar. A painted bike lane on El Camino leads you through yet another piece of prime San Francisco real estate. The magnificent homes here are large by San Francisco standards. Pedaling the gentle up and down grade makes it easy to take in the sites.

At 4.1 miles, the bike lane ends; continue riding on El Camino Del Mar. Go pass 30th Avenue, stay straight as you follow a sign to the Palace of Legion of Honor. El Camino gently weaves through the affluent neighborhood, gradually climbing and at 4.4 miles, you enter Lands End Park. This is a pleasant park with wide-open lawns and splendid views of the Golden Gate and the Marin Headlands. Carry on with your ascent on El Camino. Watch out for parked car doors opening as well as cars parking and pulling out.

When you arrive at the Palace of Legion of Honor at almost 5 miles, you've reached the high point of the ride, approximately 400 feet. (Be sure to lock up your bike if you decide to check out the museum.) Continue on the same road as it curves left in front of the museum. At this point, the road you're pedaling becomes Legion of Honor Drive, and begins a fast descent to its intersection with Clement Street. At 5.2 miles, turn right onto Clement and gear down for a 4% climb up, still sharing the road with motorists. Not to worry; the hill becomes fairly level in about a quarter mile. Go past 36th Avenue and stay on Clement past the Department of Veteran Affairs—Medical Center at 42nd Avenue. When you reach 45th Avenue at 5.9 miles, Clement curves to the left and becomes Seal Rock Drive. With the Pacific Ocean partially in view straight ahead, continue on Seal Rock which begins a short and steep downhill run. At 6.1 miles, at a stop sign intersection, your path reconnects with El Camino Del Mar. Go left onto El Camino for a few yards and then hang a right onto Point Lobos Avenue. (El Camino on your right is signed "Not A Through Street.")

Point Lobos Avenue curves and descends toward the Pacific as it carries you through Sutro Heights Park, which is a part of the Golden Gate National Recreation Area. This is a favorite tourist spot so watch out for cars backing out of parking spaces and related commotion. Sidewalks are often congested with pedestrians and so you may find it easier to stay on the street. There are a couple of eateries at this dramatic spot: the famous and elegant Cliff House and Louie's "Family Owned Since 1937." If you want to grab a bite to eat, try Louie's. If the Cliff House attracts you, don't be surprised if they deem your cycling clothing unacceptable. Back in the saddle, continue following Point Lobos Avenue as it curves southward and descends to sea level, becoming the Great Highway at 6.5 miles.

The Great Highway parallels the Pacific Ocean, about 200–300 yards on your right, and it's another popular stretch of beach. You can either ride the narrow shoulder on the Great Highway, sharing the road with frequent traffic, or ride the wide sidewalk, dodging pedestrians, strollers, and even rollerbladers. Conditions here are likely to be breezy with the wind rushing pass your ears. At 7 miles, when you see the Dutch Windmill on the left side of the highway, you're skirting the far western edge of Golden Gate Park. A few yards farther is the Beach Chalet, a casual eatery with great window views of the ocean, also on the left side of the highway.

When you reach the signal light intersection with Lincoln Way at 7.5 miles, you have a choice to make here. Continuing straight on the Great Highway for just over 2 miles will lead you to the San Francisco Zoo. Then, it's another 2 miles to return to this point.

If you decide to skip the zoo, turn left onto Lincoln Way. Make your way across the highway at the signal light and look for signed Martin Luther King, Jr. Drive leading into the park on your left. Hop onto MLK Drive. Say good-bye to the ocean wind and the traffic noise and hello to the more calm surroundings of Golden Gate Park. At about 7.8 miles, near the junction with Bernice Rodgers Way, look for a narrow paved bike path on the left side of MLK Drive.

At this point, let me make a general comment about Golden Gate Park since you may want to venture off the described bike route and explore this outstanding park. The park is basically 0.5 mile deep and a little over 3 miles across, shaped in a nearly perfect rectangle, running west to east. You can't really get lost in the park but keeping track of the main streets and narrow roadways that crisscross the park can be a bit challenging, mainly because intersections are not always signed. Fortunately, detailed park maps are permanently displayed on kiosks planted throughout the park and many landmarks are easily referenced. Rest rooms, drinking water, and telephones are scattered throughout the park too. Note also that some paved and unpaved paths are off-limits to bikes so pay attention to posted signs or restrictions painted on the path. Also, you will see signs pointing to the Golden Gate Bridge — these signs are meant for motorists, not cyclists. Though you can certainly blaze your own way, the route I describe aims to avoid heavy traffic and killer hills.

That said, hop on the bike path and follow it basically due east. In a few yards, the paved path forks. The right fork leads you past a small exercise corral for horses. (The left fork leads through a stand of trees and emerges out on John F. Kennedy Drive, near the Bison Paddock [yes, a couple of buffaloes live in the City!]. There, you can pick up another paved bike path which follows JFK Drive or you can follow the bike path as described below. Either way, both bike paths rejoin just before the Highway One (CA 1) overpass.) Assuming you take the right fork, go past the corral, cross a minor street and pick up the marked bike path again. Follow the paved route over mostly level terrain, spiced with a couple of steep but extremely brief uphill sections. Go past the Park Stadium (a huge clearing for soccer, polo, and football) on your left. Shortly thereafter, continue past a wide-open picnic area with BBQ pits and expansive playground. Beyond that on the far side is John F. Kennedy Drive. At about 9.5 miles, across from small Lloyd Lake, your bike path merges with another and skirts JFK Drive. Continue due east and in a few yards, go underneath Highway One (CA 1). On Sundays, this portion of JFK Drive after the underpass is closed to vehicular traffic for the next mile and you're likely to find the most congestion of bikers (adults and kiddies), bladers, and walkers here. Of course, being San Francisco, this is the perfect people-watching spot, especially if it's sunny. On this stretch, you ride behind the M.H. de Young and Asian Art Museums and, in the distance on your right, past the Japanese Tea Garden, the Academy of Sciences, Steinhart Aquarium, Morrison Planetarium and Shakespeare Garden. At 10.7 miles is the Conservatory of Flowers. If you ride on Sunday, definitely check out the scene immediately in front of the Conservatory. Here, a tiny portion of closed JFK Drive becomes the impromptu stage for an informal bunch of roller skaters, line-dancing their synchronized routine to the beat of funky, unending music blasting from a set of huge speakers.

Continuing on JFK Drive, at 11 miles, look for a "65 Golden Gate Bridge" sign pointing to the left. Take the left and ride up a smaller vehicle road. In almost a half mile, go right at an intersection and follow the "65 Golden Gate Bridge" sign. You're now exiting the park. Descend a few yards to the intersection of Fulton Street and Arguello Boulevard. Both roads see lots of car traffic so take care when turning left onto Fulton. Follow it for one block to Second Street. (Though Second parallels Arguello, it has much less traffic.) Turn right onto Second and begin riding through the neighborhood, going straight through about eight intersections. *But stay alert at all intersections because the cross traffic has no stop whereas your street does.*

When you reach Lake Street at 12.4 miles, hang a right, climb a short block to Arguello Boulevard. Go left onto Arguello and grind up a steep hill. At 12.7 miles, go through Jackson Street, then West Pacific Avenue—two streets that intersect Arguello. Follow Arguello on a narrow shoulder as it curves right and then left into the Presidio grounds. The climb mellows a bit and at 12.9 miles, you reach Inspiration Point, a perfect place for a breather if you want. Continue on Arguello, as it descends, following the signs to the Presidio Visitor Center. It's a fast downhill and streets Thomas Lane and Infantry Terrace are a blur as you zip past. The route levels as you reach the intersection with Moraga Avenue at 13.4 miles. Continue straight through, staying on Arguello toward the direction of the Visitor Center. In a few yards, go left onto Sheridian Avenue, then right onto Montgomery Street. Go past the Visitor Center, housed in a row of handsome old red brick buildings. Follow Montgomery as it curves right into Lincoln Boulevard. Go through the intersections of Graham Street and Keyes Avenue. Immediately after Keyes, hang a left onto Hellic Street. At 14 miles, go underneath US 101. In a few yards, you reach the intersection with Mason Street where you're facing Crissy Field and the San Francisco Bay beyond it. As of March, 1999, the renovation of Crissy Field was still underway. If the field is still being renovated, look right a few yards down and you should see a temporary vehicle road through the construction zone. Your goal at this intersection is to make your way across Crissy to a walkway near the water's edge.

Once on the water side of Crissy Field, follow the popular promenade west toward the Golden Gate Bridge and Fort Point. At 15.5 miles, the path leads you right to the pier and small white warehouse structures that once served as Fort Point Mine Depot. It's worth a short stop to read the interpretive sign that briefly describes the use of underwater mines in and around the Golden Gate Bridge from 1910 through World War II. The pier has no great historical value, and fishing and crabbing from it is allowed. From this location, you have a great sea level view of Angel Island and Alcatraz Island. Rest rooms and a drinking faucet are available here.

From the Mine Depot, Long Avenue climbs steeply but briefly on your left. Follow this road and in just over 0.25 mile, it intersects with Lincoln Boulevard. Turn right onto Lincoln and continue climbing an easy hill for a few yards to Fort Point National Historic Site gravel parking lot on your right. Here is where you close the loop and retrace your path back over the Golden Gate Bridge to your car. Ending mileage is 18.1 miles, excluding the out-and-back to the zoo. If you parked your car here at Fort Point and have not yet ridden over the Bridge, you owe it to yourself to do so—it's the most outstanding part of a ride that already has lots of memorable moments.

RIDE 82 · Sawyer Camp Trail

AT A GLANCE

Length/configuration: 12-mile out-and-back (6 miles each way); paved multi-use path

Aerobic difficulty: Easy; elevation gain almost imperceptible

Technical difficulty: Not technical

Scenery: Views of the Montara Mountain Range across Lower Crystal Springs Reservoir, especially beautiful in the summer when the fog creeps down the ridge; Jepson Bay Laurel, one of the largest laurel trees in the state.

Special comments: Great trail for young families. A good alternative when nearby trails are still wet and muddy from rain.

Though Sawyer Camp Trail is all pavement, it's immensely popular with all kinds of trail users, especially when the nearby dirt trails are still wet and muddy from rain. You don't even need a map to follow it, so long as you stay on the paved path. This 6-mile path (12 miles round-trip) is mostly flat, running south to north, paralleling I-280 and a golf course on the east and part of Lower Crystal Springs Reservoir on the west. Starting off in exposed terrain, the trail leads through shady forest near its end at the San Andreas Lake and Dam. Being completely closed to vehicular traffic, it's a great outing for young families—just be prepared to share the trail with lots of other trail users. There are benches along the way as well as a picnic area at the featured natural attraction: the Jepson Laurel Tree, the oldest, biggest laurel tree in the state. It's huge and you're bound to be amazed.

Located within the San Francisco Watershed, water captured by the San Andreas Lake and the Lower and Upper Crystal Springs Reservoirs provide clean and pure drinking water to over 2.5 million households and businesses in the counties of San Francisco, San Mateo, Santa Clara, and Alameda. Most of the water is snow run-off from the Sierra Nevada, funneled into these lakes via gravity through the Hetch Hetchy Reservoir system in Yosemite National Park. As for the name, the trail was named after Leander Sawyer in the 1850s. He grazed cattle in the San Andreas valley and later trained performing horses for circuses. An enterprising man, Sawyer eventually opened an inn for folks traveling by stagecoach. Sawyer Camp Trail was renamed San Andreas Valley Road when it was the main road between San Francisco and Half Moon Bay. In 1888, Crystal Springs Reservoir was created, flooding the road. Eventually, in 1978, with the reservoir's water line maintained at a lower level, San Mateo County closed the road to vehicular use, allowing only recreational use.

RIDE 82 · Sawyer Camp Trail

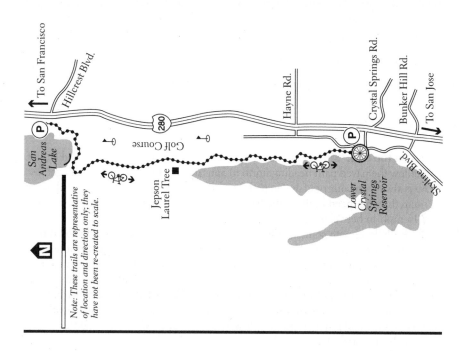

General location: About 27 miles south of San Francisco, adjacent to I-280.

Elevation change: 300 feet; starting elevation and low point 200 feet; high point 500 feet. Fairly flat except for a gradual rise at the northern end.

Season: Year-round.

Services: Drinking water available at both ends of the paved path as well as the Jepson Laurel picnic area. Portable toilets and park benches spaced throughout the route. All other services on the east side of I-280.

Hazards: Stay alert and be prepared to share the path with other trail users. Because this is an immensely popular path, the constant hazard is folks moving along at different speeds. The trail is often crowded on weekends with walkers (with or without baby-strollers), joggers, roller- and in-line skaters, and equestrians. Cyclists (road and mountain bikers) vary from young kids on training wheels to speedsters riding thousand dollar bikes and decked with the latest accoutrements. (The enforced speed limit is 15 mph and 5 mph at the first 0.8 mile on both ends of the route.

Rescue index: In case of an emergency, you're likely to meet other trail users who may be of help. Both ends of the route are easily accessed by vehicles and the roads there are well-traveled.

Land status: San Francisco Watershed (within the Golden Gate National Recreation Area), managed by the San Mateo County Parks and Recreation Department and the San Francisco Water Department.

Maps: USGS Montara Mountain and San Mateo 7.5 minute series.

Finding the trail: From San Francisco, travel south on I-280 for about 27 miles to Bunker Hill Road exit. Bear right and almost immediately turn right onto Skyline Boulevard. Drive a half mile to Crystal Springs Road and look for a small parking area on the left (reservoir side of Skyline Boulevard). There are interpretive displays here. Park and access the paved Sawyer Camp Trail from here by entering through the gate.

Sources of additional information:

> San Mateo County Parks and Recreation Department
> 590 Hamilton St.
> Redwood City, CA 94063
> (415) 363-4020

Notes on the trail: Since this is an easy trail to follow, you really don't need a map. Just follow the paved path heading north to San Andreas Dam and you won't get lost. I-280 is always on your right as you pedal to the northern end of the paved trail. Keep in mind that the speed limit for the first 0.8 mile at either ends of the route is 5 mph and 15 mph in between—and it's enforced.

Basically level with some gentle ups and downs along the way, the exposed path becomes shady near the northern end. There, many varieties of trees including oak, laurel, cypress, pine, and eucalyptus, offer welcome shade during hot, sunny outings. Of particular interest and certainly worth a stop is at 3.5 miles where the state's oldest and biggest laurel tree of its species stands. Named after California botanist Willis Laurel in 1923, it is an impressive 600-plus-year-old living organism worthy of a photo. Picnic tables here make it a pleasant spot to take a snack break, unless someone else beats you to it.

At about 4.8 miles, (there are mile markers posted along the way), you might have to gear down for a slight climb to the top of the San Andreas Dam. The view of San Andreas Lake from here, as well as the landscape southward is rewarding. Not that it's noticeable, the bike path parallels the San Andreas Fault Line. The dam's claim to fame is that it survived the 1906 earthquake that leveled San Francisco. Not bad for a man-made structure built in 1869. From the dam, continue another mile of gentle uphill to the northern terminus. When you're good and ready, return the way you came—and remember the speed limits.

RIDE 83 • Purisima Creek Redwoods—Short Loop

AT A GLANCE

Length/configuration: 7.3-mile loop, counterclockwise; wide single-track and old logging road

Aerobic difficulty: Moderately strenuous thanks to steep and mean climbs

Technical difficulty: Mildly technical with some walkable intermediate sections due to rocky, loose terrain and steepness

Scenery: This is the forest of our childhood daydreams: lush, cool, and shady tree-covered creek canyons with overlooking views to distance ridges, the Pacific Ocean and Half Moon Bay. Populated by mostly young-growth redwoods with a few old-growth trees.

Special comments: Beginners with strong endurance who don't mind walking over brief rugged terrain will enjoy the trails here. Other, more technically challenging trails here allow bikes. Some trails are closed after a heavy rain; call the park rangers for status.

This 7.3-mile loop gives you a taste of the terrain and beauty here at Purisima Creek Redwoods Open Space Preserve. Though this counterclockwise route is short, using mostly wide single-track trails (old logging roads), it's a great workout due to the climbs found in the second half of the loop. The first half is nearly 100% downhill, dropping 1,580 feet in four sweet miles over usually hard-packed dirt. As opposite as day and night, the second half of the loop is mean and nasty as it climbs back up to the north entrance, regaining every inch in less distance—3.3 miles to be exact. The only real technical challenge on the uphill is staying on your bike despite the steepness. And parts of it are steep, up to 15% grade.

By all means stop and catch your breath if you must. Tucked on the western slope of the northern end of the Santa Cruz Mountain range, Purisima Creek Redwood Open Space Preserve enjoys a cool, moist forest environment, sustained by coastal fog, deep canyons, and mild winters. The scents of this serene, peaceful forest are glorious and it's hard to believe that bustling Silicon Valley is less than a half hour away. Redwood trees are an incredible old, living organism. They were here when dinosaurs roamed the land. Though the redwoods here are not nearly as ancient, most of the remaining trees are estimated to be at least 100 years old. It is surmised that 1,000-year old trees used to grow here. Unfortunately, logging operations during the late 1800s and early 1900s fell many of them as evident by stumps measuring between 10 and 20 feet in diameter. Locations of several old logging mills can still be seen—look for cleared areas along Purisima Creek Trail, particularly near the junction of Whittemore Gulch and Purisima Creek.

General location: Located along Skyline Ridge on the San Francisco peninsula, about 30 miles north of San Jose and 15 miles west of Woodside, west of I-280.

Elevation change: 1,580 feet; starting elevation and high point 2,000 feet; low point 420 feet. Begins with one long and deep descent, followed by one seemingly unrelenting torturous climb back up to the trailhead.

Season: Year-round, though many trails are subject to closure after heavy rain.

Services: None on the route. Bring plenty of water. Any water taken from creeks should be treated before drinking. Located at the north entrance parking lot and trailhead (gate PC01) is a portable toilet, a pay phone, and ample parking. Mountain House Country Store, a privately owned and operated coffee shop is adjacent to the north entrance. Picnic tables and portable toilet also located at the south parking area and trailhead (gate PC03A). All other services can be found to the east in Menlo Park, Palo Alto, and other nearby communities.

Hazards: Be alert for rattlesnakes and poison oak. Ticks are active here and may carry diseases, so stay on designated trails and frequently check yourself and friends. In addition to other bikers, watch out for hikers and equestrians, especially on narrow trails.

RIDE 83 · Purisima Creek Redwoods—Short Loop

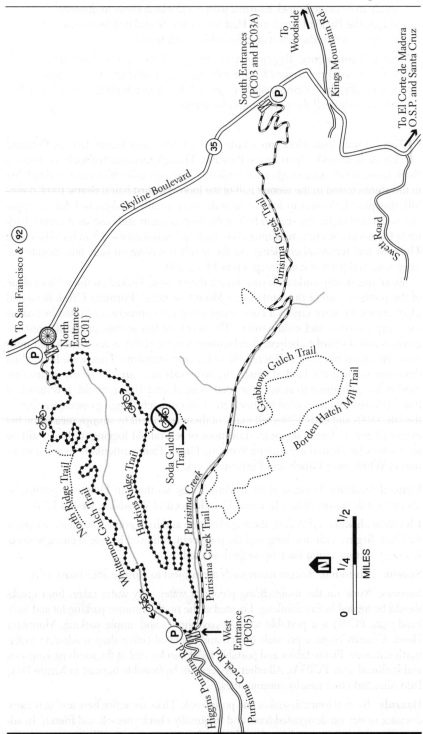

Rescue index: The preserve is fairly popular on weekends and weekday evenings. That means if you ride during those times, your chances are good of meeting another trail user who may be of help in an emergency. Otherwise, you should make your own way to the nearest park entrance adjacent to a road, preferably the north or south entrances which are both adjacent to heavily traveled Skyline Boulevard. You can flag down a passing motorist at either entrance. There's also a pay phone at the north entrance. Purisima Creek Road, where the west entrance is located, is not as well traveled. A fire station is located on Skyline, in between the north and south entrances.

Land status: Purisima Creek Redwoods Open Space Preserve, maintained by the Midpeninsula Regional Open Space District.

Maps: The official park trail map is free and can be found at the north entrance (gate PC01).

Finding the trail: To reach the north parking lot and main entrance from San Francisco: Travel southbound on I-280 to the Half Moon Bay/Skyline Boulevard/CA 92 exit, reached in about 26 miles. Go west onto CA 92 for almost 3 miles to Skyline Boulevard; turn left here. Follow Skyline for 4.3 miles and immediately after passing Mountain House Country Store, turn right into the dirt parking lot (west side of Skyline). Begin pedaling from here.

To reach the north parking lot and main entrance from San Jose: Travel northbound on I-280 toward Woodside. Take the Woodside Road/CA 84 exit. Follow CA 84 west through the quaint town of Woodside about 1.7 miles. Turn right onto Kings Mountain Road and proceed up the shady, twisty road toward Huddert County Park and Skyline Boulevard (CA 35). At almost 4 miles from the I-280 exit, bypass the entrance to Huddert County Park and go another 3 miles to Skyline Boulevard, reached at 6.8 miles. Hang a right onto Skyline and drive 2.4 miles to the north entrance, passing the south entrance along the way. Turn left into the dirt parking lot just before Mountain House Country Store. Begin pedaling from here.

Sources of additional information:

Midpeninsula Regional Open Space
  District
330 Distel Circle
Los Altos, CA 94022-1404
(650) 691-1200
mrosd@openspace.org
www.openspace.org

Trail Center
3921 E. Bayshore Rd.
Palo Alto, CA 94303
(650) 968-7065
Info@trailcenter.org
www.trailcenter.org/maps.htm
A great retail source for biking maps
of the Bay Area and California
State Parks.

Notes on the trail: This is a great little preserve, well-signed at all trail junctions and, unless the box at the entrance is empty, the free maps are extremely useful and accurate. Trails that are off-limits to bikes are signed.

Begin your ride by following North Ridge Trail, a wide single-track, as it gradually drops down a south-facing canyon slope toward the confluence of Purisima Creek and Whittemore Gulch. The trail is moderately technical with scattered semi-buried rocks and rain ruts combined with the mild descent—just enough to keep you awake as you zip downhill. It can be shady here, depending on the time of day, and though the trail is wide, stay alert for other trail users. Almost immediately, intersect Harken Ridge Trail leading off on your left. Bypass it, staying on North Ridge Trail. (Your return will be up Harken Ridge to this intersection.) The descent is fun as you cruise past mixed conifer trees, some covered with moss, a few young redwoods, and thick understory of ferns, nettles, and other bushes. Your view is not totally obscured by the forest because every so often, you catch a far-reaching glimpse of the Pacific Ocean as well as the nearby canyon sides and ridges.

At 0.8 mile, you reach a signed intersection with Whittemore Gulch Trail. Go left onto Whittemore and continue the downhill run. The trail is narrower than North Ridge and the steepness is gentler. A number of tight turns, some of which are best described as hairpins, force you to control your speed as you descend in and out of the shady forest and open terrain. You begin to see more young-growth redwoods and the aromas of the forest are delightful, making you glad just to be here.

As you drop farther, the sweet trickling sound of Whittemore Gulch becomes louder. At 2.8 miles, cross the tiny creek on a well-made footbridge. You may see the sawed stumps of what used to be huge redwoods, measuring over 5 feet in diameter in this vicinity. Rising above the creek, this is probably the first time you need to crank your pedals. Still, you have some elevation to lose as the trail resumes it descent toward Purisima Creek. You're back at creek level at 3.8 miles. A few yards farther, you reach the lowest point of the loop at about 420 feet, near the Higgins–Purisima Creek Road west entrance, located on the other side of a wide bridge. Converging here are Purisima Creek and Whittemore Gulch, and several trails. Don't go over the bridge. Instead, hang a left here onto Harkins Ridge Trail. (If you have time and want to see some old-growth redwoods and/or just want more mileage, proceed over the bridge and go left onto Purisima Creek Trail. This trail leads through impressive groves of giant redwood trees along the fern-covered creek. It also leads to Borden Hatch Mill and Grabtown Gulch Trails, both open to bikes, weather conditions permitting.)

Okay, it's payback time. Here is where the aerobic workout begins, and your technical ability to climb up spots of steep, loose, and rocky terrain tested. Harkins Ridge Trail is a fairly wide single-track and climbs 1,580 feet in 3.3 miles. Many of the brief but very steep sections measure from 3% to 15%-plus grade. Level stretches throughout the climb offer welcome relief to your muscles and lungs though they never seem long enough. Initially paralleling Purisima Creek for about 0.3 mile, try to enjoy your surroundings as you grind up Harkins Ridge. The redwoods are majestic and the forest smells are glorious. Stop and take a breather and look behind you. If it's a clear day, you may have a beautiful view of the Pacific.

At about 6 miles from the north entrance, just over 2 miles from the west entrance, bypass Soda Gulch Trail (hiking-only). Continue on Harkins Ridge Trail and almost a half mile farther, Harkins Ridge curves left atop an open little knoll while a lesser traveled trail continues straight, bearing right. A trail sign here indicates that the trail veering right leads to the park boundary in about 0.2 mile while the left leads to the North Ridge parking area at the north entrance in 0.9 mile. Follow Harkins Ridge as it curves left, becoming a narrow single-track. Though you're still climbing, the worst is over. The trail may be a bit more technical here with deep rain ruts and semi-buried tree roots and rocks.

Harkins Ridge Trail intersects North Ridge Trail at about 7 miles. You close the loop at this familiar spot. Hang a right onto North Ridge and retrace your path back to the parking area. Pat yourself on the back for having grinded up a steep and rugged slope.

RIDE 84 · El Corte de Madera Creek Loop

AT A GLANCE

Aerobic difficulty: 8-mile loop, counterclockwise; dirt fire roads and single-track

Aerobic difficulty: Moderately strenuous due to steep ups and downs

Technical difficulty: Intermediate, though a short stretch is suitable for beginners and youngsters

Scenery: Canyons and ravines comprised mostly of second-growth redwood and conifer trees. Shady, cool environment with typical understory.

Special comments: Except for a 1.2-plus-mile stretch of fire road suitable for beginners and young families, the park is generally enjoyed by riders with at least intermediate bike handling skills. Helmets required.

Ask locals who have been pedaling El Corte de Madera (ECdM) Creek Open Space Preserve since the late 1980s and they will tell you it has the best, most awesomely gnarly single-track trails in the Greater Bay Area. Today, well-signed ECdM is known for its challenging network of trails, and truth be told, it's not a great place to introduce mountain biking to a true novice. Though there are several slightly smooth fire roads which are suitable for beginners and young families, most trails and fire roads are rugged with rocks and boulders, and their steepness is enough to scare off any neophyte. The eight-mile loop described includes some of the easier trails, comprised of dirt fire roads and single-tracks. Even so, the terrain on this loop is still challenging and aerobically strong riders with solid intermediate technical skills will find this loop a lot of fun. Completely enveloped by a lush, young redwood forest and encompassing several deep canyons carved by creeks, ECdM, to this day, enjoys a reputation as being a park naturally geared for accomplished riders.

Though El Corte de Madera Creek Open Space Preserve is still loved and enjoyed by the heartiest of bikers, it used to offer better, much more technical single-tracks. In the past, as recent as 1996, ECdM was the kind of place that was known only by die-hard mountain bikers. Deviating from old logging roads, many trails were created by off-road motorcyclists and, later, local mountain bike enthusiasts. They graced the trails with names that were colorful as well as expressive: Faceplant, Nosebreak, Pipeline, Whoops!, Porsche 914 (so named for an abandoned Porsche hidden here), Dave's Wet Dream, and Devil's Staircase. In the mid-1980s, the Midpeninsula Regional Open Space District (MROSD) acquired over 2,790 acres of this area bounded by Skyline Boulevard on the east and Star Hill Road on the west. The initial policy of the District was to manage the preserve with "benign neglect," leaving the area wild. Fallen trees were left undisturbed, trails and logging roads were minimally maintained. ECdM became an avid mountain biker's dream come true. Then, in 1996, despite the objections of the local biking community, the MROSD moved forward with their comprehensive new trail plan. Much to the horror of many bike supporters, a number of the outstanding single-tracks and fire roads were "sanitized," that is, cleared of obstacles and debris, and the steepness of some trails softened. It was a

RIDE 84 · El Corte de Madera Creek Loop

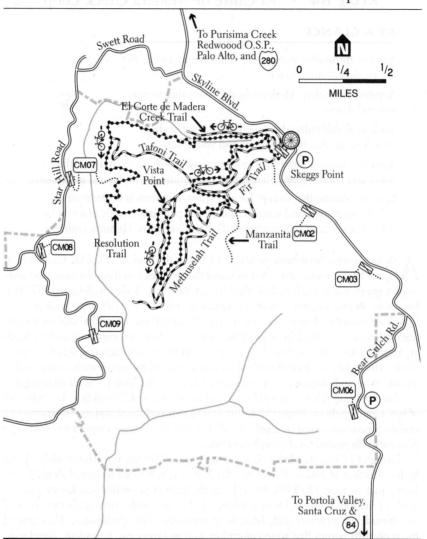

sad day when bulldozers were brought in instead of volunteers dedicated to the creation and restoration of trails by hand. Today, the political battle continues and every little victory counts. So when you ride ECdM, give thanks to the passionate local mountain bike community for protecting the park for our recreational use.

General location: Located along Skyline Ridge on the San Francisco peninsula, about 30 miles north of San Jose and 15 miles west of Woodside, west of I-280.

Elevation change: 560 feet; starting elevation and high point 2,310 feet; low point 1,750 feet. Lots of ups and downs.

Season: Year-round, though after heavy rain most of the trails are likely to remain muddy for days.

Services: None on the trail. Portable toilets available at Skeggs Point parking lot. Maps available at gate CM01 near Skeggs Point. Limited services can be found in the tiny town of Woodside. All services available in Palo Alto, some 20 miles away.

Hazards: This is a popular park used by bikers, hikers, and equestrians. Watch out for oncoming trail users, especially bikers on narrow single-track trails that hug steep slopes; pass with care. Encountering mountain lions and bobcats are rare though not unheard of. Stay on marked trails as the park boundary is not completely marked and it's easy to unknowingly venture into private property.

Rescue index: Weekend and early evening weekdays see lots of trail users, improving your chances of finding others who may be of help in an emergency. Otherwise, on less popular days, make your way either to Skyline Boulevard, Star Hill Road, or Bear Guch Road in order to flag down a passing motorist. There is an emergency call box located on the west side of Skyline Boulevard almost a half mile north of Skeggs Point parking lot.

Land status: El Corte de Madera Creek Open Space Preserve, managed and administered by the Midpeninsula Regional Open Space.

Maps: The official park trail map is free and can be found at the CM01 gate and trailhead near Skeggs Point.

Finding the trail: From either northbound or southbound I-280, travel northbound on I-280 toward Woodside. Take the Woodside Road/CA 84 exit. Follow CA 84 west through the quaint town of Woodside about 1.7 miles. Turn right onto Kings Mountain Road and proceed up the shady, twisty road toward Huddert County Park and Skyline Boulevard (CA 35). At almost 4 miles from the I-280 exit, bypass the entrance to Huddert County Park and go another 3 miles to Skyline Boulevard, reached at 6.8 miles. Hang a left onto Skyline and drive 1.5 miles to El Corte de Madera Creek Open Space Preserve, going a few yards beyond the first gate (CM01) to Skeggs Point parking lot located on the east side of Skyline. Note that southbound traffic on Skyline is not permitted to turn left into the lot. You'll need to drive past the parking lot in order to make a U-turn where it's safe and legal. Park and begin riding from Skeggs Point.

Sources of additional information: See sources of additional information for Ride 83.

Notes on the trail: If you usually ride with eye protection, I suggest you ride with amber or clear lens since most of the trails are cloaked in shade by the thick forest and deep canyons.

From the parking lot, proceed cautiously north on Skyline Boulevard. There isn't much of a shoulder here and the traffic can be frequent and fast at times. Fortunately, you're on Skyline for about 0.2 mile at which point gate CM01 appears on the west side of the road. There's a bulletin board here as well as free maps next to the gated fire road.

Say good-bye to Skyline Boulevard by going through the gate onto the fire road. In a few yards, having dropped below Skyline, you reach a signed fork. The left fork is Tafoni Trail and is your return route at the end of this loop ride. Take the right fork signed El Corte de Madera Creek Trail and enjoy a rolling descent into the lush, forested canyon. This trail is really a dirt fire road that starts off as mildly technical terrain, gradually becoming a bit more challenging with occasional deep rain ruts, and scant spots of mud and loose gravel. The nearby riparian environment is lush with thick understory and ferns, including many young redwood trees. Several redwood stumps alongside the trail tell you that old-growth trees once towered overhead.

This sweet fire road ends at a fork, about 0.8 mile from the gate. The straight ahead fork goes a few yards but is essentially a closed trail. Take the left fork and go over a wooden bridge over tiny El Corte de Madera Creek and continue on ECdM Creek Trail, now a single-track. And what a gorgeous single-track it is! The trail hugs a steep, forested slope as it begins climbing out of the creek canyon. Trees are heavily moss-covered and the canyon is cool and dark. Several brief stretches of open drop-offs on your right and a couple of hairpin turns keep you alert. Be aware of oncoming trail users on this narrow path as one person will have to step aside to let the other pass. Generally ascending, the trail dips down and pops up over twisty terrain spiced with semi-buried chunks of rocks and loose dirt.

ECdM Creek Trail intersects Tafoni Trail at about 1.8 miles. Follow the sign directing to Resolution Trail by bearing right here. Still on ECdM Creek Trail, the terrain is more of the same—twisty ups-and-downs within the shady forest. At 2.4 miles, you reach a signed junction and the beginning of Resolution. (The trail gets its name from a light airplane that crashed here years ago, named Resolution.) The right trail is the continuation of ECdM Creek Trail and leads to paved Star Hill Road and gate CM07 in 1 mile. Take the left trail signed Resolution and continue the gradual climb out of the creek canyon. Like ECdM Creek Trail, Resolution has its share of ups and downs, twists and turns, semi-buried and loose rocks, and steeply sloping drop-offs. Throw in a couple of hairpin turns and the terrain is definitely suited for riders who are strong intermediates or better.

After a mile of Resolution, you reach the signed T intersection with Fir Trail, about 3.9 miles from the gate. Hang a left onto Fir and pedal a quick 0.3 mile to the Vista Point. Turn left off of Fir and continue a few more yards to the Vista Point. Consider yourself very lucky if you have a crystal clear day because you'll be able catch a good glimpse of the Pacific Ocean from here. Trace your path back down Fir to Resolution Trail at the T intersection. Bypass Resolution and continue straight downhill on Fir Trail. From this intersection, Fir Trail becomes quite a bit more technically challenging. In fact, of the entire loop, this is the most challenging portion but very brief, about 0.3 mile. Here, the terrain is rocky, covered with loose, small chunks of rock, dirt, and gravel. Combine that with its steepness—from 6% to 18% in some spots—and you'll have a slip-sliding run on which you can really pick up speed. Not for the faint of heart, this adrenaline-pumping portion of Fir definitely requires nerves of steel and strong intermediate, if not advanced technical skills. Walking is always an option.

After the difficult section, another trail tapers into your trail from behind your right shoulder. It's unsigned but the forward direction, which is still Fir Trail, is signed, indicating the direction to Methuselah and Timberview Trails. (If you're hungry for more challenging terrain and additional mileage, you could take this hard right trail which is the continuation of Methuselah. It'll take you to the southern part of the preserve where there are more gnarly single-tracks and fire roads.) Stay straight bearing left, now on fire road Methuselah Trail and begin a moderate climb.

At just over 6 miles, you come to a major signed intersection. Methuselah Trail continues straight ahead to Skyline Boulevard and Skeggs Point. Running left and right is Manzanita Trail. (A right turn onto Manzanita Trail will take you to the southern half of the park where there are many more trails worth exploring.) Go left onto Manzanita toward Fir Trail. This tiny section of Manzanita easily and quickly takes you to Fir Trail. Go left onto Fir and in 0.2 mile, intersect Tafoni Trail, a dirt fire road. (If you're interested in checking out the geologically interesting Sandstone

Formation, go straight through the intersection onto Tafoni for a few yards. Look for a hiking-only trail on your right. Leave your bike here with a friend or throw a lock on it before walking about 0.1 mile to the site.)

At this intersection, having pedaled about 6.7 miles from the gate, take the hard right turn onto Tafoni Trail and enjoy a gentle rolling traverse across the canyon slope. In just over a mile, you close the loop at the fork with El Corte de Madera Creek Trail, just 0.1 mile from the gate. Retrace your path back to the gate. Use caution as you pedal Skyline Boulevard back to your car at Skeggs Point.

Of special note for young families: Tafoni Trail, a somewhat wide fire road, is mildly technical and suitable for youngsters and kid trailers. Tafoni is 2.2 miles in length and can be ridden as an out-and-back (4.4 miles round-trip), turning around when the kiddies get good and tired. A visit to the Sandstone Formation might hold the fascination of young minds, an added bonus to a short but pleasing bike ride.

OTHER AREA RIDES

MONTARA MOUNTAIN IN MCNEE RANCH S.P.: These routes are located along the Pacific coast side of northern San Mateo County, near Devil's Slide between Half Moon Bay and Pacifica, 25 minutes south of San Francisco. The general consensus of riders who enjoy McNee Ranch and neighboring San Pedro Valley County Park is that the bike routes here rock! Other descriptive phrases used by riders include "not for the timid," "death climb section," and "for experts only." Fire roads and single-tracks here are formidable, due to extreme steepness and technical trail conditions. Granite rocks, as well as loose sand and gravel, dominate the trails. Combine that with incredibly — even dangerously — steep ascents and descents, and you have some of the most extreme single-tracks and fire roads in the Greater Bay Area. So steep that keeping your front tire on the ground and your butt on the saddle will be challenges in themselves. And then there's the fog. A cyclist who often rides Montara Mountain stresses being extra careful if you're tackling the single-track when it's foggy — finding your way back to the main fire road can be an interesting challenge. All trails are not marked. The park is only 700 acres, and riders who keep coming back do so for the quick and intense workout. Scenery is an added bonus. The reward for all the pain is the spectacular 360-degree view of the Bay Area and Pacific Ocean, on clear days, of course, and equally stunning if the fog line is below the peak. The main artery through this small area is the abandoned, slowly eroding Old San Pedro Road, also known as the Old Coast Road since Highway 1 was built. Pedaling Old San Pedro Road from the Highway 1 gate to Pacifica as an out-and-back is a favorite route, measuring 11 miles round-trip (5.5 miles one way). That's usually enough of a workout for many bikers since the elevation gain is from sea level to roughly 1,600 feet in 2 to 4 miles. Superhumans usually climb a bit farther by taking the trail to the North Peak of Montara Mountain, sitting at elevation 1,898 feet, adding 4.6 miles (2.3 miles one way). Be prepared for wind, fog, and hot sun. Bring plenty of water.

Finding the trailhead: There are two access points to McNee Ranch State Park. One is from Highway 1 at Montara State Beach. To get there from I-280 and Belmont, take CA 92 west to Highway 1. Go north about 8 miles to Montara State Beach. Parking is on the ocean side of Highway 1, just before Martini Creek, which roughly delineates the south edge of McNee Ranch. Park here and pedal a bit further on Highway 1 to a white metal gate marking a dirt road leading into the park. This is the south end of Old San Pedro Road. The other access point is from within Pacifica. To get there, find the intersection of Highway 1 and Linda Mar Boulevard near the south edge of town. Follow Linda Mar inland to Adobe Road. Hang a right onto Adobe and follow it to Higgins Road. Go left on Higgins to its end at a gate. Park in this vicinity. Begin your ride by pedaling past the gate and onto Old San Pedro Road. This old, eroding road leads into McNee Ranch in about 2 miles and to Montara Mountain Trail about a mile farther.

Maps: USGS Topo Montara Mountain 7.5 minute series, or *Hiking, Bicycling & Equestrian Trail Map of Pacifica,* published by Pease Press (415) 221-0487.

For more information, contact:

Montara State Beach and McNee Ranch State Park
District State Park office in Half Moon Bay
(650) 726-8819

WATER DOG LAKE PARK: An oasis in a sea of houses, condos, and apartments, this tiny park is a wooded canyon and is mostly used by locals looking for a very quick and technically challenging workout. Managed by the city of Belmont, the main dirt road that runs through the park is about 2 miles. The technical single-tracks are the attraction here, even though you have to cross several paved residential streets to access them. A popular route is often described as two parts. The first part is to enter at the bottom of the park, that is, at the bottom of Lake Drive at Lyall Way. Pedal up the dirt road along the top of the ridge for about 2 miles toward the Hallmark Road gate. This portion is a fairly unremarkable mile or so except for panoramic views of the bay on clear days. Go left into a canyon and then climb up a single-track. Follow the single-track behind a bunch of homes for about a mile. After a short, steep climb beside a wooden fence, hop off the dirt trail and onto pavement in a cul-de-sac. Please respect private property by staying on public streets. This is the beginning of the more exciting second part. Head out of the cul-de-sac, and follow the pavement around, keeping an eye out for a wood chip–covered trail that provides public access to the trails behind the residences. Here is where you find a mile or so of fun, narrow, twisty, single-tracks that run mostly downhill, reportedly very technical in spots. Heads up for several small but challenging jumps. At the bottom of a steep but short descent is a cement culvert. After that, follow more single-track and wind your way through a couple of tiny creeks. The network of trails here offer many configurations, giving you 6 to 8 miles of fun.

Finding the trailhead: From US 101 in Belmont, follow CA 92 west past El Camino Real and Alameda de las Pulgas. Watch for Lyall Way on your left (south side of CA 92). Turn left onto Lyall and follow it to a stop sign intersection with Lake Drive. Park in the vicinity of this intersection and hop your bike. Water Dog Lake Park entrance is at this corner.

Maps: Detailed maps of the area don't exist.

For more information, contact:

City of Belmont
(415) 595-7441

RUSSIAN RIDGE/COAL CREEK OPEN SPACE PRESERVES: Located across Skyline Boulevard (CA 35) from one another, Russian Ridge and Coal Creek offer 8 miles and 5 miles of trails, respectively. Bikers looking for more distance—even a full day of riding—always have the convenient option of biking into adjacent MROSD parks (Midpeninsula Regional Open Space District) including Los Trancos, Skyline Ridge, Monte Bello, and Long Ridge Open Space Preserves. Like many other parks in this district, most of the single-tracks and dirt roads are open to cyclists. Located along a dominant ridge of the Santa Cruz Mountains, you can expect lots of descents and ascents into canyons, which means bikers need decent endurance. Strong beginners and intermediate riders will enjoy these trails. A popular route in Russian Ridge is pedaling up Ridge Trail to Borel Hill where Mt. Tamalpais to the north is visible on a clear day. In Coal Creek, Crazy Pete's Trail is the single-track favorite of accomplished riders.

Finding the trailhead: From I-280 near Palo Alto, take Page Mill Road west and up into the hills. When Page Mill intersects Skyline Boulevard, continue straight through to Alpine Road and park immediately on the right in the parking area. This is one of the popular entrances to Russian Ridge Open Space Preserve. Coal Creek Open Space Preserve is across Skyline Boulevard.

Maps: Both preserves offer free maps at Skyline Boulevard trailheads.

For maps and more information about these parks and others in the district, contact:

Midpeninsula Regional Open Space District
330 Distel Circle
Los Altos, CA 94022
(650) 691-1200
www.openspace.org

SOME LOCAL BICYCLE SHOPS & ORGANIZATIONS

City Cycle of San Francisco
3001 Steiner St.
San Francisco, CA 94123
(415) 346-2242

Start to Finish Bikes
939 Howard St.
San Francisco, CA 94103
(415) 920-6700
599 Second St.
San Francisco, CA 94107
(415) 243-8812

Noe Valley Cyclery
4193 24th St.
San Francisco, CA 94114
(415) 647-0886

Bicycle Outfitter
963 Fremont Ave.
Los Altos, CA
(415) 948-8092

Trail Center
3921 E. Bayshore Rd.

Palo Alto, CA 94303
(650) 968-7065
www.trailcenter.org/maps.htm
Sells maps of nearly all Bay Area parks in all jurisdictions.

Bay Area Ridge Trail Council
26 O'Farrell St., Suite 400
San Francisco, CA 94108
(415) 391-9300
www.ridgetrail.org
ridgetrail@aol.com
Like the Bay Trail system, this will also be a continuous 400-mile recreational trail that encircles the entire Bay Area. "Wilder" than the urban, sea-level Bay Trail system, the Bay Area Ridge Trail connects paths high on the ridges and in the hills surrounding the San Francisco Bay Area. Not every section of the trail system allows bikes, so please heed posted signs.

THE SOUTH BAY AND
SANTA CRUZ COUNTY

A t one time, the Santa Clara Valley was an agriculturally rich region, covered by acres of apple, peach, almond, pear, apricot, cherry, and plum orchards. But that was before anyone really knew—much less cared—about this itty-bitty thing called a silicon computer chip. Welcome to the heart of "Silicon Valley" where computers and its ancillary products have replaced orchards as the cash crop. The Santa Clara Valley, defined by the Santa Cruz Mountains in the west, the San Francisco Bay in the north, the foothills of the Diablo Range in the east, and the Gabilan Range in the south, has been transformed into the largest metropolitan area in all of northern California. And people keep coming. Jobs in the high-tech sector exceed available housing. Poor air quality and traffic congestion are just some of the consequences. San Jose, the largest city in the entire Bay Area, is sprawling with a reputation of being without character or community. By contrast, just on the other side of the Santa Cruz Mountains, is remarkably laid back Santa Cruz County, home of more state parks than any other county in California.

Fortunately, the mountains and foothills found in both Santa Clara and Santa Cruz Counties provide an escape-hatch for mountain bikers who live in the South Bay Area. All within an hour's drive from San Jose, trails for riders of all abilities abound. To the east and south, in the Diablo and Gabilan Range, all the way down to the San Luis Reservoir, scattered oak trees dot steep hills. The area is especially attractive in the spring when a thick and fresh grassy green carpet blankets the hillsides. Summer can be unbearably hot, transforming the hills to parched yellows and browns. The riding season extends well into the winter, particularly when it's dry. The Santa Cruz Mountains, on the other hand, are a completely different environment, being mostly covered by fog-loving redwood forests, some of which are now protected ancient growths. When the summers are scorchers in the Santa Clara Valley, Santa Cruz County offers cool, shady rides in its mountains and along the bluffs overlooking the Pacific Ocean. So, if you wonder how can anyone live in the rat-race world of Silicon Valley, it's because there are plenty places of solitude in which to ride, all within an hour's drive.

RIDE 85 · Monte Bello–Stevens Creek Loop

AT A GLANCE

Length/configuration: 17-mile loop, clockwise; single-track, dirt road, and pavement

Aerobic difficulty: Moderately strenuous with a very strenuous section

Technical difficulty: Intermediate, due to wet creek crossings and some up and downhill sections of single-track

Scenery: Dense forest and riparian corridor along Stevens Creek. Great views of the valley created by the San Andreas Fault. From atop Black Mountain, expansive view of rolling grasslands, the Santa Clara Valley, the entire South Bay, and the Santa Cruz Mountain range towards the Big Basin area.

Special comments: Several other trails tie into this trail, leading to other rides in the neighboring preserves. Loop can be ridden in reverse, that is, counterclockwise, which allows you to descend an extremely steep portion instead of climbing it.

The Stevens Creek–Monte Bello Loop ride starts in Stevens Creek County Park and leads into Monte Bello Open Space Preserve. One of a number of preserves and county parks clustered here, Monte Bello OSP encompasses the headwaters of Stevens Creek in the Santa Cruz Mountain range. This popular 17-mile loop can be ridden in either direction, depending on how you want to tackle a 1.3-mile steep section, either as an ascent or descent. The combination of dirt roads, rugged single-tracks, and pavement requires intermediate technical skill. A beginner with strong endurance and the right attitude will have a good time, too. Starting at Stevens Creek Reservoir, the clockwise direction begins by heading gradually uphill along the San Andreas Fault Line, through a cool forest to Indian Creek Trail, a narrow fire road. Though only 1.3 miles long, Indian Creek is sure to stick in your mind because it's steep, ranging from 7% to 10%-plus grade. Walking is perfectly acceptable. When you reach the top of Monte Bello Ridge, the remaining short uphill to Black Mountain sitting at 2,797 feet is a piece of cake. The panoramic view is worth the effort and on clear days, you can see San Francisco to the north, Mt. Hamilton to the southeast, and the Loma Prieta peak to the south. And even if it's not clear, seeing the fog roll in over the coastal ridges is a stirring sight in itself. From this vantage point, you can check out the landscape as shaped and influenced by the San Andreas Fault which runs through Monte Bello OSP.

While catching your breath on Black Mountain, notice the different vegetation and terrain on both sides of the fault line. That's because the underlying rock is geologically different. The Pacific plate (the western land mass) was originally a part of the southern Sierra Nevadas and with each quake, it moves north a few feet, sliding and pushing against the North American plate (the eastern land mass). In time, the Pacific plate will become a part of Alaska.

Something to ponder as you ride through Monte Bello OSP is the fact that this portion of the San Andreas Fault Line is predicted to be the catalyst for "The Big

One." Some geophysicists have identified the rift zone near Black Mountain as "high risk" due to the fact that the last quake—the 1989 "World's Series" quake that was centered in Loma Prieta just south of here in the Santa Cruz Mountains—did not release much of the tension and strain that's been building near Black Mountain. There's much scientific speculation about whether the Loma Prieta quake was the expected "Big One." Viewed from an airplane, much of the San Francisco Peninsula contains a nearly perfectly straight, narrow valley paralleling the San Andreas Fault Line, running south from Point Reyes in the north, down to San Juan Bautista and beyond. The valley is the result of the two plates slipping passed each other. The region around Black Mountain, however, is the kicker. Instead of a valley, we have a mountain, which suggests that the two land masses crash, get crumpled and uplifted at this point instead of just quietly slipping by. That, according to some geophysicists, is evidence of increasing tension along the fault line. So, as you head out the door for this ride, you could tell everyone you're going on a scientific field trip. Sincere thanks to my cousin Bob Gong who contributed the trail notes for this great ride.

General location: About 3.5 miles west of Cupertino, just west of San Jose in the South San Francisco Bay Area.

Elevation change: 2,247 feet; starting elevation and low point 550 feet; high point 2,797 feet.

Season: Year-round. Be prepared for a little mud in the winter months.

Services: Ample parking, rest rooms, and water at many parking areas at the south end of Stevens Creek Reservoir, the recommended starting point. Except for portable toilets at the northwest entrance at Page Mill Road and near Black Mountain, there are no services on the route. Primitive campsites available near Black Mountain; for reservations and permits, call (650) 691-1200. All services available in Cupertino and metropolitan San Jose.

Hazards: Though rarely seen, beware of rattlesnakes, bobcats, and mountain lions. Watch out for vehicular traffic while riding the paved portions of Monte Bello and Stevens Canyon Roads, especially near the reservoir. While riding the single-track section, stay alert for on-coming bikers and hikers.

Rescue index: Even though this preserve is fairly popular, especially during the weekends, you should be self-reliant at all times. Parts of the loop are remote and you may wait a long time before anyone passes by. You're likely to find help from a passing motorist along the paved portion of the loop (Monte Bello Road or Stevens Canyon Road), or along Page Mill Road at the northern preserve entrance. A phone is located about a half mile northwest of Black Mountain on dirt Monte Bello Road. There is a fire station at Stevens Creek Reservoir, which you pass while driving to the parking area and starting point.

Land status: Monte Bello Open Space Preserve (Page Mill and Picchetti Ranch Areas), managed by the Midpeninsula Regional Open Space District.

Maps: The official park trail map is free and can be found at the north entrance and parking lot (gate PC01).

Finding the trail: Even though the bulk of the ride is within Monte Bello Open Space Preserve, the recommended parking spot is in Stevens Creek County Park, at the corner of Stevens Canyon Road and Mt. Eden Road, on the south end of Stevens Creek Reservoir. (Note: Upper Stevens Creek County Park is a separate chunk of park

RIDE 85 · Monte Bello–Stevens Creek Loop

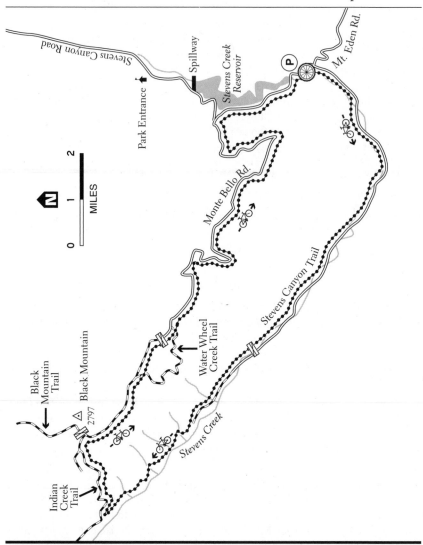

northwest of plain old Stevens Creek County Park.) To reach this starting point, drive west on I-280 out of San Jose. As you approach Cupertino, take the Foothill Expressway exit and go west by southwest for about 3 miles to the county park entrance. Foothill becomes Stevens Canyon Road as it crosses McClellan Road. Continue toward the spillway and on around the west side of the reservoir. Go pass Monte Bello Road leading off on your right at about 0.25 mile from the spillway. Stay on Stevens Canyon Road for another 1.25 miles to the intersection of Stevens Canyon and Mt. Eden Road, passing a fire station along the way. There are five parking lots near this intersection—choose one. Parking here will give you a nice warm-up before getting into the heart of the ride. Parking in a designated lot gives you the opportunity to fill your water bottles as well as take a bio-break prior to heading off into Stevens Canyon. (Parking in pulloffs along Stevens Canyon Road is limited and not permitted at the Monte Bello OSP boundary.) One final word before you start pedaling: The park is open from sunrise to sunset and rangers will issue citations to vehicles that remain in the lot after dark.

Sources of additional information:

Midpeninsula Regional Open
  Space District (MROSD)
330 Distel Circle
Los Altos, CA 94022-1404
(650) 691-1200
mrosd@openspace.org
http://www.openspace.org

Trail Center
3921 E. Bayshore Road
Palo Alto, CA 94303
(650) 968-7065

Info@trailcenter.org
http://www.trailcenter.org/maps.htm
This is a great retail source for biking maps of the Bay Area and California State Parks.

Topo!™ Interactive Maps
  on CD-ROM
Wildflower Productions
(415) 282-9112
http://www.topo.com/california

Notes on the trail: Begin by heading southwest on paved Stevens Canyon Road, away from the reservoir. Watch out for cars as you'll be sharing the road on this stretch. Begin a gentle climb over "roller" hills with Stevens Creek flowing in the opposite direction, taking turns running on either side of you. If you ride here after a rain or during an El Niño year, you're likely to see spectacular sections of whitewater along the creek. Bypass Redwood Gulch Road after about 2 miles from the intersection where you've parked your car. The traffic thins and for about 1.5 miles, Stevens Canyon Road continues its gradual climb out of Stevens Creek County Park towards Monte Bello Open Space Preserve, legally running through private land. Mind the neighbors and hoist your bike over the gate. Continue riding as the pavement becomes a gravel and hard-packed fire road. At 0.7 mile later, you reach the actual boundary of Monte Bello OSP. A map is posted here so you can get your bearings. If you're lucky, there may be a free map waiting for you in the signboard box, compliments of the preserve.

Stevens Canyon Road becomes Canyon Trail and narrows. After a creek crossing (try to keep your feet dry!), the dirt road becomes a single-track with some dipsy-doodles for about 0.3 mile. Be alert for other cyclists coming in the other direction. The landscape here is typical of a creek environment: cool forests populated by Douglas firs, oaks, pines, ferns and other understory. Continuing along Canyon Trail, two other trails intersect your path within the next 1.5 miles. Both Table Mountain Trail–Charcoal Road and the Grizzly Flat Trail (listed in order of appearance) are challenging climbs that take you nearly 2 miles to Skyline Boulevard, Long Ridge Open Space Preserve, and Upper Stevens Creek County Park. For this ride, though, continue on the Canyon Trail—save your energy because there's a challenging climb ahead! The trail once again widens for several people to ride abreast.

After another 2 miles of gradual climbing, you reach the fork of Canyon Road and Indian Creek Trail. Gear down, take a deep breath, and hang a right onto Indian Creek. This is one heck of a climb and the next 1.4 miles will test your strength. Walking and coaxing your bike uphill is an acceptable technique. During this stretch, try to admire the landscape while your leg muscles are screaming. Indian Creek gains nearly 850 feet in 1.2 miles on a nontechnical fire road. Ignore the pain and focus on your surroundings. The hills are covered with grassy meadows and populated with oak and madrone trees. Keep your eye out for deer, especially if you're fortunate enough to be one of the first ones out on the trail. As you climb above the timberline you begin to see spectacular views of the Santa Cruz Mountains to the west and Skyline Ridge with its Christmas tree farms across the narrow valley as you match its elevation. Take a moment to take in the view.

When you finally top the ridge—Monte Bello Ridge—and meet Monte Bello Road, turn right. Continue climbing but not as steeply. At about 0.3 mile, bypass Black Mountain Trail leading off on your left and in a few yards beyond it, you reach the high point of this ride, Black Mountain at 2,797 feet. [Incidentally, primitive camp sites very close to this point on Black Mountain can be reserved three days ahead by calling MROSD. at (650) 691-1200. Permits are required and rangers do check cars and people. This is a great place to catch a sunset the night before a full-day of riding Monte Bello OSP and the surrounding preserves. About 2 miles down Black Mountain Trail is the Page Mill Road entrance to Monte Bello OSP. It's another popular trailhead, especially recommended for campers.] The sweeping vista is magnificent here. Notice the nearly straight valley running north and south. That's caused by the San Andreas Fault Line which runs through Monte Bello along Stevens Creek which is now below to the west. If it's a clear day, you can see Crystal Springs Reservoir to the north as well as metropolitan San Jose to the southeast.

If your goal is to get back home today, continue on the trail to the right, toward the microwave towers. Stop at the towers for another great view. This time, take a look on both sides of the ridge you're on. Looking north by northwest, you can see San Francisco on a clear day. In fact, the entire Bay Area can be seen from this vantage point. The other side of the ridge looks out towards the Santa Cruz Mountain and the Pacific Ocean.

Follow Monte Bello Road almost 2 miles or so, generally descending towards a vineyard and the gate marking the reserve boundary. Pass Water Wheel Creek Trail on your left. (On the other hand, check it out if you'd like. Water Wheel Creek Trail is a fire road and offers a slightly longer alternate route. It rejoins Monte Bello Road near the preserve gate.) From the gate, Monte Bello Road resumes pavement and is a rapid, 5-mile descent which includes several tight, hairpin turns. Watch out for occasional vehicular traffic. (This is a popular hill-climb for road bikers too.) The road ends on Stevens Canyon Road at the reservoir's edge. A right turn at the bottom, followed by a mile on Stevens Canyon Road returns you to your car. Congratulations! Another spectacular ride under your belt.

RIDE 86 · Henry Coe Middle Ridge Loop

AT A GLANCE

Length/configuration: 11-mile loop, clockwise; dirt roads and single-track

Aerobic difficulty: Very strenuous due to steep climbs

Technical difficulty: Intermediate to advanced; single-track portion is narrow, sometimes rugged and twisty

Scenery: Remote ridges and deep canyons, oak woodlands, meadows, and forests of ponderosa pine. You can find lots of solitude here.

Special comments: Not recommended for beginners. In recent years, Coe State Park has grown to over 81,000 acres. Future trails will be constructed, most of which undoubtedly will allow bikes. Currently, there are about 200 miles of dirt roads and trails open to bikes. The Fall TarantulaFest is unique to this park.

Mention Henry W. Coe State Park to local bikers and you're likely to get a response along these lines: "Ooooh, that place is tough. Lots of steep climbing. You gotta be in great shape to ride there." The other refrain is "Awesome technical single-tracks there." They're right. Henry Coe is both. It's widely revered as the most challenging mountain biking area in the South Bay Area. The easiest access point is its western area, where the canyons are deep and the ridges high. Park rangers rate most of the bikeable roads and trails in the entire park from moderately difficult to extremely difficult (that's their combined aerobic and technical assessments). "There are practically no easy trails for bikes," as declared by the park's Web site and printed materials—and it's no joke. If you want to discourage beginning bikers, bring 'em here.

That said, the Middle Ridge Loop as described below is one of the least punishing rides available, relatively speaking. Definitely not for the weak of heart or mind. This loop will give you a good taste of what the park has to offer. The terrain of this route is varied, mixed with brutally steep long and short climbs, equally steep descents, interspersed with rolling stretches through oak woodlands. Technically, the loop consists of somewhat rugged fire roads with scattered loose rocks and an almost 3.5-mile stretch of very narrow, sometimes twisty single-track, parts of which skirt shallow drop-offs. You don't need to be an expert bike handler but you do need to have strong stamina and climbing legs. Dirt roads and trails are well-marked. (Please obey signs prohibiting bikes on hiking-only trails.)

Spring is arguably the best time to ride because temperatures are comfortable, grasslands lush and green, and wildflowers dazzling. Summer is typically blazingly hot, especially since many parts of the route are not shaded, and anything over 100 degrees feels a lot hotter when you're huffing and puffing up a steep, exposed hill. In the fall, temperatures are moderate and though not known for brilliant autumn color, the late afternoon sun illuminates the parched yellow hills, creating a golden atmosphere. Winter is typically cold and wet, interspersed with mild sunny days. (After substantial rain, the park often closes trails for several days to prevent excessive erosion and trail damage. If you plan to ride during the wet season, call ahead to find out which trails, if any, are closed. Trails may be closed after at least a half inch of rain.) This ride begins at the main entrance, next to the visitor center, on the western edge of the park, located 13 miles from US 101 in Morgan Hill via a winding road. Another popular entrance for bikers and equestrians is Hunting Hollow. Other than these two entrances, all other access points are lightly used.

Coe Park is one of the Bay Area's best backyards, offering acres of solitude. In addition to oak woodlands and scattered gray pine trees, there are areas of oak savannah, chaparral, and forests of ponderosa pine. While on Middle Ridge Trail, be sure to stop and check out the unusually large manzanita bushes which look more like trees. Their bark is reddish-chocolate color and often look like peeling paint, revealing a blonde core. Run your hand over the core—it's incredibly smooth and sensual. Wildlife thrive here and a short list include black-tailed deer, gray foxes, bobcats, wild pigs, wild turkeys, raccoons, and rarely seen mountain lions and golden eagles.

RIDE 86 · Henry Coe Middle Ridge Loop

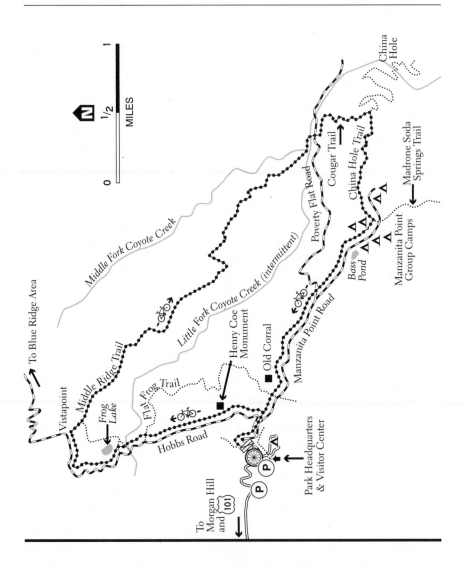

At least 137 kinds of birds have been spotted, from the majestic bald eagle to the tiny Anna's hummingbird. Another park creature worthy of mention is the tarantula. Don't be alarmed if you see any of them on the trail. They exist in great numbers here and these nonpoisonous eight-legged residents are honored by the annual "Fall TarantulaFest and Barbecue." (No, tarantulas are not the BBQ fare.) Sponsored by the Pine Ridge Association, a nonprofit organization dedicated to the well-being of Henry Coe State Park, this event includes a slide show, guided nature walks in search of tarantulas for observation, displays, music, food, and raffle drawings for

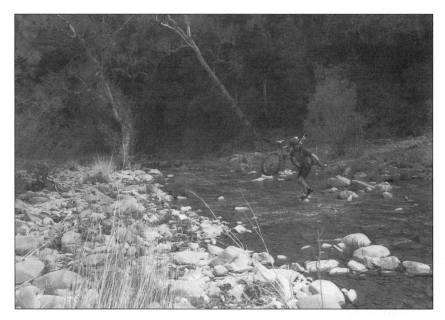

Crossing the Middle Fork of Coyote Creek.

prizes. You can even have one of these furry little guys crawl over you as you pose for the festival photographer. So, as you approach the main entrance in your car, keep a sharp eye out and try not to run over any of these celebrated creepy critters that might be crossing the road. Likewise when you're pedaling on the trails.

General location: About 35 miles south of San Jose; 13 miles east of Morgan Hill.

Elevation change: 1,800 feet; starting elevation 2,600 feet; high point 3,000 feet; low point 1,200 feet. Lots of ups and downs, some of which are very steep and long.

Season: Year-round. Spring and fall are the best times. Summer can be unbearably hot and winter is often wet, forcing brief trail closures.

Services: Water, rest rooms, picnic tables, phone, and Visitor Center at the park's main entrance. Water taken from lakes, ponds, creeks, and springs throughout the park need to be treated before consumption. Maintained campgrounds available near the main entrance. (The campground is located on an exposed hilltop—an ideal star-gazing spot.) Ample parking available in several lots and fees for day-use and camping are collected. All other services can be found in Morgan Hill and the nearby suburban cities of south San Jose.

Hazards: Before riding, inquire about the safety of Coyote Creek's Middle Fork at the Middle Ridge Trail junction. Stay alert for rattlesnakes, poison oak, and stinging nettles as well as rarely seen mountain lions. Watch out for ticks especially if you ride during the cool, moist months. Winter storms are likely to swell creeks, making them extremely hazardous, if not impossible to cross. If you ride in the summer, carry plenty of water. Heat exhaustion and heat stroke are real dangers, especially when you're out among remote steep, rugged, and exposed terrain. This warning applies to even the strongest riders who are visiting Coe Park for the first time. Ranger(s) and uniformed volunteers on duty year-round (every weekend and intermittently on weekdays) at the park headquarters as well as on patrol in the backcountry.

Rescue index: Steep trails discourage many trail users, hikers and bikers alike. For that reason, expect to see fewer people as you ride farther from the Visitor Center. You might get lucky and find someone who may be of help during an emergency. However, because other access points are lightly used, most of Coe Park is remote. That said, you need to be self-reliant. Bring enough food and water, and ride with a buddy. In case of an emergency, you'll most likely have to make your own way back to the Visitor Center/headquarters or send your buddy for help.

Land status: Henry W. Coe State Park.

Maps: *Henry W. Coe State Park, Trail & Camping Maps*, published by Buddha-Nature Maps & Books (P.O. Box 1736, Flagstaff, AZ 86002), also available at the visitor center at the park headquarters.

Finding the trail: From San Jose, drive south on US 101 to the East Dunne Avenue exit in Morgan Hill. Go east through a residential section of town, about a 3-mile stretch. Look for a sign, "Henry W. Coe State Park, 10 miles" at the top of the first hill. Continue on East Dunne as it winds up the narrow mountain road, past Anderson Reservoir. You reach the main park entrance approximately 13 miles from US 101. Continue past the lower overflow dirt parking lot to the main gate, Visitor Center/headquarters, and main parking lots. Park and begin pedaling from here.

Sources of additional information:

Henry W. Coe State Park
P.O. Box 846
Morgan Hill, CA 95038
(408) 779-2728

www.coepark.parks.ca.gov
The Pine Ridge Association can also
be reached at this address and
phone.

Notes on the trail: [Before pedaling off, ask a ranger at the Visitor Center/headquarters about the passibility of Coyote Creek's Middle Fork , specifically at the junction of Middle Ridge Trail and Poverty Flat Road. Is it safe to ford the creek?] After filling your water bottles at the Visitor Center, ride up Manzanita Point Road, (starts as a paved road just past the ranger's residence, eventually becomes gravel). Immediately bypass Monument Trail (hiking only) on your left. Go through a gate and continue heading towards Hobbs Road, Poverty Flat Road, Manzanita Point Group Camps, Bass Pond, and China Hole Trail. About 0.3 mile from the Visitor Center, turn left onto Hobbs Road, a gravel fire road, and begin a sometimes grueling climb towards Henry Coe Monument and Frog Lake. The gravel soon becomes dirt and in almost a mile from the Visitor Center, you reach the monument site and the high point of the ride, sitting at about 3,000 feet. Continue rolling along the dirt fire road through oak woodlands and in a short while, Hobbs leads you down a steep section towards the Little Fork of Coyote Creek. At almost 2 miles, in the vicinity of the creek crossing, bypass Flat Frog Trail on your right. (Flat Frog allows bikes and is an easy grade which ultimately leads back up to the Visitor Center in about 1.5 miles, making it a great little 5-mile loop, roughly.) Stay on Hobbs and begin a steep, half-mile climb towards the intersection with Middle Ridge Trail, bypassing a lesser trail on your right which leads to Frog Lake. Continue on Hobbs around the west side of the lake (on your right a few yards in the distance). When you reach Middle Ridge Trail, take a breather by continuing a few yards farther to an unmarked view point overlooking the canyon of Coyote Creek's Middle Fork and across to Mt. Sizer (3,216 feet) and Blue Ridge.

After your break, retrace your path back to Middle Ridge Trail and get ready for a sweet, slightly technically challenging 3.2-mile single-track. The intersection here sits at about 2,800 feet. Following Middle Ridge, the first 2 miles descends gently, rolling up and down oak woodlands, punctuated by several steep and loose stretches. Sections of the trail become narrower and the turns tighter. There are several stretches that skirt shallow drop-offs in some places as it weaves through stands of oak, ponderosa pine, and huge manzanita trees. Then, the last 1.5 miles of single-track becomes intense as it plunges you down almost 1,000 feet. At the bottom, sitting at 1,200 feet is the Coyote Creek Middle Fork at the junction of Middle Ridge Trail and Poverty Flat Road.

When you reach the Middle Fork, you've pedaled about 6.8 miles from the Visitor Center. Most of the year, you're faced with a wide, wet creek crossing, about 20–40 feet across and 2–4 feet deep. (The creek is normally dry in summer and early fall.) Portage your bike to the other side and pick up Poverty Flat Road. Head east (left) on Poverty Flat, a narrow dirt road. (For a shortcut back to the Visitor Center, go right onto Poverty Flat and immediately begin climbing the steep and somewhat rocky terrain. The road connects to Manzanita Point Road in about 1.4 miles. Then, go right onto Manzanita and follow it back to the Visitor Center, closing the loop at 9.5 miles.) I hope you truly enjoyed Middle Ridge Trail because it's payback time. In a few yards, turn right onto Cougar Trail, a single-track and begin an extremely steep climb back up to Pine Ridge. Switchbacks throughout and open views over chaparral bushes help ease the pain as you grind—or walk—up the mountainside, about 680 feet gain in less than a half mile. When you reach the ridge sitting at 1,880 feet, go right onto China Hole Trail. (If you need a reason to do more cussin' and climbin', hang a left instead and follow the trail down to China Hole, a great summertime swimming hole sitting at 1,160 feet. You reach it in about a half mile after losing 720 feet. After a refreshing swim, retrace your tracks, which means climbing back out.) Follow China Hole Trail basically due west and begin a moderate climb over rolling terrain. In about a mile, when you cruise past the Manzanita Point Group Camps, the trail becomes Manzanita Point Road, a wide dirt road. You're likely to past folks walking along, fishing poles and tackle boxes in hand, going to and from Bass Pond, a popular fishing hole. Continue west on Manzanita over wide-open, rolling hills, gradually gaining elevation. You close the loop by reaching the Visitor Center in about 2.5 miles from the group camps. Total distance is about 11 miles.

RIDE 87 · Pacheco State Park Loop

AT A GLANCE

Length/configuration: 9.6-mile clockwise loop; single- and double-track and dirt road

Aerobic difficulty: Moderate with some short, very steep sections

Technical difficulty: Intermediate; some spots of rocky creek crossing and a stretch of oddly banked, narrow trail traversing an exposed slope

Scenery: Rolling, grassy hills are incredibly green against a clear blue sky in the spring. Wildflowers cover the hillsides with a profusion of color. Other times of the year, the hills are parched and the temperatures can be scorching. Wind turbines can be seen on nearby hillsides.

Special comments: Not suited for very young children or kid-trailers. Not yet a well-known park, escape the crowds and enjoy the solitude while it's still available.

Pacheco State Park is a relatively young park having been opened in 1997 and not yet well-known or frequently used. Well, okay, equestrians know about the park and enjoy it frequently but mountain bikers are relatively few. Not only does the park offer incredible vistas of the rolling hills (especially gorgeous in the spring with ex-plosions of colorful wildflowers), all the trails allow bikes! Amazing. Imagine a park that's favored by equestrians that hasn't closed any trails to bikers. The routing de-scribed here gives you a taste of what this little park has to offer. Wide single-track trails make up this ride, and generally speaking, strong beginners with basic techni-cal skills are sure to love this ride. That's not to say more skilled riders will find this park boring. Who could not enjoy a jaunt amid rolling, green hills covered with wildflowers and 360-degree views of the hills and valleys in the distance? Punctuated by several very steep but short hills, even the most highly skilled riders are chal-lenged—riding up a 45-degree slope without falling off your bike is not easy.

Though the park encompasses 6,890 acres, only 2,600 acres is currently open to the public. The eastern section adjoining the San Luis Reservoir will be open once additional trails and safety issues are resolved. Currently there are 28 miles of trails now open with new trails planned. Lots of configurations can be achieved and you could spend an entire day exploring.

Pacheco State Park represents the last remaining section of the 1843 Mexican land grant of Francisco Pacheco. Owned by five generations of Pacheco's since the mid-nineteenth century, we have Paula Fatjo, a direct descendant of Francisco Pacheco, to thank for donating the land to the state. Her requirement was that her ranch land be kept intact for the pleasure of people who shared her enjoyment of horses and the surrounding unspoiled environment. (See, this park was born with equestrians in mind. We should consider ourselves lucky that bikes are even allowed, let alone on all trails. So, let's protect our biking privilege by exercising proper trail etiquette when we meet other trail users.) In addition to incredible vistas, you may see tule elk, deer, bobcat, coyote, fox, hawks, and eagles during your visit.

General location: About 90 miles southeast of San Jose, 33 miles west of Los Baños, on the west edge of San Luis Reservoir.

Elevation: 820 feet; starting elevation 1,350 feet; high point 1,920 feet; low point 1,100 feet. A variety of short hills, both mellow and steep; a few long, gradual hills.

Season: Year-round; early spring to mid-spring is the best, when the hills are green and the temperatures just right. Summers parch the hills and it gets bloody hot here, especially since there's very little shade en route. Fall months are comfortably warm months.

RIDE 87 · Pacheco State Park Loop

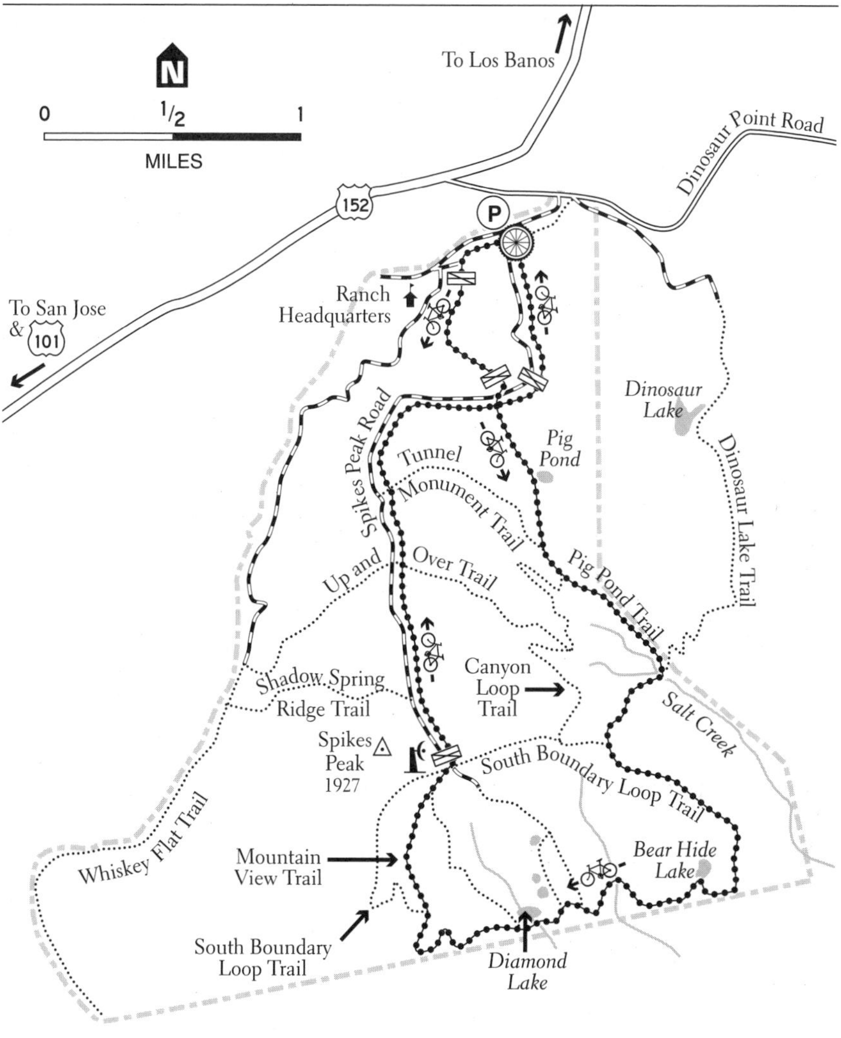

N

To Los Banos

Dinosaur Point Road

0   1/2   1
MILES

152

P

To San Jose
& 101

Ranch
Headquarters

Spikes Peak Road

Tunnel

Monument Trail

Pig
Pond

Dinosaur
Lake

Dinosaur Lake Trail

Up and Over Trail

Shadow Spring
Ridge Trail

Canyon
Loop
Trail

Pig Pond Trail

Salt Creek

Spikes
Peak
1927

South Boundary Loop Trail

Whiskey Flat Trail

Mountain
View Trail

Bear Hide
Lake

South Boundary
Loop Trail

Diamond
Lake

Services: None on the trail. Any water found on the route must be treated before consuming. No drinking water for humans at the trailhead at this time. There are a couple of picnic tables and while there are no BBQ facilities, portable ones are permitted. Parking fee is about $5. No camping allowed but there are a number campgrounds next door in the San Luis Reservoir State Recreation Area.

Hazards: Stay alert for scattered poison oak, ticks, and rattlesnakes. Equestrians frequent the park and have right of way. If you ride in the spring, expect some stretches of all trails to be a bit overgrown, effectively obscuring an otherwise obvious path. Armed with a park map and some route finding skills, you won't get completely lost, especially since occasional signs mark the trails. A section on Spikes Peak Road parallels an electric cattle fence—watch out for a related gate across the trail.

Rescue index: The route is essentially in remote territory and the back country beyond the boundaries is even more remote. And being a relatively young park, it doesn't attract many trail users. If you ride during the week, don't be surprised if the parking lot is empty. The park is popular with equestrians and you're likely to met a few on weekends. So, in the event of an emergency, don't wait for someone to come by. Make your own way back to the parking area where you may find a spartan park staff on duty. The fastest way back to the parking area is Spikes Peak Road which runs through the middle of the park. The nearest phone is at the Dinosaur Point Visitor Center, about a mile east of the state park on US 152. You can always try flagging down a motorist on heavily traveled US 152—traffic is fast here and many drivers will probably blow past you.

Land status: Pacheco State Park.

Maps: *Pacheco State Park*, a little flyer with map and mileages usually found in a box on the parking lot bulletin board.

Finding the trail: From San Jose, drive south on US 101 to US 152. Follow US 152 through Gilroy and go about 20 miles east towards the San Luis Reservoir. Take the Dinosaur Point exit to the right. (If you see the Romero Visitor Center turn-off and the reservoir, you've gone too far.) That road runs along the south side of the highway for about a half mile before entering Pacheco State Park. Continue almost another half mile to the parking area. Park and begin pedaling here.

From Los Baños, follow US 152 west for about 24 miles, going past the reservoir and the Romero Visitor Center. As soon as you past the western edge of the reservoir, watch for the Dinosaur Point Road exit which is accessed via a left turn lane on US 152. Turn left and follow the road into the park entrance and about a half mile further to the parking area. Park and begin pedaling here.

Sources of additional information:

Pacheco State Park
31426 Gonzaga Rd.
Gustine, CA 95322-9737
(209) 826-6283

Notes on the trail: This gem of a park is relatively small and the boundaries are well-marked. Be sure to take a free map with you, usually found in a box on the parking area bulletin board. Many signs planted at trail junctions furnish clues as to where you are, if not identify the exact trail you're on. If you ride in the spring, the trails near the south boundary may be overgrown and faint. Nevertheless, a few trail markers along the way assure you that you are indeed following a trail.

Starting from the parking area, pedal west on the gravel road, past the horse corral and several park buildings. (The trail directly south of the parking area is Spikes Peak Road and you'll be returning on it.) In a few yards, hang a left onto Pig Pond Trail, a wide, dirt single-track. Go through a gate and begin following the trail due south over gently rolling, wide-open hills. Cross Spikes Peak Road and continue on Pig Pond Trail. After a mile, you begin to see the wind turbines (tall windmills) on the nearby hills in the east. At about 1.5 miles, you reach Pig Pond. The wide trail on the right side of the pond is the one you want to follow. On the left side of the pond, however, is a narrow single-track and if you want to check out numerous garter

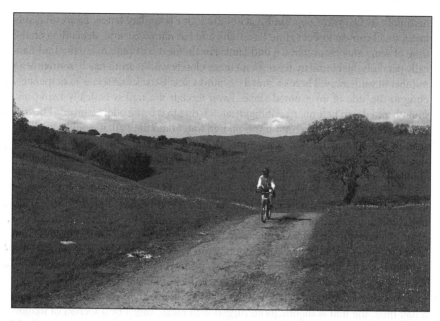

The best time to enjoy this ride is in the spring when the trails have dried and the hills are covered by a thick carpet of fresh green grass and dotted with wildflowers.

snakes that seem to gather here, by all means follow that trail. When you're finish gawking at the snakes, follow the trail on the west side of the pond and tackle a steep but short uphill followed by a sweet downhill. Go past Tunnel Monument Trail and continue straight, sort of bearing left still on Pig Pond Trail. (Remember what I said about the trail markers—not all of them identify the trail you're pedaling; sometimes they just indicate which direction the trail goes.) The wind turbines appear in the distance ahead of you.

At about 2 miles, your trail intersects Canyon Loop Trail which run both right and left. Ignore the right trail that leads towards Up and Over Trail. Instead, bear left and go through a gate. Now, you begin skirting the eastern boundary of the park as evident by a fence on your left. Here, you can actually hear the wind turbines if they're operating. And if you're riding in the spring, you'll see a hillside of wildflowers. Enjoy a long descent then cross tiny Salt Creek (beginners may want to walk over the somewhat rocky creekbed). Still on Canyon Loop, the trail parallels the stream for a few yards before heading up a steep but short hill on your right. You're now pedaling away from the fence, it now being directly behind you. If the ground is a bit moist from the last rain, expect the going to be a bit tough, especially if horses have left hoof prints deep in the soft, somewhat muddy trail. This is where you experience the most shade from a clump of trees and understory (a welcome respite if it's blazing hot). When you reach the top, the trail becomes generally packed dirt and gravel, and is a wide single-track, sometimes looking like a double-track.

You reach the South Boundary Loop Trail at just over 3 miles. The trail runs both left and right. A sign indicates that the left trail leads to Bear Hide Lake. Follow the left trail and continue the gradual climb up a sparsely forested hill. The trail then begins cruising up and down towards Bear Hide Lake. Eventually, you're forced to make a hard right as Canyon Loop Trail reaches the south boundary fence. Descend gently into a small canyon to Bear Hide Lake. The trail has narrowed, and, depending on the time of year, may be overgrown and faint. For the next half mile or so, the trail basically parallels the boundary fence, sometimes closely within arm's reach, sometimes a number of yards away. There's a stretch of narrow single-track that seems to desperately cling to the side of an exposed slope. Even though the trail is basically hard-pack, smooth and doesn't climb, it's a difficult stretch due to it being oddly banked. The trail itself is not level; it's angled and if you poured water onto the trail, it would run off the side. Beginners may find this a bit unnerving, especially if they're not accustomed to single-track riding. Walking is an acceptable technique and this odd stretch is short, about 0.2 mile.

At about 5 miles, go through a gate (remember to leave it as you found it: opened or closed). Here, Spike Peak Road leads uphill on your right. This road is the main trail through the heart of Pacheco State Park and it's essentially a narrow dirt road that is the quickest way back down to the parking area. Good to know if you're running out of time or you need to bail out due to foul weather or an emergency. But for this ride, continue straight, bearing left on the wide single-track, still on South Boundary Loop Trail. As you drop down into the Diamond Creek drainage amid open space, tiny Diamond Lake comes into view and the boundary fence is on your left. For less than a half mile, the trail is slightly more rugged with rocks, edged by a section of shallow drop-offs. Continue past the lake and cross a tiny creek. Depending on past usage and recent rains, the trail may peter out a bit then reappear. Even if you seem to lose the trail, you'll be able to spot a trail marker nearby. There is a trail marker that indicates a trail leading up and over a rise on your right. According to the map, this is Diamond Lake Trail. Bypass it and stay on South Boundary Loop Trail, still following the fence.

At about 6 miles, the trail veers right and heads north away from the fence. The single-track trail is still South Boundary Loop Trail and at 6.2 miles, it intersects Mountain View Trail (the first junction after turning your back to the boundary fence). Shift into low gear, hang a right onto Mountain View and begin climbing a steep but short open hill, practically devoid of trees. If the trail is faint, look up the hill to a lone oak tree and ride or walk in that direction. The trail becomes more obvious next to the tree amid a 360-degree view of the rolling hills. As you continue uphill, short radio towers begin to come into view on your left. Several signs that simply indicate a trail are planted here and there.

At about 7 miles, you reach a major four-way intersection with an impressive view of the wind turbines and the San Luis Reservoir in the distance. The signs here identify Canyon Loop Trail and Spikes Peak Road. At this point, go left through a gate and onto Spike Peak Road. Take note: the fencing adjacent the gate is an electric cattle fence. In a few yards, you reach the top of the climb with the radio towers directly nearby on your left. This is the highest point in the park. From here, following Spikes Peak Road is mostly a downhill run punctuated by several steep but short hills. As you bomb down this road, watch out for a cattle gate with a small solar panel looming over it. The gate is not obvious from a distance and if you're intoxicated by the fast descent, you might run right into it. So, heads up. Bypass other trails (or explore them if you wish!) and keep following Spikes Peak Road as it runs over hill and dale. The 360-degree views are exhilarating along this stretch and before you know it, you reach the intersection with Pig Pond Trail. Look familiar? You rode through this intersection at the beginning of your ride. Continue through Pig Pond Trail and stay on Spikes Peak. In a few yards, go through a gate and coast the last half mile back to the parking area.

RIDE 88 · Big Basin: Gazos Creek– Chalk Mountain Ride

AT A GLANCE

Length/configuration: 21.7-mile combination [12.9-mile loop with an 8.8-mile out-and-back (4.4 miles one-way)]; dirt fire roads. China Grade option: 26.2-mile ride with some pavement.

Aerobic difficulty: Moderately strenuous due to steep but brief climbs

Technical difficulty: Mostly mild; some intermediate stretches of short, steep descents over gravel

Scenery: Shady forests of old- and young-growth redwoods, conifers, and tan oaks, as well as exposed, arid, chaparral-covered terrain. Glimpses of the Pacific Ocean as you approach Chalk Mountain and on clear days, you can see all the Marin Headlands.

Special comments: Several configurations of varying length can easily be made, all of which are suitable for strong beginners. Strong adults with kid-trailers can ride Gazos Creek Road from the park headquarters as an out-and-back.

Despite being next door to the heavily populated Bay Area, general consensus declares Big Basin Redwoods State Park as one of California's finest parks. And being the first state park inducted into the State Parks System in 1927, it is the oldest. Within its 17,000-plus acres are majestic old-growth redwoods (some over 1,500 years old), four waterfalls, marshlands, rocky peaks, and both lush riparian and arid chaparral ecosystems. This bike route is composed of fire roads that lead through the heart of the park, along high ridges, up and down creek drainages, and through several starkly contrasting environments (Ridge, Gazos Creek, Johansen, White House Canyon, and Chalks Roads). Essentially, the ride described is a 12.9-mile loop, ridden counterclockwise with a 4.4-mile out-and-back (8.8 miles round-trip) mid-way in the loop for a total distance of 21.7 miles. Because the ride starts and ends on the loop, you can easily skip the out-and-back ridge ride to Chalk Mountain. But consider this before you dismiss it: on clear days, the short ride to the top rewards you with a splendid view of the Pacific, up to the Marin Headlands, and even the Farallon Islands. Using easy, wide fire roads, the elevation gain is a mere 300 feet with some healthy ups and downs thrown in to get you breathing heavy—even strong beginners can ride it. (Unlike the cool redwood forest, the ridge can be very hot and dry. Be sure to bring plenty of water.) Optionally, you can lengthen this ride to 26.2 miles by pedaling North Escape Road and China Grade (two rarely used paved vehicle roads) and a short stretch on CA 236. But why ride pavement when you can ride all dirt? This paved road option is quite a bit more scenic because it runs through the park's best display of old-growth redwoods, some as tall as 300 feet and 40–50 feet in diameter. (This China Grade Option is described briefly at the end of the main ride.)

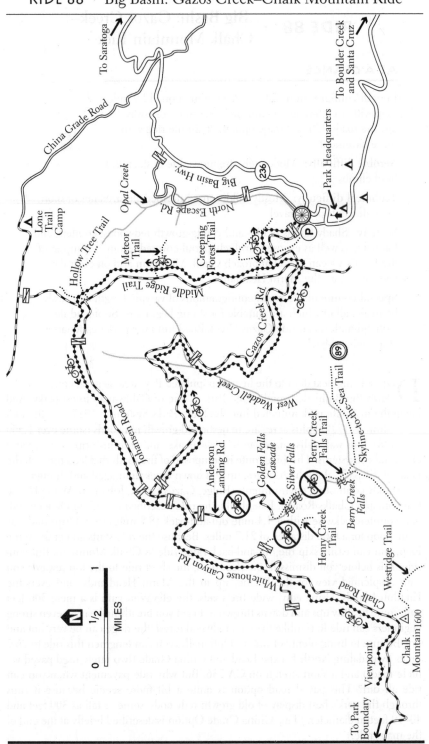

Whichever route you choose, solid, basic bike handling skill are all that's required, making this a mildly technical ride. Some spots may be a bit more rugged, sandy, or steep but it's nothing that dismounting and walking a couple of steps can't overcome. Strong stamina, however, is required, thanks to lots of steep but brief climbs.

So what's the big deal about redwoods? Well, they're bigger and older than you and me for starters. And they're the closest thing to being immortal on this planet. Though some of the redwoods standing in Big Basin are 1,500 to 2,000 years old, it's estimated they are offshoots of older trees which were offshoots of still older trees, many of which date way back to the Jurassic period when dinosaurs were roaming the earth. The ones that grow here are lucky, having been saved just in the nick of time from hungry loggers in the late-1800s when the Gold Rush was setting off a population explosion. Demand for lumber soared and numerous lumber mills were established from Monterey up to the Oregon border. Soon, loggers began salivating over Big Basin. In 1900, a movement of educators and community leaders to save the redwoods was launched. By 1902, after intense campaigning, a legislative bill created the California Redwoods Park that encompassed a small portion of the park we now have today. Though slated to open for public enjoyment shortly thereafter, a fire broke out at a nearby sawmill and ultimately consumed almost the entire park. The park finally recovered in 1911. In 1927, the California State Park System was born. Becoming the first park in the system, California Redwoods Park was renamed Big Basin Redwoods State Park. Today, acquisition of privately held parcels of land in the Big Basin watershed is the goal of the Sempervirens Fund working in conjunction with the State Department of Parks and Recreations. As an example, Gazos Creek is one of three streams south of San Francisco that is still blessed with a native run of coho salmon. Because cohos are sensitive to silt and water temperature, its survival is dependent on the stream gradient and thick tree canopy. Logging practices that strip trees from a mountainside that drains into a creek results in unchecked soil runoff, ultimately clogging streams and disrupting riparian and aquatic habitat. Completely securing the watershed protects the life-blood of all ecosystems within the park and guarantees the integrity and preservation of the forest community.

General location: About 23 miles north of Santa Cruz.

Elevation change: 1,000 feet; starting elevation and low point 1,000 feet; high point 2,000 feet. Outbound mostly sustained ascents, interspersed with a few level sections.

Season: Year-round. Winter may see lots of rain though some years have been relatively dry. Summer attracts the most use. Fall is the best time, when the temperatures are moderate and most of the tourists have left.

Services: Water, phone, rest rooms, visitor center, showers, and small grocery store can be found at the main entrance near the park headquarters. Maintained campground and tent cabins available. Even though there are over 100 campsites, this is one of the prettiest campgrounds in all of California. Eateries, gas, grocery stores, shops, and other services located in nearby Boulder Creek. All other services in Santa Cruz.

Hazards: Rattlesnakes, particularly in dry, chaparral terrain. Mountain lions live here but are rarely encountered. The 26-mile option pedals China Grade, a lightly used vehicle road, and CA 236, a slightly busier but very short stretch of road. Watch out for other trail users (hikers, bikers, and equestrians), especially on popular Gazos Creek Road.

Rescue index: You can always find help and a phone at the park headquarters. Summer sees the most use and you're likely to encounter other trail users who may be of help, especially on Gazos Creek Road. Chalk Road and White House Canyon Road are not as popular and you're likely to wait a long time for someone to come along. In the off-season, especially during the week, expect to make your own way back down to the park headquarter or send a buddy for help.

Land status: Big Basin Redwoods State Park.

Maps: *Big Basin Redwoods State Park Map,* published by Mountain Parks Foundation in conjunction with the California State Park System.

Finding the trail: From Santa Cruz, go north on CA 9, a windy mountain road through dense forests. Follow it for 12 miles to Boulder Creek and the CA 236 intersection. Turn left (west) onto CA 236 and drive 9 miles to the main park entrance and headquarters. Go left onto North Escape Road and park in a day-use space, near the headquarters. Be sure to stop off at the headquarters and pay a use fee, about $6 (and be sure to display the receipt on your car).

Sources of additional information:

Big Basin Redwoods State Park
21600 Big Basin Way
Boulder Creek, CA 95006
(831) 338-8860

Mountain Parks Foundation
525 N. Big Trees Park Rd.

Felton, CA 95018
(831) 335-3174

Sempervirens Fund
Drawer BE
Los Altos, CA 94023-4054
(650) 968-4509

Notes on the trail: Trails and dirt roads are fairly well marked throughout the park. The only real big challenge is finding your way from where you've parked around the park headquarters area to the trailhead. From the intersection of CA 236 and North Escape Road where the headquarters is located, pedal north on North Escape. Look left for a paved road leading over Opal Creek via a vehicle bridge. Follow this left across the bridge and through a large gate—this is Gazos Creek Road that is closed to unauthorized vehicles. A sign at the gate says "Authorized vehicles only" but bikes are allowed. Pavement soon turns to gravel as it begins to climb gently. You're among the fragrant forest now. Keep your eyes and ears open and you may be lucky enough to spot an endangered marble murrelet flittering from tree to tree. Cruise past Creeping Forest Trail and Dool Trail, (hiking only). In less that a mile from the bridge, Middle Ridge Road, a fire road, leads off on your right.

Hang a right onto Middle Ridge, go through the gate and begin the climb up to Johansen Road at Berry Creek Ridge. Views are not terrific from this road with only glimpses of nearby ridges. If you look closely, you may have a glimpse of the ocean from a rocky knoll. View or not, it's a peaceful stretch among a shady forest of redwoods, mixed conifers, and tan oaks. The road is interspersed with lots of steep but brief ups and downs. Let your bike zip down the hill and ride the momentum up to the top of the next rise. Trail condition is mildly technical with a few patches of sand and semi-buried slabs of boulders to keep you awake. Go pass Meteor Trail (hiking only) at 2.4 miles and Hollow Tree Trail at 3.5 miles, adjacent to a metal gate across Middle Ridge Road. Continue through the gate and in a few yards, you reach the intersection with Johansen Road running both left and right. There's an interpretive signboard here which talks about Berry Creek Ridge, its headwaters which sustains the nearby 1,000 year-old redwoods, and the Johansen Family who immigrated from Denmark and operated three log mills in the area.

Hang a left onto Johansen Road and begin a gradual descent punctuated by steep but brief ups and downs along the forested ridge. The road condition is fairly mild with some rough spots, similar to Middle Ridge Road. Go through another gate at about 4 miles. Stay on the main, well-traveled road, ignoring any roads or trails that lead off on your right—they run outside the state park boundary which Johansen Road closely parallels. At 6.3 miles, go through another gate located at Sandy Point. There's not much to see here and if not for a small wooden sign nailed to a tree, you wouldn't know this is Sandy Point. A trail on your left makes a sharp hairpin turn and it connects to Gazos Creek Road in a few yards. Bypass it and continue on Johansen Road for a few yards to a major intersection within the shady forest. The dirt road due straight, bearing right is White House Canyon Road, which leads to Chalks Road and eventually to the top of Chalk Mountain in 3.8 miles. The road on the left is the top of Gazos Creek Road, the same road you originally pedaled at the beginning of the ride. (If you're running out of time or lack the steam to push on to Chalk Mountain, you can turn left onto Gazos and follow it all the way down to the park headquarters. From here, you reach the headquarters in 6.5 miles.) From this intersection, the ride out to Chalk Mountain is a 4.4-mile out-and-back (8.8 miles round-trip).

If the day is crystal clear, like after a rain, you have to ride out to Chalk Mountain because you'll be able to see up the coast to the Marin Headlands and the Farallon Islands. To the south, you'll see the Monterey Peninsula. If not, the ride is still a good add-on for more mileage. Though the elevation gain is a mere 300 feet, approximately, there are plenty of ups and downs to push your endurance. To reach Chalk Mountain, bear right onto White House Canyon Road, a wide, fairly smooth fire road, and proceed through a gate. In a short ways, go past gated Anderson Landing Road on your left (signed off-limits to bikes and horses). Look through the trees on your right (west) and glimpses of the Pacific Ocean come into view—if you're lucky, there won't be a fog bank obscuring the horizon.

The landscape soon changes and you emerge from the cool, dense redwood forest to exposed, arid terrain covered with chaparral bushes and a scattering of conifer and tan oak trees. The easy, wide fire road skirts a few spots of drop-offs and you have far reaching views of the inland ridges and valleys. Road composition becomes fine gravel and yellowish-white in color, like chalk. In fact, the road leads you past a mound that looks like a huge, loose sand pile of this chalk-colored gravel, completely devoid of vegetation. Ignore a lesser, unsigned road on your right marked by a dilapidated gate. As you gradually climb past the sand pile on your right, Henry Creek Trail (hiking only) appears on your left. Stay on the main, wide, exposed road. On your right, bypass another dirt road (which is actually the continuation of White House Canyon Road leading into private property). At this point, as you go through a gate, your road now becomes Chalk's Road. The next 1.5 miles to Chalk Mountain is a push up several long stretches of steep terrain. Mellow sections here and there give you some respite while wide open views offer you a good reason to stop and catch your breath. Bypass Westridge Trail (hiking only) on your left. In a few yards, go past a dirt road on your right and stay on the main road as it curves to the left. From within the curve, there's another road on your left leading to the top of Chalk Mountain in a few yards. There's not much here except a short radio tower, a concrete shack and an outhouse hidden in the bushes. For the prize viewing spot, however, continue through the curve, staying on the main road to the next rise about 0.5 mile further.

When you're finished enjoying your break, turn around and retrace your path back to the Gazos Creek Road and Johansen Road intersection. When you reach the intersection, hang a right onto Gazos Creek Road and begin a gradual descent towards the creek through the cool redwood forest. Along the way, there are stumps of huge redwoods, evidence that old-growth trees once lived here. Almost 3 miles from the previous intersection, you cross the creek running through a culvert under the trail and begin climbing out of the drainage. About 0.7 mile from the creek, go through a gate and continue on the road, cruising past young-growth redwoods, mixed conifers, ferns, and lush understory. Just over 2 miles from the creek, after a series of gradual ups and downs interspersed with level sections, you close the loop by reaching the junction with another gated fire road on your left. That road should look familiar because it's Middle Ridge Road. From this point, stay right and retrace your path on Gazos Creek Road toward the vehicle bridge and park headquarters. Approximate mileage including the out-and-back to Chalk Mountain is about 21.7 miles.

China Grade Option: This routing skips Middle Ridge Road entirely. Starting from the same parking area as above, begin pedaling north on North Escape Road. Instead of turning left towards the bridge, continue on the paved road. In a few yards, go through a gate that closes the road to unauthorized vehicles. Go through a second gate after about a mile. The road begins a gradual climb and at almost 3 miles from the first gate, go through another gate at the junction with CA 236 (Big Basin Highway). Stay alert for traffic as you turn left onto CA 236. Follow the highway for about a mile to China Grade, another paved road. Say good-bye to the traffic as you cautiously turn left onto China Grade. A little over 3 miles up China Grade, the pavement becomes dirt. But along the way, as you grind up the moderate grade, you'll be rewarded with some of the best views in the park. About 100 yards past Skyline-to-the-Sea Trail, on your left, is the only view of Moss Landing and the Monterey Bay. Also on this stretch are outstanding views overlooking a forest of ancient, old-growth redwoods. About a mile after the dirt road begins, look for gated Johansen Road on your left. Go through the gate and follow Johansen to its intersection with Middle Ridge Road. Bypass Middle Ridge and, as previously described, continue on Johansen to Chalk Mountain and returning on Gazos Creek Road. Total distance for this option is about 26.2 miles. [Many thanks to David Jones, park aid at Big Basin Redwoods State Park, for recommending this option.]

RIDE 89 · Big Basin: Skyline-to-the-Sea Trail (Waddell Creek)

AT A GLANCE

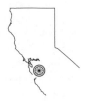

Length/configuration: 11-mile out-and-back, (5.5 miles each way); mostly dirt road

Aerobic difficulty: Easy; mostly smooth, graded fire road

Technical difficulty: Mildly technical with deep rain ruts

Scenery: Shady ride through young-growth redwood and conifer forests along a lush creek environment. A short, half-mile hike leads to Berry Creek Falls, a 70-foot waterfall in a lush, mossy, forest environment.

Special comments: Suitable for youngsters and adults with kid-trailers.

H ere's a gem of a bike route that everyone can enjoy, including youngsters and adults pulling kid-trailers. This 11-mile out-and-back (5.5 miles each way) is the only portion of the magnificent Skyline-to-the-Sea Trail that allows bikes. Starting at sea level, near the Rancho del Oso Nature and History Center, the route gently gains about 450 feet in over five leisurely miles on a well-graded fire road through the Waddell Creek valley. The last quarter-mile or so steepens slightly but is still an easy pedal. A mostly smooth trail bordered by riparian habitat and meadows, and shaded by tall Douglas fir, Monterey pine, and second-growth redwood trees, the route closely follows the creek for the entire bikeable distance. In the spring, this stretch is blessed with over 20 species of wildflowers, including a profusion of forget-me-nots. Severe winter storms may leave a couple of rain-rutted spots which require portaging your bike—and kid-trailer—for a couple of steps. A footbridge spans Waddell Creek so you needn't get your tootsies wet, unless you want to, of course. The creek does swell, typically in the winter and spring, and sometimes fording it can be a risky undertaking. Highlighting the ride is Berry Creek Falls, a 70-foot free fall tumbling into Waddell Creek, surrounded by towering redwoods, ferns and sorrel, and moss-covered rocks. Though the bike route ends at Berry Creek Falls Trail, it's a short hike to the falls, about a half-mile of easy hiking. That trail is hiking-only and a bike rack is conveniently provided. There's an observation deck at the base of the falls and if the day is warm, it's a nice spot for a picnic. If you hike roughly one mile beyond Berry Creek Falls, you'll see Golden Falls Cascade and Silver Falls.

The creek is named after William Waddell, either because as a logger in the 1800s, he brought down some of the biggest redwood trees in the area, or because he was mauled to death by a grizzly bear near the creek. (Perhaps the Native Americans who revered the ancient redwood forest with religious superstition were on to something.) Grizzlies once roamed these parts, particularly along the creek, until the late 1880s when they were completely wiped out by hunters in the name of protection. If you'd like more information about the natural and social history of the region, visit Rancho del Oso Nature and History Center located near the trailhead at Highway 1 (CA 1). "Rancho del Oso" is Spanish for Ranch of the Bear.

General location: About 20 miles north of Santa Cruz on Highway 1 (CA 1).

Elevation change: 450 feet; starting elevation and low point is sea level; high point 450 feet. Berry Creek Falls observation deck is at 600 feet, approximately.

Season: Year-round. Winters tend to be wet, sometimes rainy.

Services: Water, pit toilets, and pay phone available near the first gate at the park office, near the horse camp, about 0.4 mile from Highway 1 on Skyline-to-the-Sea Trail. Pit toilets are generally available at all 4 trail camps within the first 3 miles of the trail. Parking available at Waddell Beach on the west side of Highway 1 across from the trailhead (fee usually charged during the summer). The public is invited to visit the Rancho del Oso Nature Center located a few yards south of the trailhead on Highway 1. (Parking at the Nature Center is not recommended because in order to access the trailhead, you'd have to ride a short stretch on Highway 1. The trail which connects the Nature Center to the bikeable trail is hiking-only.) Though this route is the "backdoor" into Big Basin Redwoods State Park, you can't pedal all the way to the park headquarters and campground on this route because after a certain point, the trail is hiking-only. All services can be found in Santa Cruz.

Hazards: Expect a few rain ruts that force you to dismount and carry your bike a couple of steps. Watch out for other trail users, especially during the popular sum-

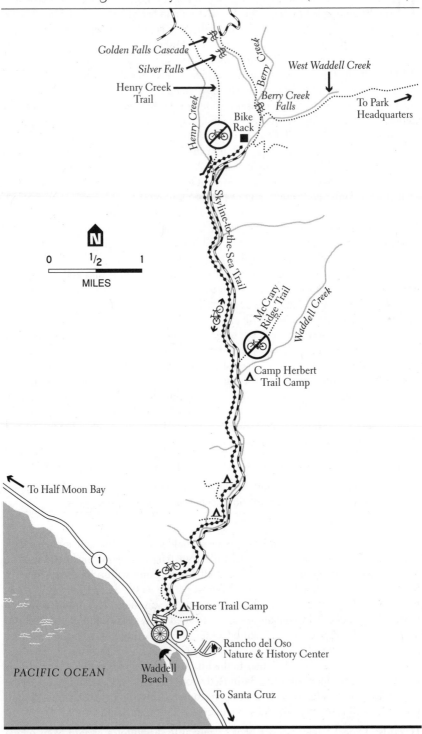

Golden Falls Cascade

Silver Falls

Henry Creek
Trail

Berry Creek

West Waddell Creek

Henry Creek

Berry Creek
Falls

To Park
Headquarters

Bike
Rack

Skyline-to-the-Sea Trail

N

0   1/2   1

MILES

McCrary Ridge Trail

Waddell Creek

Camp Herbert
Trail Camp

To Half Moon Bay

1

Horse Trail Camp

P

Rancho del Oso
Nature & History Center

PACIFIC OCEAN

Waddell
Beach

To Santa Cruz

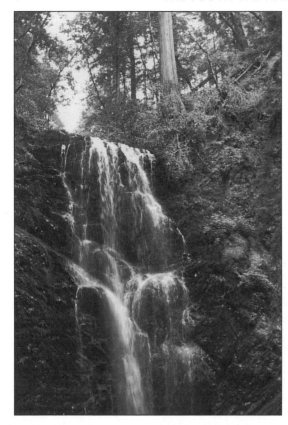

Berry Creek Falls is worth the short hike from the end of the bikes-permitted portion of Skyline-to-the-Sea Trail.

mer months. Though the trail is wide, youngsters should be comfortable with sharing the trail with others. Mountain lions live here but are rarely encountered.

Rescue index: During the popular summer months, chances are good you'll meet other trail users who can offer assistance. The trail sees fewer use all other times of the year, especially on weekdays. A pay phone is located at the horse camp, about 0.4 mile from the trailhead at Highway 1. You can always flag down a passing motorist on Highway 1 who may be of help.

Land status: Big Basin Redwoods State Park.

Maps: *Big Basin Redwoods State Park Map*, published by Mountain Parks Foundation in conjunction with the California State Park System.

Finding the trail: From Santa Cruz, drive north on Highway 1 (CA 1) for about 18 miles, going through the tiny town of Davenport along the way. After passing Rancho del Oso Nature Center on your right, you'll immediately go across the Waddell Creek bridge. After the bridge is a small parking area on the right side, directly across from Waddell Beach on your left. The beginning of Skyline-to-the-Sea Trail is adjacent to the small dirt lot—look for a gate across the trail which is actually a paved road at the trailhead. Park in either this lot or across the highway at Waddell Beach. (A parking fee is often charged at the beach parking lot.) Begin pedaling from here.

Sources of additional information:

Big Basin Redwoods State Park
21600 Big Basin Way
Boulder Creek, CA 95006
(831) 338-8860

Mountain Parks Foundation
525 N. Big Trees Park Rd.
Felton, CA 95018
(831) 335-3174

Notes on the trail: [Before pedaling off, be sure to bring a bike lock.] It's easy to follow and you really don't need a map; just stay on the main, well traveled road. From the highway parking area, go through the gate which controls vehicle access onto Skyline-to-the-Sea Trail. The pavement becomes dirt in a short ways, after you pass the ranger office and horse camp. The first 3 miles closely parallels the park boundary and leads you past a few homes and farms along the way. At 3.2 miles, just after Camp Herbert, you leave civilization behind as you continue to follow Waddell Creek into the heart of Big Basin Redwoods State Park. Stay on the main, wide dirt road, bypassing all lesser trails. Incidentally, all the trails that intersect your road are hiking-only. Expect a couple of deep rain ruts to force you to dismount and portage your bike a few yards. At about 5.3 miles, you reach a point where you need to cross Waddell Creek. You can either ford the 20- to 30-foot-wide creek—and probably get your shoes wet—or you can use the footbridge which is reached in a few yards by a single-track trail. After the crossing, continue on Skyline for about a 0.5 mile to its junction with Berry Creek Falls Trail. This is the end of the bikeable trail, as evident by the bike rack. Lock your bike and hike about 0.5 mile to Berry Creek Falls and its observation deck. Silver Falls and Golden Falls Cascade is about a mile further up the hiking trail. The hike is a lovely jaunt and worth every inch. When you've had your fill of the serene surroundings, retrace your path back to the trailhead and your car.

RIDE 90 · Henry Cowell State Park Ramble

AT A GLANCE

Length/configuration: 8.5-mile out-and-back with spur (4.25 miles each way); paved multi-use path and dirt roads

Aerobic difficulty: Moderate overall due to some climbing; paved path is easy

Technical difficulty: Mild; some sandy patches

Scenery: Shady redwood and mixed conifer forest; lush riparian habitat along San Lorenzo River; chaparral vegetation at the higher elevations; distance view of the Monterey Bay and surrounding Santa Cruz Mountains from atop the Observation Deck. Of special note is Cathedral Redwoods, site of giant redwood trees.

Special comments: Great place for family camping and bicycling weekends. The Roaring Camp and Big Trees Railroad Line with trips to the Santa Cruz Boardwalk is accessible from the park.

Looking for a great outdoor adventure with the youngsters? Load up the car with camping gear, marshmallows for roasting over the campfire, and, of course, your bikes. Henry Cowell State Park is just the ticket. (To be exact, the state park is divided into two huge, unconnected chunks of land. The ride described here is in the southern unit.) This 8.5-mile out-and-back with spur (4.25 miles each way) route follows a paved multi-use path and dirt roads. While hardcore, highly skilled riders would be bored by this ride, it's perfect for the kiddies.

The park is a repository of great wilderness diversity, offering parents and children a first-hand educational experience. Here you'll find magnificent, fog-loving giant redwoods, rich riparian habitat along the San Lorenzo River, a grassy meadow which serves as a natural gathering place for wildlife, and a chaparral community of sun-worshipping shrubs in the higher elevations. Not to be missed is the Redwood Loop, an easy one-mile hiking-only trail that threads through a forest of giant redwoods. (Kids don't want to walk? Tell 'em the grove is similar to a location in the movie *Return of the Jedi*, in which the Ewok's forest was the site of a flying battle scene. That location is actually along the Howland Hills–Stout Grove Ride, Ride 8.) Continue to subject your child to an educational adventure by taking them to the park's nature center which offers exhibits on the natural and human history of the park. And to get your kids to visit the center, bribe them with a choo-choo train ride on the adjacent historic Roaring Camp & Big Trees Railroad line. The line's old-fashioned steam-powered train chugs through the scenic redwood forest on the steepest narrow-gauge railroad grade in North America. During the summer, you can even take the train to the Santa Cruz beach and Boardwalk, home of the Big Dipper Roller Coaster. Now is this a great family outing or what?

General location: 6 miles north of Santa Cruz, just south of Felton. Note: this ride takes place in the southern unit of the state park; the northern unit is less than a mile north of Felton.

Elevation change: 505 feet; starting elevation 700 feet; high point 800 feet; low point 295 feet. Gently rolling terrain.

Season: Year-round though winter and early spring tend to be wet.

Services: Water, rest rooms, and showers available at the Graham Hill campground entrance. Water spigot with potable water located at the Observation Deck. Visitor Center along with rest rooms, water, and picnic tables can be found at the Park Head-quarters entrance off CA 9. Plenty of parking available at both entrances. Steelhead fishing along San Lorenzo River is allowed (permit required) in the winter months on Wednesdays and weekends. All other services found in nearby Santa Cruz.

Hazards: Youngsters should be comfortable sharing the path with other trail users. The bikeable trails in the park are generally wide, allowing ample room for passing. If you ride the brief River Trail out-and-back section alongside the grassy meadow near the park headquarters expect to encounter some vehicular traffic in the main entrance parking lot. If you follow trails leading down toward San Lorenzo River, there are no bridges at any crossings.

Rescue index: You may find other trail users who may be of help, especially in the summer when the park is popular.

Land status: Henry Cowell Redwoods State Park (southern unit).

RIDE 90 · Henry Cowell State Park Ramble

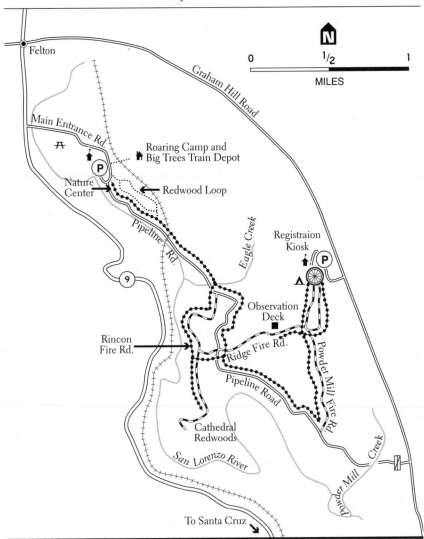

Maps: *Henry Cowell Redwoods State Park,* published by Mountain Parks Foundation (525 N. Big Trees Park Road, Felton, CA 95018), available at visitor center and campground entrance.

Finding the trail: From within Santa Cruz, follow Highway 1 (CA 1) north and take the Ocean Street/Central Santa Cruz exit. Hang a right onto Graham Hill Road and head inland for about 3 miles uphill and turn left into the campground at the park entrance. (The park headquarters and nature center is located at the main entrance on CA 9, about 6 miles north of the intersection of Highway 1 and CA 9 in Santa Cruz.)

Sources of additional information:

Henry Cowell Redwoods State Park
101 N. Big Trees Park Rd.
Felton, CA 95018
(408) 335-4598
Camping info: (408) 438-2396

Roaring Camp & Big Trees Narrow
  Gauge Railroad
P.O. Box G-1
Felton, CA 95018
(831) 335-4484

http://www.roaringcamp.com
Train schedule: Runs daily during
the spring, summer, and fall, though
frequency varies depending on peak
months. Off-season hours are generally limited to weekends and holidays. Call ahead for schedule, fees,
and planned activities. Round-trip
fares start at about $11 for kids and
$15 for adults.

Notes on the trail: [Before hopping on your bike, be sure to bring a bike lock with you. Consider bringing a camera, too, as there are many photo opportunities, especially if you have kids along.] From the park campground off Graham Hill Road, pedal south through the campground to Ridge Fire Road, a dirt road. Bypass several hiking-only trails along the way. (Single-track trails are tempting. Sorry, bikes are only allowed on dirt roads throughout the park.) About 0.3 mile from the campground, bear right at the signed junction with Powder Mill Fire Road (this is the spur portion of the ride). In about 0.2 mile further, you reach the Observation Deck. The deck is a modern structure, (not exactly architecturally attractive). But no matter— you're not here to view the deck but rather the Monterey Bay and Pacific Ocean, which is especially gorgeous on a clear day. After soaking in the view, retrace your path back to the junction with Powder Mill Fire Road. (You could continue due west from the deck on Ridge Fire Road, but I wouldn't recommend it. That portion of the road is deep sand punctuated by tall planks much like mini-retaining walls used to stabilize the trail. Follow this portion of Ridge and I guarantee you'll carry your bike more than you'll ride. Not much fun, especially if you're accompanied by whining youngsters.) From the intersection, bear right onto Powder Mill and follow it down a slight descent to Pipeline Road, reached in about 0.5 mile.

Pipeline Road is a fairly level, paved multi-use path. Go right onto it and continue past Ridge Fire Road and Rincon Fire Road (we return to explore them later). Begin skirting San Lorenzo River, and cruise underneath a railroad track trestle. In about 2.3 miles, Pipeline ends in the vicinity of the park headquarters, near a grassy meadow, the Environmental Education Center and Bookshop, the Nature Center, and main park entrance. Across the parking lot from the Bookshop is the Roaring Camp & Big Trees Narrow-Gauge Railroad. The train depot located on the other side of the tracks can be accessed via a short walking path, even though the railroad line is not part of the state park and is not on park property. Riding your bike on the tracks is not only stupid, it's prohibited! (The good folks that run the railroad line asked me to stress that because, despite the obvious reason to stay off, occasionally dim bikers pedal the tracks and trestles, and then complain that the train's running!) Also, not to be missed near the end of Pipeline is the Redwood Loop, a 1-mile hiking-only trail that threads through magnificent giant redwoods. It's a worthwhile stroll and the kiddies might even get a kick out of the size and age of these living organisms. A lovely picnic area is available near the grassy meadow.

When you're finished exploring this portion of the park, turn around and retrace your path on Pipeline Road back to the Rincon Fire Road junction. Hang a right onto Rincon, a dirt road, and begin a gentle climb. Follow the road as it curves through the shady redwood forest. Bypass a dirt road leading off on your left (that's Ridge Fire Road though it's not signed as such). In almost a mile, you reach Cathedral Redwoods, site of towering redwoods. The trees' elevated canopies enclose the area, creating a sense of great reverence, much like the awe induced by a sacred cathedral. After sufficient oohing and ahhing and checking out the trees, turn around and retrace your path on Rincon Fire Road. (If you continue out on Rincon, the road quickly loses elevation as it leads down to the river. Bikes are allowed but bear in mind that you'll have to climb back up the hill—an especially grueling challenge for most youngsters.) Retrace your tracks about a half-mile from the Cathedral and make a right onto an unsigned dirt road—this is Ridge Fire Road and it intersects Pipeline Road in about a few yards, about 0.2 mile.

Hang a right onto Pipeline and retrace your path back to Powder Mill Fire Road. (You can continue on Pipeline about 0.3 mile further, at which point the road descends steeply to the creek. Just like the Rincon Fire Road mentioned above, the return is somewhat steep and likely to not be much fun for kids.) Go left onto Powder Mill and begin a gradual climb back up toward the campground. About a half-mile from Pipeline, Powder Mill forks; bear right and follow it all the way back to the campground and your parked car. (You know you've missed this turn if you reach the Ridge Fire Road intersection. Ridge runs both left and right. You can turn right here and retrace your path back to the campground.)

RIDE 91 · Wilder Ranch: Gray Whale Loop

AT A GLANCE

Length/configuration: 12-mile figure-8 loop; dirt road, single- and double-track and pavement

Aerobic difficulty: Moderate with a mix of brief gentle and steep climbs

Technical difficulty: Mostly intermediate with some mild sections; smooth and wide dirt roads; single-tracks provide the most challenge being narrow, sometimes strewn with loose rocks, exposed tree roots and lined with poison oak

Scenery: Shady forest along creek ravines; fragrant forests of young-growth redwood, eucalyptus, conifer, and laurel trees; wide-open rolling meadows; occasional hilltop views of the Pacific Ocean and the Monterey Bay

Special comments: The park contains about 33 miles of trails, all of which are open to bikers. Strong youngsters may enjoy the dirt road portions of this loop as an out-and-back.

How many state parks in northern California allow bikes on all trails? Not many. Wilder Ranch State Park is one of those rarities. (Pacheco State Park, Ride 87, is another one described earlier in this chapter.) The landscape at Wilder is diverse and its trails are terrific. Hard to believe that us mountain bikers have the run of the place. This figure 8-loop gives you a good taste of the terrain and trails as it meanders for 12 miles round-trip through shady, cool creek habitat and fragrant forests of redwoods, laurel, conifer, and eucalyptus. The ride uses plenty of dirt roads and single- and double-tracks, typically hard-packed dirt with scattered shallow patches of sand. Sections of the single-tracks are tasty, mostly in the shady forest, spiced with abrupt dips, short climbs, exposed tree roots, and poison oak. Adventurous beginners who know when to dismount and walk can still enjoy the single-tracks.

Blessed with over 33 miles of trails, the park encompasses over 6,200 acres, from the coastal bluffs edging the Pacific Ocean on the south side of Highway 1 (CA 1) to the rolling meadows and ravines of the Santa Cruz Mountains on the north side. In late 1997, the Gray Whale Ranch area was added, extending the northern boundary all the way to Empire Grade Road, making use of old ranch roads which run through open, rolling meadows and redwood canyons. Immediately on the other side of the road is the University of California–Santa Cruz campus, site of a network of fun single-track trails open to bikes.

Like many other parts of the state, this area was home to Native Americans. The Ohlone Indians lived here for over 4,000 years, living off the bounty of the land and sea. In the late 1700s, livestock raising was introduced by the padres of the Santa Cruz Mission. In the late 1830s, Rancho Refugio (now present-day Wilder Ranch) was created and named by a Mexican land grant. In addition to raising cattle, subsequent owners began dairy farming and cheese-making. Jose and Maria Bolcoff (daughter of the original owner of the ranch) raised 14 children in their adobe home. Built in 1830, the adobe is the oldest structure on the ranch and still stands today. In 1871, the ranch was purchased by D. D. Wilder and L. K. Baldwin. They continued dairy farming and frequently introduced equipment which were deemed innovative for that time, including the water-driven Pelton wheel. By the turn of the century, "Wilder's Dairy" was considered one of the finest "cream dairies" in California. New structures were built and included a dairy barn, a new horse barn, a bunkhouse, and the grand Victorian home where descents of Wilder lived. In the late 1960s, the Wilder family sold the ranch to a developer who was intent on constructing houses and commercial buildings. Public opposition prevailed and the state purchased the property in 1975. In 1989, the park was open to public use. Today, a variety of historical and cultural events indigenous to the area are sponsored throughout the year, including a barn dance and barbeque, roping demonstrations, historic children's games, and docent-led tours.

General location: About 2 miles north of Santa Cruz on Highway 1 (CA 1).

Elevation change: 890 feet; starting elevation and low point 85 feet; high point 975 feet. Lots of brief ups and downs.

Season: Year-round. Some trails develop deep pockets of mud during the wet months. Summer finds the trails hot and dusty.

Services: Water and rest rooms available at the state park parking lot; parking fee charged. Pay phone located near the park entrance booth. Picnic tables and pit toilets available at the Wilder Ranch Cultural Preserve historic area. Docent-led tours of the site offered during certain times of the year.

Hazards: This is a popular park, especially during the weekends. Expect to share the road with other trail users, including equestrians. Watch out for on-coming traffic while on single-track trails. Wagon Wheel Trail, a single-track, is designated one-way. Shady, narrow paths alongside creeks are prone to erosion after a storm, punctuating intermediate trails with extremely difficult spots. Dismounting and carrying your bike over these rugged spots may be the safest option. Poison oak can be found in shady, forested areas. Cars parking for free along Highway 1 outside the park are prone to vandalism.

Rescue index: Though the park's popularity can be considered a drawback, it also means you're likely to meet other trail users who may be of help during an emergency. If you ride early in the day during the week, you're sure to find solitude on these trails. Should you need help, make your way to the Empire Grade Road on the northern boundary and flag down a passing motorist. Directly across from Empire, in the near distance, are the dormitories of University of California–Santa Cruz. Otherwise, make your way back down to Highway 1 or the park office on the southern boundary where phones are located at the Cultural Preserve and near the park entry booth.

Land status: Wilder Ranch State Park.

Maps: *Welcome to Wilder Ranch*, published by Southeast Publications USA, Inc., available at park office entry booth.

Finding the trail: From the intersection of Highway 1 and CA 17 in Santa Cruz, follow Highway 1 north. Traffic gets a bit gnarly through this part of town so keep an eye out for signs indicating Highway 1. Go through CA 9/River Street, High Street, Bay Street, and Western Drive. About 2 miles after Western Drive, turn left (toward the ocean) at the brown state-park sign. At the park entry booth, stop to pay the parking fee (about $6) and pick up a map. Park in the paved lot and begin pedaling from here. (Free parking along the dirt pull-offs along Highway 1, just before and after the left turn into the park, is permitted. However, because vandalism has been known to occur in these free lots, I highly recommend leaving your car in the park's paved lot—the fee is a small price to pay. Besides, Wilder Ranch uses the revenue to maintain the park for your enjoyment).

Sources of additional information:

Wilder Ranch State Park
1401 Old Coast Rd.
Santa Cruz, CA 95060
(831) 423-9703; (831) 426-0505

Notes on the trail: From the paved parking lot, pedal north through the lot and hang a right on the same road you drove in on; you're now riding away from the park entry booth. (If you're riding with a cyclometer, start it here as you leave the parking lot.) The paved road descends towards the Cultural Preserve, marked by several old, simple Victorian houses and barns. You reach the preserve in about a half-mile, at which point, turn left into the historic site. Please obey the signs to dismount and walk your bike through the site towards Highway 1. In a short distance, bear left and then right past an old barn that houses antique farm equipment. Hop back on your bike and follow the road as it leads through a tunnel under Highway 1. Now on the north side of the highway, amid a clearing surrounded by rolling hills, continue on the dirt road, bypassing Wilder Ridge Loop Trail on your left.

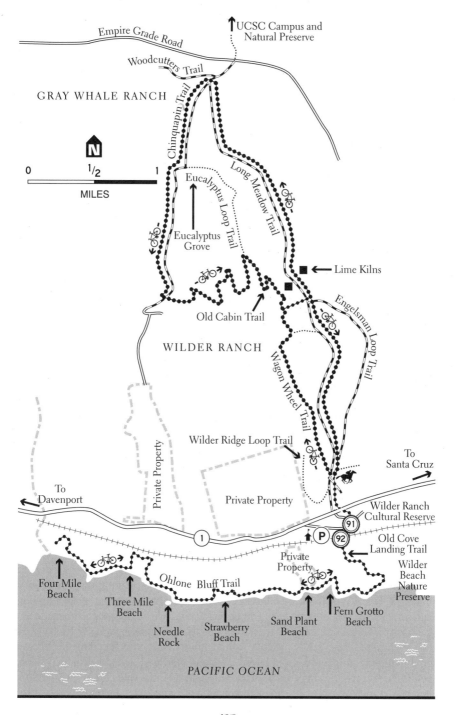

A few yards farther, you reach a signed intersection of five trails. Take Wagon Wheel Trail by staying left. (Wagon Wheel is designated one-way, the direction you're headed.) The trail begins as a hard-packed, single- and double-track trail. Soon, the trail is marked by scattered patches of soft dirt and some loose rocks. The trail leads you into the shady forest and you find yourself among moss-covered trees, redwoods, ferns, and thick patches of green sorrel. The trail narrows and hugs a tiny creek, occasionally skirting a shallow drop-off of about 10–20 feet on your left. Portions of Wagon Wheel are highly prone to erosion after a storm or a long season of wet weather. Stay alert for potholes and washouts, especially since the trail is dark and shady for the next 1.7 miles. This stretch is the most technically challenging of the entire figure-8 loop. You gain elevation as Wagon Wheel leads you up sometimes very steep but brief sections over patches of loose rock the size of softballs and cantaloupes. The single-track trail seems more like a narrow trough at times, with tall grasses and bushes on both sides. Watch out for poison oak which grow profusely along this stretch. Eventually, Wagon Wheel veers away from the creek and out of the deep shade. Bypass several unmarked trails leading off your path; stay left. At 2.5 miles, you reach the junction with Old Cabin Trail on your left. Bear right, still following Wagon Wheel, now a wide, hard-packed trail heading east. From this point, the rest of the ride is not nearly as challenging.

In a short distance, about 0.3 mile farther, at 2.8 miles, you come to another major four-way intersection in a small clearing. A sign here indicates Old Cabin Trail is reached by the trail you've been riding. Hang a left onto an unidentified wide single-track (sometimes masquerading as a double-track) and begin riding north. In a few yards, after going through a metal gate (leave it as you found it—open or closed), you see a sign identifying this road as Long Meadow Trail. The sign also tells you that Chinquapin Trail is reached in 2.2 miles. In the near distance, the remains of several limekilns can be seen. Follow Long Meadow towards Chinquapin as the trail leads you between the two widely placed limekilns. After a steep and brief hill climb, the terrain opens up more dramatically, revealing rolling grassy hills.

Welcome to the meadow. The trail continues to run up and down, sometimes steeply, but, in general, over easy terrain. Look behind you once in a while and, if the fogbank has dissipated a bit, you'll see the ocean. At about 3.6 miles, underneath a huge tree within all this open space is a pit toilet. Long Meadow Trail continues its gradual climb. At 4 miles, go through an opening in a fence. The meadow begins to diminish as redwoods and conifer trees appear. Soon, you reach the junction with Chinquapin Trail at about 5 miles, roughly the high point of the figure-8 loop.

Hang a left onto Chinquapin Trail (a right takes you to Empire Grade Road and the north access gate of Wilder Ranch in 0.3 mile). The trail begins a gradual descent interspersed with some level sections. Cruise through small open meadows and a few stands of trees. At about 6 miles, after passing a large fragrant Eucalyptus Grove on your immediate left, Chinquapin ends at Eucalyptus Loop Trail. The trail runs in both direction but for this ride, go right. (Explore this area later, creating your own configurations.) Eucalyptus is a wide hard-pack trail dotted with occasional spots of erosion and soft dirt, just the thing to keep you alert. Keep an eye out for a signed narrow single-track trail on your hard left—it's the continuation of Eucalyptus Loop Trail and it's located next to a deep sandy patch near the bottom of a short descending hill. (If you go through the sand and reach a paved road and a dirt trail signed Enchanted Loop, you've just missed the single-track.) Hop onto narrow Eucalyptus Loop Trail and follow it as it rolls over open meadows, becoming a double-track in some places. Like most of the trails in Wilder Ranch, this trail is mostly hardpack with some patches of sand—all very rideable. Eventually, the trail leads you back into the shady forest filled with redwoods, conifers, and laurel as well as ferns. At 7.8 miles, the single-track becomes a bit technical with exposed tree roots as it leads you down towards a creek. Cross the creek and climb a very short, steep and rugged stretch spiced with more tree roots. Poison oak lining the trail may persuade you to dismount and walk this brief, difficult portion. After a sharp left turn running uphill, the trail mellows somewhat and the poison oak is not as threatening. Amidst the redwoods, cross another tiny creek and climb a short hill out of the ravine. When you emerge from the forest and into an open meadow, the single-track widens. At 8.7 miles, signed Old Cabin Trail leads off on your right from Eucalyptus Loop Trail.

Turn right onto Old Cabin Trail, a generally easy, narrow single-track punctuated by a few deeply rutted sections. Descend into the redwood forest again, toward another tiny ravine. Expect exposed tree roots and abrupt dips in the trail. Stay alert to dodge tree limbs and more poison oak. At 9.4 miles, grind through a tiny creek and then climb steeply out of the ravine. The trail soon levels. Take a breather if you wish—your surrounding is beautiful and peaceful, and the smells of the forest are pleasantly earthy. About 0.3 mile from the last creek, you reach the intersection with another trail. Though not signed here, it's a familiar spot—you're at the top of Wagon Wheel Trail again.

Bear left onto Wagon Wheel and retrace this portion to the wide-open intersection just before the limekilns. (Behind you, Wagon Wheel is off-limits to bikes in that direction.) Go right onto Engelman Loop Trail and head south. Engelman is a wide, mostly hard-packed trail with some patches of soft dirt. In this direction, the trail gently descends over wide-open meadows, interspersed with some level stretches. At 10.3 miles, a wide-open view of the Pacific Ocean looms far ahead of you. About a mile farther, at 11.5 miles, Engelman leads you back to the five-way intersection at the bottom of Wagon Wheel Trail. If you're still yearning for more riding, by all means explore any of these other trails. Otherwise, continue straight, heading south towards Highway 1 and the tunnel. Retrace your path back through the Cultural Preserve and to your car. Total distance for this figure-8 configuration is about 12 miles.

RIDE 92 · Wilder Ranch: Old Cove Bluff Trail

AT A GLANCE

Length/configuration: 15-mile out-and-back (7.5 miles each way); wide dirt trail

Aerobic difficulty: Easy

Technical difficulty: Mildly technical

Scenery: The Pacific Ocean, crashing surf on the bluff walls, sandy beaches, and ferns growing from the ceiling of a hidden cave. Dramatically shaped natural bridges and cliff walls shaped by the pounding tides. Harbor seals enjoy hanging-out on a gigantic flat rock clearly visible from the path. Gray whale migration occurs between late October to January and February to June.

Special comments: The first 2.3 miles is suitable for youngsters and kid-trailers. Parents: don't be surprised to see nude sunbathers in secluded beach coves.

Unlike the other trails in Wilder Ranch State Park, both Old Cove Landing and Ohlone Bluff Trails are easy, flat, wide-open paths. Often referred to jointly as the Old Cove Bluff Trail, this 15-mile out-and-back (7.5 miles each way) follows the edge of the coastal headlands, ranging in elevation from sea level to about 50 feet. What these two connecting paths lack in technical challenge, they make up with spectacular ocean views. Centuries of pounding sea shaped the jagged cliff edges and a number of beaches, some of which lie within sheltered coves, are easily accessible. If the wind isn't blowing too hard, picnicking can be a splendid affair. It's no surprise that riders of all ages and abilities love this route.

In addition to the scenery, a wide variety of animals hang out here. There's the endangered snowy plover, pigeon guillemot, and cormorants to name a few birds. In the sea, you'll see harbor seals, sea otters, and migrating gray whales. (The whales can be seen typically between late October to January, and February to June.) Underwater, just out of view, are pond turtles in the estuaries, shellfish, and other mollusks. The coastal bluff itself is described by geologists as a marine terrace. The trail atop the bluff was the ocean floor at one time. Look beneath your tires as well as the cliff walls along the beaches and you'll see broken bits of shell. Look inland, away from the ocean. Notice the terrain is shaped by several step-like formations. Created by geological forces over time, the landscape is a combination of ancient sea cliff (the steep portions) and marine terrace (the flatter sections). Carved by pounding surf, changes in sea level, wind, rain, and erosion and uplifted by earthquakes, the terraces are especially noticeable between Santa Cruz and Half Moon Bay, where Wilder Ranch lies.

Young families can make Wilder Ranch a full day of fun. Docent-led tours of the historical farm and cultural events — some of which are geared specifically for kids — are often held during the summer. For more information about Wilder Ranch, see the introduction to the previous ride as well as contacting the state park.

General location: About 2 miles north of Santa Cruz on Highway 1 (CA 1).

Elevation change: Negligible change; consistently about 0–50 feet elevation.

Season: Year-round. Often foggy and wet during the winter and early spring, particularly in the morning.

Services: Water and rest rooms available at the state park parking lot; parking fee charged. Pay phone located near the park entrance booth. Picnic tables and pit toilets available at the Wilder Ranch Cultural Preserve, a historic area, as well as docent-led tours of the site.

Hazards: This is an immensely popular trail, especially during the summer and on sunny weekends year-round. The greatest hazard is watching out for other trail users. Riders, especially youngsters, need to be comfortable sharing the wide path with other trail users. The edge of the bluff is generally well-insulated with low shrubs, leaving only a few exposed spots. Still, the trail is flat and wide, and youngsters will generally have no difficulty staying safely on the trail. If you venture out into the ocean, stay alert for strong undertows and supervise children at all times. The trail crosses a single set of railroad tracks; it's not signal-controlled and odds are you won't encounter a passing train. Still, keep your eyes and ears open, especially if you're accompanied by children.

Rescue index: Though the park's popularity can be considered a drawback, it also means you're likely to meet other trail users who may be of help during an emergency, especially during the summer and on sunny weekends year-round. The nearest phone is at the park entry booth.

Land status: Wilder Ranch State Park.

Maps: *Welcome to Wilder Ranch,* published by Southeast Publications USA, Inc., available at park office entry booth.

Finding the trail: From the intersection of Highway 1 and CA 17 in Santa Cruz, follow Highway 1. Traffic gets a bit gnarly through this part of town. Keep an eye out for signs indicating Highway 1. Go through CA 9/River Street, High Street, Bay Street, and Western Drive. About 2 miles after Western Drive, turn left (toward the ocean) at the brown state-park sign. At the park entry booth, stop to pay the parking fee (about $6) and pick up a map. Park in the paved lot and begin pedaling from here. (Free parking along the dirt pull-offs along Highway 1, just before and after the left turn into the park is permitted. However, because vandalism has been known to occur in these free lots, I highly recommend leaving your car in the park's paved lot—the fee is a small price to pay. Besides, Wilder Ranch uses the revenue to maintain the park for your enjoyment).

Sources of additional information:

Wilder Ranch State Park
1401 Old Coast Rd.
Santa Cruz, CA 95060
(831) 423-9703; (831) 426-0505

Notes on the trail: [Before pedaling off, pack a bike lock. Consider bringing a camera too.] From the parking lot, head west towards the farm fields and ocean via the "Nature Trail." The path soon turns to dirt as it leads you over the railroad tracks. (Stay alert for trains.) Follow the flat, sometimes rain-rutted ranch road as it cuts through agricultural fields of yummy, smelly brussel sprouts. (Incidentally, this area produces 60% of the U.S. crop) As you approach the ocean on the bluff edge, you cruise past a platform overlooking the Wilder Beach nature preserve. Being a protected habitat for the endangered snowy plover, the preserve is designated off-limits to the public. Not to fret—there are many other beaches along the route that invite your presence.

About 0.3 mile farther, notice a narrow inlet shaped by the rocks and cliffs. This tiny cove was the landing site for small schooners hauling supplies to and from the ranch. A few yards farther, keep your eyes peeled for an enormously flat rock just barely exposed above the ocean. Chances are, there's a party of barking or sleeping harbor seals hanging out on it. (The best vantage point from this direction is to look behind you. If you miss it on the way out, you're likely to see it on your return.)

At almost 2 miles from the parking lot, look for a trail marker labeled "8." A few yards beyond it is a narrow footpath that leads down to Fern Grotto Beach. Hidden from view is a sea cave worth checking out. Leave your bike on the main path (locked by itself or to another bike) and hike down to the beach. Check out the ferns in the caves—they're growing upside down from the ceiling. An intriguing site. How do these water-loving plants survive? There's an abundance of fresh water seeping through the permeable layers of rock overhead. The source of the water is unconfirmed; it might be field run-off but the constancy of the water implies natural seepage.

Continue pedaling on the trail and at about 2.4 miles, the trail drops steeply down to Sand Plant Beach. If you're towing a kid-trailer, you'll have to leave it and your bike on the trail. (Various maps may show this area as private property but actually, the land immediately inland on the headlands is private. The beach is public property.) This is a great, sandy beach albeit small. If you seek shelter from the wind for a nice picnic, you may find a calm spot along the base of the cliff walls. This is the recommended turn around point for youngsters.

To continue on the trail, carry or push your bike across the sandy beach to the far side. There, a narrow, rocky trail hugs the cliff wall for a few yards as it rises to the top of the bluff. As you portage your bike up this section, watch out for stinging nettle and poison oak scattered along the trail. Once back on top, the number of other trail users is fewer. The wide, exposed, easy path continues to skirt the cliff edge on your left and farmlands on your right. Along this stretch, the trail leads you above and around several more isolated beaches, some of which are favored by occasional nude sunbathers. You cruise past unsigned Strawberry, Three Mile, and Four Mile Beaches. (The mile references some point in Santa Cruz and is not a measure of distance from the state park parking lot.) Keep an eye out for Needle Point Rock sitting a few yards off shore. Constant wave action has worn away soft portions of mudstone, creating holes and natural bridges. At about 7.6 miles, you reach the western boundary of Wilder Ranch State Park at Four Mile Beach, also known as Baldwin Beach. There aren't any signs identifying the beach but it's generally popular on the weekends, a favor site for surfers. This is the end of the road, more or less and you can return to your car via busy Highway 1. The better and preferred route is to simply turn around and return the way you came along the bluff trail. This will give you a chance for ocean views from a different perspective.

RIDE 93 · Nisene Marks–Sand Point Ride

AT A GLANCE

Length/configuration: 17.6-mile out-and-back (8.8 miles each way); dirt fire road. [Optional mileages can be found in adjacent Soquel Demonstration State Forest and is briefly described at the end of this ride.]

Aerobic difficulty: Moderately strenuous due to long stretches of climbing

Technical difficulty: Mildly technical

Scenery: Thick, shady forest of second-growth redwoods and Douglas fir. Epicenter of the 1989 Loma Prieta Earthquake.

Special comments: Strong children can usually ride about the first 3–4 miles. To shorten the ride for youngsters, park at several picnic areas farther up on the bike route. Super-strong adults towing kid-trailers will surely impress everyone.

On any given weekend when the weather is dry, this 17.6-mile out-and-back (8.8 miles each way) in the Forest of Nisene Marks is an immensely popular and pleasant workout. And if you're single and want to meet other cyclists, this is a great ride for that purpose. Close to town and quickly accessed, this is such an easy route to follow that many locals don't think twice about riding alone—there's bound to be other bikers on the trail. The route follows Aptos Creek Fire Trail for its entire uphill journey to Sand Point Overlook. Nearly 100% in a shady, young-growth redwood forest along the cool riparian environments of Aptos and Bridge Creeks, the trail is actually a wide dirt road, generally smooth and hardpacked. The first 3.8 miles or so is a gentle grade, almost imperceptible and young families may enjoy it as a shortened out-and-back (about seven miles round-trip), stopping for a picnic at any of three designated picnic areas along the way. (Parents, you can shorten the ride by parking at any of these picnic sites.) Thereafter, the road steepens from 7% to 9% grade and the rest of the way is a moderately strenuous grind, interspersed with a few brief gentle stretches. When you reach Sand Point Overlook—and you're blessed with a fairly clear day—terrific views of Monterey Bay, the city of Santa Cruz, portions of Big Basin Redwoods State Park, and surrounding ridges are your reward. This is a popular gathering place for bikers as it is the turn around point for the 17.6-mile out-and-back. From here, returning to the trailhead is a fast and fun downhill flight all the way back to your car.

Remember the 1989 Loma Prieta Earthquake that collapsed freeway structures in Oakland and on the San Francisco–Oakland Bay Bridge, and interrupted the World Series game? The epicenter of that quake is located about a half-mile off this route. At almost four miles from the trailhead, Aptos Creek Trail, a moderately easy hiking-only footpath, leads off the bike route to the exact center. A sign marks the spot but keep a sharp eye out for small remnant fissures nearby.

Like many other areas once covered by acres of massive, old-growth redwood trees, the Forest of Nisene Marks has a history of logging and capitalism. Acquired in 1883, the Loma Prieta Lumber Company collaborated with the Southern Pacific Railroad Company. The largest lumber mill in Santa Cruz County was built, creating the small mountain town of Loma Prieta. The rail company, backed by strong financial and technological resources, constructed a broad-gauge railroad line from this region down to the Southern Pacific tracks in Aptos, stretching a little over seven miles. And so began the deforestation of every canyon in the watershed. Within 40 years, a staggering 140 million board feet of redwoods had been removed, leaving only a handful of first-growth trees. (Keep your eyes peeled: two of these ancient ones still stand along the Aptos Creek Road. Large flaws saved them from the loggers.) In 1923, having stripped the land clean, the railroad was removed and the lumber mill ceased operation. Evidence of this unfettered era of industry can still be seen throughout the park, including rusting rails, discarded cable and still thriving non-native eucalyptus trees planted by logging families that lived here. The most noticeable reminder of that era which you see on this ride are huge redwood stumps, some diameters the size of new Volkswagen Beetles. In the 1950s, the Marks family, an active farming family in the Salinas Valley southeast of here, purchased the lumber company's 9,600 acres. In 1963, with assistance from the Nature Conservancy, the Marks children donated the land to the State of California in memory of their mother, Nisene Marks. The Marks children stipulated that the property be kept free from development so that the redwood forests could recover and regenerate naturally. In 1963, with the help of the

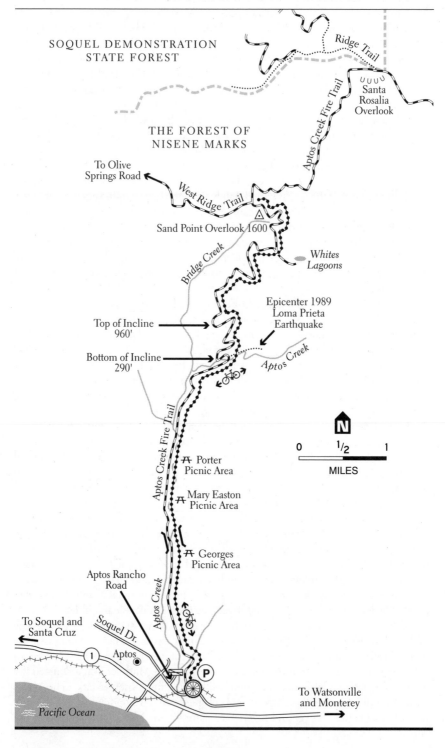

SOQUEL DEMONSTRATION
STATE FOREST

Ridge Trail

Santa
Rosalia
Overlook

Aptos Creek Fire Trail

THE FOREST OF
NISENE MARKS

To Olive
Springs Road

West Ridge Trail

Sand Point Overlook 1600

Whites
Lagoons

Bridge Creek

Epicenter 1989
Loma Prieta
Earthquake

Top of Incline
960'

Aptos Creek

Bottom of Incline
290'

Aptos Creek Fire Trail

Porter
Picnic Area

Mary Easton
Picnic Area

N

0   1/2   1
MILES

Georges
Picnic Area

Aptos Rancho
Road

Aptos Creek

To Soquel and
Santa Cruz

Soquel Dr.

1   Aptos

P

To Watsonville
and Monterey

Pacific Ocean

Save-the-Redwoods League, more properties downstream from the Marks land was acquired, expanding the protection and restoration of the canyon. Thanks to the Marks family and the Nature Conservancy, the forest ecosystem is healing and we have a peaceful and beautiful environment in which to enjoy.

General location: About 4 miles south of Santa Cruz off Highway 1 (CA 1).

Elevation change: 1,400 feet; starting elevation and low point 200 feet; high point at Sand Point Overlook 1,600 feet.

Season: Year-round. Best time is spring to late fall. Winter can be wet and muddy.

Services: Other than pit toilets at several picnic grounds near the trailhead, there are no services on the route. Bring your own water. A pay phone is available in the tiny shopping center near the intersection of Soquel Drive and paved Aptos Creek Road (which becomes the dirt fire road leading up to Sand Point Overlook) in the village of Aptos. Some services, including eateries and small grocery store available in Aptos; all other services in Santa Cruz.

Hazards: An immensely popular trail with mountain bikers, try not to run over other trail users, especially when bombing downhill on the return trip from Sand Point. Likewise, stay alert for speedsters as you grind uphill. Watch out for occasional poison oak and ticks, particularly if you take a hiking sidetrip to the check out the Epicenter of the 1989 Loma Prieta earthquake.

Rescue index: It's possible to meet other trail users who may be of assistance in an emergency, especially during the weekends and late in the afternoon, year-round.

Land status: The Forest of Nisene Marks State Park.

Maps: *The Forest of Nisene Marks State Park*, published by Advocates for Nisene Marks State Park

Finding the trail: From Santa Cruz, follow Highway 1 (CA 1) south toward Monterey. Take the Seacliff Beach/Aptos exit which is State Park Road. Proceed to the north (inland) side of Highway 1 and make a right onto Soquel Drive. Move into the left lane and follow Soquel Drive for about 0.6 mile and go left onto Aptos Creek Road. Immediately after crossing the railroad tracks, park in the large dirt turnout on the right and begin your ride from here.

Sources of additional information:

The Forest of Nisene Marks
    State Park
600 Ocean St.
Santa Cruz, CA 95060
(831) 429-2850

Soquel Demonstration State Forest
4750 Soquel–San Jose Rd.
Soquel, CA 95073
(831) 475-8643

Notes on the trail: [Before pedaling off, consider bringing a bike lock.] If you want to hike the short trail to the Epicenter of the 1989 Loma Prieta Earthquake, you must leave your bike at the trailhead. If you're more comfortable riding with eye protection, consider clear or yellow glasses because this ride is nearly 100% in the shade. This forest, after all, is thick with young-growth redwoods and evergreens.

This route is a no-brainer to follow: you simply stay on Aptos Creek Fire Road all the way to Sand Point Overlook, reached in about 8.8 miles. All other lesser trails that intersect the fire road are hiking-only. If you plan to continue farther, especially to explore the single-tracks in the Soquel Demonstration State Forest, a map is recommended.

Begin by pedaling north on paved Aptos Creek Road. In a few yards, the road becomes a dirt fire road. Cruise past Georges Picnic Area and over the Steel Bridge. Here at the bridge, you have a splendid view of the deep and narrow canyon carved by Aptos Creek. After the bridge, bear right, staying on the fire road and continue past Mary Easton and Porter Picnic Areas. Though you're gaining elevation, the climbing is gentle, almost imperceptible. At about 3 miles, you reach the Loma Prieta Mill Site, its foundation timbers being the only remains. Continue past Mill Pond and Trout Gulch Trails. About a mile beyond the mill site, go past Aptos Creek Trail, a hiking-only path which leads to the Epicenter of the 1989 Loma Prieta Earthquake. (There's a bike rack here—a big clue that bikes are not allowed on the hiking-only trail. Check out the trail now or on your return trip back to your car.)

When you pass the Epicenter trailhead, the grade on Aptos Creek Fire Road steepens significantly. Bear down as this is the toughest section of the ride. You're now making an assault on China Ridge. This portion of the route is called "The Incline," so named for the fact that in 1910–18, the Molino Timber Company made use of the grade and a steam donkey to lower rail car loads of split wood down to Aptos Creek. At just over 5 miles from your car, you reach the "Top of the Incline," elevation 962 feet. You will have climbed about 600 feet in about 1.4 miles beyond the Epicenter trailhead. From that point, the road levels significantly for nearly 0.7 mile. After that, the remaining 2.9 miles to Sand Point Overlook climbs again though not as steeply as the "Incline."

At about 8.8 miles, you reach a major intersection of dirt roads within a small clearing. This is Sand Point Overlook, the obvious clue being several fallen logs popularly used as benches. If the sky is clear, free of fog and haze, you have a terrific view down Bridge Creek Canyon, the Monterey Bay, the town of Santa Cruz, the Ben Lomond Ridge, and portions of Big Basin Redwoods State Park. This is favorite stopping place for riders (and hikers) and if you're looking to make biker-friends, this is the place.

After enjoying the view and catching your breath, get ready for a fun, 8.8-mile downhill blast all the way back down to your car. Stay alert and courteous and try not to flatten other riders or hikers grinding up the hill. Total distance for the out-and-back to Sandy Point Overlook is 17.6 miles.

Option for more mileage: For those of you aching for more riding, you can continue into the Soquel Demonstration State Forest. The area contains 2,700 acres of redwoods, mixed hardwoods, and riparian and chaparral ecosystems. All the dirt roads and single-tracks there are open to bikes, and moderate to intermediate technical skills are required. The terrain is rugged and the trails are more in harmony with nature as opposed to the graded, smooth fire road you just rode up on. Biking is allowed so long as you stay on trails and roads—please don't cut through virgin ground. Riders must be self-reliant as the area is fairly inaccessible, and for that reason, riding alone is highly discouraged. Stay alert—poison oak and ticks are scattered throughout the forest. You must bring enough drinking water as it is not available here. Any water taken from creeks needs to be treated before consumption. To reach the Demonstration Forest, continue following Aptos Creek Fire Trail, bearing right. (If you veer left, you'll be on West Ridge Trail, heading slightly downhill toward the trail camp and eventually out of the park and onto paved road.) From Sand Point,

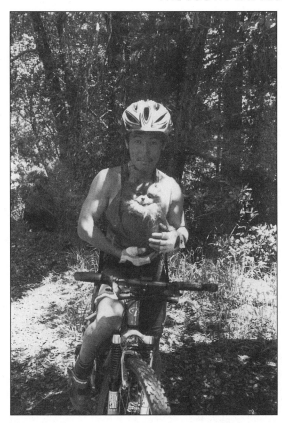

This cyclist at Sand Point
was giving new meaning
to "riding partner" and
"taking out the dog."

you'll climb about 800 feet elevation for about 3 miles before reaching Ridge Trail
that leads into the Demonstration Forest. Aptos Creek Fire Trail intersects Ridge at
the Santa Rosalia Overlook, another great viewpoint of the Monterey Peninsula and
the Bay. To return to your car parked in Aptos, re-enter the Forest of Nisene Marks
at the Santa Rosalia Overlook and retrace your path on Aptos Creek Fire Trail.
Enjoy!

OTHER AREA RIDES

SARATOGA GAP/LONG RIDGE OPEN SPACE PRESERVES: This 12-mile loop is in a class by itself. A frequent refrain is that "this is what mountain bikes were made for." Rated moderately strenuous for riders with mild to intermediate technical skills, the route is a combination of fire roads and single- and double-track trails, some of which are exhilaratingly—almost dangerously—fast. Though some climbing is involved, steep ups and downs and mellow rolling terrain provide variety, and the trails are generally described as a blast. Can't complain about the scenery either, which consists of shady forest, views of the ocean, Santa Cruz Mountain ranges, and Big Basin State Park. Rangers have been known to ticket speedsters. The general direction of the ride is this: Begin on Saratoga Gap Trail following it to a four-way intersection with Charcoal Road (a steep, one-way fire road that's legal for bikes going uphill). Bear left onto Long Ridge Road (primarily a fire road) and very soon cross Skyline Boulevard (watch out for cars!). Continue on Long Ridge pedaling away from Skyline, riding into Long Ridge Open Space and past a scenic viewpoint. The trail winds through the forest, gradually making its way back toward Skyline, and merges into Peters Creek Loop Trail. Follow Peters Creek, eventually passing a pond and meadow before hitting Skyline Boulevard again. Cross Skyline into Monte Bello Open Space and hop on Grizzly Flat Trail. Grizzly starts off as a fire road, then becomes single-track. Cross a creek and climb out of the drainage via switchbacks, still on single-track. When you reach Canyon Trail, go right for a short while, and then make another right onto Table Mountain Trail. After about a mile, it merges into Charcoal Road (the one-way fire road previously mentioned). Bear down and grind your way up the steep grade for about 2 miles. At the familiar intersection with Saratoga Gap, go left and retrace your path back to the trailhead and your car.

Finding the trailhead: From Los Gatos, follow CA 9 through the town of Saratoga all the way to its intersection with Skyline Boulevard (CA 35). Park in the lot on your left, just before the intersection. The trailhead is across CA 9, before Skyline.

Maps: Contact the MROSD. USGS topo maps Mindego Hill and Cupertino 7.5 minute series (not all trails are depicted).

For more information, contact:
Midpeninsula Regional Open Space District (MROSD)
330 Distel Circle
Los Altos, CA 94022
(650) 691-1200
www.openspace.org

FREMONT OLDER OPEN SPACE PRESERVE: This is one of the best places for beginners. Intermediate and better riders will probably be bored. Trails are mostly mild fire roads and includes some fun single-tracks. Initial climb up to the ridge means you need decent endurance. You can configure your own ride, creating loops and out-and-backs, riding as many miles as you like. Watch out for hikers, equestrians, dog-walkers, and ticket-writing rangers.

Finding the trailhead: From I-280 in Sunnyvale/Cupertino, go south on Foothill Expressway, which soon turns into Stevens Canyon Road. Stay on Stevens Canyon Road to Stevens Creek Park. At an intersection before the spillway, near the park entrance, turn left, and follow the road down for a brief distance, bearing left into the first parking lot (the "sunken" lot). Pedal into Fremont Older Open Space by going past the Villa Maria picnic area and hopping onto Coyote Ridge Trail.

Map: Contact the Midpeninsula Regional Open Space District (MROSD).

For more information, contact:
Midpeninsula Regional Open Space District (MROSD)
330 Distel Circle
Los Altos, CA 94022
(650) 691-1200
www.openspace.org

SIERRA AZUL—LEXINGTON LOOP: Starting in Los Gatos, this 15-mile loop through wooded and steep Sierra Azul Open Space and Lexington County Park is considered one of the best workouts in the South Bay. After a mellow 0.25-mile start, the next 4 miles is a grueling climb (1,800 feet gain) on Kennedy Trail, a fire road. When you reach the top, go right onto Priest Rock Trail and hold on for about 2 miles on a fast "killer" downhill (rocky with some loose chunks and dusty red clay dirt). When you reach an intersection, leave Priest Rock and hang a right onto Limekiln Trail (also known as Overgrown). Follow this wide gravel trail, and continue descending. Switchbacks on this stretch can sneak up on you if you're not expecting them. When you reach Alma Bridge Road, go right and follow it alongside Lexington Reservoir. Go across the dam face toward CA 17, but just before the highway, look for a fenced area with a dirt road on your right. Hop onto this dirt road and follow it down to a bridge over Main Street in Los Gatos. Make a right on Main Street and continue on it as it becomes Los Gatos Boulevard. Be careful of motorists. Stay on Los Gatos Boulevard all the way to Kennedy Road and eventually to your parked car.

Finding the trailhead: Before hopping on your bike, check with a local bike shop (in Los Gatos) for trail and accessibility conditions. From San Jose, head south on CA 17 (I-880 becomes CA 17). Take the CA 9 exit and go left for about a mile to Los Gatos Boulevard. Go left again on Los Gatos Boulevard and proceed about a half mile, then hang a right on Kennedy Road. Head up to the top of the hill and park near the trailhead (gated fire road). Bring plenty of water. It can be brutally hot in the summer.

Maps: Consult local bike shops listed at the end of this chapter.

For more information contact:
Midpeninsula Regional Open Space District (MROSD)
330 Distel Circle
Los Altos, CA 94022
(650) 691-1200
www.openspace.org

JOSEPH D. GRANT PARK: Of all the places to ride in the Greater Bay Area, Grant Park is one of the few where you can ride for hours and see very few people, if any. Like an oasis in the sky, this 9,500-acre-plus park ranges from 1,600 to 2,900 feet and is located about 10 miles east of San Jose. Blessed by rolling grasslands and majestic oak trees, Grant Park has over 40 miles of trails, nearly half of which welcome mountain bikes. An effectively laid network of trails allows for many routing configurations, which translates into several hours of riding over diverse terrain. Bikers of all abilities and all ages will find trails that match their skills and stamina. There are single-tracks and fire roads, mostly moderately technical, and some which are very steep and strenuous. Paved Mt. Hamilton Road (CA 130) bisects the park into northeast and southwest halves and leads to Lick Observatory atop Mt. Hamilton at 4,213 feet. Summers are often hot and dry. Spring is the best time to ride, when the temperatures are comfortable and wildflowers cover the rolling hills. Fall is nice too, though the hills are parched and yellow-brown. Winter is rideable, since the sandy composition of the terrain generally drains well. Cattle and lots of wildlife are here too, including herds of wild boar, bobcats, and rarely seen mountain lions. Here's a strenuous 9 to 10 mile ride favored by intermediate-skilled cyclists: From the parking area near the main entrance, gradually ascend Hotel Trail past Circle Corral to Eagle Lake. At the lake, go left onto Foothill Pine Trail and then north on Bonhoff Trail. Cross Mt. Hamilton Road and continue rolling north on a ridge following Canada de Pala Trail. When you reach Los Huecos, go left onto it and have a rollicking good time descending to Grant Lake. Close the loop by returning to the parking area where you began. Heartier riders can add about 5.2 miles more—and more climbing—by adding on the following: Bypass Los Huecos. In a short time, bypass Halls Valley Trail. Bear right at an intersection and proceed on Pala Seca Trail. Be sure to take a short side trip to Antler Point (2,995 feet) for a superb view of the sprawling Santa Clara Valley and beyond. Backtrack a short distance to Pala Seca, and go right toward Line Shack where the trail becomes Canada de Pala Trail. Follow Canada de Pala back to the Pala Seca Trail intersection to close this little loop, then retrace your path back to Los Huecos Trail. Hop onto Los Huecos and descend to Grant Lake and your parked car.

Finding the trailhead: From downtown San Jose, go north on US 101 or I-680 to Alum Rock Avenue. Follow Alum Rock east toward the hills and turn right onto Mt. Hamilton Road (CA 130). Proceed on Mt. Hamilton for about 8 miles to the park entrance.

Map: Available at the park entrance ranger station.

For more information, contact:

County of Santa Clara
Parks & Recreation Department
298 Garden Hill Dr.
Los Gatos, CA 95032
(408) 358-3741
www.parkhere.org

SOME LOCAL BICYCLE SHOPS & ORGANIZATIONS

Calmar Cycles
2236 El Camino Real
Santa Clara, CA 95050
(408) 249-6907

Cupertino Bike Shop
10493 S. De Anza Blvd.
Cupertino, CA 95014
(408) 255-2217

Los Gatos Cyclery
15954 Los Gatos Blvd.
Los Gatos, CA 95032
(408) 356-1644

Mikes Freedom Bicycles
1805 Freedom Blvd.
Freedom, CA 95019
(408) 722-8650

Midpeninsula Regional Open Space
District (MROSD)
330 Distel Circle
Los Altos, CA 94022
(650) 691-1200
www.openspace.org

THE MONTEREY PENINSULA
AND BIG SUR

About 90 minutes south of sprawling San Jose is the stunningly beautiful Monterey Peninsula, jutting out into the Pacific Ocean. A decidedly slower, less populated area, Monterey County is the "Salad Bowl" of the entire country with its bountiful patchwork of agricultural farmlands in the Salinas Valley. Poised on the ocean's edge is well-known Pebble Beach, a gated community which caters to celebrities and the affluent, and boasts world-famous golf courses and the famed 17-Mile Drive. Snaking south of the peninsula along the rugged coastline is the most photographed portion of Highway 1, clinging to high cliffs overlooking the sea. Sandwiched by the ocean and Los Padres National Forest, Highway 1 is a fitting entryway into that elusively defined area called Big Sur, where the Santa Lucia Range abruptly and dramatically crashes into the water. High fog is a frequent occurrence, from late spring through summer, often burning off by the afternoon. Locals claim that the best times of the year are fall and spring, when the days are less foggy and the temperatures are on the warm side. Less than 20 minutes inland, the climate is considerably hotter, drier, and the skies more blue than hazy. Rain wets the entire greater peninsula area, for a day or two at times, typically late fall through winter.

Truth be told, this region offers few dirt roads and trails that are bike-legal. The northern portion of Los Padres in Monterey County is dominated by the Ventana Wilderness and, like all designated wildernesses, does not allow bikes. Bikes are permitted in the forest land outside the Ventana boundary but trails and roads found there are insanely steep and rugged, and anyone attempting to pedal them will undoubtedly do more hiking than biking. However, the peninsula does has one of the best-paved trails in all of Northern California: the Monterey Recreation Path, a nearly 30-mile multi-use path that closely follows the edge of the Pacific. Combine that with the 17-Mile Drive to Carmel Road Ride and you have an exceptionally worthy 55-mile-plus trip despite being completely paved. Dirt routes in this region can be ridden year-round, except after a soaking rainstorm in which case Old Coast Road and trails in Andrew Molera State Park become muddy and impassable. In contrast, inland trails such as those in Fort Ord Public Lands and Toro Regional Park drain and dry quickly, thanks to porous and packed sand conditions. So if you're seeking decent trails for a leisurely ride or a hard workout, you'll be pleased with what you find here.

RIDE 94 · Toro Park–Ollason Peak Loop

AT A GLANCE

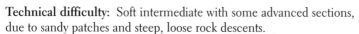

Length/configuration: 9-mile loop, counterclockwise; mostly narrow dirt road, including some single-track and paved road

Aerobic difficulty: Mostly moderate with a short half-mile strenuous stretch

Technical difficulty: Soft intermediate with some advanced sections, due to sandy patches and steep, loose rock descents.

Scenery: Panoramic views of the Monterey Bay, the patchwork agricultural fields of the Salinas Valley and a portion of Los Padres National Forest

Special comments: When the cities of Monterey, Carmel, and Pacific Grove are shrouded by high fog and cool temperatures, go about 15 minutes inland to Toro Park where the sun is usually shining, even blazingly hot at times.

Toro Park is one of the few places on the Monterey Peninsula where mountain biking is welcomed. Covering 4,700 acres, the park only offers roughly 18 miles of bikeable trails. The 9-mile loop described below forms the longest loop in the park. But it is a worthy ride. The route consists of semi-hardpacked dirt roads spiced with some loose gravel and deep ruts created by rain runoff, punctuated with a smattering of soft dirt and sandy patches. Throw in some roller coaster steep but short hills, ridge top riding replete with sweeping views of wooded canyons, grassy hills and the Salinas Valley—even a glimpse of the Monterey Bay—and you have one heck of a ride.

Most of the riding is moderately technical with a few short advanced sections. A novice biker who has great endurance and attitude and is just beginning to develop technical skills will enjoy this challenge. (Knowing when to dismount and walk is a skill, too!) That's not to say intermediate skilled riders will find this ride boring. Beginning at about 150 feet elevation, the trail climbs 1,650 feet in 4.9 miles to Ollason Peak sitting at 1,800 feet. Big deal, you say? Think you can climb up nearly vertical walls like Spiderman on two wheels? Here's your chance to test your technical climbing skills: Take the Simas Peak test, offered as an optional out-and-back off this loop. It's an incredibly steep trail graded at over 16%, rising over 100 feet in 0.25 mile. See if you can climb it without popping a wheelie.

Toro Park is one of three chunks of public regions on the peninsula that allows biking (the other being Fort Ord with about 50 miles of bikeable trails and Garland Park which hiking groups have effectively managed to make off-limits to bikers except for a measly 1.5-mile loop). Many trails and signs at Toro suffered significant damage during the 1998 El Niño winter and repairs have been slow. According to the one-and-only full-time park ranger, any funding that the park acquires is generally funneled toward maintaining the huge and immensely popular picnic grounds, located just inside the park. Apologetically, he stated that repairing trails, replacing

RIDE 94 · Toro Park–Ollasson Peak Loop

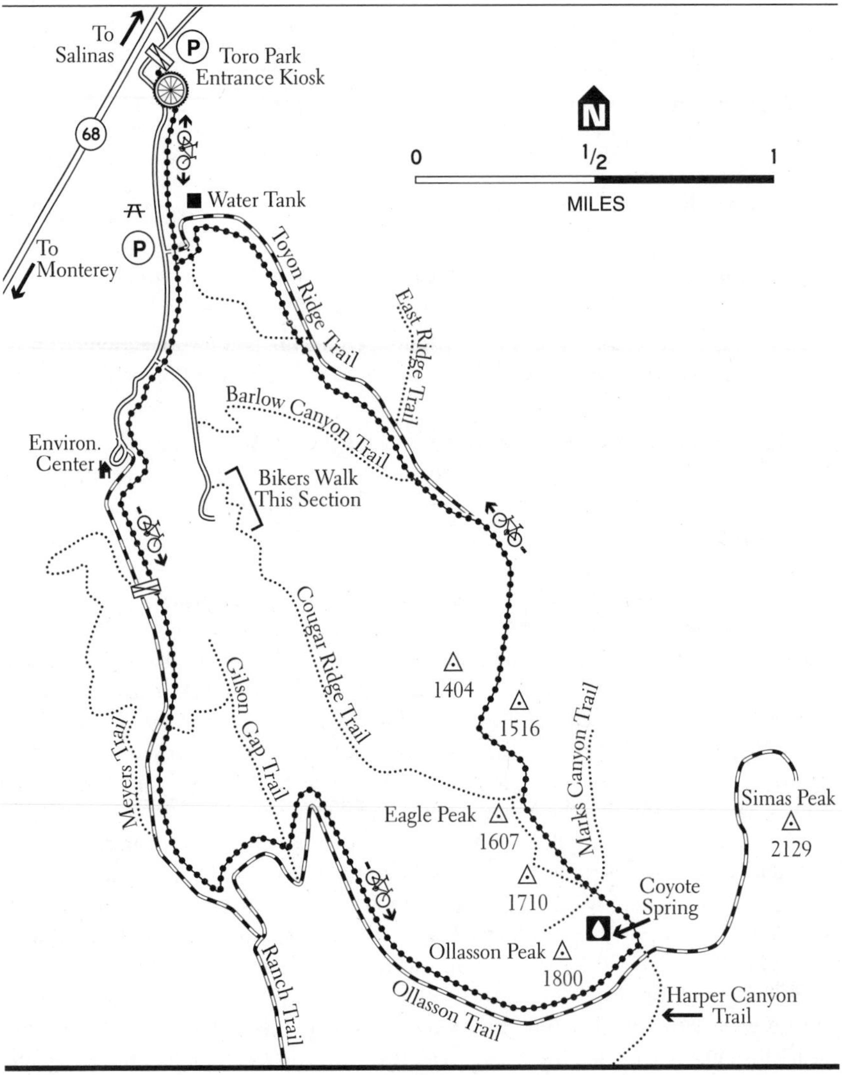

To Salinas

P Toro Park Entrance Kiosk

68

N

0   1/2   1

MILES

■ Water Tank

To Monterey **P**

Toyon Ridge Trail

East Ridge Trail

Barlow Canyon Trail

Environ. Center

Bikers Walk This Section

Cougar Ridge Trail

Gilson Gap Trail

Mevers Trail

△ 1404

△ 1516

Marks Canyon Trail

Eagle Peak △ 1607

△ 1710

Simas Peak △ 2129

Coyote Spring

Ollasson Peak △ 1800

Ranch Trail

Ollasson Trail

Harper Canyon Trail ←

damaged signs and generating a super-accurate park map are not high priority. That's OK , I said, citing that part of the sport of mountain biking is dealing with varied terrain and figuring out which way to go.

General location: About 13 miles east of Monterey and about 5 miles west of Salinas on CA 68.

Elevation change: 1,650 feet change; starting elevation and low point 150 feet; high point 1,800 feet. Begins with ascent on gentle terrain, then steep and long toward Ollason Peak, followed by a long, mostly gradual downhill.

Season: Year-round, though it can get hot during the summer. Trails are frequently closed after a significant amount of rainfall (call ahead). Splendid green-carpeted rolling hills and wildflowers from March through May.

Services: Located just inside the entrance are well-maintained picnic grounds, complete with drinking water, picnic tables, BBQ pits, horseshoe pits, volleyball courts, rest rooms, ball fields, and paved parking lots. All other services in Salinas or Monterey.

Hazards: Carry enough water, especially during the warm months, typically June through October. Creeks and springs that flow in the winter are typically dry during the summer. Any water found in the backcountry should first be treated before drinking as cattle grazing is permitted in portions of the park. Watch out for poison oak. Mountain lions are rarely encountered.

Rescue index: The route is somewhat popular with other trail users on the weekends, especially in the summer. Weekday users are fewer. Otherwise, for emergency help, you'll have to make your own way back down the trail to the picnic grounds near the park entrance to find help.

Land status: Monterey County Parks.

Maps: *Toro Park Trails*, as produced and printed by the Monterey County Parks Department, (available at park entrance booth, but only if park personnel is on duty).

Finding the trail: From Monterey, travel east on CA 68 (also called the Monterey-Salinas Road) for about 13 miles. From downtown Salinas, drive west on CA 68 for about 6 miles. From either direction, take the Portola Road exit and follow signs to the park entrance that is located immediately on the south side of CA 68. This is the one and only main paved entrance to Toro Park and it's located on the far northern end of the park. You can park outside the entrance in the dirt parking lot across the road from the entrance and pedal in, thereby avoid paying the entry fee. Otherwise, drive about a half mile into the park and park in any of the parking lots next to the picnic grounds.

Sources of additional information:

Monterey County Parks Department
P.O. Box 367
Salinas, CA 93902
(831) 755-4895 or (831) 755-4899

Notes on the trail: You can ride this loop in either direction, but I think counterclockwise is the most fun and rewarding. I prefer descending Toyon Ridge instead of ascending because the downhill cruise is sweetened by sweeping panoramic views of the Salinas Valley, wooded and grassy hills and canyons, and the Monterey Bay. The loop described here is pedaled in a counterclockwise direction.

Starting from the entrance, pedal into the park on the paved main road, heading south. Our first destination is the dirt road trailhead at the Environmental Center about 1.3 miles from the entrance. Cruise past the picnic grounds and parking areas. Bypass all trails leading off the road on both sides, including one that's signed Olasson Trail at about 0.7 mile from the entrance. Continue straight through a T intersection, staying on the pavement and following the brown sign pointing up a steep but short hill toward the Environmental Center. After climbing about 130 feet in 0.3

mile, you reach the top of the hill and the road becomes the parking lot for the Center. There are rest rooms and a drinking fountain here.

Here is where you pick up Ollason Trail, which is actually a one-car-width dirt road. Go past the rest rooms and immediately on your right, follow the paved asphalt walkway as it curves around the small residences, heading south. After a few yards, where a yellow fire hydrant is planted, the dirt road begins. The road is not signed but it's the Ollason Trail. For the next 3.4 miles to the peak, stay on Ollason, a one-car-width, semi-hardpacked dirt road with quite a bit of loose dirt and sand. In fact, expect to find some deep sandy patches that will want to suck your wheel to a dead stop. Persevere, as they are short and rideable for the most part. The trail begins climbing gradually, leading you through shady, contorted stands of live oak alongside a tiny creek. Bypass all lesser trails leading off Ollason.

At about 1.6 miles, you reach a large metal locked gate across the trail. Adjacent to the gate is a C-shaped walk-through wooden structure. The best way to get you and your bike through this narrow structure is to stand your bike upright on its back wheel and walk it through the structure. (Incidentally, here is where Meyers Trail, a wide single-track, takes off on your right. If you want, you can take this trail, following it as it weaves and climbs up and down through the trees and eventually reconnecting with Ollason Trail in about a mile. Watch out for poison oak.)

Still pedaling on Ollason, the trail begins to alternate between sun and shade. Follow the trail as it continues to climb gradually, leading you past grazing cattle and over more soft dirt patches. Bypass several lesser trails at around 2.1 miles, one of which is signed Gilson Gap Trail and is off-limits to bikes. In a few yards, peer through the trees and across the tiny creek on your right and you begin to see Meyers Trail paralleling your trail. Shortly thereafter, it rejoins Ollason. Stay on Ollason as it curves through a shady stretch where a cattle water trough is located.

At about 3 miles, you reach an intersection in which only Ollason Trail is signed. Follow the sign, making a hard left to stay on Ollason. (According to the map, the other wide trail leading off to the right through an opening in the fence is Ranch Trail. This trail leads down to Ollason Canyon and eventually to where the biking trail ends and the hiking-only trail continues. If you choose to explore this trail, it adds about 2 miles round-trip and includes some steep terrain.)

Ollason Trail begins to climb more steeply up a north-facing slope, rising above the ravine in which you initially pedaled. At almost 3.5 miles, Gilson Loop Trail joins Ollason on your left. You've just climbed about 860 feet since beginning the ride from the park entrance. Continue following Ollason as it curves north, emerging from the cover of the oak trees and revealing the patchwork pattern of agricultural fields in the Salinas Valley. The landscape becomes more open with fewer trees and your view more expansive. Trail conditions become more demanding as the pitch steepens significantly and deeper, longer stretches of soft dirt and sand slow your progress. The technical challenge here is maintaining traction on your back tire while grinding through the deep sand. Hang in there, the sand pit is just under 200 yards. The trail becomes rideable once again and the steepness alternates between short sections of easy and arduous terrain. If you're here on this ridge during the spring and your timing is keen, your huffing and puffing will be rewarded with a glorious display of wildflowers, amid open fields of rolling green hills. Otherwise, you'll have to settle for sweeping views of sun-parched grassy hills and the piquant smell of wild sage under foot and wheel.

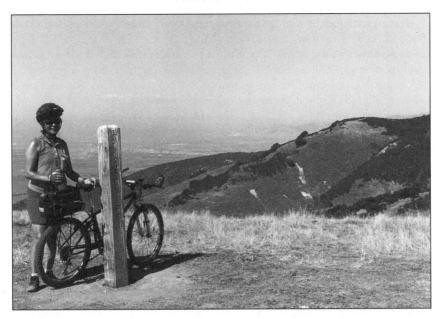

Linda takes a breather at the top of Ollason Peak, overlooking parts of Monterey and Salinas.

Pushing on, you finally reach Ollason Peak, about 4.7 miles since beginning the ride. A 360-degree view and a single wooden signpost declaring "Ollason Peak, elevation 1800" greets you. If you're lucky to be here on a truly clear day, you can see Santa Cruz across the Monterey Bay in the north, as well as the Salinas Valley to the northeast, and a portion of Los Padres National Forest to the south. In the near distance, immediately on your right is Simas Peak. From Ollason Peak, you can see an incredibly steep trail running almost straight up into the sky and another steep trail leading off the hill to the left of it. Decide now if you want to test your Spiderman abilities on this wall of a hill because if you do, you'll want to get a running start. Start by continuing on Ollason Trail as it dives down an extremely steep and rugged descent for about 200 yards, before going straight up again. Stay with the momentum and let it catapult you up the wall. Believe me, if you stop at the base of the wall, you won't want to tackle it because it looks steeper than when viewed from Ollason Peak.

For the rest of us mere mortals, continue on the loop by following the same steep descent that Spiderman would take, down to the base of the wall. There, you come to a major intersection. This is where the signs in the field don't quite jive with the map. Straight ahead, facing east, is the trail to Simas Peak, up the wall. The narrow hiking trail shooting down the hill on your right, leading south, is Harper Canyon Trail, incorrectly signed here as "Ollason Trail" and bikes are not allowed. On your left, to the north, is a trail misleadingly signed "Toyon Ridge." According to the map, this trail should be Coyote Springs Trail (because it leads right past Coyote Springs) and then intersects Toyon Ridge Trail shortly thereafter. And to add further confusion, there are three trails leading off in the direction of "Toyon Ridge." The trail you want is the middle, narrow, faint trail, sitting at the base of the V formed by two converging slopes. The other narrow trails higher up on both slopes are cattle trails that ultimately peter out.

Hang a left onto the middle, faintly defined, hard-packed, single-track trail and follow it gently down into a ravine, riding north. The trail skirts a deeply eroded section resembling a baby Grand Canyon, then continues into a small stand of oak trees with sparse underbushes. In a few yards, still within the trees, cross over a culvert semi-buried in a deeply eroded section of the trail. You've just passed Coyote Springs, or what's left of it, depending on the time of year.

Emerge from the shady ravine and after a few yards of level, easy riding, you come to a major intersection, sitting at 1,560 feet elevation and about 5.2 miles from the start of the ride. Eagle Peak, elevation 1,710 feet, lies just beyond the hill ahead. Marks Canyon Trail, a hiking-only trail, takes off on the right; Whale Trail/Redtail Canyon leads off on the left (and is not indicated on the park map). Straight ahead, toward Eagle Peak and paralleling each other are two trails: Toyon Ridge and Coyote Springs. Toyon Ridge climbs steeply to the top of Eagle Peak in less than a half mile while Coyote Springs traverses its eastern slope. (You can follow either of these two parallel trails because they rejoin in about a mile.) Take the trail on the right signed Coyote Springs and begin a very steep but short climb over rutted and soft dirt conditions. After about 200 yards, you reach the top of the rise, back in the bushes and trees. Here, the trail resembles a wide single-track and double-track rather than a dirt road. The climbing continues on a gentler pitch as the trail traverses the eastern slope. In a few more yards, Toyon Ridge Trail rejoins Coyote Springs Trail on your left. At this intersection, look left, up the slope a bit and you can see several other signposts. These signs mark the beginning of Cougar Ridge Trail (bikes allowed). Bypass Cougar Ridge, saving it for another time. Continue straight, due north, as the single-track trail now becomes Toyon Ridge Trail. It's nearly all downhill from here as the fun roller-coaster ride begins. The panoramic views of the Monterey Bay, the grassy hills of Fort Ord and the Salinas Valley spread below you like welcoming, opened arms.

In less than a half mile, come to a signed fork in a small clearing. The trail signs here are a bit confusing. The left fork points to Toyon Loop Trail. Another sign and arrow here indicates that you've been riding Toyon Ridge, yet, continuing straight ahead on the same trail—the right fork—it's not signed. So where does your trail, Toyon Ridge, continue—straight ahead on the unsigned right fork toward a big metal gate? (I suspected that the right fork is a continuation of Toyon Ridge. However, the only way around the locked gate was to squeeze through the narrowly spaced barbed wire fencing. I decided to follow the left fork, Toyon Loop.)

Follow Toyon Loop trail, a slightly technical, wide single-track, as it traverses the western slope of a hill, skirting a steep and bushy drop-off on your left. About 400 yards from the confusing intersection, Toyon Loop leads you through a narrow, metal gate. The trail then becomes very narrow thanks to lots of overgrown bushes. A few yards later, you reach the intersection with Toyon Ridge Trail. (You can take Toyon Ridge or stay on Toyon Loop—they reconnect in just over a half mile.) Veer left onto Toyon Ridge and climb a short distance to the next little hill, then continue the roller-coaster descent along the ridge top. Though the trail is much wider and hard-packed, intermediate technical skill is required due to a few extremely rutted, steep sections strewn with loose gravel. In fact, for the next 2 miles, this trail is interrupted with some rather deep man-made rain runoff ruts, some of which require walking if you're not adept at jumping and flying.

As you continue the moderately steep descent on Toyon Ridge Trail, bypass all other trails: Barlow Canyon (no bikes) at 7 miles, East Ridge Trail (no bikes) at 7.2 miles, Bessie Canyon Trail (yes bikes) at 7.6 miles and then, Bessie's Loop (maybe bikes, not indicated on the map) at 7.7 miles. At 8.1 miles, near the bottom of the hill, you reach an intersection that's signed Toyon Ridge Trail shooting off on the right while the main wide trail that you've been on continues straight toward a huge water tank. Head for the water tank and in a few yards, the trail ends in the overflow dirt parking lot. Go past the gate, hang a right, and go through the lot toward the paved road, at which point you close the loop. Turn right onto the paved road and retrace your path back to your car, or check out some of the other trails which you previously bypassed.

RIDE 95 · Fort Ord: Guidotti–Goat Trail Loop

AT A GLANCE

Length/configuration: 13-mile loop, clockwise; dirt roads, single- and double-tracks

Aerobic difficulty: Moderate due to some gradual climbing and a few steep but short sections

Technical difficulty: Mild to intermediate; occasional patches of sand, few rocky and rough sections; an extremely rocky section can easily be avoided or walked

Scenery: Wide-open, rolling hills with glimpses of the Salinas Valley. Hidden tiny valleys make you feel like you're in a remote area even though a busy highway and residential community is within 5 miles at any given time during the ride.

Special comments: One of the few areas on the Monterey Peninsula with legal single-track trails. Each March, the Sea Otter Classic, a NORBA-sanctioned race, is held here. Expect patches of soft dirt and deep sand.

The Fort Ord Public Lands, managed by the Bureau of Land Management (BLM), is one of the last wild, undeveloped areas on the Monterey Peninsula. And get this: Unlike other BLM land in the country, this one doesn't allow off-road vehicles. That means no blaring, solitude-shattering whines of motorbikes and vehicles. The exception is certain times of the year when the popular Laguna Seca Recreation Area, on the western boundary of the BLM land, is hosting a noisy event and you may hear the roar of engines in the distance. This 13-mile, clockwise loop gives you a good taste of the varied terrain that makes up the public lands that's open to bikers, hikers, and equestrians. You'll ride along high ridges, through maritime chaparral, grasslands, oak woodlands, shallow valleys, and wetlands. The trails that make up this loop are a combination of dirt roads and single- and double-track trails. Climbs come in a variety of grades, from long, gradual ascents to very steep but short roller-coasters thrills. Though the trails are mostly hardpack, expect to find stretches of sand that can be either rideable or wheel-swallowing. But don't let the mention of sand discourage you from this wild landscape. While the land is basically arid with few trees—hence, little shade—spring finds the rolling hills lush with tall, green grass, dotted with colorful wildflowers. Summer can be hot, leaving sun-parched hills and dusty conditions, at which time riding late in the afternoon—or in the evening during a full moon—is a fun option favored by locals. Throughout the year, when the chilly, coastal fog lingers in Monterey, you can drive a few miles inland and find a big difference in the weather. At Fort Ord, the climate tends to be warmer, drier, and sunnier than along the shore. And you can find solitude here, in the hidden valleys or along the ridge tops. The views are simply expansive and it's easy to let your soul soar. Technically speaking, the single-track trails are mostly intermediate, spiced with a few advanced sections, while the major dirt roads are non- to mildly rated. With over 50 miles of bikeable trails, numerous configurations can be made, from easy to challenging. In fact, the nationally popular Sea Otter Classic, a NORBA-sanctioned mountain bike race is held every March, using the single-track trails located on the southwest area of Fort Ord Public Lands, next to Laguna Seca. Thanks to AmeriCorps, the youth service organization established in 1994, many of the trails have been signed and documented on a free map published by the Bureau of Land Management. (Maps can be found at all park gates.)

Got the urge to break out in song as you ride? How about "Over hill, over dale, we will hit the dusty trail, and the caisson keep rolling along. . . ." Originally built in 1917, Fort Ord was an Army military base occupying over 28,000 acres. The terrain was ideal for training infantry. Military maneuvers were staged and parts of the property were used as an artillery range. During World War II, the base was a primary staging area for the Pacific Theater of Operations, causing the population to grow to over 50,000. Though the base closed in 1991, the last of the troops were finally withdrawn in 1994. The Bureau of Land Management has since officially received 16,000 acres, but only 7,200 acres have been safely converted to public use. Scouring every inch of the land for unexploded ordnances and other old military hardware is a slow, ongoing, and arduous process. For that reason, all trail users—hikers, equestrians, and bikers—are warned to stay out of closed areas that have not been cleared. Those areas are clearly posted with warning signs. The Public Lands currently open to the public by the Bureau of Land Management still offer plenty of terrain to explore.

General location: About 9 miles east of Monterey, about 115 miles south of San Francisco.

Elevation change: 600 feet change; starting elevation 200 feet; high point 800 feet; low point 160 feet. Great mix of gentle, long hills along with some steep but short ups and downs.

Season: Year-round. Spring is the best time to ride because the hills are green with new grass and dotted with wildflowers. Summer can be very hot, especially since most of the trails are without shade. Autumn is cooler and in the early evening, when the sun is low on the horizon, a golden light illuminates the sun-parched hills.

Services: None on the trail. Be sure to bring plenty of water, especially during the summer when temperatures can reach the 90s and little shade is found. Water found in the public lands must be treated before consumption. Water, food, and rest rooms in the nearby 7-Eleven convenience store in Toro Creek Estates, a residential community. Maintained campground with rest rooms, showers, and water available at Laguna Seca Recreation Area, outside the western boundary of Fort Ord Public Lands. All other services available in Monterey and Salinas.

Hazards: The Fort Ord Public Lands is only a portion of the former military base. Of all the undeveloped, still natural land within the base, this area managed by the BLM is the only area deemed safe for recreational used by the public. The huge

RIDE 95 · Fort Ord: Guidotti–Goat Trail Loop

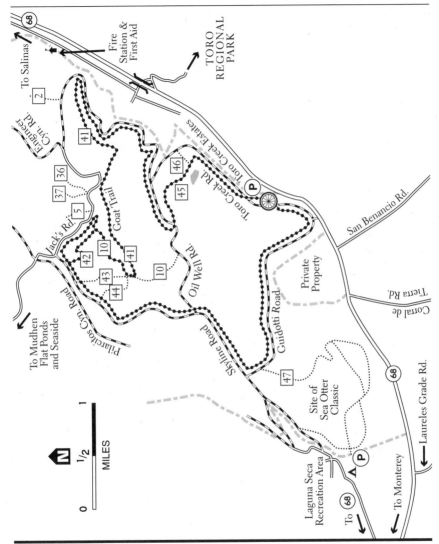

chunk of land west of the Public Lands, specifically west of Barloy Canyon Road, is off-limits to the public due to the existence of scattered unexploded ordnances. Unless you want to get your bike blown apart, among other things you value, obey all "Danger! Keep out!" signs throughout Fort Ord. The Public Lands is designated safe from unexploded ordnances but do stay alert for unfamiliar objects, metal and otherwise. If you spot a suspicious object, don't touch it but do mark it's location and contact the BLM office at Fort Ord (now referred to as "The Annex") at (831) 394-8314 or the BLM main office in Hollister at (831) 630-5000. Be ready to share the trail, especially the narrow single-tracks with other trail users, such as hikers and equestrians. Watch out for poison oak. Mountain lions live here and while attacks are rare, do stay alert. Expect hard-packed trails to be patched with deep sand that can quickly halt your momentum.

Rescue index: On weekends, especially during the pleasant dry months, the trails are patrolled by staff and volunteers of the Bicycle/Equestrian Trail Assistance Unit. They're generally equipped with two-way radios and first-aid kits. A fire station at which you can find emergency help is located on Portola Drive, near CA 68 outside the southeastern boundary of the public land. The southern edge is also bordered by Toro Creek Estates, a residential development.

Land status: Fort Ord Public Lands, managed by the Bureau of Land Management.

Maps: *Fort Ord Public Lands Trail Map*, published by the Bureau of Land Management.

Finding the trail: Fort Ord Public Lands are located on the north side of CA 68 (also known as the Monterey-Salinas Highway) between Monterey and Salinas. From US 101 in Salinas, head south on CA 68 toward the Monterey Peninsula for about 13 miles. The east entrance to the Fort Ord Public Lands is off Reservation Road/River Road (County Road G17) but for this ride, continue past it by staying on CA 68. After passing Toro Park Regional Park located immediately on the south side of CA 68, look right for a dirt parking area (not within the residential development). A BLM signboard marks the trailhead and it's posted on the west edge of the dirt lot, about 200 yards from the highway. If you reach San Benancio Road intersection, you've just passed it. This parking area is immediately adjacent to the back side of homes in the Toro Creek Estates. Park and begin riding from here. From Monterey, from the intersection of Highway 1 (CA 1) and CA 68, go north (by northeast) on CA 68 for about 6 miles. Go past the entrance to Laguna Seca Recreation Area and through the intersections of Laureles Grade Road, Corral de Tierra, and San Benancio Road. Immediately look for the same dirt parking area on your left. Caution: Turning left and crossing the opposing lane may be a challenge if there's a lot of traffic. You may have to continue past the dirt lot, turning left into the residential community and doubling back on CA 68.

Sources of additional information:

Fort Ord Public Lands
Bureau of Land Management
20 Hamilton Court
Hollister, CA 95023
(831) 394-8314

The Annex office at Fort Ord
Located on Eucalyptus Road
(831) 394-8314

Laguna Seca Recreation Area
Highway 68, west of Laureles Grade
(831) 422-6138 or (831) 755-4899

Notes on the trail: Be sure to pick up a map at the BLM signboard adjacent to the dirt parking lot. A word about the map and the identification of the trails out in the field: Most of the lesser trails throughout Fort Ord are signed and identified by numbers, and most—not all—accurately correspond to the map. On the other hand, the main, obvious dirt roads such as Guidotti, Skyline, and Jack's Roads are named as such on the map but are actually unsigned in the field. Expect to see a few unsigned single-track trails in the field that are not indicated on the map; they are not official trails as identified by the BLM. All trails are open to bikers unless signed otherwise.

Here, near the signboard, there are numerous single-track trails running in several directions. Follow an unsigned single-track just to the left of the signboard and leading away behind it. The trail is a fairly level stretch through tall grasses. In a few yards, the single-track joins Guidotti Road, a wide dirt road, which runs both left and right. Hang a left here. Guidotti is likely to be patched with deep, wheel-swallowing sand and riding through it is almost impossible. You can usually get past some of the sand traps by riding an occasionally narrow trail paralleling the road that many riders before you have blazed. Otherwise, endure drudging through the sand for about 200 yards. On your far left is the highway. A clue to knowing you're on Guidotti Road is a metal gate on your left, next to the highway. Bypass the gate, staying on Guidotti which at this point looks like a double-track trail as it leads through a sparse forest of oak, laurel, and deciduous trees as well as chaparral. A few yards further, the trail leads over an old cement bridge. For the next 1.8 miles, Guidotti snakes over a series of treeless, wide open, rolling hills on its way up to the highest point of this ride. Trail conditions improve, becoming hard-packed dirt with fewer patches of shallow sand. The steepness varies, nothing more than 9% grade. As you gain elevation, your view becomes more and more expansive. Eventually, the highway and residential homes of Toro Creek Estates behind you become totally hidden and the landscape all around you seems devoid of civilization. Off on your right, you get a glimpse of the farm fields of the Salinas Valley, the famed salad bowl of the entire country. At 2.2 miles, a few yards before Guidotti intersects Skyline Road, trail 47 leads off on your left. (For those of you interested in riding the single-tracks of the Sea Otter Classic mountain bike race course, 47 will take you to them. The trails connected by 47 are typically challenging and fun for intermediate- to expert-level riders.)

At the wide open, unsigned intersection of Guidotti and Skyline Road, go right onto Skyline. Skyline is a wide, smooth, generally hard-packed dirt road with occasional loose gravel and cruises the top of a long ridge. The riding is fast, fun and easy. Bear left at 3.1 miles, bypassing another unsigned dirt road (that's Oil Well Road which leads back down toward CA 68 and the Toro Creek Estates residential community). At 3.7 miles, bypass a minor dirt road and a lesser single-track on your right. Almost a half mile further, continue past signed trail 44 which comes in on your right. At about 4.4 miles, ignore an unsigned road on your left (it's a connector road to Pilarcitos Canyon Road, another smooth, wide dirt road much like Skyline Road). Stay on Skyline, bearing right, and continue past trails 43 and 42. [Trail 42 is also called Redrock Ridge Trail on the map. It's a highly technical single-track that's popular with technically skilled riders. If you want to tackle this challenge, the better approach is to hop on 42 at the top instead of here at the bottom. To reach the top, continue on the following trail description.] When you reach paved Jack's Road, hang a right. Pedal the pavement for about 0.75 mile to trail 10, a dirt trail. Go right onto 10, across from 5. Climb up 10 for about 0.2 mile to 42 which leads off on your right. Continue straight, bearing left on 10. [As promised, technically skilled riders looking for a single-track challenge can access 42 from this point. Going down 42 is decidedly more fun in this direction. This way, you tackle the twisty, rocky, narrow trail as a downhill instead of a climb. Expect the trail to be occasionally extremely steep but brief, resembling a narrow trough in spots, with abrupt drops and a few sand traps. Stay alert for other trail users. This gnarly single-track is less than a mile long and it dumps you back onto Skyline Road. Once back on Skyline, just go right to Jack's Road, and retrace your path to the top of 42 on 10. Unless you want to ride this little technical stretch again, continue on the ride by following 10 past 42.]

Trail 10 is a mildly rugged trail with some loose sand. Follow it up and down several very steep, short hills. Fly down those hills and let your momentum carry you up to the top of the next rise. About a half mile from the top of 42, you reach a four-way intersection. Not all the trails are signed here. Stay on 10, bearing left, then make a hard left onto signed trail 41. [To shorten the overall ride, stay on 10, bypassing 41. Trail 10 will eliminate about 5 miles of this loop.] Also called Goat Trail on the BLM map, 41 is a narrow single-track that hugs and traverses a steep, exposed slope as it heads east. This is one of the best trails in all of Fort Ord and the direction you're riding—west to east—is decidedly more fun than the opposite way. Goat Trail is moderately technical and beginners with an adventurous attitude who know when to dismount and walk can handle it. Though the narrow trail begins a bit ruggedly with short ups and downs, it quickly mellows into a fairly level path as it cuts through meadows of tall grass, becoming double-track in some stretches. In a little more than a half mile from leaving 10, Goat Trail nearly intersects paved Jack's Road, coming within 20 yards. Stay on Goat Trail, bearing right. For the next 1.5 miles, the path becomes a bit more technical with a few steep dips and rutted trail conditions, interspersed with a mellow stretch through a through a wide open meadow with a 360-degree view. [Riders who find Goat Trail thus far too difficult have the opportunity to skip the upcoming tougher section. Simply follow Jack's Road downhill, continuing on it when the road becomes dirt. Jack's Road and Goat Trail intersect and end near a tiny lake—a perfect place to re-group.] Follow Goat Trail past a tiny little lake, weaving around a small stand of oak trees, riding in and out of the shade. (There's a picnic table here near the trail at the lake.) Just after the lake, the trail ends at Jack's Road, now a wide dirt road. In fact, Jack's Road terminates here, too. At this point, the residential houses of the Toro Creek Estates is close by, about 200–300 yards away. Make a hard right onto unsigned Oil Well Road, another wide, smooth dirt road.

After a few yards on Oil Well Road, go past a BLM signboard. [Here, too, is another bail-out opportunity. Go left toward the houses, exiting the BLM property and onto paved Anza Drive. Pedal through the residential neighborhood and make your way back to your car.] You can cruise or ride hard on Oil Well as it traverses the hills up and above the homes. There are several more bail-out trails leading down out of BLM land and into the neighborhood. Bypass them all. Eventually, the road curves northwest and you begin a gradual climb back toward Skyline Road. About 2.4 miles from the BLM signboard, keep an eye out for a narrow single-track signed 45 on your left. If you reach trail 10, you've just passed 45. Hang a hard left onto 45, a narrow trail that can, at times, appear to disappear under the tall, overgrown grass. The trail leads you over and down a wide open hill toward two ponds and the housing development. After passing the ponds, 45 ends at Toro Creek Road, a dirt road. Go right and the road immediately drops down into the dry, sandy creek bed. Portage your bike about 30–40 yards over the deep sand toward a softball field on the other side of the creek. Toro Creek Road becomes rideable again as it skirts the ball field and the backyards of a bunch of homes. Soon, after passing the last house, bear right onto a single-track and follow it back to your car at the trailhead. Total distance of the loop as described is about 13 miles.

RIDE 96 · Fort Ord: Mudhen Lake–Rim Trail Ramble

AT A GLANCE

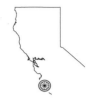

Length/configuration: 11.5-mile ramble (out-and-back with 2 loops)

Aerobic difficulty: Moderate

Technical difficulty: Mild to intermediate; mostly smooth dirt and paved road with dirt trails of irregular conditions

Scenery: Magnificent views of the agriculturally rich Salinas Valley from the rim of a ridge; peaceful, sparsely wooded sandstone canyons and rolling hills of tall grasses in a former military base.

Special comments: Suitable for confident young riders and strong beginners. Kid-trailers not recommended. If you ride the short single- and double-track trails in this description, route-finding ability is recommended.

W hile the previous ride may not be suited for all beginners, Mudhen Flats–Rim Trail Ramble is perfect for fairly strong riders with basic technical skills. This 11.5-mile meandering route is mostly mildly technical, using abandoned paved roads, dirt roads and single- and double-track trails. Not many places offer such easy access into acres of peaceful, hidden canyons and hills like the Fort Ord Public Lands. Except for a one-mile 8–9% grade hill, all other climbs are generally brief, ranging from gentle to steep. If you really want to make it a truly easy ride, you can skip the narrow dirt trails and simply ride the route as an out-and-back, using only wide dirt and paved roads.

While the Monterey Peninsula attracts over seven million tourists annually, only about 16,000 of them ever visit the Fort Ord Public Lands. Why is that? Truth be told, most of the terrain at Fort Ord is not exceptionally spectacular and the trails have a reputation of being sandy. The land, being predominantly sandstone and arid, is mostly chaparral country with seasonal tall grasses with stands of oak and evergreen trees scattered over rolling hills. Those conditions make for shadeless, dusty trails, especially when the weather's hot. While the trails are mostly hardpack, there are frequent patches of deep sand just waiting to swallow your wheel and suck the fun out of riding. But there are immensely enjoyable routes to be found at Fort Ord, and this—like the previous description—is one of them. Though locals have been riding Fort Ord for the last 10 years, it wasn't until 1994 that the trails began to be officially scouted, documented, and signed. With the help of AmeriCorps volunteers, most but not all of the confusion of trails at Fort Ord has been sorted out. On this ride, a short, almost two-mile stretch is a convoluted network of criss-crossing trails, a mess of signed and unsigned paths. Don't let that discourage you, though. You can't really get lost on that portion. While this section can be easily avoided, I recommend riding it because the view of the Salinas Valley from the canyon rim is glorious.

Locals know that Fort Ord and neighboring Toro Park is as good as mountain biking gets in the Monterey Peninsula. They also know that when the rest of the peninsula is shrouded in chilly, depressing fog (which is often, even in the summer), Fort

RIDE 96 · Fort Ord: Mudhen Lake–Rim Trail Ramble

To Salinas

68

River Rd.

Firehouse &
First Aid

TORO REGIONAL PARK

To Laguna Seca
Recreation Area
& Monterey

Reservation Road

P

Delapidated
Log Cabin

Toro Creek Estates

Toro Creek Estates

68

30

31

33

33

2

41

4

33

Old Reservation Road

Private Property

Engineer Cyn. Rd.

35

Goat Trail

Private Property

G17

To Marina

FT. ORD PUBLIC LANDS

36

37

5

41

7

Jack's Rd.

10

FT. ORD PUBLIC LANDS

Skyline Rd.

Pilarcitos Cyn. Rd.

8

9

11

Crescent Bluff Rd.

Mudhen Flat Ponds

49

Eucalyptus Rd.

To Seaside

N

1/2

MILES

0

1

Ord is likely to be warm and sunny. Though not spectacular when compared to other areas of the state, the undeveloped foothills, canyons, and valleys that make up Fort Ord Public Lands has its own quiet beauty, devoid of hordes of people. What Fort Ord lacks in impressive scenery, it makes up in abundant solitude. You just have to know which trails to follow.

General location: About 9 miles east of Monterey, about 115 miles south of San Francisco.

Elevation change: 410 feet change; starting elevation and low point 90 feet; high point 500 feet. Lots of rolling, gentle hills.

Season: Year-round. Spring is the best time to ride because the hills are green with new grass and dotted with wildflowers. Summer can be very hot, especially since most of the trails are without shade. Autumn is cooler and in the early evening, when the sun is low on the horizon, a golden light illuminates the sun-parched hills.

Services: None on the trail. Be sure to bring plenty of water, especially during the summer when temperatures can reach the 90s and little shade is found. Water found in the public lands must be treated before consumption. Water, food, and rest rooms in the nearby 7-Eleven convenience store in Toro Creek Estates, a residential community. Maintained campground with rest rooms, showers, and water available at Laguna Seca Recreation Area, outside the western boundary of Fort Ord Public Lands. All other services available in Monterey and Salinas.

Hazards: The Fort Ord Public Lands are only a portion of the former military base. Of all the undeveloped, still natural land within the base, this area managed by the BLM is the only area deemed safe for recreational used by the public. The huge chunk of land west of the Public Lands, specifically west of Barloy Canyon Road, is off-limits to the public due to the existence of scattered unexploded ordnances. Unless you want to get your bike blown apart, among other things you value, obey all "Danger! Keep out!" signs throughout all of Fort Ord. The Public Lands is designated safe from unexploded ordnances but do stay alert for unfamiliar objects, metal and otherwise. If you spot a suspicious object, don't touch it but do mark it's location and contact the BLM office at Fort Ord (now referred to as "The Annex") at (831) 394-8314 or the BLM main office in Hollister at (831) 630-5000. Be ready to share the trail, especially the narrow single-tracks with other trail users, such as hikers and equestrians. Watch out for poison oak. Mountain lions live here and while attacks are rare, do stay alert. Expect hard-packed trails to be patched with deep sand that can quickly halt your momentum.

Rescue index: On weekends, especially during the pleasant dry months, the trails are patrolled by staff and volunteers of the Bicycle/Equestrian Trail Assistance Unit. They're generally equipped with two-way radios and first-aid kits. A fire station at which you can find emergency help is located on Portola Drive, near CA 68 outside the southeastern boundary of the public land. The southern edge is also bordered by Toro Creek Estates, a residential development.

Land status: Fort Ord Public Lands, managed by the Bureau of Land Management.

Maps: *Fort Ord Public Lands Trail Map*, published by the Bureau of Land Management.

Finding the trail: Fort Ord Public Lands is located on the north side of CA 68 (also known as the Monterey-Salinas Highway) between Monterey and Salinas. From Salinas, head south on CA 68 toward the Monterey Peninsula for about 6 miles. The east entrance to the Fort Ord Public Lands is off Reservation Road/River Road (CR G17). Take the Reservation Road exit. On the north side of CA 68, make the first left onto Portola Drive, then bear right as it curves into Creekside Terrace Road. Follow Creekside Terrace for about 0.3 mile to its end at the east gate. Park and begin pedaling from here. From Monterey, take CA 68 due north (by northeast) for about 13 miles. Along the way, you'll go past Laguna Seca, Portola Drive turn-off, Toro Creek Estates, and Toro Regional Park. When CA 68 becomes a four-lane highway, watch out for the Reservation Road/River Road exit. Take this exit and go north underneath CA 68. Hang a left onto Portola Drive, then a right onto Creekside Terrace Road.

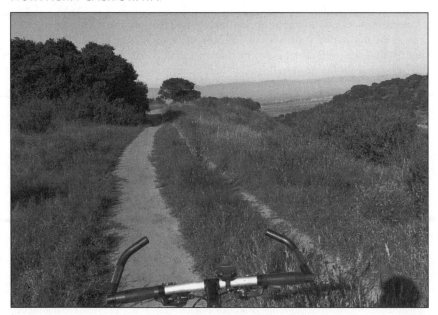

An eastward view of the agricultural fields down in Salinas Valley, as seen from the Rim Trail.

Follow Creekside Terrace for about 0.3 mile to its end at the east gate. Park and begin pedaling from here.

Sources of additional information: See sources of additional information for Ride 95.

Notes on the trail: Be sure to pick up a map at the BLM signboard adjacent to the dirt parking lot. A word about the map and the identification of the trails out in the field: Most of the lesser trails throughout Fort Ord are accurately signed and identified by numbers, and most—not all—accurately correspond to the map. The narrow plateau between Engineer Canyon Road and the canyon rim is a mess of single-track trails; the map is slightly incorrect and trail markers in the field can be confusing. But not to worry—given several landscape features, it's hard to truly get lost in that region (more details below). Also note that the main, obvious dirt roads such as Engineer Canyon and Jack's Roads are named as such on the official map but are actually unsigned in the field. Jack's is mostly paved, becoming dirt near the southern boundary of the public land. Expect to see a few unsigned single-track trails in the field that are not indicated on the map; they are not official trails as identified by the BLM. All trails are open to bikers unless signed otherwise.

From the eastern parking area, go north through the gate and follow Old Reservation Road, an abandoned paved road. After a level start, the road drops gently, then gradually begins to climb, becoming slightly steeper as it approaches a notch in the sandstone hill up ahead. Along the way, go past several dirt paths—trails 30, 2, and 3. When you reach the notch and the crest of this initial climb, continue past the other end of trail 30 as well as trail 3. About a mile from the gate, you reach the intersection with Engineer Canyon Road, a wide, smooth dirt road on your left. (Old Reservation Road essentially dead ends at Engineer.) Hang a left onto Engineer and follow it as it rolls along just below a ridgeline. Bypass all other dirt trails.

At about 2.5 miles, a few yards after passing trails 3, 33 and 36, Engineer Canyon Road intersects Jack's Road. This is where Jack's Road changes from pavement to dirt. Turn right onto Jack's Road and follow the paved portion. (A left onto the dirt road will lead you back out of the BLM land and into Toro Creek Estates.) Jack's Road is a wide road, totally free of motor vehicles. Continue on Jack's as it climbs gently, becoming steeper as you reach the high point of the ride about 0.7 mile from Engineer. (Just before the crest, look for trail 36 on your right. That's an optional dirt trail you can take on your return.) After reaching the top of the climb, the next mile is a sweet and fast downhill cruise. Zip past Skyline Road and in a few yards further, Pilarcitos Canyon Road (both of which are wide, smooth dirt roads that lead to Laguna Seca—something to keep in mind if you're looking for more miles to pedal). Let your momentum down the hill carry you up another short rise. In no time, you reach Mudhen Lake (really two big ponds).

Jack's Road intersects paved Eucalyptus Road on the left and dirt Crescent Bluff Road on the right, next to the lake at about 2.8 miles from Engineer Canyon Road. Hang a left onto Eucalyptus and ride along the north edge of the lake. This is a peaceful spot for a picnic where birds sing and hoot. How convenient that there's a picnic table nearby along Eucalyptus. Just beyond the lake, check out the huge sand slide—about 40 yards across—on the right. The road looks like it has been snow-plowed. (Of course, over time, the sand shifts and disperses and by the time you visit, it may not look like much of a sight.) If you'd like, you can ride around both lakes by taking a dirt trail (unsigned 49 turning into 71) leading away from the paved road. Go through the dried marsh flatland, following the trail around to the left and even-tually back toward Jack's Road.

Begin your return by turning left onto Jack's. Retrace your path up to the high point on Jack's. In this direction, the road steepens significantly just before the crest, but per-severe—it's over in less than a mile. Remember trail 36 near the crest? If you're want-ing to ride a slightly more rugged and technical trail, go left onto 36. (If not, just con-tinue down Jack's to the end of the pavement. Then, hang a left onto Engineer Canyon Road and continue to retrace your steps back to Old Reservation Road and eventually your car.) But for those seeking a bit more of a challenge, follow 36 as it climbs up a short rise. The brief climb rewards you with an expansive view of the lower hills behind your left shoulder and the Salinas Valley straight ahead. The trail soon lev-els and semi-buried rocks, boulders and some patches of sand continue to wake up your technical skills. Bypass trail 38 and begin a somewhat steep but short descent down to Engineer Canyon Road. When you reach Engineer, continue across the dirt road and pick up trail 3 or 33. Both trails weave in and out of one another as they cruise along the flat terrain along the rim of a canyon. Unofficially dubbed the Rim Trail by locals, the trail heads east by northeast skirting a rim of a canyon on your right. From this vantage point, looking ahead to the east, the views of the Salinas Valley are mag-nificent, its cultivated farmlands resembling a patchwork of salad greens and other cash crops. Indeed, what you're looking at is the northern edge of the nation's "salad bowl." Expect to find a mess of single-tracks, criss-crossing along this narrow strip of land between the rim and Engineer Canyon Road. Follow either trails 3 or 33 but def-initely stay off of trail 4 and any other trail that leads down the rim. As a guide, keep the rim about 20 to 50 yards on your right and the Salinas Valley ahead of you due east. (If you reach Engineer Canyon Road, you've veered off the rim, having descended and gone a bit too far north. No matter. You can just retrace your path back up the rim or just continue cruising on Engineer heading east and eventually intersect Old

Reservation Road. Then go right and follow the now familiar paved road back to the trailhead where your car is parked.) As you follow the dirt trails along the rim, trail 33 intersects trail 3 for the last time about 0.2 mile from Old Reservation Road. Continue on trail 3 as it descends to paved Old Reservation Road. Turn right onto the now familiar road and enjoy an easy cruise back to the trailhead and your car.

RIDE 97 · Monterey Recreation Trail

AT A GLANCE

Length/configuration: 29.4-mile out-and-back (14.7 miles each way); mostly well-separated paved multi-use recreation trail with a few short stretches on quiet streets. Trail can be accessed at numerous points, allowing you to determine your own length.

Aerobic difficulty: Easy; mostly flat riding

Technical difficulty: Mildly technical; being able to share the trail with many other trail users is a critical bike-handling skill

Scenery: Gorgeous Monterey Bay shoreline, beaches, and parks despite the trail's close proximity to popular tourists attractions

Special comments: Suitable for kids and kid-trailers (though some sections can be very congested). Lots of side attractions.

The completely paved, 14.7-mile Monterey Recreational Trail (29.4-mile round-trip) is the jewel of the towns of Pacific Grove, Monterey, Sand City, Seaside, and Marina. Enjoyed by riders of all ages and abilities, it's an immensely popular path that hugs the gorgeous Monterey Bay shoreline, 95% of it being Class 1, that is, a path that's completely separated from vehicle roads. (Heartier riders can extend their journey into Pebble Beach and Carmel via the famed 17-Mile Drive route. See Ride 98.) The year-round trail is used by walkers (some with baby strollers), dog walkers, joggers, skaters, both fast and leisurely bikers (road, hybrid, and mountain bikes), and rental pedal carriages (those goofy, but fun contraptions that seat four to five passengers). The most popular length is between Pacific Grove and Sand City, nearly all flat, about zero to 30 feet above sea level. From Sand City through Marina, the Rec Trail gently rolls up and down, and though not as scenic, this portion has much fewer trail users. Beach access, parks, picnic tables, drinking fountains, and rest room facilities are scattered throughout the length of the path, especially along the Pacific Grove and Monterey stretches. On the north and northwest side of the trail is the magnificent natural scenery of the Monterey Bay National Marine Sanctuary, stretching from Rocky Point in Marin County in the north down to Cambria in San Luis Obispo County in the south. Home to the most expansive kelp forests and one of the deepest underwater canyons on earth, hundreds of varieties of birds, fish, invertebrate species and marine mammals live in these waters. The other side of the Rec Trail (the inland side), is dominated by many man-made attractions, including the world-class Monterey Bay Aquarium, historic Cannery Row (now bustling with tourists shops), Fisherman's Wharf, Monterey Bay Kayaks rentals, and Seaside/Del Monte Beach where hordes of kite flyers often congregate on sunny Sundays. Stores, eateries, and hotels are within easy access to the Rec Trail.

In 1975, the California Coastal Conservancy was formed with the intent of improving public access to coastal lands as well as to protect agricultural lands and coastal resources. As part of the California Coastal Plan, the Conservancy launched the California Coastal Trail, an ambitious project that will ultimately link the entire 1,100-mile California coast line. Today, that dream is only about half realized. According to the agency, no completion date is scheduled. As you can probably guess, when it comes to valuable coast property in California, lots of funding is required. When the project began in 1976, roughly half of the state's coastline was public property while the other half was private property or held by the military. Always envisioned as a long-term project, coughing up the money has never been easy. Funding in the early 1990s has been lean. In an effort to leverage their money, the agency is constantly forging meaningful partnerships with communities, local governments, and private property owners. In 1984, the first stretch in Monterey County—the section between Lovers Point in Pacific Grove and Fisherman's Wharf in Monterey—was officially opened. Though disconnected, subsequent stretches between the Wharf and Marina were soon built. In order to connect the paved paths, riding busy streets around Sand City and through Seaside was required. In 1998, the crucial Sand City link was constructed, making the 14.7-mile long Rec Trail from Pacific Grove to Marina nearly 100% Class 1 status. (As of 1999, several short but temporary sections in Sand City are class 2 and 3, that is, painted bike lane on the shoulder of a road and shoulderless road designated a bike route, respectively.)

General location: About 85 miles south of San Jose.

Elevation change: Negligible; mostly at sea level.

Season: Year-round. On rare occasions, a grey whale may be seen in the Monterey Bay during migration season, typically late October to January and February to June.

Services: All services available throughout the trail.

Hazards: The greatest hazard is sharing the path with other trail users. Children should be confident with their bike handling skills. Because of the trail's popularity, all riders, especially children, need to exercise proper and safe bicycling etiquette, such as pulling off to the side when stopping, not making abrupt turns across the trail, and riding on the right side of the path. Expect to encounter bikers that ride much too fast, and weave in and out of pedestrians, baby strollers, and pedal carriages. The paved trail is designated for bikers and skaters. Though pedestrians are asked to walk on the dirt alongside the paved trail whenever possible, many who are tourists are oblivious to such sign postings. They force those of us on wheels to go around them, veering into the on-coming lane. Passing is generally not a big deal except on congested popular stretches. So, when passing, watch out for on-coming speedsters and other pedestrians. Also, the Rec Trail crosses many streets and busy intersections—stay alert and don't expect motorists to stop. Brief stretches on lightly traveled Roberts, Tioga, and Metz Streets actually share the pavement with vehicles. Roberts and Metz Streets use painted bike lanes; Tioga is a shoulderless road. Metz runs along the backside of a big shopping center, where the loading docks and dumpsters are located. When on Metz, stay alert for huge shipping trucks; also expect speeding motorists using the lightly traveled road as a shortcut.

RIDE 97 · Monterey Recreation Trail

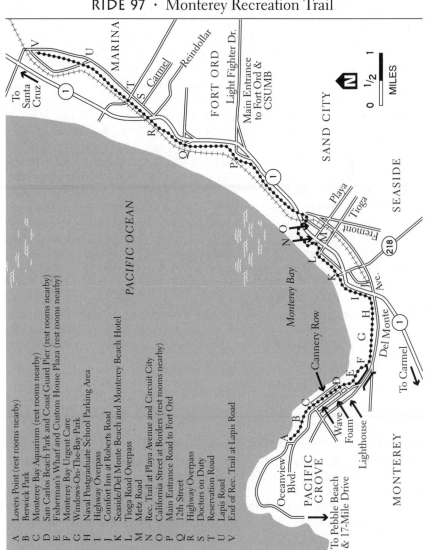

A Lovers Point (rest rooms nearby)
B Berwick Park
C Monterey Bay Aquarium (rest rooms nearby)
D San Carlos Beach Park and Coast Guard Pier (rest rooms nearby)
E Fisherman's Wharf and Custom House Plaza (rest rooms nearby)
F Monterey Bay Urgent Care
G Windows-On-The-Bay Park
H Naval Postgraduate School Parking Area
I Highway Overpass
J Comfort Inn at Roberts Road
K Seaside/Del Monte Beach and Monterey Beach Hotel
L Tioga Road Overpass
M Metz Road
N Rec. Trail at Playa Avenue and Circuit City
O California Street at Borders (rest rooms nearby)
P Main Entrance Road to Fort Ord
Q 12th Street
R Highway Overpass
S Doctors on Duty
T Reservation Road
U Lapis Road
V End of Rec. Trail at Lapis Road

Rescue index: Except for the two stretches south and north of Marina, you're likely to meet other trail users who may be of help. A phone is never too far away thanks to the many businesses and residents that line the path. Two emergency medical clinics, Monterey Bay Urgent Care and Doctors on Duty, are located on the path, near Fisherman's Wharf and in Marina, respectively. The entire trail is never far from a major highway, businesses, and homes.

Land status: Property of the cities of Pacific Grove, Monterey, Sand City, Seaside, and Marina.

Maps: As of the end of 1999, maps have yet to be updated to show the new Sand City stretch. The map included with this description is the most accurate and up-to-date.

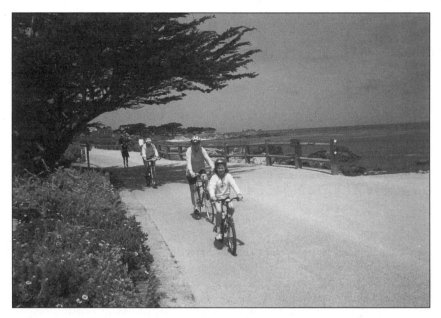

Mary Lou and Keely share the immensely popular Monterey Recreation Trail with others while pedaling the Pacific Grove portion of the shore-hugging 14.7-mile path

Finding the trail: Where do you want to access the Rec Trail? I suggest you read through the description and familiarize yourself with the map. To reach the Monterey Peninsula from San Jose, drive south on US 101 to its intersection with the second CA 156 exit (to Monterey Peninsula), just north of Salinas. Head west on CA 156 for about 5 miles to Highway 1 (CA 1). CA 156 merges onto southbound Highway 1. In about 4 miles, after crossing the Salinas River, the first Del Monte Avenue exit appears. This exit leads you the northern-most end of the Rec Trail. If you want to access the least crowded, least interrupted stretch, take this exit and make your way to the east side of Highway 1 via an overpass. Here, a few yards beyond the overpass, cross the railroad tracks and look for Lapis Road on your right. There's a rough dirt parking lot at the intersection of Lapis and Del Monte. Park here as close to the edge of the lot or the stop sign as possible (many huge commercial trucks hauling trailers of vegetables use this lot as a turnaround). Adjacent to the lot, paralleling Del Monte is the beginning of the paved path, marked by a simple bike trail sign.

To access the more popular and scenic sections of the trail in Sand City, Monterey, or Pacific Grove, where the tourist attractions are located, continue south on Highway 1 toward Monterey. You can see the paved trail immediately on the right side of the highway as you approach Sand City. A little over 8 miles from the first Del Monte Avenue exit, another exit appears, signed "Sand City, Seaside, Fremont Boulevard." This is the site of another convenient parking area. To park here, take this exit and at the end of the off-ramp, go left and underneath Highway 1. Located at the next intersection is Borders bookstore within a huge shopping center. Go right and park in the Borders parking lot. The bike trail runs alongside this intersection. Pick up the Rec Trail here, and pedal due west, toward Monterey.

The western-most end of the Rec Trail is at Lovers Point in Pacific Grove. There are many other places to park near the trail between Borders and Lovers Point.

Note: If you park in residential neighborhoods, be sure to check for street signs that may indicate "Residential Parking" which means if you don't live there, your time is limited typically to one hour. To reach the west end trailhead and other suitable parking areas in between, ignore the Sand City exit and continue on Highway 1 for almost 3 miles to the Pacific Grove exit—it's the first exit after the "CA 218, Del Rey Oaks" exit. (Incidentally, located at bottom of the CA 218/Del Rey Oaks exit is the Monterey Beach Hotel adjacent to the Seaside/Del Monte Beach. Colorful kites which you can see from Highway 1 may be flying. Parking is available here, too—just be aware of any posted parking regulations.) The Pacific Grove off-ramp dumps you onto Del Monte Avenue in a west-bound lane. (The Rec Trail parallels Del Monte and from this point on, you can easily access it from anywhere you like.) Continue west on Del Monte and in 0.3 mile at a signal light intersection surrounded by a grove of tall, eucalyptus trees, you reach a small parking lot adjacent to the trail and across from the main entrance to the Naval Postgraduate School. (This is a popular and convenient parking spot—and it's free of charge. If you want to park here, you'll need to bear right just before the intersection.)

To continue on to Lovers Point, stay on Del Monte Avenue and go past Windows-On-The-Bay Park, Monterey Bay Kayaks, Fisherman's Wharf, and several parking lot entrances to the Wharf (fee charged in these lots). You can see the Rec Trail on your right paralleling your road. After the second Fisherman's Wharf entrance (next to Monterey Bay Urgent Care), stay in the right lane and go through the tunnel. As you emerge from the tunnel, stay in the right lane and immediately bear right onto Foam Street, toward Cannery Row and the aquarium.

As soon as you turn onto Foam, San Carlos Beach and parking area appear on your right. (There are metered parking spaces as well as a timed lot. Here you'll also find rest rooms, water, and picnic tables next to a wide open grassy park with a great view of the bay.) Foam parallels Wave Street and Cannery Row, which are two blocks to the right toward the bay. Sandwiched in between Wave Street and Cannery Row is the Rec Trail, which from Foam is obscured from view. You can access the trail at any point along this stretch. (While you may find parking in this vicinity, be aware that it's metered or timed and enforcement is everyday into the evening, including Sundays and some holidays.) Follow Foam to its end at a T intersection with David Street. Go right onto David for one block and then a left onto Oceanview Boulevard (called Wave Street on your right). At this intersection are located the Monterey Bay Aquarium and the American Tin Cannery (factory outlet stores with public rest rooms and water available). Lovers Point is 1 mile from this intersection. As you drive along Oceanview, you'll find many places which allow extended parking at no charge. You can usually find free, untimed parking up any number of side streets, but do look for posted signs regulating parking. Rest rooms and a grassy park are located at Lovers Point.

Sources of additional information:

Transportation Agency for Monterey
    County (TAMC)
312 E. Alisal St.
Salinas, CA 93901
(831) 755-8961

Pacific Grove Recreation
    Department
515 Junipero Ave.
Pacific Grove, CA 93950
(831) 648-3130

Monterey Bay Aquarium
886 Cannery Row at David Ave.
Monterey, CA 93940-1085
(831) 648-4888 or (800) 756-3737
  for tickets
Admission: about $16 adults,
  $7 children

Pacific Grove Chamber of
  Commerce
Forest and Central Ave.
Pacific Grove, CA 93950
(831) 373-3304

Monterey Peninsula Visitors &
  Convention Bureau
401 Camino El Estero
Monterey, CA 93942-1770
(831) 649-1770

City of Sand City
1 Sylvan Park
Sand City, CA 93955
(831) 394-1451

City of Seaside Recreation
  Administration
986 Hilby Ave.
Seaside, CA 93955
(831) 899-6270

Marina Parks & Recreation
211 Hillcrest Ave.
Marina, CA 93933
(831) 384-4636

Notes on the trail: If this is your first time riding the Rec Trail, be sure to bring a bike lock. There will undoubtedly be places you'll want to stop and check out. You can begin and end your ride at any point along the Rec Trail, making your outing as long or as short as you desire. The paved path is well-marked with signs and a painted stripe divides the trail into left and right lanes. Always stay right except when passing. Get into the habit of saying "Passing on your left." Better yet, put a bell on your handlebars—it's a friendly way to announce your presence, unless you're mean-spirited and like scaring the daylights out of unsuspecting pedestrians. Here are some highlights and noteworthy places found along the trail, starting at Lovers Point and riding toward Marina. Letters correspond to the locations on the map.

From Lovers Point (A) to the Monterey Bay Aquarium (C), the distance is 1 mile. At Lovers Point, there's a sheltered little beach where the kiddies can splash in the water, free from undertows and crashing waves. Also located here is a snack-bar, kayak rentals, a volleyball court, and rest rooms. This stretch is a scenic and very popular section that follows the rugged shoreline. A frequent sight are lazy California seals, draped over seemingly uncomfortable rocks protruding above the water. Look closely and you're likely to spot playful sea otters frolicking in the kelp forest canopies. Quaint, modest homes line this stretch, as well as the magnificent Seven Gables Bed & Breakfast Inn, a beautifully maintained yellow Victorian. Many wooden benches overlooking the bay invite you to sit a while. Roughly half-way between Lovers Point and the Aquarium is Berwick Park (B), a small but lovely grassy park—a pleasant place for a picnic (no tables here, though). The world-class Monterey Bay Aquarium is a worthwhile visit and you easily spend two hours and not see everything. This portion sees lots of use so expect some congestion.

From the Aquarium (C) and San Carlos Beach Park (D), the distance is 0.7 mile. Along this stretch is historic Cannery Row. Immortalized by Nobel Prize-winning author John Steinbeck in his 1945 book of the same title, Cannery Row was populated by industrious fish canneries, hard-working laborers, and colorful characters. Sardines and its accompanying stench was the life-blood of Monterey at that time.

With the disappearance of sardines from the bay, the canneries were eventually shut down and abandoned. Today, replaced by souvenir shops, eateries, and art galleries, the Row attracts thousands of tourists every year. That said, you can imagine the place being a "zoo" during the tourist season. Fortunately, the Rec Trail is separated from the streets although it crosses them numerous times. Stay alert: many sightseeing motorists are unaware and don't always stop at Rec Trail crossings. This stretch through Cannery Row sees tremendous use, especially during the summer months. It's a wonder that more collisions involving cyclists and pedestrians don't occur. San Carlos Beach Park is a great place for a picnic. You'll find picnic tables, benches, a nice grassy lawn, drinking fountains, and rest rooms here. The pier jutting out into the bay next to this beach is the Coast Guard Pier. If looking at hordes of noisy California seals give you a thrill, take a short side trip and ride out to the end of the pier (it's fenced closed at the end). There, almost 100 of these furry mammals sometimes lounge on the rock pilings, sleeping, sunning, and barking up a storm.

From San Carlos Beach (D) to Fisherman Wharf's at the Custom House Plaza (E), the distance is 0.5 mile. Outdoor events are staged at the Plaza throughout the year and if that's the case, expect lots of pedestrians. If you venture off the path, heading inland, you'll be in the heart of old Monterey. If you're into historical adobe buildings, you can find plenty of them here, some with guided tours offered. (For more information, contact the Monterey Visitors Bureau listed in "Sources of Additional Information.")

From Fisherman's Wharf (E) to Windows-On-The-Bay Park (G), the distance is 0.5 mile. The paved Rec Trail leads through the Plaza (the faded painted bike lane may be hard to see) and skirts the edge of a huge public parking lot. About 0.2 mile from the Wharf, the trail leads you across a vehicle road that leads into the public parking lot. Stay alert for cars turning into the lot. The path immediately leads up the sidewalk, pass Monterey Bay Urgent Care (F), an emergency medical clinic, and then makes a hard left. The paved trail skirts busy Del Monte Avenue on your right. Watch out for turning vehicles as the Rec Trail crosses another parking lot entry way. About 0.3 mile from Urgent Care, Windows-On-The-Bay Park is reached. Directly across Del Monte from the park is another park, complete with a tiny lake, paddle boats and a playground for kids. (Good to know if you have youngsters who are bored with riding.) This short portion between Urgent Care and the Windows Park is often busy with other trail users and is one of the least pleasant stretches on the entire trail. Fortunately, it's brief.

From Windows-On-The-Bay Park (G) to the Naval Postgraduate School (NPGS) parking area (H), the distance is 0.7 mile. Turn away from busy and noisy Del Monte Avenue by making a hard left as soon as you reach the Windows Park. The trail approaches the beach and then goes around the backside of the park. There are a few picnic tables here, a water fountain, several volleyball courts, and a splendid grassy lawn. (In late 1999, the park was undergoing major relandscaping. When the trail is reopened in early 2000, this description may vary slightly.) From here on out, the Rec Trail becomes much less congested and you can safely pick up speed now. This stretch to the NPGS parking area cruises between businesses, fenced homes, and tall sand dunes. Immediately before the parking area, the trail leads through an intensely fragrant eucalyptus grove.

From the NPGS parking area (H) to the intersection of Roberts Road and the Rec Trail at the Comfort Inn hotel (J), the distance is 1 mile. The trail leads underneath a Highway 1 overpass (I) before reaching the intersection. Instead of following the bike sign pointing straight, turn left onto Roberts Road and follow the well-painted bike lane toward Highway 1. The bike lane runs around small Roberts Lake, going through a small parking lot before connecting to the paved Rec Trail again. The separated trail soon resumes alongside Roberts Road, going right toward the busy intersection of Canyon del Rey Boulevard and Highway 1 on- and off-ramps, in front of K-Mart. After making a hard left, the path leads underneath the overpass toward the Monterey Beach Hotel. Located next to the hotel is Seaside/Del Monte Beach (K), a favorite place for kite-flyers on sunny Sunday afternoons. The numerous creative contraptions soaring in the sky are a delightful and colorful sight to behold.

From Seaside Beach (K) to Tioga Road overpass (L), the distance is 0.7 mile. The separated Rec Trail continues east, skirting Sand Dunes Drive. Tall dunes temporarily obscure your view of the bay. Surprise, there's a hill on this short stretch! It's a moderately steep rise—about 80 yards—to the Tioga Avenue overpass.

From the top of the Tioga overpass (L) to the resumption of the separately paved Rec Trail at Circuit City (N), the distance is 0.5 mile. This stretch of the bike route is class 3 (using a narrow vehicle road) as it descends shoulderless Tioga Avenue 0.2 mile to Metz Road (M). At that intersection, the route makes a hard left onto Metz and follows the vehicle road as it curves around the back side of huge stores. This is loading dock dumpster land and the scenery is fairly unattractive. Watch out for commercial trucks and speeding motorists looking for a shortcut. Fortunately, this portion is brief. (This is the temporary route for the Rec Trail and Sand City plans to some day re-route the path to the other side of Highway 1.) Before you know it, Metz intersects Playa Avenue next to Circuit City (N). Playa dead ends into the sand dunes on your left and there, the class 1 separately paved Rec Trail resumes.

From the resumption of the Rec Trail (N) to the California Street/Monterey Road intersection (O), the distance is 0.6 mile. The trail immediately goes underneath Highway 1 toward the bay. The tall sand dunes muffle the sound of the traffic noise, and the waves crashing on the beach below can be easily heard. This stretch is arguably the most spectacular stretch of the entire Rec Trail. The trail rises moderately and briefly and yields an expansive view of the bay. (One day when my husband and I rode this stretch, we witnessed a swarm of about 5,000 birds flying in a huge circle just above the water. After about 20 minutes, they commenced dive-bombing into the water. It was dinner time. Even from our vantage point about 500 yards away, their gleeful gawking was incredibly loud.) The trail soon leads you underneath Highway 1 near the busy California Street intersection. There's a Borders bookstore (O) near this corner in a big shopping center. Vehicular traffic is heavy but not to worry—the Rec Trail makes a hard left and never crosses the busy road.

From the Borders/California Street intersection (O) to a Highway 1 overpass in Marina (R), the distance is 4.8 miles, mostly uninterrupted. You won't see many trail users on this stretch, and that's just great if you want to ride hard and work up a bit of a sweat. This stretch rolls moderately up and down—go ahead, power up the rises without shifting gears. The scenery is not splendid as it follows Highway 1 sometimes closely, other times distantly. This section of the Rec Trail is sandwiched between the highway and the abandoned Fort Ord military property. Along the way, bypass the "Main Entrance" road to Fort Ord (P) as well as 12th Street (Q), both of which lead east over Highway 1 and into Fort Ord. The trail enters Marina city limits as it runs underneath the Highway 1 overpass. (If you have plenty of time, there are many intermediate mountain bike trails worth exploring. The 12th Street overpass is highly recommended instead of tremendously busy "Main Entrance." Then, you'll need to ride about 9 miles of paved and dirt vehicle roads in order to reach the Fort Ord Public Lands that is the designated off-road biking area. See the previous two trail descriptions.)

From the overpass (R) to the end of the Rec Trail at the second Lapis Road intersection (V), the distance is 3.3 miles. The trail skirts Del Monte Avenue once again and cruises through town, passing Doctors on Duty (S) (an urgent medical clinic), and eventually crosses Reservation Road (T). The final stretch to the end of the Rec Trail leads you past the first Lapis Road junction (U) and then terminates at its second junction (V) in 2.7 miles from Reservation Road. From there, turn around and return the way you came.

RIDE 98 · 17-Mile Drive to Carmel Road Ride

AT A GLANCE

Length/configuration: 29-mile out-and-back (14.5 miles each way); paved vehicle roads

Aerobic difficulty: Easy to moderate; mostly flat with some moderate rises

Technical difficulty: Mildly technical; some stretches of designated bike lane. Being accustomed to sharing sometimes narrow, shoulderless road with motorists is required.

Scenery: The wild Pacific Ocean crashing against a rugged shoreline; the famed golf courses and million-dollar estates of Pebble Beach; resident flocks of deer; the quaint village of Carmel; white-sand beaches

Special comments: Not recommended for children. This popular route sees a fair amount of traffic. On weekends and holidays, intial point of entry is allowed only at the Pacific Grove gate.

Never mind that this is a road ride. The famed 17-Mile Drive is a ride that's rated as one of the Top 100 routes to pedal in America. If this is your first time to the Monterey Peninsula, this ride is an outstanding way to see a variety of sights. Described as a 29-mile out-and-back (14.5 miles one-way), this ride includes only a nine-mile stretch of the 17-Mile Drive loop (by far the most stunningly scenic portion of that entire loop). Ranging from zero to 150 feet above sea level, the entire route rises and fall over such a wide range that you could easily say it's mostly flat. Rises are moderate with a few slightly steeper but short hills. The first seven miles is graced with a comfortably wide bike lane. The last 7.5 miles follows narrow and often shoulderless roads. Fortunately, the roads are curvy and that effectively helps to keep speeding motorists at bay. Starting from Lovers Point in unpretentious Pacific Grove, the route follows the rugged shoreline on Oceanview Boulevard and Sunset Drive before turning into the gated community of 5,300-acre Pebble Beach. Your journey through this golfer's paradise leads you past many impressive million-dollar estates, through the grounds of the Lodge (the main lodging and gathering place of the resort), pass the famed, oft-photographed Lone Cypress (a weathered cypress tree growing out of a rock outcropping which juts into the ocean). Eventually, the route veers off 17-Mile Drive and runs into the quaintly upscale village of Carmel. There, the route follows Scenic Drive, leading you past the white sands of Carmel Beach and cozy beachfront homes, including a Frank Lloyd Wright house before ending at Carmel River State Beach.

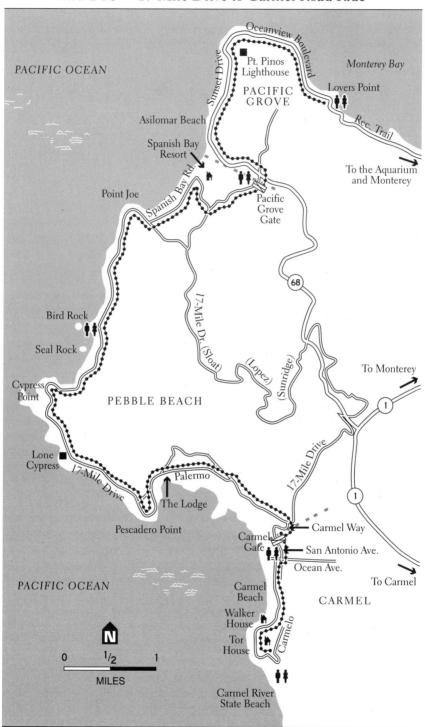

PACIFIC OCEAN

Oceanview Boulevard

Sunset Drive

Pt. Pinos Lighthouse

PACIFIC GROVE

Monterey Bay

Lovers Point

Asilomar Beach

Spanish Bay Resort

Rec. Trail

To the Aquarium and Monterey

Point Joe

Spanish Bay Rd.

Pacific Grove Gate

68

17-Mile Dr. (Sloat)

(Lopez)

(Sunridge)

Bird Rock

Seal Rock

To Monterey

1

Cypress Point

PEBBLE BEACH

Lone Cypress

17-Mile Drive

Palermo

The Lodge

17-Mile Drive

1

Pescadero Point

Carmel Way

Carmel Gate

San Antonio Ave.

Ocean Ave.

To Carmel

PACIFIC OCEAN

Carmel Beach

CARMEL

Walker House

Tor House

Carmelo

N

0   1/2   1

MILES

Carmel River State Beach

Enough talk of the high-priced real estate. The real draw to this ride is the wild, restless Pacific Ocean. The majority of the route closely follows the water's edge, past inviting beaches and rocky tidepools. As you ride along, imagine you're skirting the rim of the Grand Canyon. Lying a few miles west in the ocean is an enormously wide and deep canyon, dropping thousands of feet in some places. There are no man-made structures like off-shore oil-drilling rigs planted here. The view west is completely uninterrupted except by the ever present distant fog-bank. This is the pristine Monterey Bay National Marine Sanctuary, stretching from Rocky Point in Marin County in the north down to Cambria in San Luis Obispo County in the south. Blessed by nature with expansive kelp forests, hundreds of varieties of birds, fish, invertebrate species, and marine mammals live within these waters. Keep your eyes peeled because you may spot California seals and sea otters playing in the surf. Better yet, if you're riding between late October and January, or February and June, you might see the spray or the tail of a diving grey whale, migrating to or from the warmer waters off Mexico.

General location: About 85 miles south of San Jose.

Elevation change: Negligible when spread out over the entire 14.5-mile length; mostly near sea level between 0 to 150 feet.

Season: Year-round.

Services: Water and rest rooms at the trailhead at Lovers Point in Pacific Grove. Eateries and several small food stores in nearby Pacific Grove. The Pebble Beach Market next to the Lodge offers gourmet sandwiches to go and picnic fixings—it's favorite turnaround point for local riders. Several public rest room areas available (see map); some hotels and restaurants along the route graciously allow you to use their facilities.

Hazards: The greatest hazard is sharing the road with motor vehicles. This is an extremely popular auto route, especially in the summer. The bike route uses a combination of class 2 and class 3 roads (that is, painted bike lanes and shoulderless roads designated as a bike route, respectively). Numerous dirt pull-outs invite motorists to slow down, hesitate, and often stop. So, expect drivers to cut you off, pull out abruptly in front of you, and to open car doors into your path. Stay alert and give yourself safe distance from parked cars. Wear layers since the weather is often breezy and chilly, even during the summer.

Rescue index: The entire route is heavily traveled by motorists, bikers, skaters, and pedestrians and you're likely to find someone who can be of assistance. Residents, places of business, and a few pay phones are located on the route.

Land status: City streets through the cities of Pacific Grove and Carmel; public access roads through privately owned community of Pebble Beach.

Maps: Other than the map shown here, separate maps are published by the communities of Pacific Grove, Pebble Beach, and Carmel. When you enter Pebble Beach and pick up 17-Mile Drive at the Pacific Grove gate, you'll be required to sign a liability waiver. The back of the waiver has a map which shows part of this route. Ask the "ranger" manning the gate for a color brochure which contains a map of the entire 17-Mile Drive loop. For a map of Carmel, most road maps (Rand-McNally, AAA, etc.) will do.

Finding the trail: To reach the Monterey Peninsula from San Jose, drive south on US 101 to its intersection with the second CA 156 exit (to Monterey Peninsula), just north of Salinas. Head west on CA 156 for about 5 miles to Highway 1 (CA 1). CA 156 merges onto southbound Highway 1. Continue on Highway 1 through the towns of Marina, Sand City, and Seaside. Take the "Pacific Grove, Del Monte Avenue" exit, (it's the one after the CA 218/Del Rey Oaks exit and the Monterey Beach Hotel). The off-ramp drops down into a westbound lane of Del Monte Avenue. Follow Del Monte toward Fisherman's Wharf and the Monterey Bay Aquarium. As soon as you pass the main entrance to Fisherman's Wharf public parking lot, move into the right lane. Continue past the second Wharf entrance (next to Monterey Bay Urgent Care) and go through a tunnel. As you emerge from the tunnel, Del Monte becomes Lighthouse Avenue. Stay in the right lane and immediately follow Foam Street. Follow Foam to its end at a T intersection with David Street. Go right onto David and then a left onto Oceanview Boulevard (called Wave Street on your right.) This intersection is directly in front of the Monterey Bay Aquarium. Lovers Point is 1 mile from this intersection. Parking immediately next to Lovers Point is time-limited. You can find free, untimed parking up any number of side streets. Note: If you park in residential neighborhoods, be sure to check for street signs that may indicate "Residential Parking" which means if you don't live there, your time is limited typically to one hour. Rest rooms and a grassy park are located at Lovers Point. Begin your ride here.

Sources of additional information:

The Pacific Grove gate to Pebble Beach (for a map)
Near the intersection of Sunset Dr. and 17-Mile Dr.
Pebble Beach, CA 93953

Pacific Grove Recreation Department
515 Junipero Ave.

Pacific Grove, CA 93950
(831) 648-3130

Pacific Grove Chamber of Commerce
Forest and Central Ave.
Pacific Grove, CA 93950
(831) 373-3304

Notes on the trail: Consider bringing a bike lock, just in case you want to spend time on a sunny beach, explore Carmel for a bite to eat, or just plain explore.

Starting at Lovers Point in Pacific Grove, go west on Oceanview Boulevard, hugging rocky shoreline. Though there's a comfortably wide shoulder all the way around to Sunset Drive, watch out for sightseers pulling in and out of parking areas as well as onto the dirt shoulder of the road. When you pass Point Pinos Lighthouse sitting a short distance from the road on a slight hill, you're at the mouth of the bay and now approaching the open sea. Continue past Asilomar State Beach at about 2.7 miles. Sunset curves inland and begins a gentle, almost half-mile climb past several restaurants, a hotel, several storefronts and warehouses. At 3.5 miles, Sunset intersects 17-Mile Drive next to the Pebble Beach Market, a small convenience store. Turn right on to 17-Mile and in less than a half mile, you reach the Pacific Grove gate. Motorists are required to stop and pay an entry fee here. Since you're on your bike, you're allowed free entry but you must stop and sign the liability waiver. (You get to keep the yellow copy as a souvenir. Keep your copy because if you ride into Carmel via the Carmel gate, you may need to show it in order to re-enter Pebble Beach at that gate.) Before proceeding, ask the "ranger" at the gate for a color brochure of Pebble Beach—it contains a slightly more detailed map than the one on the back of your waiver.

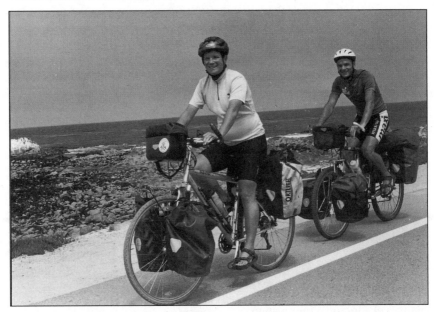

Due to an unexpected pregnancy, Emmanuelle and Dominique end their South America–to–Alaska cycling honeymoon on the 17-Mile Drive bike route into Carmel and then on down to Big Sur.

Proceed on 17-Mile Drive and about 0.7 mile from the gate, make a hard right onto Spanish Bay Road. (Don't miss this turn, even though a 17-Mile Drive sign points to the left. That direction will lead you up steep hills and into a convoluted network of residential streets.) Spanish Bay Road descends gradually toward the water and the ocean comes into view again. There are picnic tables here and the beach is inviting. At about 5.3 miles, Spanish Bay Road intersects another portion of 17-Mile Drive again. Bear right onto 17-Mile. As you approach Point Joe, power up a slight hill before curving south, still following the rugged coastline. This stretch leads you past the Monterey Peninsula Country Club and you're likely to see flocks of docile deer grazing on the golf courses. At 7 miles, Bird Rock appears, a huge rock outcropping about 100 yards from the shore. Take a guess why it's called Bird Rock. Public rest rooms and picnic tables are located at this turnoff to the Rock. Maybe you'll be lucky and miss sharing the site with a tourist bus of sightseers.

The next 2 miles to the Lone Cypress rolls up and down, weaving through the pine forest, passing magnificent mansions and Cypress Point Golf Course along the way. Stay alert for cars on this stretch, as the shoulder is practically non-existent. A half mile before the Lone Cypress, you have a clear view of the ocean again. Keep an eye peeled toward the ocean—you can actually see whales spouting during migration season.

From the Lone Cypress, continue following 17-Mile Drive around Pescadero Point and at 10.6 miles, bear right onto Cypress Drive to the Lodge. Welcome to the world-famous Pebble Beach Golf Course. Here you'll find plenty of boutiques with breathlessly priced items. Hungry? The Pebble Beach Market offers tasty gourmet sandwiches to go, café lattes, and other goodies as accompaniments. (How convenient that there's an ATM machine nearby.) Afterward, continue on Cypress Road and in about 0.2 mile, stay straight onto Palermo Way where Cypress turns right. Follow Palermo pass the tennis club and in about 0.3 mile, bear right onto Whitman Lane, staying on it for about 0.1 mile to it's intersection with 17-Mile Drive. Hang a right onto 17-Mile and watch out for traffic—the road is very narrow and there's no shoulder. In almost a mile since turning off Whitman, bear right onto Carmel Way and follow the curvy road toward the Carmel gate. Exit Pebble Beach via the manned gate and Carmel Way becomes San Antonio Avenue. This is Carmel-by-the-Sea (or simply Carmel).

Cruise through a neighborhood of quaint cottages and homes. In about 0.2 mile, you reach Ocean Avenue, the main street of town lined with upscale shops, eateries, and restaurants. Go right on Ocean for one block to Scenic Drive. (Ocean Avenue ends at Carmel Beach, a splendidly clean beach of white sand.) For the first several blocks, Scenic Drive is tightly lined on both sides by charming homes. The right side soon opens and the ocean and Carmel Beach comes into view once again. You'll undoubtedly think, "Wow, I'd sure like to have a house on this street." At the intersection of Scenic Drive and Martin Street is the Walker House, a stone dwelling designed and built by Frank Lloyd Wright in 1948. It sits on the beach side of Scenic Drive and was used in the 1959 film *A Summer Place*. Several blocks ahead is another architectural gem. Located on Ocean View Avenue between Scenic Drive and Stewart Way is Tor House, a medieval-looking stone dwelling and tower built by Irish-American poet Robinson Jeffers. Both places are privately occupied so please don't go peeking inside the windows. Continue following Scenic Drive around and at 14.5 miles, you reach Carmel River State Beach. This is my recommended turnaround point. On your return, consider checking out Carmel (I recommend locking up your bike and walking). When you've had your fill of this charming village, make your way back to the Carmel gate and retrace your route all the way back to Lovers Point. (I don't recommend riding the inland portion of 17-Mile Drive. Though there are signs posted, following the route is fairly convoluted as it twists, turns, and climbs through modest residential neighborhoods.) Seeing the spectacular Pacific shoreline in the opposite direction is guaranteed to be just as pleasing.

RIDE 99 · Old Coast Road

AT A GLANCE

Length/configuration: 10.6-mile point-to-point or 21.2-mile out-and-back or 19-mile loop, clockwise; dirt road (loop includes pavement)

Aerobic difficulty: Strenuous due to long gradual climb up several ridges

Technical difficulty: Mildly technical; all smooth dirt road with loose gravel on descending portions

Scenery: Old-growth redwoods, shady forest habitat along Bixby Creek, and grass-covered open hills. Some stretches offer expansive views of the Pacific Ocean and rolling hills and valleys.

Special comments: Suitable for strong beginners. This ride can be enjoyed as a short or long out-and-back, a point-to-point ride requiring a shuttle vehicle, or a loop. During the summer, public buses equipped with bike racks run along Highway 1, stopping at the north and south trailheads and two popular restaurants a few miles further south.

L ong before Bixby Bridge was constructed, the only way around the deep gap carved by Bixby Creek was an old dirt logging road. Today, the county road, referred to as Old Coast Road, is still well-traveled, mainly by residents who live in a handful of secluded, modest homes tucked within a few remaining old-growth redwood groves. This beautiful dirt road is anchored by Highway 1 (CA 1) at its north and south trailheads. Running 10.6 miles long, its condition is smooth, hard-packed dirt and wide enough for a single vehicle. It winds steeply up and down several ridges and ravines, and through redwood forests thick with lush understory, and over dry, open grassy hills. Occasional views of the Pacific Ocean and the rugged coastline are spectacular—just rewards for riders with strong endurance and climbing strength. Basic technical skills are all that's needed to enjoy this ride. Several climbs range from two to three miles while steepness is mostly 7% grade with a few steeper sections. Fortunately, the route is interspersed with gentle stretches and fun, long descents. All in all, Old Coast Road is quite a workout, especially if you ride it as a 21.2-mile out-and-back (10.6 miles each way). Of course, you can shorten it by turning around and going back whenever you're good and ready. On the other hand, you can lengthen your riding adventure by adding the Creamery-Ridge Ride in Andrew Molera State Park, located across the highway from the south trailhead (see Ride 100).

A marvel of engineering, graceful Bixby Bridge is one of the most photographed sites along the Pacific Coast Highway (CA 1). Numerous car commercials have been filmed here. After several years of construction, it was completed in October 1932, making it one of the largest single-arch concrete bridges in the world. Spanning a canyon over 100 feet in width, the central arch of Bixby is 320 feet long and 260 feet high. Though the bridge may appear to be simple and fragile when compared to massive cable and steel suspension bridges elsewhere, arch bridges remain one of the oldest forms of bridge that have tremendous natural strength. Supported by two abutments on both ends of the bridge, the weight of the Bixby Bridge arch itself—as well as crossing traffic—is distributed outward along the arch's curve. Every inch of the arch is subjected to great compression, deriving its stability from the pressure. One of the most famous examples of this phenomenon is the Pont du Gard aqueduct in southern France, built by the Romans before the birth of Christ. Constructed of enormous stone blocks, the towering structure is held together not by mortar but by the sheer force of its own weight.

General location: About 15 miles south of Monterey on Highway 1 (CA 1).

Elevation change: 1,000 feet change; starting elevation 100 feet; high point 900 feet; low point 50 feet. Several ridges make for long, moderately steep hills interspersed with mellow stretches.

Season: Year-round. Winter tends to be cool and wet. After a heavy rain, the road is likely to be muddy and road closure is a possibility.

Services: None on the dirt road. You can find a phone, pit toilets, water, and a maintained campground at Andrew Molera State Park, located at the south trailhead

RIDE 99 · Old Coast Road

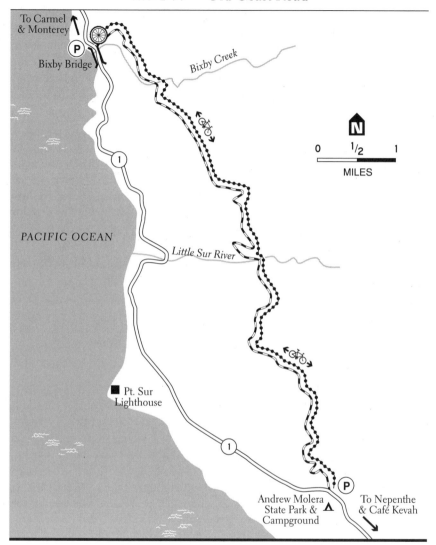

across Highway 1. Within 3 miles further south are several privately run campgrounds as well as eateries and tourist shops. Nepenthe and Café Kevah restaurants, both well-known Big Sur establishments, are both 7.5 miles south of the south trailhead. Between Memorial Day and Labor Day, public buses run twice daily between the north trailhead at Bixby Bridge and Nepenthe/Café Kevah.

Hazards: Old Coast Road is used by a handful of local residents as well as occasional sightseers. Unless the day is damp, expect traffic to kick up a fair amount of dust. When flying down long, curvy portions of the route, stay alert for on-coming vehicles and loose gravel. When you venture off the road to commune with nature, watch out for poison oak.

Rescue index: The road is easily accessible by passenger vehicles and you might get lucky with a sightseeing motorist who may be of help. If you need immediate emergency assistance, you may find someone at home in one of the few secluded residences along the route—but proceed at your own risk, for these folks like their privacy and not all residents have phones. Otherwise, make your way back down to Andrew Molera State Park located at the south trailhead and seek help or use the phone there. You can always attempt to flag down a passing motorist on Highway 1.

Land status: County road permitting public access; bounded by private property.

Maps: USGS Point Sur and Big Sur 7.5 minute series.

Finding the trail: From Monterey, follow Highway 1 (CA 1) south through Carmel. From Rio Road in Carmel, drive about 12.6 miles and go over Rocky Point Bridge, a small concrete arch bridge. Continue about a half mile further (13.4 miles from Rio Road) to Bixby Bridge, a bigger, more picturesque arch concrete structure. Immediately before the bridge, park in the dirt pulloff on the ocean side of the highway. This is a popular tourist spot overlooking the bridge. Directly across the highway is the beginning of Old Coast Road, a wide dirt road. Cautiously cross over to the other side of the highway and start pedaling up the dirt road, away from the ocean and bridge.

Sources of additional information:

Andrew Molera State Park
c/o Pfeiffer Big Sur State Park #1
Big Sur, CA 93920
(831) 667-2315 or (831) 649-2836

Monterey-Salinas Transit (MST)
One Ryan Ranch Rd.
Monterey, CA 93940

(831) 899-2555
www.mst.org

Big Sur Natural History Association
P.O. Box 189
Big Sur, CA 93920

Notes on the trail: Following Old Coast Road is a piece of cake. You can even ride without a map. Just stay on the main dirt road for the next 10.6 miles to its southern end at Highway 1. Creek crossings are facilitated by a bridge or culverts so you won't be getting your feet wet. All other lesser roads that intersect the main road lead to private property so don't even think about exploring them. You can start at either the north or south trailhead—at Bixby Bridge or Andrew Molera State Park, respectively. A point-to-point ride requires a shuttle arrangement, which is quick and easy to set up since the distance on Highway 1 between the two trailheads is 8.4 miles. The ride described below begins at Bixby Bridge.

From the bridge, the dirt road begins by leading up a gradual climb heading inland. The road hugs the slope with Bixby Creek flowing down below on your right. Soon, after about a mile, the road descends steeply into the drainage and small redwood groves begin casting a cool shade over the road. After crossing the creek, the road leads you up Sierra Grade. Along the way, tiny trickling tributaries follow you as it weaves to the left and right side of the road. The vegetation becomes thick with a variety of ferns, sorrel and other lush flora. Lovely clover meadows blanket edges of the creek and you might even feel the eyes of stealth leprechauns watching you.

At about 4 miles, as you emerge from the cover of the redwood forest, you reach the top of the first major climb. Coastal grassy hills spread out before you, and your effort is rewarded with the first sighting of the ocean since leaving Bixby Bridge. If the weather is cool, consider zipping up your jacket because the next 2.2 miles is a fast and fun downhill flight into the drainage of Little Sur River. You lose almost 1,000 feet. Milk it for all it's worth because after reaching the river, the road winds up another ridge. The next several miles are much drier and exposed. Along the way, watch out for motor vehicle—you're approaching popular Little Sur Trail trailhead (hiking-only). At about 6.6 miles, bypass the hiking trail and continue grinding up to the ridge. Level stretches give you some respite from the arduous climbing and at almost 8 miles, you finally reach the summit of the second ridge. Once again, you're rewarded by splendid views of the Pacific Ocean, the rugged coastline, Point Sur Lighthouse, and Highway 1. The remaining 2.6 miles to the south trailhead at Highway 1 is a sweet descent and you can really pick up speed. As you fly down this stretch, expect loose gravel, especially as you round the curves.

You reach Highway 1 at 10.6 miles, across the highway from Andrew Molera State Park. If you're riding this route as a point-to-point, your end-shuttle vehicle should be parked here at the dirt pulloff across from the state park entrance. If not, you can return to your car at Bixby Bridge in one of three ways. Option 1: Return the way you came on Old Coast Road, making the total round-trip out-and-back 21.2 miles. This is the most scenic and safest option. Option 2: Make a loop by taking Highway 1 north back up to Bixby Bridge. Riding Highway 1, however, means you have to share the road with often unfriendly and unaware motorists for 8.4 miles while climbing up a few long grades on narrow and sometimes non-existent shoulders. Option 3: Wait for the Monterey-Salinas Transportation (MST) bus to come along and give you a lift. Both trailheads are bus stops for the MST bus. The only catch is that the bus runs only twice a day during the summer. The bus stops generally around 12:30 p.m. and 4:30 p.m., fare is about $2, and exact change required. (Before committing to this plan, call MST for current information.) If you miss the first bus, you can kill time by riding the trails in Molera State Park (see the next trail description) or hanging out at Nepenthe/Café Kevah, which is the end of the line for the bus. To reach Nepenthe/Café Kevah, pedal south on Highway 1 for 7.5 miles. Expect to ride up several arduously steep stretches while hugging the narrow shoulder. If the day is sunny and warm, reward yourself with lunch at Café Kevah. It's a great place—the food is reasonably priced, creative and tasty, and their only seating is on a huge outdoor deck overlooking the Pacific.

RIDE 100 · Andrew Molera: Creamery-Ridge Ride

AT A GLANCE

Length/configuration: 7.3-mile round-trip (a loop with an out-and-back); single- and double-tracks

Aerobic difficulty: Moderately strenuous (the loop is easy; the out-and-back climbs considerably)

Technical difficulty: Intermediate (the loop is mildly technical due to the narrow single-track bordered by lots of poison oak; the steepness of the out-and-back challenges you to stay on your bike)

Scenery: Spectacular panoramic view of the Big Sur coastline

Special comments: Due to the amount of poison oak along narrow stretches, the flat, easy loop is not recommended for young children. See the optional Cooper Cabin Trail at the end of this description for another easy out-and-back.

Though the bike trails in Andrew Molera State Park are short and are generally out-and-backs, at least mountain biking is allowed here. Other nearby state parks within the Big Sur area is off-limits to bikes and much of the property on both sides of CA 1 (fondly referred to as Highway 1), is fiercely private. Alas, this state park is the best opportunity we mountain bikers have to pedal legendary Big Sur, where the greatest meeting of land and sea is anything but subtle.

The Creamery-Ridge Trails are a combination loop and out-and-back, measuring 7.3 miles total, round-trip. The Creamery Loop is about 1.7 miles, easy, flat, non-technical, and suitable for beginners who have no trouble staying on narrow single-track (or else suffer the consequences of poison oak). The Ridge Trail out-and-back is 2.8 miles one-way (5.6 miles round-trip), rated moderately strenuous due to several steep climbs. Technically, the Ridge Trail requires intermediate bike handling skills since the challenge is staying on the bike and not popping wheelies while grunting and groaning up the steep but brief terrain, about 11% grade in some stretches. Gaining over 1,200 feet in just over 2 miles, the reward is the spectacular panoramic view of the Big Sur coastline.

General location: 22 miles south of Carmel along CA 1.

Elevation change: 1,200 feet gain and loss. Starting elevation and low point: near sea level; high point 1,100 feet. Several long hills with some very steep but brief sections on the outbound.

Season: Year-round, depending on the water level of Big Sur River.

Services: Drinking water, walk-in campground, and pit toilets available in the park. Day-use fee (about $3) required. Gas, quaint restaurants, small grocery stores, public phones, and boutiques nearby, within 4-7 miles south of the park on CA 1. All other major services, including medical help can be found in Carmel and Monterey, 22 miles north.

Hazards: Watch out for poison oak. There's of lots of it, everywhere, even entwined in shoulder-level bushes. Encounters with bobcats and rattlesnakes are possible though infrequent; mountain lions and wild pigs are rarely seen. If you ride between winter and early spring, foot bridges that cross Big Sur River will not be in place. Wading through the river is possible, though you need to gauge the depth and swiftness. If you venture down to the beach, stay alert for deadly sleeper waves. Do not, repeat, do not take them for granted, even the little gentle waves. Each year, many people are literally swept away, off rocks and beaches, and carried out to sea.

Rescue index: During the summer months, the park is extremely popular—you're apt to meet other people enjoying the trails. That said, getting help from other trail users is likely. Park use during the week and in the off-season is reduced so in case of emergency, you should make your way back to the main park entrance instead of waiting for someone to come along.

RIDE 100 · Andrew Molera: Creamery-Ridge Ride

Land status: Andrew Molera State Park.

Maps: Adequate map and general information about the park available for 50¢ at the park entry booth, published in cooperation by California Department of Parks and Recreation. USGS Big Sur 7.5 minute series.

Finding the trail: From the intersection of Rio Road in Carmel, drive 22 miles south on CA 1. The park entrance is immediately on the right. Enter, pay the day use fee and park in the big dirt lot.

Sources of additional information:

California Department of Parks and
    Recreation
P.O. Box 942896
Sacramento, CA 94296-0001

Big Sur Natural History Association
P.O. Box 189
Big Sur, CA 93920

Andrew Molera State Park
c/o Pfeiffer Big Sur State Park #1
Big Sur, CA 93920
(831) 667-2315 or (831) 649-2836

Notes on the trail: Trails are fairly well-marked in the field and all trails are shown on the park map. The Creamery Loop is a bit ambiguous in that it's labeled as such on the map but not in the field. That said, begin by finding the trailhead that leads over Big Sur River, sort of directly across the parking lot from the entry kiosk. If the seasonal bridge is not in place, find a shallow section and wade through the river, about 30 feet wide. (You may have to abort your ride if the water is too high or swift.) Continue on the hard-packed dirt single-track trail through a narrow stretch, bounded on both sides by tall grass and bushes. Try not to brush up against the bushes, as poison oak is everywhere. A few yards after crossing the river, you reach a signed fork. Take the fork, signed "Beach Trail" with an arrow pointing to the right single-track. The trail leads you through a flat meadow. The trail is basically wide, mostly hardpack with some small semi-buried boulders, thin spots of loose sand, and occasional potholes. If you're riding in the spring, you can expect portions of this trail to be overgrown in some places with tall grass. Trail maintenance is not year-round, so watch out for poison oak encroaching on the trail.

At about 0.8 mile, you reach another trail at a signed junction. The trail to the right leads to the mouth of the river and ultimately the ocean. Go left, instead, onto the Ridge Trail. From here, look left and you can see your challenge: a portion of the Ridge Trail as it climbs steeply up an exposed slope. Take a deep gulp and say a sincere "Thank you!" that you have 21 gears. Pedal a few yards on single- and double-track to the next signed fork. Though the left fork is unsigned, the right one is signed Ridge Trail. Bear right and begin climbing a steep (about 7% grade), wide single-track. The terrain may be rutted and the angle will test your ability to stay on your bike. For the next 2.7 miles to the high- and turnaround point, the trail varies from 1–5 feet wide, from single- to double-track, and climbs over 1,200 feet. The first mile on the Ridge Trail climbs steeply, about 8% to 11%, mercifully interspersed with a few flatter stretches and a couple of short descents. Most of the terrain is exposed, covered by coastal scrub plants, and spectacular views of the ocean quickly emerge on your right. On your left, the tall mountain ridges obstruct your view and Pico Blanco, a gray-white barren peak watches over you.

After a welcomed but short descent, bypass Hidden Trail leading off on your left (no bikes allowed), about 2.1 miles from the parking lot. From this intersection, the steepness of Ridge Trail may appear daunting but once you begin pedaling the incline, you'll discover that it's not as steep and arduous as the initial climbs. Around 2.6 miles, as you round the inland side of a small mound, the ocean is obscured from view, blocked by tall and thick vegetation. Look left and down and you can see Highway 1, snaking along the foot of the eastern mountain range. (If you're riding in the spring, your huffing and puffing up Ridge Trail is likely to be rewarded with clumps of purple wild irises, bright red indian paintbrush, golden poppies, wild lilac bushes, and tiny wild flowers.) After a short distance, glimpses of the ocean appear and at 2.9 miles, bypass South Boundary Trail. Continue following Ridge Trail. Go through a shady forest populated by strikingly snarly live oak trees. A bit further and you begin cruising through a stand of young-growth redwood trees. You reach the end of Ridge Trail with a final, short climb to the park's south boundary. There's a comfortable wooden bench here, perfectly positioned to view the crashing waves of the Pacific far below you. The trail leading downhill toward the ocean is Panorama Trail and, unfortunately, bikes are not allowed. Take a snack break and drink in the view before heading back down the way you came.

Flying downhill on the return is a scream and makes the climb all worthwhile. The Big Sur coastline is in fairly constant view all the way down. At 6.4 miles, you reach the intersection with Bluff Trail. (Bikes are allowed on this easy 1.5-mile out-and-back, 3.0-mile round-trip, and it's worthy of a side trip if you have time). Bypass Bluff Trail, staying straight on the Ridge Trail. The next intersection is in a few yards, at about 6.5 miles. Does this spot look familiar? This is where the tough bikers separated from the less adventurous ones. Say good-bye to Ridge Trail by hanging a sharp right here, almost like a hairpin right turn. You're now back on the Creamery Loop. Follow this flat trail as it skirts the meadow on your left. The trail width varies from narrow to wide single-track interspersed with brief double-track. At about 7.2 miles, follow a trail on your right signed "Parking Lot." (A few yards straight ahead and on the right is River Trail, another short out-and-back trail that's open to bikes.) Follow another "Parking Lot" sign at the next junction and a few yards further, you close the loop at the junction with Beach Trail. Bear right and proceed across Big Sur River, finishing at the parking lot at 7.4 miles.

Optional easy trail: The Cooper Cabin and Trail Camp Trail. This trail is located on the north side of Big Sur River. It's a 1-mile out-and-back (2 miles round-trip) trail and is a combination single-track and fire road. This easy trail is opened to bikes and leads out to Molera Point and the Headlands Trail (no bikes allowed). The short walk on the headlands offers a spectacular view of the Big Sur coastline and beach, and is a great place to watch the semi-annual whale migration, from October to January and February to July. Oh yes, the sunsets can be awesome here, too.

OTHER AREA RIDES

COAST RIDGE ROAD: Like the Old Coast Road (described earlier in this chapter), the Coast Ridge Road is one of the few bikeable routes in Los Padres National Forest. This 27.2-mile out-and-back maintained dirt road (13.6 miles one way) skirts the southwest edge of the Ventana Wilderness and offers some of the best views of the Big Sur coastline. The bikeable portion of the Coast Ridge Road starts behind Ventana Inn and climbs roughly 3,000 feet in 13.6 miles to the turnaround point at the Anderson Peak southwest ridge. The journey leads you through four gates and past Deangulo and Cold Springs Road (Big Sur Trail) before reaching Anderson Peak. (Past the peak, the road continues a short distance, bounded by private property as it enters the wilderness where bikes are not permitted.)

Finding the trailhead: From Carmel and the intersection of Carmel Valley Road and Highway 1, drive about 27 miles south on Highway 1 to the celebrated Ventana Inn. Turn left (inland) to the inn and continue about 260 yards from the highway. On your right, there's a public parking area for day-users. Do not park higher up at the inn or restaurant. Hop on your bike and follow the paved road east for about 0.1 mile. The road makes an abrupt left turn at a fork and climbs past the restaurant. Proceed straight ahead from the fork and go through a gate. This is the beginning of the Coast Ridge Road. Note: you may encounter signs or irate homeowners declaring the road to be off-limits, citing private property. Truth is, the Coast Ridge Road is maintained by the forest service (with our tax dollars) as a fire road and is considered a public easement. Just remember that you must turn around at Anderson Peak, which essentially marks the wilderness boundary.

Maps: USGS Partington Ridge 7.5 minute series.

For more information, contact:

Los Padres National Forest
Monterey Ranger District
406 South Mildred Ave.
King City, CA 93930
(831) 385-5434

ARROYO SECO–INDIANS ROAD TO MEMORIAL PARK: Enjoy this oddity while you can. Wilderness areas are off-limits to mountain bikes. However, this 16 mile stretch of graded dirt road (32 miles round trip) located in the Ventana Wilderness is an exception (and a phone call to the Monterey District Ranger office confirmed it). Arroyo Seco–Indians Road cuts through the Wilderness and the Santa Lucia mountain range in the northernmost section of the Los Padres National Forest. Indeed, both sides of the road are wilderness-designated land and bikers are required to stay on the road; trails leading off the road are strictly prohibited. The road is actually a county road that was in place before the wilderness was created. Currently managed by the forest service, foul weather since 1995 has resulted in landslides, washouts, and other damage which has forced the road's closure to motorized vehicles and motorbikes. Lucky for us, use by hikers, equestrians, and mountain bikers is still permitted year-round, at least as of January 2000. The local chapter of the Sierra Club is pushing for full compliance of the wilderness area, which means mountain bikes would be prohibited. Technically mild to intermediately rated, this 16-mile stretch offers westward views of the Ventana Wilderness. The dirt road begins at Arroyo Seca Recreation Area, runs through Escondido Campground at 14 miles, and basically ends at the Indians Memorial and Campground at 16 miles, the turnaround point. Pavement resumes beyond this point. Wet weather often produces a few muddy sections, but the rock-based road is generally rideable. The stretch between Escondido and Memorial is especiallly popular in the sommer where beach access to the Arroyo Seco River is enjoyed. As the name implies, the area was inhabited by the Costanoans and Essalen Indians. In the vicinity of the Memorial is the Indians Guard Station, a restored cabin originally built in 1929 by the Civilian Conservation Corps. (Thanks to my friend Ted Walters, who calls this ride his favorite mountain bike trail in all of Monterey County. After you've ridden it, visit his creative little restaurant, Passionfish, in nearby Pacific Grove and tell him what you think.)

Finding the trail: From Carmel, drive east by southeast on Carmel Valley Road County Road G 16) about 40 miles to Arroyo Seco Road (also known as Jamesburg Road). Go right (south) on Arroyo Seco and follow the paved road about 4 miles into the Los Padres National Forest and Arroyo Seco Recreation Area (a campground). There the paved road ends at a locked gate and becomes a the dirt road which you'll be pedaling. Expect to pay a day-use fee to park here. From the town of Soledad on US 101, head west by southwest on Arroyo Seco Road for about 20 miles to the junction with Carmel Valley Road. Continue as directed above, heading south to the Arroyo Seco Recreation Area.

Maps: USGS Junipero Serra Peak 7.5 minute series.

For more information, contact:

Los Padres National Forest
Monterey District Ranger
406 South Mildred Ave.
King City, CA 93930
(831) 385-5434

SOME LOCAL BICYCLE SHOPS

Sports Center Bicycles
1576 Del Monte Blvd.
Seaside, CA 93955
(831) 899-1300

Aquarian Bicycles
486 Washington St.
Monterey, CA 93940
(831) 375-2144

Joselyn's Bicycles
398 E. Franklin St.
Monterey, CA 93940
(831) 649-8520

Adventures-By-The-Sea
299 Cannery Row
Monterey, CA 93940
(831) 372-1807
(Bike and kayak rentals)

Bay Bike Rentals
Cannery Row
640 Wave St.
Monterey, CA 93940
(831) 646-9090

Bay Bike Rentals
Fisherman's Wharf
99 Pacific St., Suite 255-C
Monterey, CA 93940
(831) 655-8687

Winning Wheels
223 15th St.
Pacific Grove, CA 93950
(831) 375-4322

Carmel Bicycle
7150 Carmel Valley Rd.
Carmel, CA 93923
(831) 625-2211

Bobcat Bicycles
141 Monterey St.
Salinas, CA 93901
(831) 753-7433

Bear Bikes
1288 N. Main St.
Salinas, CA 93906
(831) 444-8460

Salinas Bicycle & Fitness
315 West Market
Salinas, CA 93901
(831) 424-1723

APPENDIX

DOES YOUR BICYCLE FIT?

Proper bicycle fit makes all the difference. Finding the right equipment means getting a bicycle that truly conforms to your body and not the other way around. Fine-tuning the geometry of the bicycle to complement the rider, is equally important to men as it is to women. It can be the start of a great, lifelong love affair with this healthy activity or be as short as a fling. I think too many people, especially women, give up on cycling much too quickly because he or she just didn't feel comfortable on a bike. I submit that if the bicycle were properly adjusted to their body, they would be one with their bike and enjoy many glorious miles together. But how do you figure out the right fit?

Whether you're shopping for a new set of wheels or already have one, your first task is to find a dedicated bicycle dealer—a dealer with a truly knowledgeable and caring staff. I won't go into all the nuances of how to fit a bike to your physique—that's a role for you and your bike dealer—but I will give you a couple of tips.

Most bicycles, by default, are built to fit the average man. Women are built differently than men: women generally have longer legs and shorter torsos while men are the opposite, though men are generally taller. Of the bicycles on the market today, most women have no trouble finding one that fits their leg length. They can even find a bicycle that gives them the required three- to five-inches of clearance between crotch and top tube. But here's the kicker: A frequent problem with women is the reach, that is, the distance between the saddle and the handlebars. Since most bikes are built with a man's longer torso in mind, many women (and some men, too) find themselves over-extended on most bikes. If left uncorrected, excruciating neck and shoulder pain may develop. As a result, the rider does one of three things: 1) endures the discomfort and pain, which eventually leads to 2) gives up on bicycling altogether, or 3) spends the time to figure out the problem and fixes it. The fact is, having a comfortable reach between saddle and handlebar is just as important as stand-over comfort and safety.

Tip 1: The reach can be corrected by replacing the handlebar stem with a suitably shorter one. The saddle can also be adjusted forward slightly but then, the alignment of the knee to the spindle (the pedal and its axle) becomes a concern. A good bike dealer should address both of these issues in your quest for an overall proper fit. (If your dealer pulls out a plumb line to measure your knee-to-spindle alignment, congratulations, you're in a seriously dedicated shop.) Women, for more bike fit advice, check out "Bike Fit a la Wombat," an insightful article at www.wombat.org. Also check out www.terrybicycles.com.

Tip 2: After many miles and numerous hours of riding, you'll inevitably feel better in a "stretched out" position. Don't be surprised if you find yourself wanting a slightly longer stem or want to scoot the saddle back—your body is gradually becoming comfortable and "one" with the bike. So, expect to continue to fine-tune your bike throughout many miles of riding. Eventually, you and your bike will fit like a hand in glove.

Tip 3: Saddles are often a sore subject for both men and women but they needn't be. Many innovative saddles have been designed with anatomically sensitive areas in mind. There are extra padded and wide seats, gel saddles and some with holes positioned for crucial spots. Georgena Terry pioneered the first women's saddle with cutaway holes. Terry saddles for both men and women have since become a name synonymous with exceptionally comfortable seats. Learn about saddle design at www. terrybicycles.com.

Tip 4: If you're a petite rider with short legs like me (26-inch inseam), you'll have trouble finding a mountain bike with the proper leg length. Several bicycle manufacturers (Trek, Cannondale, GT Bikes, as well as Terry) have been building bikes with innovative frames that accommodate the smaller rider. For extremely short riders, bicycles with 14-inch frames or smaller and 24-inch wheels may be your only option. Though these small bikes may look like a "kid bike," many reputable manufacturers are recognizing the petite adult market. There are small mountain bikes out there that use high quality components and materials and are constructed to withstand adult weight and more aggressive riding styles.

BASIC SPECIFICATIONS OF MY MOUNTAIN BIKE

Manufacturer: Terry Precision Cycling
Model: Jarcaranda
Tires: 24" tires
Speed: 21-speed
Front fork suspension: Anti-Gravity
Front and back derailleurs: Shimano Deore LX
Chainrings: 48/38/28

Regrettably, the Jarcaranda is no longer manufactured. Terry has replaced it with Flora, the only mountain bike in the Terry line. The Flora is available in these frame sizes: 11" and 14" (24" wheels); 16" and 18" (26" wheels). Though this 28-speed bike is considered a hybrid by some, the Flora is capable of much more rugged terrain. To make her a mud-and-obstacle-loving bike, change her tame tires to more knobby ones and add a front suspension fork or suspension stem.

For more information, contact:

Terry Precision Cycling
1704 Wayneport Rd.
Macedon, NY 14502
(800) 289-8379
talktous@terrybicycles.com

GLOSSARY

This short list of terms does not contain all the words used by mountain bike enthusiasts when discussing their sport. But it should serve as an introduction to the lingo you'll hear on the trails.

ATB — all-terrain bike; this, like "fat-tire bike," is another name for a mountain bike

ATV — all-terrain vehicle; this usually refers to the loud, fume-spewing three- or four-wheeled motorized vehicles you will not enjoy meeting on the trail—except, of course, if you crash and have to hitch a ride out on one

blaze — a mark on a tree made by chipping away a piece of the bark, usually done to designate a trail; such trails are sometimes described as "blazed"

blind corner — a curve in the road or trail that conceals bikers, hikers, equestrians, and other traffic

blowdown — see "windfall"

BLM — Bureau of Land Management, an agency of the federal government

bollard — a post (or series of posts) set vertically into the ground that allow pedestrians or cyclists to pass but keep vehicles from entering (wooden bollards are also commonly used to sign intersections)

braided — a braided trail condition results when people attempt to travel around a wet area; networks of interlaced trails can result and are a maintenance headache for trail crews

buffed — used to describe a very smooth trail

Carsonite sign — a small, thin, and flexible fiberglass signpost used extensively by the Forest Service and BLM to mark roads and trails (often dark brown in color)

catching air — taking a jump in such a way that both wheels of the bike are off the ground at the same time

cattle guard	a grate of parallel steel bars or pipes set at ground level and suspended over a ditch; cows can't cross them (their little feet slip through the openings between the pipes), but pedestrians and vehicles can pass over cattle guards with little difficulty
clean	while this may describe what you and your bike won't be after following many trails, the term is most often used as a verb to denote the action of pedaling a tough section of trail successfully
combination	this type of route may combine two or more configurations; for example, a point-to-point route may integrate a scenic loop or an out-and-back spur midway through the ride; likewise, an out-and-back may have a loop at its farthest point (this configuration looks like a cherry with a stem attached; the stem is the out-and-back, the fruit is the terminus loop); or a loop route may have multiple out-and-back spurs and/or loops to the side; mileage for a combination route is for the total distance to complete the ride
cupped	a concave trail; higher on the sides than in the middle; often caused by motorcycles
dab	touching the ground with a foot or hand
deadfall	a tangled mass of fallen trees or branches
decomposed granite	an excellent, fine- to medium-grain, trail and road surface; typically used in native surface road and trail applications (not trucked in); results from the weathering of granite
diversion ditch	a usually narrow, shallow ditch dug across or around a trail; funneling the water in this manner keeps it from destroying the trail
double-track	the dual tracks made by a jeep or other vehicle, with grass, weeds, or rocks between; mountain bikers can ride in either of the tracks, but you will find that whichever one you choose, no matter how many times you change back and forth, the other track will appear to offer smoother travel
dugway	a steep, unpaved, switchbacked descent
endo	flipping end over end
feathering	using a light touch on the brake lever, hitting it lightly many times rather than very hard or locking the brake
four-wheel-drive	this refers to any vehicle with drive-wheel capability on all four wheels (a jeep, for instance, has four-wheel drive as compared with a two-wheel-drive passenger car), or to a rough road or trail that requires four-wheel-drive capability (or a one-wheel-drive mountain bike!) to negotiate it
game trail	the usually narrow trail made by deer, elk, or other game

gated	everyone knows what a gate is, and how many variations exist on this theme; well, if a trail is described as "gated" it simply has a gate across it; don't forget that the rule is if you find a gate closed, close it behind you; if you find one open, leave it that way
Giardia	shorthand for *Giardia lamblia,* and known as the "back-packer's bane" until we mountain bikers expropriated it; a waterborne parasite that begins its life cycle when swallowed, and one to four weeks later has its host (you) bloated, vomiting, shivering with chills, and living in the bathroom; the disease can be avoided by "treating" (purifying) the water you acquire along the trail (see "Hitting the Trail" in the Introduction)
gnarly	a term thankfully used less and less these days, it refers to tough trails
graded	refers to a dirt road that has been smoothed out by the use of a wide blade on earth-moving equipment; "blading" gets rid of the teeth-chattering, much-cursed washboards found on so many dirt roads after heavy vehicle use
hammer	to ride very hard
hammerhead	one who rides hard and fast
hardpack	a trail in which the dirt surface is packed down hard; such trails make for good and fast riding, and very painful landings; bikers most often use "hardpack" as both a noun and adjective, and "hard-packed" as an adjective only (the grammar lesson will help you when diagramming sentences in camp)
hike-a-bike	what you do when the road or trail becomes too steep or rough to remain in the saddle
jeep road, jeep trail	a rough road or trail passable only with four-wheel-drive capability (or a horse or mountain bike)
kamikaze	while this once referred primarily to those Japanese fliers who quaffed a glass of sake, then flew off as human bombs in suicide missions against U.S. naval vessels, it has more recently been applied to the idiot mountain bikers who, far less honorably, scream down hiking trails, endangering the physical and mental safety of the walking, biking, and equestrian traffic they meet; deck guns were necessary to stop the Japanese kamikaze pilots, but a bike pump or walking staff in the spokes is sufficient for the current-day kamikazes who threaten to get us all kicked off the trails
loop	this route configuration is characterized by riding from the designated trailhead to a distant point, then returning to the

trailhead via a different route (or simply continuing on the same in a circle route) without doubling back; you always move forward across new terrain but return to the starting point when finished; mileage is for the entire loop from the trailhead back to trailhead

multipurpose a BLM designation of land that is open to many uses; mountain biking is allowed

off-camber a trail that slopes in the opposite direction than one would prefer for safety's sake; for example, on a side-cut trail the slope is away from the hill—the inside of the trail is higher, so it helps you fall downhill if your balance isn't perfect

ORV/OHV a motorized off-road vehicle (off-highway vehicle)

out-and-back a ride where you will return on the same trail you pedaled out; while this might sound far more boring than a loop route, many trails look very different when pedaled in the opposite direction

pack stock horses, mules, llamas, etc., carrying provisions along trails

point-to-point a vehicle shuttle (or similar assistance) is required for this type of route, which is ridden from the designated trailhead to a distant location, or endpoint, where the route ends; total mileage is for the one-way trip from the trailhead to endpoint

portage to carry your bike on your person

pummy soil with high pumice content produced by volcanic activity in the Pacific Northwest and elsewhere; light in consistency and easily pedaled; trails with such soil often become thick with dust

quads bikers use this term to refer both to the extensor muscle in the front of the thigh (which is separated into four parts) and to USGS maps; the expression "Nice quads!" refers always to the former, however, except in those instances when the speaker is an engineer

runoff rainwater or snowmelt

scree an accumulation of loose stones or rocky debris lying on a slope or at the base of a hill or cliff

side-cut trail a trail cut on the side of a hill

signed a "signed" trail has signs in place of blazes

single-track a single, narrow path through grass or brush or over rocky terrain, often created by deer, elk, or backpackers; single-track riding is some of the best fun around

skid road the path created when loggers drag trees through the forest with heavy equipment

slickrock	the rock-hard, compacted sandstone that is great to ride and even prettier to look at; you'll appreciate it even more if you think of it as a petrified sand dune or seabed (which it is), and if the rider before you hasn't left tire marks (from unnecessary skidding) or granola bar wrappers behind
snowmelt	runoff produced by the melting of snow
snowpack	unmelted snow accumulated over weeks or months of winter—or over years—in high-mountain terrain
spur	a road or trail that intersects the main trail you're following
squid	one who skids
stair-step climb	a climb punctuated by a series of level or near-level sections
switchback	a zigzagging road or trail designed to assist in traversing steep terrain; mountain bikers should not skid through switchbacks
talus	the rocky debris at the base of a cliff, or a slope formed by an accumulation of this rocky debris
tank trap	a steep-sided ditch (or series of ditches) used to block access to a road or trail; often used in conjunction with high mounds of excavated material
technical	terrain that is difficult to ride due not to its grade (steepness) but to its obstacles—rocks, roots, logs, ledges, loose soil.
topo	short for topographical map, the kind that shows both linear distance and elevation gain and loss; "topo" is pronounced with both vowels long
trashed	a trail that has been destroyed (same term used no matter what has destroyed it . . . cattle, horses, or even mountain bikers riding when the ground was too wet)
trialsin	highly technical riding over natural and artificial obstacles at low speeds, with points assessed for putting down a foot, or "dab" (to complete a section without dabbing it is to "clean" it)
two-track	see "double-track"
two-wheel-drive	this refers to any vehicle with drive-wheel capability on only two wheels (a passenger car, for instance, has two-wheel drive); a two-wheel-drive road is a road or trail easily traveled by an ordinary car
waterbar	an earth, rock, or wooden structure that funnels water off trails to reduce erosion
washboarded	a road that is surfaced with many ridges spaced closely together, like the ripples on a washboard; these make for very rough riding, and even worse driving in a car or jeep

whoop-de-doo   closely spaced dips or undulations in a trail; these are often
                    encountered in areas traveled heavily by ORVs

wilderness area   land that is officially set aside by the federal government to
                    remain natural—pure, pristine, and untrammeled by any ve-
                    hicle, including mountain bikes; though mountain bikes had
                    not been born in 1964 (when the United States Congress
                    passed the Wilderness Act, establishing the National
                    Wilderness Preservation system), they are considered a "form
                    of mechanical transport" and are thereby excluded; in short,
                    stay out

windchill   a reference to the wind's cooling effect on exposed flesh; for
                    example, if the temperature is 10 degrees Fahrenheit and the
                    wind is blowing at 20 miles per hour, the windchill (that is,
                    the actual temperature to which your skin reacts) is minus 32
                    degrees; if you are riding in wet conditions things are even
                    worse, for the windchill would then be minus 74 degrees!

windfall   anything (trees, limbs, brush, fellow bikers . . .) blown down
                    by the wind

INDEX

Abbreviations, road designations, 3
Academy of Sciences, San Francisco, 423, 427
Aerobic level ratings, *xv. See also* specific rides
Alpine Meadows Road, Western States Trail, 223, 224
American River, Western Sierras, 142–63
American River Bike Path, Folsom Lake State Recreation Area, Western Sierras, 142–46
Andrew Molera State Park, Monterey Peninsula, 525–29
Angel Island State Park, North Bay, 379–84
Angora Lakes Out-and-Back, El Dorado National Forest, Lake Tahoe Area, 241–44
Annadel State Park Loops, Wine Country, 131–37
Ansel Adams Wilderness, Eastern Sierras, 322
Anthony Chabot Regional Park, East Bay, 372
Aptos Creek Fire Trail, Forest of Nisene Marks State Park, 480–85
Arcata Community Forest, North Coast, 24–28
Around Lake Tahoe, 199–277
Arroyo Seco Recreation Area, Los Padres National Forest, Monterey Peninsula, 530–31
Asian Art Museum, San Francisco, 423, 427
Auburn State Recreation Area, Western Sierras, 151–63
Auburn-to-Cool Trail (ACT), Olmstead Loop, 151–55

Avenue of the Giants Road Ride, Humboldt Redwoods State Park, North Coast, 20–24

Baccharis Trail, East-West Ridge Loop, 366
Backdoor Trail, Backside Loop at Northstar, 211
Back Ranch Fire Trail, China Camp State Park, 416
Backside Loop at Northstar, Lake Tahoe Area, 208–12
Bald Hills Road, Lost Man Creek-Holter Ridge Bike Trail, 35, 38
Bald Mountain Loop at Sugarloaf Ridge State Park, Wine Country, 138–39
Baldwin Estate, Pope Baldwin Bike Path, 245
Barnabe Peak, Samuel P. Taylor Park, North Bay, 400–405
Barry's Trail, Boggs Mountain Demonstration Forest, 122
Bay View Trail, China Camp State Park, 415, 416
Beach Cruiser Trail, Mammoth Mountain Bike Park, 320, 323
Beach Trail, Andrew Molera State Park, 528
Bear Basin Butte Lookout, Smith River National Recreation Area, North Coast, 54–55
Bear Bones Trail, Boggs Mountain Demonstration Forest, 122–23
Bear Creek Trail, Briones Crest Loop, 355
Bear Trap Basin, Stanislaus National Forest, Western Sierras, 196
Belgum Trail, Wildcat Canyon Regional Park, 361–62

Berry Creek Falls, Big Basin Redwoods State Park, 465, 468

Bicycle Trails Council Of the East Bay (BTCEB), 374

Big Basin Redwoods State Park, South Bay, 459–68

Big Boulder Trail Loop, Tahoe National Forest, Western Sierras, 169–73

Big Meadows, El Dorado National Forest, Lake Tahoe Area, 261–73

Big Ring, Mammoth Mountain Bike Park, 324–27

Big Springs Trail, Backside Loop at Northstar, 211–12

Big Springs Trail, Boggs Mountain Demonstration Forest, 122–23

Big Sur, 490–532

Big Trees Trail, Joaquin Miller Park, 374

Bike compatibility, 533–34

Bill's Trail, Samuel P. Taylor Park, 404

Bison Paddock, San Francisco, 423, 426

Bizz Johnson Trail, Lassen National Forest, Shasta Cascade, 91

Black Diamond Mines Loop, East Bay, 346–51

Black Mountain Trail, Monte Bello-Stevens Creek Loop, 448

Black Point, Mono Tufa State Reserve, Eastern Sierras, 286–91

Blithedale Ridge Road, Mt. Tamalpais State Park, 395

Bluff Trail, Andrew Molera State Park, 529

Bobcat Trail, Tennessee Valley Double Loop, 390

Bodie Historic State Park, Eastern Sierras, 331

Boggs Mountain Demonstration Forest, Wine Country, 119–24

Bolinas Ridge Fire Road, Golden Gate National Recreation Area, North Bay, 396–400

Bonhoff Trail, Joseph D. Grant Park, 488

Boondock Trail, Backside Loop at Northstar, 211

Boulder Creek Loop, Whiskeytown–Shasta–Trinity National Recreation Area, Shasta Cascade, 69–72

Boy Scout Tree Trail, Howland Hill, 48

Breeze, Joe, 377, 391, 406

Brewery Gulch Road, Van Damme State Park, 106

Briceberg Loops, Western Sierras, 195–96

Bridle Trail, East-West Ridge Loop, 366

Briones Crest Loop, Briones Regional Park, East Bay, 351–56

Briones-to-Mount Diablo Trail, Shell Ridge Recreational Area, 344, 345

Brockway Summit, Tahoe Rim Trail, 221

Bruce Lee Trail, Mount Diablo State Park, 340–41

Brunswick Canyon Ride, Lake Tahoe Area, 278–79

Buckeye Ravine Trail, Shell Ridge, 345

Buker Ridge Loop, Klamath National Forest, Shasta Cascade, 90

Bullards Bar Loop, Tahoe National Forest, Western Sierras, 177–80

Burnside Lake Out-and-Back, Toiyabe National Forest, Lake Tahoe Area, 247–51

Burton Creek State Park, Lake Tahoe Area, 212–17

Cal-Ida Road, North Yuba River Trail, 187

California Coastal Trail, Monterey Peninsula, 509

California Trail, Arcata Community Forest, 27, 28

Camp Reynolds, Angel Island, 381, 383

Canada de Pala Trail, Joseph D. Grant Park, 488

Cannery Row, Monterey Recreation Trail, 508, 513–14

Canyon Creek, Klamath National Forest, Shasta Cascade, 90

Canyon Loop Trail, Pacheco State Park, 457, 458

Canyon Trail, Annadel State Park Loops, 135–36, 137

Canyon Trail, East-West Ridge Loop, 366

Canyon Trail, Long Ridge Open Space Preserve, 486

Canyon Trail, Monte Bello-Stevens Creek Loop, 447

Carmel, Monterey Peninsula, 516–21

Carruthers Cove Trail, Ossagon–Gold Bluff Loop, 32, 33–34

Carson Ridge, Lake Tahoe Area, 249

Carson River Ride, Lake Tahoe Area, 278–79

Carson Valley, Lake Tahoe Area, 253, 261, 268, 276

Cascade Canyon Trail, North Bay, 405–11

Caspar Creek–640-630 Loop, Jackson Demonstration State Forest, Mendocino Coast, 99–101

Castle Peak, Lake Tahoe Area, 200–205

Cathedral Road, Fallen Leaf Lake Easy Loop, 239, 240–41

Cell phones, 9

Chabot Observatory, East-West Ridge Loop, 367

Chalk Mountain, Big Basin Redwoods State Park, 459–64

Charity Valley, Lake Tahoe Area, 247

Charlie's Trail, Boggs Mountain Demonstration Forest, 123

Chimney, Whiskeytown–Shasta–Trinity National Recreation Area, Shasta Cascade, 76–79

Chimney Rock Trail, Tahoe National Forest, Western Sierras, 180–83

Chimney Sierra Trail, Sly Park Recreation Area, 168

China Camp State Park, North Bay, 411–16

China Grade, Big Basin Redwoods State Park, 459, 464

China Hole Trail, Henry W. Coe State Park, 453

Chinquapin Trail, Wilder Ranch State Park, 476

Christmas Valley Trail, TRT: Big Meadows to Round Lake, 269–73

Cinder Cone Loop, Tahoe National Forest, Lake Tahoe Area, 212–17

Cinderella Trail, Joaquin Miller Park, 374

Clear Creek Vista Trail, El Dorado Mine Loop, 83–89

Clikapudi Trail, Shasta–Trinity National Forest, Shasta Cascade, 62–65

Climbing rides, xix

Coal Creek Open Space Preserve, West Bay, 441–42

Coastal Trail, North Coast Last Chance Section, 38–44

Ossagon–Gold Bluff Loop, 32, 33–34

Coast Ridge Road, Los Padres National Forest, Monterey Peninsula, 530

Combination rides, 3

Community Forest Loop Road (11), Arcata Community Forest, 28

Comptche–Ukiah Road, Van Damme State Park, 106

Conservatory of Flower, San Francisco, 423, 427

Contra Loma Trail, Black Diamond Mines Loop, 350–51

Cooper Cabin Trail, Monterey Peninsula, 529

Corcoran Mine Trail, Black Diamond Mines Loop, 350, 351

Cougar Ridge Trail, Toro Park, 496

Cougar Trail, Henry W. Coe State Park, 453

Cow Mountain Recreation Area, Mendocino Coast, 115

Coyote Ridge Trail, Tennessee Valley Double Loop, 384–90

Coyote Springs Trail, Toro Park, 496

Coyote Trail, Backside Loop at Northstar, 211

Crater Flats, Inyo Craters Loop, 302

Crazy Pete's Trail, Coal Creek Open Space Preserve, 442

Creamery Loop, Andrew Molera State Park, 525–29

Creekside Trail, Backside Loop at Northstar, 212

Creek Trail, Boggs Mountain Demonstration Forest, 123–24

Crest Trail, Briones Crest Loop, 355

Cryptosporidiosis prevention, 8

Cultural Preserve, Wilder Ranch State Park, 474

Culvert Trail, Stagecoach–Lake Clementine Loop, 163

Curran Trail, Tilden Regional Park, 362

Damnation Creek Trail, Coastal Trail– Last Chance Section, 43

Dardanelles Lake, Lake Tahoe Area, 270, 272

Darrington Trail, Salmon Falls Out-and-Back, 151

Deadman Creek Road, Inyo Craters Loop, 302

Dead Man's Elbow, Lower Ice Box Loop, 82

Deadmans Pass, Inyo National Forest, Eastern Sierras, 331–32

Deer Flat Road, Mount Diablo State Park, 338

Deer Mountain, Eastern Sierras, 300

Del Norte Coast Redwoods State Park, North Coast, 29, 38–44

Devil's Gulch, Samuel P. Taylor Park, North Bay, 400–405

Devil's Pulpit, East Bay, 340

Dirt Road rides, xix

Divide Trails (1st, 2nd and 3rd), Big Boulder Trail Loop, 173

Dollar Point Trail, Tahoe City Bike Paths, 229–34

Donner Canyon Trail, Mount Diablo State Park, 340

Donner Pass Road, Hole-In-The-Ground Trail, 200

Donner Ski Ranch Mountain Bike Park, Lake Tahoe Area, 218

Donner Summit, Lake Tahoe Area, 200

Downieville, CA, Western Sierras, 169–70

Drunken Bear Trail, Paige Meadows Ride, 225, 228

Drury Parkway, Ossagon–Gold Bluff Loop, 28–34

Dun Trail, East-West Ridge Loop, 366

Eagle Mountain Cross-Country Ski Area and Mountain Bike Park, Lake Tahoe Area, 217–18

Earthquake Fault, Mountain View, 315–19, 323

Earthquake Walk, Bolinas Ridge, 398

East Bay Area, 334–76

East Bay Skyline Trail, Wildcat Canyon Regional Park, 361–62

Eastern Sierras, 281–333

East Ridge Trail, Redwood Regional Park, East Bay, 362–67

Easy rides, xviii

Easy Shade Rest Ride, Inyo National Forest, Eastern Sierras, 304–7

Echo Lift, Backside Loop at Northstar, 211, 212

Eel River, Avenue of the Giants Road Ride, 23–24

Ehrman Mansion, Lake Tahoe Area, 233, 235, 238

8-Ball Trail, Bullards Bar Loop, 178

El Capitan, Eastern Sierras, 283, 286

El Corte de Madera Creek Open Space Preserve, West Bay, 435–39

El Dorado Mine Loop, Whiskeytown–Shasta–Trinity Recreation Area, Shasta Valley, 83–89

El Dorado National Forest, Lake Tahoe Area, 238–44, 261–73, 279–80

Eldridge Grade, Mt. Tamalpais State Park, 390–95

Elk Camp Ridge Trail, Gasquet Toll Road, 48–53

Elk Prairie, Prairie Creek Redwoods State Park, 28–34

Emerald Lake, Lake Tahoe Area, 242

Empire Creek Trail, Chimney Rock Trail, 183

Enderts Beach Overlook, Coastal Trail–Last Chance Section, 39

Engelman Loop Trail, Wilder Ranch State Park, 477

Engineer Canyon Road, Fort Ord Public Lands, 506–7

Epic rides, xix

Etiquette, trail, 5–7

Eucalyptus Loop Trail, Wilder Ranch State Park, 476–77

Eucalyptus Road, Fort Ord Public Lands, 507

Fallen Leaf Lake Easy Loop, El Dorado National Forest, Lake Tahoe Area, 238–41

Family rides, xviii

Feather Falls Out-and-Back, Plumas National Forest, Western Sierras, 194

Fern Canyon Bike Path, Mendocino Coast
Russian Gulch State Park, 106–10
Van Damme State Park, 102–6

Fern Canyon Trail, Ossagon–Gold Bluff Loop, 34

Fiddle Creek Trail, North Yuba River Trail, 183–87

Fireboard Trail, TRT

(Tahoe Rim Trail), 223

Fire Iron Road, Mt. Tamalpais State Park, 395

Fire road rides, *xix*

First-aid kit, 9

Fir Trail, El Corte de Madera Open Space Preserve, 438

Fisher, Gary, 391, 406

Fisherman's Wharf, Monterey Recreation Trail, 508, 514

Flat Frog Trail, Henry W. Coe State Park, 452

Follow Me Trail, Mammoth Mountain Bike Park, 327

Folly Trail, Backside Loop at Northstar, 211

Folsom Lake State Recreation Area, Western Sierras, 142–51

Foothill Pine Trail, Joseph D. Grant Park, 488

Forest City, CA, Western Sierras, 187–93

Forest City Trail Council (FCTC), 188–89

Forest History Trail, Manly Gulch Loop, 98

Forest of Nisene Marks State Park, South Bay, 480–85

Forsyth, Greg, 220–21, 226

Fort Bragg, CA, Mendocino Coast, 94

Fort McDowell, Angel Island, 381, 384

Fort Ord Public Lands, Monterey Peninsula
Goat Trail, 497–502
Guidotti Road, 497–502
Mudhen Lake, 503–8
Rim Trail Ramble, 503–8

Fort Point, San Francisco, 421, 425

Fort Point Mine Depot, San Francisco, 427

Fountain Place Road, TRT: Big Meadows to Kingsbury Grade, 267

Freel Meadows, Lake Tahoe Area, 266, 267

Fremont Older Open Space Preserve, South Bay, 487

Friendship Trail, Ossagon–Gold Bluff Loop, 33

Gasquet Toll Road, Smith River National Recreation Area, North Coast, 48–53

Gazos Creek, Big Basin Redwoods State Park, 459–64

General Creek Easy Loop, Sugar Pine Point State Park, Lake Tahoe Area, 234–38

Geological landscape rides, *xviii*

Gerbode Valley, North Bay, 385

Giardiasis prevention, 8

Ginger Gap Trail, Shell Ridge Recreational Area, 344

Glory Hole Recreation Area, Western Sierras, 194–95

Goat Trail, Toro Park, 502

Gold Bluffs, Prairie Creek Redwoods State Park, North Coast, 28–34

Golden Falls Cascade, Big Basin Redwoods State Park, 465, 468

Golden Gate Bridge, West Bay, 421–28

Golden Gate National Recreation Area, 384–90, 396–400

Golden Gate Raptor Observatory (GGRO), North Bay, 385

Gold Rush Country of the Western Sierras, 141–98

Gold Valley Road, Big Boulder Trail Loop, 172

Gong, Bob, 445

Goodyears Bar, North Yuba River Trail, 186

Graham Trail, East-West Ridge Loop, 366

Granite Chief Wilderness, Lake Tahoe Area, 226

Grasshopper Peak Loop, Humboldt Redwoods State Park, North Coast, 12–16

Gravy Train Trail, Mammoth Mountain Bike Park, 323

Gray Pine Trail, Bald Mountain Loop, 138

Great Water Ditch Trail, Whiskeytown–Shasta National Recreation Area, Shasta Valley, 83–89

Grizzley Trail, Bogg's Mountain Demonstration Forest, 122

Grizzly Flat Trail, Long Ridge Open Space Preserve, 486

Grizzly Flat Trail, South Bay, 447

Grover Hot Springs, Lake Tahoe Area, 247, 250–51

Gunsight Peak, Klamath National Forest, Shasta Cascade, 90–91

Half Dome, Eastern Sierras, 282, 286

Halls Ranch Trail, North Yuba River Trail, 183–87

Happy Camp Campground Rides, Six Rivers National Forest, North Coast, 55–56

Harkins Ridge Trail, Purisima Creek Redwoods Open Space Preserve, 433–34

Hart, Keith, 273–74

Hartley Springs Loop, Inyo National Forest, Eastern Sierras, 294–99

Haunted Deer Forest, El Dorado Mine Loop, 83, 88

Hawkins Peak, Lake Tahoe Area, 247, 250

Henness Pass Road, Forest City's Pliocene–Sandusky Loop, 191–93

Henry Cowell Redwoods State Park, South Bay, 468–72

Henry Creek Trail, Big Basin Redwoods State Park, 463

Henry W. Coe State Park, South Bay, 448–53

High Country of the Eastern Sierras, 281–333

High Point Trail, Boggs Mountain Demonstration Forest, 123

Hobbs Road, Henry W. Coe State Park, 452–53

Hobergs Loop Trail, Boggs Mountain Demonstration Forest, 122

Hole-In-The-Ground, Tahoe National Forest, Lake Tahoe Area, 200–205

Holter Ridge Bike Trail, Redwood National and State Parks, North Coast, 34–38

Homestead Valley Trail, Briones Crest Loop, 355–56

Hope Creek Ten Taypo Trail, Ossagon–Gold Bluff Loop, 32

Horse Canyon/Silver Lake Loop, Lake Tahoe Area, 279–80

Horseshoe Lake Loop, Inyo National Forest, Eastern Sierras, 311–14

Hot Creek Hatchery Road, Inyo National Forest, Eastern Sierras, 327–30

Hotel Trail, Joseph D. Grant Park, 488

Hot Springs, Inyo State Forest, Eastern Sierras, 327–30

Houghton, Ray, 95, 99

Howland Hill, Jedediah Smith Redwoods State Park, North Coast, 44–48

Humboldt Redwoods State Park, North Coast, 12–24

Humbug Creek Loop, Klamath National Forest, Shasta Cascade, 90–91

Humbug Trail, South Yuba Primitive Camp Loop, 177

Indian Creek Trail, Monte Bello–Stevens Creek Loop, 444, 447–48

Indians Memorial, Los Padres National Forest, Monterey Peninsula, 530–31

International Mountain Bicycling Association (IMBA), Rules of the Trail, 5–6

Inyo Craters Loop, Inyo National Forest, Eastern Sierras, 299–303

Inyo National Forest, Eastern Sierras, 294–330, 331–33

Jackson State Demonstration Forest, Mendocino Coast, 94–101, 114

Jack's Road, Fort Ord Public Lands, 506, 507

Jammer Chair Flat, Sardine Valley Loop, 208

Janes Creek Trail (7), Arcata Community Forest, 28

Japanese Tea Garden, San Francisco, 423, 427

Jaynes Lane, Bullards Bar Loop, 178

Jedediah Smith National Recreation Area, Western Sierras, 142

Jedediah Smith Redwoods State Park, North Coast, 29, 44–48

Jelmini Basin, Stanislaus National Forest, Western Sierras, 196

Jenkinson Lake Loop, Sly Park Recreation Area, Western Sierras, 164–69

Jethro's Trail, Boggs Mountain Demonstration Forest, 121, 122

Joaquin Miller Park, East Bay, 374–75

Johansen Road, Big Basin Redwoods State Park, 462, 463

John Muir Wilderness, Eastern Sierras, 304, 310, 312, 314, 322

Jones, David, 464
Joseph D. Grant Park, South Bay, 488–89
June Lake, Eastern Sierras, 298

Kamikaze Downhill (race), Mammoth Mountain Bike Park, 323
Karen's Trail, Boggs Mountain Demonstration Forest, 122
Kingsbury Grade, El Dorado National Forest, Lake Tahoe Area, 261–69
Kings Range National Conservation Area, North Coast, 16
Kirkwood Resort, Lake Tahoe Area, 218–19
Klamath National Forest, North Coast, 55, 90–91
Knolls Loop, Inyo National Forest, Eastern Sierras, 307–11

Lady Bird Johnson Grove, North Coast, 38
Lafayette–Moraga Trail, East Bay, 368–71
Laguna Point, MacKerricher Ten Mile Coastal Trail, 110–13
Lake Clementine Loop, Auburn State Recreation Area, Western Sierras, 159–63
Lake Cleone, Mackerricher Ten Mile Coastal Trail, 110–13
Lake Ilsanjo, Annadel State Park Loops, 131–37
Lake Natoma, American River Bike Path, 146
Lake Shasta, Shasta Cascade, 62–68
Lake Tahoe Area, 199–277
Lands End Park, San Francisco, 425
Lassen National Forest, Shasta Cascade, 91
Last Chance Section, Coastal Trail, 38–44
Lava Beds National Monument, Shasta Cascade, 93
Lavezzola Road, Big Boulder Trail Loop, 173
Ledson Marsh, Annadel State Park Loops, 131–37
Letts Lake Recreation Area, Mendocino Coast, 116
Level ratings
  aerobic, xv
  technical skills, xv–xvi

Lexington County Park, South Bay, 487–88
Link Trail, Backside Loop at Northstar, 211
Little Alkali Lake, Eastern Sierras, 330
Little Bald Hills Road, Howland Hill, 48
Little Lake Road, Manly Gulch Loop, 96
Little Mt. Hoffman Lookout, Medicine Lake Highlands, Shasta Cascade, 92–93
Little River, Mendocino Coast, 102–6
Long Meadow Trail, Wilder Ranch State Park, 476
Long Ridge Open Space Preserve, South Bay, 486
Lookout Lift, Backside Loop at Northstar, 211, 212
Look Prairie Road, Peavine Road Loop, 18, 19
Loop rides, 3
Loop Trail, Tilden Regional Park, 360
Los Huecos Trail, Joseph D. Grant Park, 488
Los Padres National Forest, Monterey Peninsula, 530–31
Lost Man Creek, Redwood National and State Parks, North Coast, 34–38
Lovers Point, Monterey Recreation Trail, 509, 513
Lower Ice Box Loop, Whiskeytown–Shasta–Trinity National Recreation Area, Shasta Cascade, 79–83
Lower Lola Montez Trail, Hole-In-The-Ground Trail, 204
Lower Loop, Angel Island, 379–84
Lower Oil Canyon Trail, Black Diamond Mines Loop, 350
Lower Rock Creek Trail, Inyo National State Forest, Eastern Sierras, 322

MacKerricher Ten Mile Coastal Trail, MacKerricher State Park, Mendocino Coast, 110–13
Mac's Trail, Boggs Mountain Demonstration Forest, 122
Malakoff Diggins State Historic Park, Western Sierras, 173–77
Mammoth Mountain, Eastern Sierras, 299, 302, 303

Mammoth Mountain Bike Park, Inyo State Forest, Eastern Sierras, 319–27

Mammoth Mountain Bike Park, Lake Tahoe Area, 219

Mammoth Scenic Loop, Inyo Craters Loop, 303

Manly Gulch Loop, Jackson Demonstration State Forest, Mendocino Coast, 95–99

Manzanita Point Road, Henry W. Coe State Park, 453

Manzanita Trail, El Corte de Madera Open Space Preserve, 438

Manzanita Trail, Stagecoach–Lake Clementine Loop, 160, 162

Maps, 3, 4–5

Marincello–Bobcat Trails, Tennessee Valley Double Loop, 384–90

Marin County, North Bay, 377–419

Markleeville Peak, Lake Tahoe Area, 247, 250

Marlette Lake, Lake Tahoe Area, 255–61

Marlin Headlands, San Francisco, 421–28

Marsh Trail, Annadel State Park Loops, 136, 137

Marysville Road, Bullards Bar Loop, 178

Mattole Road
 Avenue of the Giants Road Ride, 20–24
 Grasshopper Peak Loop, 12–16
 Peavine Road Loop, 17–20

Maurer, Julie, 206

Mayacmas Mountains, Mendocino Coast, 115

McCurdy Trail, Bolinas Ridge Fire Trail, 400

McNee Ranch State Park, West Bay, 440–41

Meadow Canyon Trail, Tilden Regional Park, 362

Medicine Lake Highlands, Little Mt. Hoffman Lookout, 92–93

Mendocino Coast, 94–117

Merced River, Eastern Sierras, 282, 285

Meridian Ridge Road, Mount Diablo State Park, 340

Methuselah Trail, El Corte de Madera Open Space Preserve, 438

Meyers Trail, Toro Park, 494

Mezue Trail, Wildcat Canyon Regional Park, 362

M.H. de Young Museum, San Francisco, 421–23, 427

Middle Ridge Road, Big Basin Redwoods State Park, 462, 463, 464

Middle Ridge Trail, Henry W. Coe State Park, 448–53

Middle Steve's S Trail, Annadel State Park Loops, 135

Middle Trail, Mount Diablo State Park, 340

Midpeninsula Regional Open Space District (MROSD), 420, 435, 441–42

Mill Creek Trail, El Dorado Mine Loop, 88

Mill Creek Trail, Howland Hill–Stout Grove, 48

Minaret Summit Vista, Eastern Sierras, 315, 323, 331, 332

Miner Ridge Loop, Letts Lake Recreation Area, 116

Miners Trail, Black Diamond Mines Loop, 350

Mirror Lake, Eastern Sierras, 282, 286

Mission Peak Regional Preserve, East Bay, 372–73

Missouri Bar Trail, South Yuba Primitive Camp Loop, 176–77

Mitchell Canyon Loop, Mount Diablo State Park, 335–41

Miwok Fire Trail, China Camp State Park, 414

Miwok Nature Trail, Sly Park Recreation Area, 168

Miwok Trail, Tennessee Valley Double Loop, 389

Modoc National Forest, Shasta Cascade, 92–93

Mokelumne Wilderness, 196, 247

Mono Lake Tufa State Reserve, Eastern Sierras, 286–94

Montara Mountain, West Bay, 440–41

Monte Bello Open Space Preserve, South Bay, 444–48

Monterey Bay Aquarium, Monterey Recreation Trail, 508, 513

Monterey Bay National Marine Sanctuary, Monterey Recreation Trail, 508

Monterey Peninsula and Big Sur, 490–532

Monterey Recreation Trail, Monterey Peninsula, 508–16

Monument Trail, Henry W. Coe State Park, 452

Moraga Trail, East Bay, 368–71

Mormon Emigrant Trail, Sly Park Recreation Area, 164, 169

Morrison Planetarium, San Francisco, 423, 427

Moss Rock Ridge, Mount Diablo State Park, 339

Mountain House Road, North Yuba River Trail, 186

Mountain View, Inyo National Forest, Eastern Sierras, 315–19

Mountainview Trail, Mammoth Mountain Bike Park, 323

Mountain View Trail, Pacheco State Park, 458

Mount Diablo State Park, East Bay, 335–45

Mount Tamalpais (Mt. Tam), North Bay, 390–95

Mr. Toad's Wild Ride, TRT: Big Meadows to Kingsbury Grade, 266, 267

Mt. Shasta Mine Loop, Whiskeytown–Shasta–Trinity National Recreation Area, Shasta Cascade, 72–76

Mt. St. Helena North Peak, Robert Louis Stevenson State Park, Wine Country, 124–27

Mt. Tam (MountTamalpais), North Bay, 390–95

Mt. Tam North Side Loop, North Bay, 417

Napa Valley, Wine Country, 118, 124–31

National Off-Road Biking Association (NORBA), Code of Ethics, 6

Nature Trail, Wilder Ranch State Park, 479–80

Navarro Ridge Road, Mendocino Coast, 114–15

Navy Beach, Eastern Sierras, 294

Negit Island, Eastern Sierras, 287

New Luther Pass Road, TRT: Big Meadows to Round Lake, 272

New Melones Lake, Glory Hole Recreation Area, 194–95

Nike Missile Site, Angel Island, 381, 383, 384

Nimbus Dam, American River Bike Path, 142, 146

Nimitz Way, Wildcat Canyon Regional Park, 362

North Bay Area–Marin County, 377–419

North Bloomfield, Ca, Western Sierras, 174

North Canyon Trail, Flume–TRT Ride, 255–61

North Coast, 11–56

North Escape Road, Big Basin Redwoods State Park, 459, 464

North Loop, Tennessee Valley Double Loop, 384–90

North Peak Trail, Mount Diablo State Park, 339–40

North Ridge Trail, Purisima Creek Redwoods Open Space Preserve, 433–34

Northstar-at-Tahoe, Lake Tahoe Area, 208–12

North Tahoe Regional Park, Lake Tahoe Area, 219

North Trail, Russian Gulch State Park, 109–10

North Yuba River Trail, Tahoe National Forest, Western Sierras, 183–87

Nortonville Trail, Black Diamond Mines Loop, 351

Noyo River, Mendocino Coast, 110–13

Oak Ridge Trail, China Camp State Park, 416

Oak Tree Trail, Pleasanton Ridge National Park, 373

Oat Hill Mine Road, Wine Country, 127–31

Obsidian Dome, Eastern Sierras, 294, 295, 298

Off The Top–Mammoth Mountain Bike Park, Inyo State Forest, Eatern Sierras, 319–23

Old Cabin Trail, Wilder Ranch State Park, 477

Old Camptonville Road, Bullards Bar Loop, 179

Old Coast Road, Monterey Peninsula, 521–25

Old Haul Road. *See* MacKerricher Ten Mile Coastal Trail

Old Luther Pass Road, TRT: Big Meadows to Round Lake, 273

Old Railroad Grade, Mt. Tamalpais State Park, 390–95

Old Reservation Road, Fort Ord Public Lands, 506, 508

Old Springs Trail, Tennessee Valley Double Loop, 385, 390

Old Town Sacramento, Western Sierras, 142–43

Ollason Peak, Toro Park, 491–97

Olmstead Loop, Auburn State Recreation Area, Western Sierras, 151–55

Onofrio Gulch, Mt. Shasta Mine Loop, 72–76

Ossagon Trail, Prairie Creek Redwoods State Park, North Coast, 28–34

Out-and-back rides, 4

Pacheco State Park, South Bay, 453–58

Pacific Crest Trail, TRT: Big Meadows to Round Lake, 270, 272

Paige Bar Road, Mt. Shasta Mine Loop, 72–76

Paige Meadows Ride, Tahoe National Forest, 224–29

Painted Rock, Lake Tahoe Area, 216, 221, 223

Palace of Legion of Honor, San Francisco, 421, 425

Pala Seca Trail, Joseph D. Grant Park, 488

Palisades, Wine Country, 130–31

Panum Crater, Eastern Sierras, 292, 294

Paoho Island, Eastern Sierras, 287

Paper Route Trail, Mammoth Mountain Bike Park, Eastern Sierras, 324–27

Patrick Creek Road, Gasquet Toll Road, 48–53

Peacock Gap Trail, China Camp State Park, 416

Peavine Road Loop, Humboldt Redwoods State Park, North Coast, 17–20

Pebble Beach, Monterey Peninsula, 516–21

Perimeter Road Loop, Angel Island, 379–84

Peters Creek Loop Trail, Long Ridge Open Space Preserve, 486

Phoenix Lake, Mt. Tamalpais State Park, 395

Pickett Peak, Lake Tahoe Area, 247, 249

Pierson Cabin, Bear Basin Butte Lookout, 54

Pig Pond Trail, Pacheco State Park, 456–57, 458

Pine Creek Trail, Shell Ridge Recreational Area, 345

Pine Mountain, North Bay, 405–11

Pine Nut Cracker (race), 273–74

Pine Nut Mountain Loops, Lake Tahoe Area, 273–77

Pioneer Trail, TRT: Big Meadows to Kingsbury Grade, 263, 269

Pipeline Road, Henry Cowell Redwoods State Park, 471–72

Pleasanton Ridge Regional Park, East Bay, 373–74

Pliocene Ridge, Tahoe National Forest, Western Sierras, 187–93

Plumas National Forest, Western Sierras, 194

Point Reyes National Seashore, North Bay, 396–400, 417–18

Point-to-point rides, 4

Pole Line Road, Peavine Road Loop, 20

Pony Peak Ride, Klamath National Forest, North Coast, 55

Pope Baldwin Bike Path, Lake Tahoe Area, 245–46

Pope Estate, Pope Baldwin Bike Path, 245

Poverty Flat Road, Henry W. Coe State Park, 453

Powder Mills Fire Road, Henry Cowell Redwoods State Park, 471, 472

Powerline Fire Trail, China Camp State Park, 415

Prairie Creek Overlook, Lost Man Creek–Holter Ridge Bike Trail, 35

Prairie Creek Redwoods State Park, North Coast, 28–34

Presidio, San Francisco, 421, 424

Prospector Gap Road, Mount Diablo State Park, 340

Prospect Tunnel Trail, Black Diamond
    Mines Loop, 350
Pudding Creek, MacKerricher Ten Mile
    Coastal Trail, 110–13
Purisima Creek Redwoods Open Space
    Preserve, West Bay, 430–34
Pygmy Forest, Mendocino Coast, 102–6

Quarry Road Out-and-Back, Auburn State
    Recreation Area, Western Sierras,
    155–59

Rails-To-Trails Conservancy
    Bizz Johnson Trail, 91
    Lafayette–Moraga Trail, 368–71
    Rams Ride, Shasta–Trinity National
        Forest, Shasta Cascade, 90
Rancho del Oso Nature and History
    Center, South Bay, 465
Ranch Trail, Toro Park, 494
Randall Trail, Bolinas Ridge Fire Road,
    400
Ravine Peak Out-and-Back, Lake Tahoe
    Area, 278
Rawhide Trail, Paige Meadows
    Ride, 228, 229
Rebel Ridge Trail, Bullards Bar Loop,
    178, 179
Red House Flume Trail, Flume–TRT
    Ride, 260
Red Oak OHV Trail, Chimney Rock
    Trail, 183
Redrock Ridge Trail, Fort Ord Public
    Lands, 501
Redwood Creek Overlook, Lost Man
    Creek–Holter Ridge Bike Trail, 38
Redwood National and State Parks, North
    Coast, 28–48
Redwood Regional Park, East Bay,
    362–67
Repack (race), 377–79
Repack Road, Pine Mountain, 405–11
Resolution Trail, El Corte de Madera
    Open Space Preserve, 438
Ride recommendations, *xviii–xix*
Ridge Fire Road, Henry Cowell
    Redwoods State Park, 471, 472
Ridge Fire Trail, China Camp State Park,
    416

Ridgeline Trail, Pleasanton Ridge
    National Park, 373
Ridge Road, Arcata Community Forest,
    25, 28
Ridge Trail
    Andrew Molera State Park, Monterey
        Peninsula, 525–29
    Annadel State Park Loops, Wine
        Country, 136
    Black Diamond Mines Loop, East Bay,
        349–51
    Russian Ridge, West Bay, 442
    Samuel P. Taylor Park, North Bay,
        400–405
Rim Trail, South Yuba Primitive Camp
    Loop, 176
Rincon Fire Road, Henry Cowell
    Redwoods State Park, 471, 472
Ritter Range, Eastern Sierras, 281, 332
River Trail, Andrew Molera State Park,
    529
Road designation abbreviations, 3
Roaring Camp & Big Trees Railroad,
    Henry Cowell Redwoods State Park,
    469, 471
Robert Louis Stevenson State Park, Wine
    Country, 124–27
Rock Creek Lake Ride, Inyo National
    State Forest, Eastern Sierras, 332
Rockefeller Forest, North Coast, 23, 24
Rockville Hills Park, Wine Country,
    139–40
Rough Go Trail, Annadel State Park
    Loops, 135, 137
Round Lake, El Dorado National Forest,
    Lake Tahoe Area, 269–73
Ruby Bluff Overlook, Western Sierras,
    187, 191, 192
Russian Gulch State Park, Mendocino
    Coast, 106–10
Russian Ridge, West Bay, 441–42
Rusty's Trail, Paige Meadows Ride, 228

Saddleback Road, Chimney Rock Trail,
    181
Salmon Falls Out-and-Back, Folsom Lake
    State Recreation Area, Western Sierras,
    147–51

Samuel P. Taylor State Park, North Bay, 400–402

San Andreas Fault Line, 396–98, 444–45, 448

San Andreas Lake, West Bay, 428–30

San Carlos Beach Park, Monterey Recreation Trail, 513, 514

Sand Harbor Overlook, Flume–TRT Ride, 261

Sand Point Overlook, Forest of Nisene Marks State Park, 480–85

Sand Ridge Lake, Hole-In-The-Ground, 204

Sandusky Loop, Tahoe National Forest, Western Sierras, 187–93

San Francisco Bay, West Bay, 421–28

San Francisco Zoo, San Francisco, 423, 426

San Geronimo Ridge Road, Pine Mountain, 410

San Joaquin Valley, East Bay, 340

San Pablo Ridge Trail, Wildcat Canyon Regional Park, 361–62

Santa Cruz County, 443–89

Saratoga Gap Trail, South Bay, 486

Sardine Valley Loop, Tahoe National Forest, Lake Tahoe Area, 205–8

Sargent Cypress Forest, North Bay, 410

Sawyer Camp Trail, Golden Gate National Recreation Area, West Bay, 428–30

Saxon Creek Trail, TRT: Big Meadows To Kingsbury Grade, 266

Scenic rides, xviii–xix

Schotzko, David, 201, 203

Sea Otter Classic (race), 498, 501

Seaside/Del Monte Beach, Monterey Recreation Trail, 508, 515

Sequoia Bay View Trail, Joaquin Miller Park, 374

7-Ball Trail, Bullards Bar Loop, 178, 179

17-Mile Drive, Monterey Peninsula, 516–21

Shakespeare Garden, San Francisco, 423, 427

Shasta Bally Road, Whiskeytown–Shasta–Trinity Recreation Area Chimney, 76–79

    Upper and Lower Ice Box Loop, 79–83

Shasta Cascade, 57–93

Shasta–Trinity National Forest, Shasta Cascade, 62–90, 92–93

Shell Ridge Recreation Area, East Bay, 341–45

Shoreline Trail, China Camp State Park, 414–15

Shuman, John, 76, 80, 85

Sierra Azul Open Space Preserve, South Bay, 487–88

Sierra Nevadas, 141–98

Signal Peak, North Coast, 53

Silver Falls, Big Basin Redwoods State Park, 465, 468

Silver Lake Loop, Lake Tahoe Area, 279–80

Sinbad Creek Trail, Pleasanton Ridge National Park, 373

Single-track rides, xviii

Siskiyou Wilderness, North Coast, 53

Six Rivers National Forest, North Coast, 54–56

Ski Resorts, Lake Tahoe Area, 217–19

Skyline-to-the-Sea Trail (Waddell Creek), Big Basin Redwoods State Park, 464–68

Skyline Trail, Toro Park, 501

Skyline Wilderness Park, Wine Country, 138

Sly Park Recreation Area, Western Sierras, 164–69

Smithneck Road, Sardine Valley Loop, 208

Smith River National Recreation Area, North Trail, 48–55

Snow Crest Road, Western States Trail, 224

Soda Gulch Trail, Purisima Creek Redwoods Open Space Preserve, 434

Sonoma Coast State Beach, Wine Country, 139

Sonoma Valley, Wine Country, 118

Soquel Demonstration State Forest, South Bay, 484

South Bay and Santa Cruz County, 443–89

South Boundary Loop Trail, Pacheco State Park, 457–58

South Camp Peak, Genoa Road–TRT Loop, 253

South End Loop, Letts Lake Recreation Area, 116

South Loop, Tennessee Valley Double

Loop, 384–90

South Shore Drive, Boulders Creek Loop, 72

Southshore Hiking Trail, Sly Park Recreation Area, 167

South Tufa Out-and-Back, Mono Lake Tufa State Reserve, Eastern Sierras, 291–94

South Upper Truckee Road, TRT: Big Meadows to Kingsbury Grade, 263, 266

South Warner Wilderness Loop, Modoc National Forest, Shasta Cascade, 92

South Yuba Primitive Camp Loop, Western Sierras, 173–77

Spikes Peak Road, Pacheco State Park, 456, 458

Spooner Lake State Park, Lake Tahoe Area, 255–61

Spring Creek Trail, Annadel State Park Loops, 137

Spur rides, 4

Squaw Creek Ridge Road, Grasshooper Peak Loop, 15–16

Squaw Leap Loop, Western Sierras, 196–97

Squaw Sky Harbor Out-and-Back, Western Sierras, 196–97

Squaw Valley Bike Park, Lake Tahoe Area, 218

Stagecoach Trail, Auburn State Recreation Area, Western Sierras, 159–63

Stage Road, Shell Ridge Recreational Area, 341–45

Stamp Mill, El Dorado Mine Loop, 85, 87

Stanislaus National Forest, Western Sierras, 196

Star Lake, Lake Tahoe Area, 267

Star Mine Trail, Black Diamond Mines Loop, 350

Stein, John, 57, 62, 66, 69

Steinhart Aquarium, San Francisco, 423, 427

Stern Trail, Bald Mountain Loop, 138

Stevens Canyon Road, Monte Bello–Stevens Creek Loop, 447, 448

Stevens Creek County Park, South Bay, 444–48

Stewartville Trail, Black Diamond Mines Loop, 346–51

Stout Grove, Howland Hill, North Coast, 44–48

Stream Trail, East-West Ridge Loop, 366

Sugarloaf Ridge State Park, Wine Country, 138–39

Sugar Pine Point State Park, Lake Tahoe Area, 229–38

Suisun Bay, East Bay, 351

Summit Road, Mount Diablo State Park, 338–39

Sunset Trail, Joaquin Miller Park, 374

Sweetwater Trail, Salmon Falls Out-and-Back, 151

Table Mountain Trail, Long Ridge Open Space Preserve, 486

Table Mountain Trail–Charcoal Road, South Bay, 447

Table Top Trail, Briones Crest Loop, 355

Tafoni Trail, El Corte de Madera Creek Open Space Preserve, 437, 438, 439

Tahoe City Bike Paths, Tahoe National Forest, Lake Tahoe Area, 229–34

Tahoe Mountain Road, Angora Lakes Out-and-Back, 244

Tahoe National Forest, Western Sierras, 169–234

Tahoe Rim Trail Association, 199

Tahoe Rim Trail (TRT), Lake Tahoe Area, 212–24, 251–73

Tahoe-to-Truckee (TNT) Road, Burton Creek State Park, 215–16

Tallac Historic Site, Pope Baldwin Bike Path, 245

Tank Turns Trail, Mt. Tamalpais State Park, 395

Technical rides, *xix*

Technical skills level ratings, *xv–xvi. See also* specific rides

Temelpa Trail, Mt. Tamalpais State Park, 394

Ten Mile River, Mendocino Coast, 110–13

Tennessee Valley Double Loop, Golden Gate National Recreation Area, North Bay, 384–90

Thermalito Trail, Pleasanton Ridge National Park, 373

Tilden Regional Park, East Bay, 356–62
Timberview Trail, El Corte de Madera
  Open Space Preserve, 438
Tish Tang A Tang Ridge, Six Rivers
  National Recreation Area, North Coast,
  55
TNT (Tahoe-to-Truckee) Road, Burton
  Creek State Park, 215–16
Toiyabe National Forest, Lake Tahoe
  Area, 247–51, 255–69
Tools for bike maintenance and repairs,
  8–9
Topographic maps, 3, 4–5
Toro Park, Monterey Peninsula, 491–97
Tour De Skunk, Mendocino Coast, 114
Tour of San Francisco and the Golden
  Gate, West Bay, 421–28
Tower House Historical District, El
  Dorado Mine Loop, 83–85, 87
Tower Irrigation Ditch Trail, El Dorado
  Mine Loop, 87
Toyon Ridge Trail, Toro Park, 496–97
Trail, defined, *xvii*
Trail Camp Trail, Monterey Peninsula,
  529
Trail etiquette, 5–7
TRT (Tahoe Rim Trail), El Dorado
  National Forest, Lake Tahoe Area
  Big Meadows, 261–73
  Kingsbury Grade, 261–69
  Round Lake, 269–73
TRT (Tahoe Rim Trail), Lake Tahoe Area
  Flume Ride, 255–61
  Genoa Road Loop, 251–55
TRT (Tahoe Rim Trail), Tahoe National
  Forest, Lake Tahoe Area
  Cinder Cone Loop, 212–17
  WST (Western States Trail), 219–24
Truckee River Bike Path, Western States
  Trail (WST), 223
Truckee River Recreation Trail, Tahoe
  City Bike Paths, 229–34
Tunnel Creek Road, Flume–TRT Ride,
  259–60, 261
Twin View Lakes, Eastern Sierras, 326
Two Quarry Road, Annadel State Park
  Loops, 135, 136

Underwood, Peter, 262, 263, 269, 271

United States Forest Service, 1, 3, 5
United States Geological Survey
  (USGS), 1
topographic maps, 3, 4–5
Upper Fire Road Loop, Angel Island,
  379–84
Upper Ice Box Loop, Whiskeytown–
  Shasta–Trinity National Recreation
  Area, Shasta Cascade, 79–83
Upper Oil Canyon Trail, Black Diamond
  Mines Loop, 350
Upper Preacher Gulch Road,
  Grasshopper Peak Loop, 15, 16

Valhalla Estate, Pope Baldwin Bike Path,
  245
Van Damme State Park, Mendocino
  Coast, 102–6
Ventana Wilderness, Monterey Peninsula,
  530–31
Vichy Springs Resort, Mendocino Coast,
  115
Village Trail, China Camp State Park,
  414

Waddell Creek, Big Basin Redwoods
  State Park, 464–68
Wagon Wheel Trail, Wilder Ranch State
  Park, 476, 477
Wall Point Road, Shell Ridge
  Recreational Area, 344–45
Warren P. Richardson Trail, Annadel
  State Park Loops, 131–37
Water Dog Lake Park, West Bay, 441
Waters Gulch Loop, Shasta–Trinity
  National Forest, Shasta Cascade, 66–68
Water supplies, 7–8. *See also* specific
  rides
Water Wheel Creek Trail, Monte
  Bello–Stevens Creek Loop, 448
Waterwheel Trail. *See* Horseshoe Lake
  Loop, Eastern Sierras
Watson Lake, Tahoe Rim Trail, 221, 223
West Bay Area, 420–42
Western Sierras, 141–98
Western States Trail (WST), Tahoe
  National Forest, Lake Tahoe Area,
  219–24
West Point Inn, Mill Valley, CA, North

Bay, 391, 394

Westridge Trail, Ossagon–Gold Bluff Loop, 33

West Ridge Trail, Redwood Regional Park, East Bay, 362–67

West Shore Bike Path, Tahoe City Bike Paths, 229–34

Whiskeytown Downhill (race), 58–61

Whiskeytown National Recreation Area, Shasta–Cascade, 58–62, 69–89

White House Canyon Road, Big Basin Redwoods State Park, 463

Whitmore Hot Springs, Eastern Sierras, 330

Whittemore Gulch Trail, Purisima Creek Redwoods Open Space Preserve, 434

Wildcat Canyon Regional Park, East Bay, 356–62

Wilder Ranch State Park, South Bay
  Gray Whale Ranch, 472–77
  Ohlone Bluff Trail, 477–80
  Old Cove Bluff Trail, 477–80

Wildflower viewing rides, *xviii*

Wildlife viewing rides, *xviii*

Williams, Greg, 170, 173, 174, 177, 180

Willow Creek Road, Wine Country, 139

Wine Country, 118–40

Yosemite Bug Hostel Lodge & Campground, Western Sierras, 195

Yosemite National Park Bike Trail, Eastern Sierras, 282–86

Zig Zag Trail, Ossagon–Gold Bluff Loop, 33

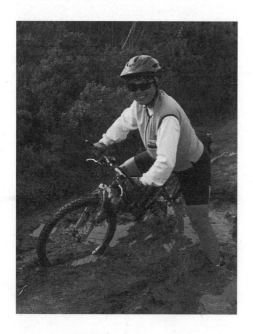

ABOUT THE AUTHOR

A native Californian, Linda Austin was bitten by the bicycling bug in the early 60s, when she discovered how to "pop wheelies" with her brothers on her little Stingray bike, complete with a pink banana seat. In the mid-80s, she became an avid recreational road cyclist after a friend introduced her to the Georgena Terry line of bicycles, specially designed for petite riders. In 1992, she found a mountain bike that accommodated her "5-foot-nothing" height. In 1994, Menasha Ridge Press and Falcon Press released *The Mountain Biker's Guide to Colorado*, a book of trails which she coauthored (as Linda Gong) with Gregg Bromka. When not riding her road or mountain bike, Linda is a graphic artist and web designer in the San Francisco Bay Area where she and her husband Bruce reside. She invites your comments via email at austinmtnbike@hotmail.com.